Cardiac PET and PET/CT Imaging

Cardiac PET and PET/CT Imaging

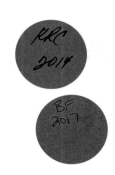

Editors

Marcelo F. Di Carli, MD
Chief of Nuclear Medicine, Co-Director of Cardiovascular Imaging, Brigham and Women's Hospital, Associate Professor of Radiology and Medicine, Harvard Medical School, Boston, Massachusetts, USA

Martin J. Lipton, MD, FACR, FACC
Director of Education, Non-Invasive Imaging, Brigham and Women's Hospital, Professor of Radiology, Department of Radiology, Harvard Medical School, Boston, Massachusetts, USA

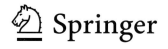

Springer

Marcelo F. Di Carli, MD
Chief of Nuclear Medicine
Co-Director of Cardiovascular Imaging
Brigham and Women's Hospital
Associate Professor of Radiology
   and Medicine
Harvard Medical School
Boston, MA
USA

Martin J. Lipton, MD, FACR, FACC
Director of Education, Non-Invasive
   Imaging
Brigham and Women's Hospital
Professor of Radiology
Department of Radiology
Harvard Medical School
Boston, MA
USA

Library of Congress Control Number: 2006927422

ISBN: 978-0-387-35275-6   e-ISBN: 978-0-387-38295-1

Printed on acid-free paper.

9 8 7 6 5 4 3 2 1

springer.com

This textbook is dedicated to our families:

Maritxu, Gilda, and Milena Di Carli
and
Jacquelyn and Sam Lipton

Foreword

When the history of medicine in the latter half of the twentieth century is written, the advances in cardiovascular diagnosis, therapy, and prevention will stand out as one of the most important achievements. Although the age-corrected death rate secondary to coronary artery disease has declined substantially in industrialized nations during this period, the prevalence of these conditions remains stubbornly high because of the aging of the population. Importantly, the incidence of coronary events and of one of their most important sequelae—heart failure—is rising alarmingly in the developing world. When viewed from a global perspective, cardiovascular disease is assuming a progressively greater importance, and it is estimated that by 2025 it will be, for the first time in human history, the most common cause of death.

Clearly, rather than resting on the laurels of our achievements, an intensification of the battle against cardiovascular disease must now be undertaken. Cardiovascular imaging will, without question, play a critical role in this battle. The appropriate selection of therapeutic measures, be they pharmacologic, catheter-based, surgical, alterations in lifestyles, or some combination of these, depends on accurate assessments of both cardiac structure and function. Increasingly, the changes that dictate management are quite subtle and require a level of precision that was not available to clinicians heretofore. Positron emission tomography (PET), especially when combined with contemporary techniques of computed tomography (CT), allows virtually simultaneous assessment of cardiac and coronary arterial structure together with myocardial perfusion and metabolism. The combination of these noninvasive approaches provides information that is an order of magnitude greater than that obtained previously.

As these new technologies move rapidly from the research laboratory to clinical practice, it is vital to train cardiologists, radiologists, and specialists in nuclear medicine in their appropriate use. To achieve this important goal, Drs. Di Carli and Lipton and their talented contributing authors have provided in *Cardiac PET and PET/CT Imaging* a most valuable resource for this training. In addition to summarizing—in a manner understandable by clinicians—the theoretical underpinnings and instrumentation of these techniques, they lay out clearly the array of clinical situations in which these two imaging modes, as well as cardiac magnetic resonance imaging, provide information that is of enormous value for clinical management. This remarkable book also has a keen eye on the future. Advances in molecular imaging, which will certainly find its way into practice in the second decade of the twenty-first century, are also discussed lucidly and are well illustrated.

The editors, Drs. Di Carli and Lipton, and the contributing authors deserve thanks and congratulations for providing this important new textbook. It will be appreciated by trainees, clinicians, and investigators in this field.

Eugene Braunwald, MD
Harvard Medical School
Brigham and Women's Hospital
Boston, Massachusetts, USA

Preface

The field of cardiovascular imaging in general, and cardiovascular nuclear medicine in particular, is witnessing dramatic change, especially with emerging new technology such as positron emission tomography/computed tomography (PET/CT). Relatively recent FDA approval of PET radiopharmaceuticals and changes in reimbursement in oncology and, more recently, in cardiology continue to fuel exponential growth in the deployment of integrated PET/CT cameras, especially throughout the United States, Europe, and Asia (Japan and Korea). As a result, clinical PET and PET/CT imaging are no longer the domain of university hospitals. This is the good news. The bad news is that there is now an enormous gap between the growth of these technologies for diagnosis and management of patients with heart disease and the limited knowledge base obtained by cardiologists, nuclear medicine specialists, and radiologists lacking clinical experience in performing and interpreting these procedures. This gap is self-evident in cardiac PET and PET/CT imaging. Although currently only a handful of teaching programs offer specialized training in cardiac PET and PET/CT, the number of these programs is expected to grow fairly rapidly.

The books on PET and, more recently, PET/CT are almost exclusively dedicated to imaging applications in oncology. In those textbooks, cardiac imaging is narrowly focused on myocardial perfusion and viability from a highly research-oriented perspective. Those isolated chapters are designed only to illustrate the possible applications of PET and PET/CT in cardiology and not to provide the trainee or imaging specialist with a systematic approach to the complexities of cardiac imaging.

Cardiac PET and PET/CT Imaging is intended to narrow the gap between technology and the practical clinical knowledge base. The goal of this book is to educate, stimulate, and serve as a resource to cardiology, radiology, and nuclear medicine trainees, as well as imaging and medical specialists, with the most up-to-date information regarding the current practice for cardiac PET and integrated PET/CT, including the advanced applications of CT coronary angiography. To this end, we have assembled a multidisciplinary group of clinical and imaging experts from cardiology, radiology, and nuclear medicine to provide a systematic, practical, and in-depth approach to imaging with PET and CT, as well as correlative imaging with magnetic resonance imaging (MRI). We hope that the thoughtful and forward-thinking conception of this text, with its 40 tables and 234 figures, will allow its content to remain current even in an era of rapid technical and scientific evolution.

Part I includes the general principles of cardiac imaging and instrumentation with chapters on PET, CT, and integrated PET/CT. In addition, this section also includes a chapter on the principles of quantification and tracer kinetic modeling with PET.

Part II includes comprehensive reviews on PET radiopharmaceuticals for cardiac imaging and iodinated contrast agents for CT angiography. It also contains unique chapters on cross-sectional anatomy of the heart and vessels and on the increasingly important issue of patient and occupational radiation dosimetry.

Part III is devoted entirely to the diagnosis of coronary artery disease, which accounts for the vast majority of heart disease in developed countries. The chapters include comprehensive reviews on patient preparation and stress protocols for perfusion imaging, myocardial perfusion imaging protocols and quality assurance, myocardial perfusion imaging with PET, and the use of quantitative myocardial perfusion imaging for evaluating coronary artery disease. This section also contains comprehensive reviews on the use of contrast and noncontrast CT for diagnosing coronary disease, a critical review of the relative merits of coronary imaging with CT and MRI, and the integration of myocardial perfusion and coronary anatomy for diagnosis and management of coronary artery disease (CAD).

Heart failure has emerged as one of the most important problems in cardiology, and imaging plays a key role in diagnosis and treatment planning. Part IV includes chapters on the principles of myocardial metabolism, evaluation of myocardial viability with PET and with MRI, a critical review of the role of imaging in evaluating ischemia and viability in diagnosis and management of heart failure, and the emerging role of imaging of cardiac innervation and receptors in heart failure.

Part V provides a forward look at the emerging role of molecular imaging in cardiology. It includes comprehensive reviews on imaging of the vulnerable plaque with PET/CT and MRI, imaging of gene products and cell therapy, and imaging of angiogenesis.

Part VI includes a library of cardiac PET/CT cases illustrating a broad spectrum of common clinical scenarios from identification of normal scans and recognition of artifacts to identification of high-risk scans, assessment of myocardial viability, integration of perfusion and coronary anatomy, and the importance of recognizing incidental findings.

We are thankful for the skilled assistance of Jeselle Gierbolini. We would also like to acknowledge the dedication and help of our technical staff in nuclear medicine, CT, and MRI. We are also grateful for the expert editorial assistance of our development editor, Merry Post, who has tolerated our frequent requests for changes that we believe made the book even better. Finally, we would also like to acknowledge our Radiology Department chair at Brigham and Women's Hospital, Steven Seltzer, for his unflagging support of innovation in imaging and his encouragement to write this textbook.

Marcelo F. Di Carli, MD
Martin J. Lipton, MD, FACR, FACC

Contents

Part V   Emerging Role of Molecular Imaging

Part VI   Case Illustrations of Cardiac PET and Integrated PET/CT
Sharmila Dorbala, Zelmira Curillova, and Marcelo F. Di Carli

Contributors

Frank M. Bengel, MD
Director of Cardiovascular Nuclear Medicine, Visiting Associate Professor of Radiology, Johns Hopkins University Medical Institution, Baltimore, MD, USA

Myrwood C. Besozzi, MD
Clinical Professor of Medicine, University of Tennessee Medical Center, Knoxville Cardiovascular Group, PC, Knoxville, TN, USA

Lawrence M. Boxt, MD
Professor of Clinical Radiology, Albert Einstein College of Medicine of Yeshiva University, Director of Cardiac MRI and CT, North Shore University Hospital, Manhasset, NY, USA

Douglas P. Boyd, PhD
Adjunct Professor of Radiology, Heartscan Headquarters, University of California at San Francisco, Walnut Creek, CA, USA

Javed Butler, MD, MPH
Associate Professor of Medicine, Cardiology Division, Emory University, Atlanta, GA, USA

Jonathan P.J. Carney, PhD
Assistant Professor of Radiology, University of Pittsburgh Medical Center, Pittsburgh, PA, USA

Frank P. Castronovo, Jr., RPh, PhD
Director of Health Physics and Radiopharmacology, Associate Professor of Radiology, Brigham and Women's Hospital, Harvard Medical School, Boston, MA, USA

Sharon E. Crugnale, MS, RCEP
Section Head, Exercise Physiology, Division of Nuclear Medicine, Brigham and Women's Hospital, Harvard Medical School, Boston, MA, USA

Zelmira Curillova, MD
Fellow in Cardiovascular Imaging, Brigham and Women's Hospital, Harvard Medical School, Boston, MA, USA

Santo Dellegrottaglie, MD
Instructor of Medicine (adjunct), Cardiovascular CT/MRI Program, The Zena and Michael A. Wiener Cardiovascular Institute, The Marie-Josée and Henry R. Kravis Cardiovascular Health Center, Mount Sinai School of Medicine, New York, NY, USA

Marcelo F. Di Carli, MD
Chief of Nuclear Medicine, Co-Director of Cardiovascular Imaging, Brigham and Women's Hospital, Associate Professor of Radiology and Medicine, Harvard Medical School, Boston, MA, USA

Frank P. DiFilippo, PhD
Director of Nuclear Imaging Physics, Department of Molecular and Functional Imaging, Cleveland Clinic Foundation, Cleveland, OH, USA

Vasken Dilsizian, MD
Professor of Medicine and Radiology, University of Maryland School of Medicine, Director, Cardiovascular Nuclear Medicine and Cardiac Positron Emission Tomography, University of Maryland Medical Center, Baltimore, MD, USA

Lawrence W. Dobrucki, PhD
Post-Doctoral Research Fellow, Section of Cardiovascular Medicine, Yale University School of Medicine, New Haven, CT, USA

Sharmila Dorbala, MD
Associate Director of Nuclear Cardiology, Brigham and Women's Hospital, Instructor in Radiology and Medicine, Harvard Medical School, Boston, MA, USA

Georges El Fakhri, PhD
Associate Professor of Radiology, Harvard Medical School, Physicist, Nuclear Medicine Division, Brigham and Women's Hospital, Boston, MA, USA

Zahi A. Fayad, PhD
Director, Imaging Science Laboratories, Director, The Eva and Morris Feld Cardiovascular Research Laboratory, Professor, Departments of Radiology and Medicine (Cardiology), The Zena and Michael A. Wiener Cardiovascular Institute, The Marie-Josée and Henry R. Kravis Cardiovascular Health Center, Mount Sinai School of Medicine, New York, NY, USA

John Finley IV, MD
Instructor in Medicine, Tufts-New England Medical Center, Tufts University School of Medicine, Boston, MA, USA

Valentin Fuster, MD, PhD
Director of the Zena and Michael A. Wiener Cardiovascular Institute, Director of the Marie-Josée and Henry R. Kravis Cardiovascular Health Center, Richard Gorlin, MD/Heart Research Foundation Professor of Medicine, Mount Sinai School of Medicine, New York, NY, USA

Robert J. Gropler, MD
Professor of Radiology, Medicine, and Biomedical Engineering, Lab Chief, Cardiovascular Imaging Laboratory, Mallinckrodt Institute of Radiology, Washington University School of Medicine, St. Louis, MO, USA

Takahiro Higuchi, MD
Research Fellow, Nuklearmedizinische Klinik der Technischen Universität München, Munich, Germany

Udo Hoffmann, MD
Co-Director MGH Cardiac MRCT PET Program, Massachusetts General Hospital, Assistant Professor of Radiology, Harvard Medical School, Boston, MA, USA

Fabien Hyafil, MD
Research Fellow, Imaging Science Laboratories, Departments of Radiology and Medicine (Cardiology), The Zena and Michael A. Wiener Cardiovascular Institute, The Marie-Josée and Henry R. Kravis Cardiovascular Health Center, Mount Sinai School of Medicine, New York, NY, USA

Raymond Y. Kwong, MD, MPH
Co-Director of Cardiac CT and MRI, Instructor in Medicine and Radiology, Brigham and Women's Hospital, Harvard Medical School, Boston, MA, USA

Martin J. Lipton, MD, FACR, FACC
Director of Education, Non-Invasive Imaging, Brigham and Women's Hospital, Professor of Radiology, Department of Radiology, Harvard Medical School, Boston, MA, USA

Josef Machac, MD
Director of Nuclear Medicine, Professor of Radiology and Associate Professor of Medicine, Mount Sinai School of Medicine, New York, NY, USA

Warren J. Manning, MD
Chief of Non-Invasive Cardiac Imaging (Cardiology), Beth Israel Deaconess Medical Center, Professor of Medicine and Radiology, Harvard Medical School, Boston, MA, USA

Stephen C. Moore, PhD
Director of Nuclear Medicine Physics, Associate Professor of Radiology, Brigham and Women's Hospital, Harvard Medical School, Boston, MA, USA

Koenraad J. Mortele, MD
Associate Professor of Radiology, Harvard Medical School, Associate Director, Division of Abdominal Imaging and Intervention, Director, Abdominal and Pelvic MRI, Director, CME Department of Radiology, Brigham and Women's Hospital, Boston, MA, USA

M. Raquel Oliva, MD
Fellow in Radiology, Brigham and Women's Hospital, Harvard Medical School, Boston, MA, USA

John A. Rumberger, MD
Medical Director, HealthWISE Wellness Diagnostic Center, Clinical Professor of Medicine, Ohio State University, Columbus, OH, USA

Javier Sanz, MD
Assistant Professor of Medicine/Cardiology, Clinical MRI/CT Program, Cardiovascular Institute, Mount Sinai Hospital, New York, NY, USA

Heinrich R. Schelbert, MD, PhD
George V. Taplin Professor, Department of Molecular and Medical Pharmacology, David Geffen School of Medicine at UCLA, Los Angeles, CA, USA

A. Robert Schleipman, RT, CNMT, MSc
Instructor, Health Physics and Radiopharmacology, Brigham and Women's Hospital, Boston, MA, USA

Markus Schwaiger, MD, PhD
Professor of Nuclear Medicine, Director, Nuklearmedizinische Klinik der Technischen Universität München, Munich, Germany

Ahmad Y. Sheikh, MD
Research Fellow, Department of Cardiothoracic Surgery, Stanford University Medical Center, Stanford, CA, USA

Albert J. Sinusas, MD
Professor of Medicine and Diagnostic Radiology, Director, Animal Research Laboratories, Section of Cardiovascular Medicine, Director, Cardiovascular Nuclear Imaging and Stress Laboratories, Yale University School of Medicine, Yale New Haven Hospital, New Haven, CT, USA

Ahmed A. Tawakol, MD
Co-Director, Cardiac MR-PET-CT Program, Co-Director, CIMIT Cardiovascular Disease Program, Instructor in Medicine, Harvard Medical School and Massachusetts General Hospital, Boston, MA, USA

David W. Townsend, PhD
Professor of Medicine and Radiology, Director, Cancer Imaging and Tracer Development Research Program, University of Tennessee, Graduate School of Medicine, Knoxville, TN, USA

James E. Udelson, MD
Associate Chief, Division of Cardiology, Director, Nuclear Cardiology Laboratory, Co-Director, Heart Failure and Transplant Center, Tufts-New England Medical Center, Associate Professor of Medicine, Tufts University School of Medicine, Boston, MA, USA

Joseph C. Wu, MD, PhD
Assistant Professor in Medicine and Radiology, Stanford University, Stanford, CA, USA

Part I
Instrumentation and Principles of Imaging

1 Instrumentation and Principles of Imaging: PET

Frank P. DiFilippo

Positron Annihilation and Tomography

Positron emission tomography (PET) is a noninvasive modality that produces tomographic images of the distribution of a radionuclide-labeled tracer injected in the body.[1] As the name suggests, PET imaging is based on radionuclides that decay by positron emission (Figure 1.1A. For example, fluorine-18 (^{18}F)decays to oxygen-18 (^{18}O), emitting a positron (β^+) and a neutrino (ν_e):

$$^{18}\text{F} \rightarrow {}^{18}\text{O} + \beta^+ + \nu_e \tag{1}$$

(The neutrino does not affect PET imaging and may be ignored in this discussion.) A positron is an elementary particle classified as antimatter and is analogous to an electron, having identical mass but opposite electrical charge. The positron is ejected from the nucleus and rapidly loses its kinetic energy through collisions with numerous nearby electrons. Since antimatter and matter are mutually unstable, the positron and an electron then undergo a process known as *positron annihilation* and are converted into a pair of gamma-ray photons. Because total energy is conserved, each gamma ray has energy of 511 keV, which is equivalent to the mass of the positron and of the electron according to the well-known relationship $E = mc^2$. Because total momentum is conserved, the two gamma rays travel in opposite directions with a relative angle very close to 180 degrees.

Thus, if a coincident pair of 511 keV gamma rays is detected, the *line of coincidence* connecting the two detected coordinates passes near the point in space where the annihilation event occurred and also where the positron decay occurred. When many such event pairs are detected, the activity distribution of the positron-emitting radionuclide within the volume of interest may be reconstructed. This process is the basis of PET imaging. Unlike single photon emission computed tomography (SPECT) imaging, which uses a collimator to define the angle of incidence of detected gamma rays, no extrinsic collimator is necessary for PET imaging, and higher count sensitivity is obtained. A typical detection efficiency for a collimated SPECT detector is on the order of 0.01%, whereas many modern three-dimensional (3D) PET scanners have detection efficiencies around 0.5% or higher.

Furthermore, since there is no loss of resolution from collimator blur in PET, its spatial resolution (4 to 8 mm) is superior to that of SPECT. The fundamental limit of PET spatial resolution depends on the average range of travel of the positron prior to

3

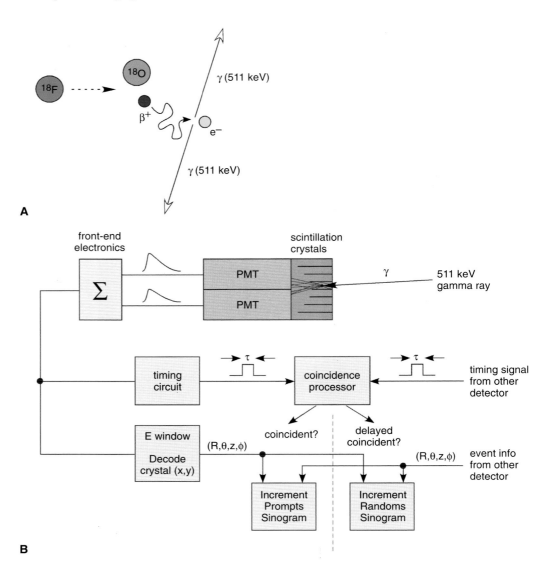

FIGURE 1.1. Overview of PET event detection. (A) Annihilation radiation (pair of 511 keV gamma rays) results from the interaction of an electron e⁻ and positron β⁺ emitted by a PET radionuclide (^{18}F in this example, which decays to ^{18}O). The positron rapidly slows down due to numerous collisions with electrons along its path, traveling only a short distance prior to annihilation. (B) Schematic of a PET scintillation detector and associated event processing (in conjunction with a coincident event recorded in an opposing detector).

annihilation (0.5 mm in the case of ^{18}F decay) and the noncollinearity of the gamma-ray pairs (approximately ±0.25°).[2,3] These effects most often are negligible compared to the spatial resolution of commercial PET detectors. However, for radionuclides that emit energetic positrons (such as rubidium-82 [^{82}Rb], whose effective positron range is approximately 5 mm), the loss of spatial resolution and image quality is noticeable.

PET Detectors

Detectors used in PET scanners[4,5] are designed for optimal detection of 511 keV coincident gamma rays under clinical imaging conditions. A schematic of a typical PET scintillation detector is shown in Figure 1.1B; it consists of several elements. First, the incident gamma ray is absorbed in a scintillation crystal and produces energetic electrons, which in turn produce a cascade of visible photons. This flash of visible light exits the crystal and is shaped by a light guide before reaching an array (often a 2 × 2 block) of photomultiplier tubes (PMTs). The PMTs convert the flash of light into electronic pulse signals that are processed by front-end amplifiers and other electronics. The integrated signal from the group of PMTs is measured and is proportional to the total energy deposited in the crystal. The scintillation event is rejected if the detected energy is outside the allowed range for 511 keV gamma rays, set by the lower-level discriminator (LLD) and upper-level discriminator (ULD) values (approximately 400 keV and 650 keV, respectively). By restricting the acceptable energy range, the number of scattered events (those interacting within the body before being detected) is minimized because the scattered gamma rays have energies lower than 511 keV. In addition, a position-weighted signal is processed in order to determine the crystal of interaction, which specifies the detected location of the event. The spatial resolution of the detector is limited largely by the physical size of the individual scintillation crystals.

After being processed by the front-end electronics, the electronic signals associated with the scintillation events are then processed by coincidence electronics. The coincidence electronics sample all detectors and accurately determine the time of each detected event, within time resolution τ. The timing pulses from all electronics banks then are compared. If two time pulses overlap, the two associated events are considered to be simultaneous and are designated as a coincidence pair. The definition of simultaneity is limited by the coincidence timing window 2τ, which is in the range of 4 to 16 ns on clinical PET scanners. The coincidence timing window is set to be as small as possible so that nearly all true coincidence events are detected and as many "random" coincidence events as possible are rejected.

Random coincidences arise when two 511 keV gamma rays originating from different positron decay events are detected by chance within the coincidence timing window. For a pair of detectors having "singles" count rates of S_1 and S_2 for individual 511 keV gamma rays, the random coincidence rate R for the pair of detectors depends linearly on the coincidence timing window and is given by:

$$R = 2\tau\, S_1\, S_2 \tag{2}$$

The random coincidence rate is proportional to the square of the source activity, whereas the true coincidence rate is linear with respect to the source activity. Thus, the relative contribution of random coincidences rises for increasing injected dose. Both random and scatter events lead to erroneous backprojection (see Figure 1.2) and should be minimized through appropriate detector design and configuration.

An important consideration in PET detector design is the scintillation crystal material, whose characteristics directly affect PET imaging performance. The crystal's mass density, elemental composition, and thickness together determine its ability to fully absorb 511 keV gamma rays. Since a pair of gamma rays must be detected to produce a coincident event, the PET coincidence sensitivity depends on the square of the detector sensitivity, and thus the crystal's "stopping power" (attenuation coefficient at 511 keV) is a significant property. The scintillation light output of the crystal affects the accuracy in determining the gamma-ray energy and crystal of interaction and thereby affects the scatter rejection and intrinsic spatial resolution. In addition, the scintillation decay time of the crystal specifies the duration of the light pulse, which impacts both the dead time and timing resolution per event. A crystal with a shorter scintillation decay time is able to sustain higher count rates without saturating the detector and allows for improved rejection of random events through a more precise coincidence window. Thus, scintillation crystals with high attenuation

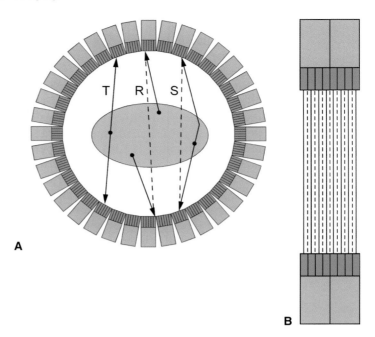

FIGURE 1.2. Detector configuration in PET scanners. (A) Front view showing a circular arrangement of block detectors around a patient cross section. Examples of true (T), random (R), and scatter (S) coincidence events are shown. For true events, the line of coincidence connecting the two points of detection passes near the point where the positron decay occurred. The random and scatter events result in erroneous lines of coincidence (dashed lines) and contribute to background counts. (B) Side view cross section (expanded view) illustrating the individual N rings and the $(2N-1)$ slices defined by the ring geometry. Solid lines denote central slices; dashed lines denote in-between slices.

coefficient at 511 keV, high light output, and short decay time are most appropriate for PET detectors. Modern commercial PET scanners utilize crystals of bismuth germanate (BGO), lutetium oxyorthosilicate (LSO), or gadolinium oxyorthosilicate (GSO).[6]

PET Scanner Design

Modern PET scanners consist of a large number of crystals (4000 to 24,000) in a cylindrical arrangement of discrete rings (Figure 1.2), with typical ring diameter of 85 cm and axial field of view of 16 cm. The N crystal rings define a total of $2N-1$ slices (at the ring centers and at the midpoints between the rings). The detector geometries of PET scanners vary: Some designs use compact block detector modules and others use fewer but larger flat-panel detector components. Most PET scanners are of full-ring design; however, some models employ partial rings of detectors with a rapidly rotating gantry in order to reduce cost, at the expense of reduced count sensitivity. The physical size of each crystal is typically 4 to 8 mm in cross section and 20 to 30 mm in thickness. The crystal arrays are backed by PMTs and front-end electronics, which connect to the remaining coincidence electronics within the temperature-stabilized gantry.

Because imaging is based on electronic collimation, the spatial resolution of the PET scanner is limited mainly by the intrinsic spatial resolution of the detectors. Since an event location is resolved to a specific crystal, the spatial resolution is approximately that of the cross-sectional size of the crystal (4 to 8 mm). While this is true near the center of the transaxial field of view, the spatial resolution does worsen slightly with increasing radius due to the unknown depth of interaction of the events within the thick crystals, typically increasing by 1 mm at a radius of 10 cm and by more at larger radii.

Many PET scanners employ axial septa to restrict the axial angle of incidence to a smaller range (Figure 1.3). The septa are tungsten or lead annuli located along the ring boundaries of the crystal array. The septa absorb most axially oblique gamma rays and provide some degree of collimation in the axial direction only. However, the septa are not true collimators in that electronic collimation still specifies the axial and transaxial angles of the coincident event pairs. In several scanner models, the septa can be in the extended position (for two-dimensional (2D)-imaging mode) or in the retracted position (for 3D-imaging mode).[7] Other scanner models operate exclusively either with fixed septa in 2D mode or without septa in 3D mode, with the latter situation being common for newer PET/CT scanners.

There are advantages and disadvantages associated with PET imaging in 2D with septa as opposed to imaging in 3D without septa. Imaging with septa means that simpler 2D image reconstruction algorithms may be used since most axially oblique events are not recorded. This is done at the expense of greatly reduced count sensitivity, however. In 3D mode, a typical fourfold increase in count sensitivity is attained by recording the axially oblique events, allowing for shorter imaging times with reduced injected dose. An unwanted side effect of imaging in 3D mode is that many random and scatter coincident events arising from outside the axial field of view, which would have been absorbed by the septa, instead are detected and recorded (Figure 1.3). Thus, use of axial septa may be warranted in imaging situations where the high background event rate would impact image quality or quantitative accuracy.

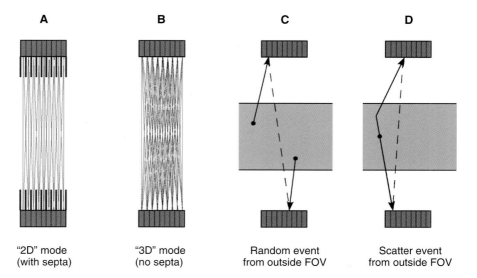

A	B	C	D
"2D" mode (with septa)	"3D" mode (no septa)	Random event from outside FOV	Scatter event from outside FOV

FIGURE 1.3. Imaging with and without axial septa. In 2D mode (A), the septa prevent most oblique events from being detected, and only coincidence events within the same ring or between adjacent rings are recorded. In 3D mode (B), the septa are removed and a much larger number of lines of coincidence are detected, greatly increasing the sensitivity of the scanner. However, the removal of septa in 3D mode allows random events (C) and scatter events (D) arising from activity outside the axial field of view (FOV) also to be recorded, thereby increasing background counts.

Image quality is often characterized by noise equivalent counts (NECs) acquired.[8] NEC is defined as:

$$NEC = \frac{T^2}{(T + S + kR)} \qquad (3)$$

where T, S, and R represent true counts, scatter counts, and random counts, respectively. The factor k depends on the method of randoms correction applied and is equal to 2 for the most common case (using the delayed coincidence method and with the object being imaged occupying most of the scanner field of view). As can be seen in this equation for NEC, true counts add beneficially to image quality, whereas random and scatter counts detract from image quality.

An important characteristic of PET scanner design is the count-rate capacity of the detectors. At low activity levels, the true coincidence rate is proportional to the activity. However, each event requires a processing time that depends on the crystal's scintillation decay time and the design of the front-end electronics. At higher event rates, an increasing fraction of events overlap in time to produce erroneous effects known as pulse pileup. Detector saturation from pulse pileup contributes to dead-time loss, thereby reducing the total counts recorded. As a result, the count rate depends nonlinearly on activity as the degree of pulse pileup increases, eventually reaching a point above which the count rate begins to decrease (Figure 1.4). Optimal imaging generally is attained when the injected dose is such that the scanner operates on the upward slope and near the peak of the NEC curve. NEC and imaging time are affected by many factors such as injected dose, body habitus, activity outside the region of interest, whether septa are used, and detector dead-time characteristics. Therefore, optimal scan protocols can vary substantially among patients, studies, and scanners. Performance tests using standard phantoms are performed to assess differences in scanner characteristics.[9,10]

Data Corrections

In addition to excellent image quality, a goal of PET imaging is to achieve a high degree of quantitative accuracy. This goal is particularly important in cardiac imaging since relative or absolute perfusion or viability, or both, are being assessed in all regions of the myocardium. PET imaging achieves quantitative accuracy

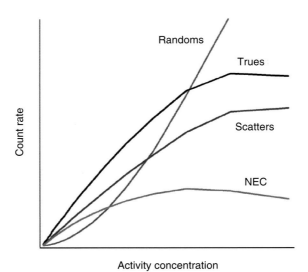

FIGURE 1.4. PET count-rate curve example. True, random, and scatter count rates are displayed, along with the resultant noise equivalent count (NEC) rate. Note the increasing randoms fraction and detector dead-time loss at higher activities.

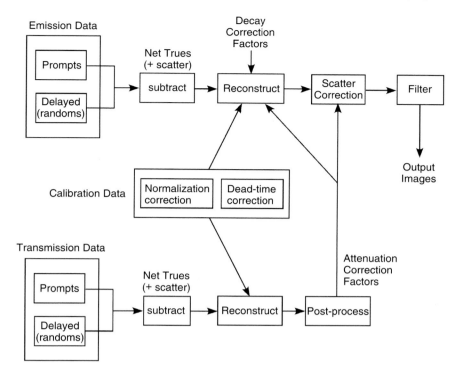

FIGURE 1.5. Flowchart of PET data processing and image reconstruction.

through applying corrections for many factors: detector normalization, dead-time loss, random events, body attenuation, and scatter events. Figure 1.5 shows a schematic of PET data processing and illustrates the steps where these corrections are implemented.

Detector Corrections

Detector normalization and dead-time loss corrections are based on scanner-specific calibrations done prior to imaging. Normalization data reflect the relative sensitivity of each scintillation crystal element in the scanner, which can differ substantially among crystal elements. A normalization calibration scan using a uniform source of known activity is performed at regular intervals and after tuning or servicing the detectors. On a daily basis, a quality assurance scan is performed and checked against the previous system normalization data to ensure that significant drift in the detector electronics has not occurred. Detector dead-time loss is the fraction of counts lost to pulse pileup and is reflected in the count-rate characteristics of the scanner (see Figure 1.4). The dead-time loss of a detector block commonly is estimated as a function of the measured singles event rate, based on prior calibration tests of the detector count-rate curve.

To achieve quantitative accuracy, the raw data must be rescaled by the appropriate normalization and dead-time loss correction factors. Applying the normalization factors ensures uniform detector sensitivity and allows the reconstructed images to be expressed in terms of activity concentration or in terms of standardized uptake values (SUV),[11,12] if data are normalized to injected dose and body weight or lean body mass. Applying the dead-time loss factors ensures a linear relationship between the actual count rate and the absolute activity in the field of view. These corrections serve to accurately reflect the true flux of gamma rays impinging on the crystal elements and are necessary for quantitative image reconstruction.

Randoms Correction

PET scanners record all "prompt" coincident events that occur simultaneously within the timing resolution of the detector electronics. The prompt events (P) consist of true (T), random (R), and scatter (S) coincident events:

$$P = T + R + S \qquad (4)$$

Since the recorded prompt events contain background events (random and scatter), they do not represent the true activity distribution. Corrections for the background events must be applied to ensure the quantitative accuracy of reconstructed images.

Correction for random events often is achieved by direct measurement using the delayed coincidence technique, which is based on the principle that events occurring at time intervals much longer than the detector response time are uncorrelated. A separate coincidence processor is configured to detect pairs of events occurring at a relatively large time difference compared to the event processing time. Unlike event pairs recorded by the prompt coincidence processor, those recorded by the delayed coincidence processor are due solely to random coincidences. For each line of coincidence (LOC), the number of delayed events (D) is subtracted from the number of prompt events, thus canceling the random events (on average):

$$(P - D)_{avg} = (T + S)_{avg} \qquad (5)$$

It is important to note that this does not exactly cancel out the random events on a specific LOC because of count fluctuations (Poisson noise). During image reconstruction, there is an averaging effect over many LOCs, and the delayed subtraction method for randoms correction becomes quantitatively accurate in the resultant image. However, the direct subtraction of delayed coincidence counts increases the relative noise level in the images because the count fluctuations in the prompt and delayed data are additive. The noise introduced by this method can be mitigated by filtering the delayed coincidence data prior to subtraction.

Attenuation Correction

A positron decay event is detected only if both 511 keV gamma rays reach the detectors and are fully absorbed by the scintillation crystals. If either of the gamma rays is scattered or absorbed by the body, then a true coincidence event is not recorded. Such count losses from body attenuation depend on the body habitus and can be surprisingly large. For example, if the total path length of the LOC through the body is 20 cm and assuming uniform attenuation equal to that of water, only 15% of 511 keV gamma-ray pairs along this LOC escape the body without absorption or scatter. If the total path length is 40 cm (as in many heavier patients), the fraction of nonattenuated gamma-ray pairs is only 2%. Because of body attenuation, regions near the edge of the body would appear much more intense in images, since the average degree of attenuation over all LOCs there is less than in the central regions of the body.

Fortunately, the body attenuation can be measured and corrected in a straightforward fashion (Figure 1.6). An interesting property of PET imaging is that the fraction of attenuated events along a specific LOC is constant, no matter where along this line the positron decay occurred (even from within a source placed outside the body). An external gamma-ray source produces a transmission shadow profile of the body, and by measuring the position-dependent transmission data, the attenuation factors along each LOC are measured. By rotating the transmission source around the body, tomographic attenuation data are acquired. By weighting the PET emission data according to the attenuation data during image reconstruction, the resultant images then are corrected for attenuation (see Figure 1.7).

FIGURE 1.6. PET attenuation and transmission attenuation correction. Both 511 keV gamma rays arising from positron decay must pass through the body without attenuation in order for the coincidence event to be recorded. In the figure, one of the gamma rays is shown to be absorbed before exiting the body. For a line of coincidence through a uniform object, the probability that neither of the rays is attenuated is independent of the point along the line of coincidence where the event occurred and is equal to $e^{-\mu*D}$, where D is equal to the total distance (D1 + D2). The attenuation probability factors may be measured based on transmission data from a point or rod source outside the body. The transmission source (shown in red) rotates around the body to measure attenuation factors at all angles of incidence in order to reconstruct an attenuation map.

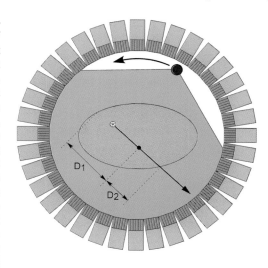

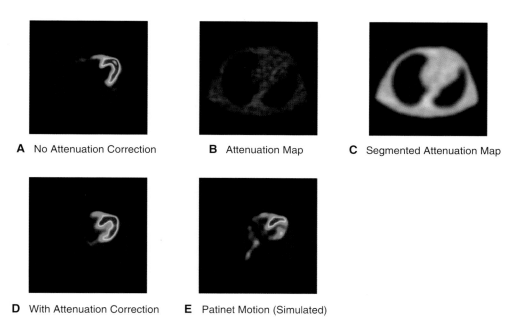

A No Attenuation Correction   **B** Attenuation Map   **C** Segmented Attenuation Map

D With Attenuation Correction   **E** Patinet Motion (Simulated)

FIGURE 1.7. Transaxial slice images from an ^{82}Rb cardiac PET study reconstructed (A) without attenuation correction. Note the abnormal myocardial distribution with higher apparent radionuclide concentration at the apex. The corresponding transmission attenuation map (B) clearly shows the lung and tissue regions. Segmentation algorithms are often used to produce a transmission map with reduced noise (C) in order to improve the study image quality. After the application of attenuation correction, the resultant image (D) shows a much more uniform myocardial distribution. It is important to note that the emission and transmission scans are performed sequentially, and the possibility exists for misregistration due to patient motion. The potential effect of patient motion is illustrated in image (E), for which the transmission image had been manually offset by 2 cm toward the left (patient's right side) prior to attenuation correction. In this situation, the lateral wall of the myocardium is incorrectly located within the lung region of the misregistered transmission data and is severely undercorrected for attenuation.

Transmission sources are present in virtually all dedicated PET scanners. Many models use germanium-68 (^{68}Ge) rod sources that emit 511 keV gamma-ray pairs from positron decay of gallium-68 (^{68}Ga, the daughter radionuclide of ^{68}Ge). The transmission data are distinguished from the emission data by knowledge of the rod source location. Other PET scanners use cesium-137 (^{137}Cs) point sources instead, which emit (noncoincident) 662 keV gamma rays. During the transmission scan, the detectors operate in singles mode instead of coincidence mode, and the higher-energy ^{137}Cs transmission gamma rays are distinguished from the 511 keV annihilation gamma rays by energy windowing. New hybrid PET/CT scanners often do not have radionuclide transmission sources and instead use the x-ray CT scanner to generate transmission data.

Count statistics in transmission scans must be considered, since noise in the transmission data propagates through image reconstruction and may affect the resultant image quality. Sufficient transmission counts must be acquired to produce an attenuation map of sufficient quality, and the transmission acquisition time should account for patient body habitus and for transmission source activity as the sources decay. Depending on scanner design, the transmission acquisition time may range from 1 to 15 minutes. To further reduce noise, segmentation image processing is often performed. The segmentation algorithm first distinguishes regions in the attenuation map as body tissue, lung tissue, air, or the patient table. The algorithm then assigns adjusted values to these regions based on the corresponding known or typical attenuation coefficients and produces a new and less noisy attenuation map (Figure 1.7).

Scatter Correction

After the delayed coincidences are subtracted, the resultant data contain both true and scatter events. Thus scatter correction is needed for quantitative imaging, and several methods and algorithms for scatter correction have been proposed and implemented.[13,14] A common implementation is to model the contribution of scattered counts based on the theory underlying Compton scatter of gamma rays. Using the transmission attenuation map and an initial estimate of the reconstructed emission images, the corresponding scatter distribution is computed. Certain approximations are made in the scatter model algorithm to accelerate computation for practical clinical use. The distribution of background counts outside the body is useful for normalizing the computed distribution with respect to the actual emission data. After subtracting the scatter contribution, the data are reconstructed once again to yield the scatter-corrected images.

The accuracy of scatter correction of course depends on the specific algorithm used and its ability to accurately model the actual scatter processes in the body. Usually better results are obtained with increasing sophistication of the scatter model in the algorithm. The absolute accuracy also depends on the scatter fraction (SF), that is, the relative contribution of scatter in the reconstructed image:

$$SF = \frac{S}{T + S}$$

(6)

A high scatter fraction has the effect of amplifying errors from scatter correction, because a larger fraction of the data must be subtracted. The scatter fraction of a particular data set depends on several factors, including the energy window (LLD and ULD values, which are set according to the energy resolution of the detectors at 511 keV), the region of the body scanned, and body habitus. In many cases, a major factor is whether axial septa are used and also the degree of side shielding of the detectors, since the septa and shielding are very effective in blocking axially oblique scatter events (Figure 1.3). For example, a standard 20 cm cylindrical phantom may exhibit a scatter fraction of 20% in 2D mode and 45% in 3D mode, and the scatter fraction in patients may be considerably higher. Furthermore, scatter in 3D mode is significantly more complex and more difficult to model because of cross-plane events and events arising from outside the axial field of view. In situations in which a high degree of quantitative accuracy is required, imaging may be better performed in 2D mode, for which scatter correction generally is more accurate.

Data Processing and Image Reconstruction

Sinogram Representations

As the PET coincidence events are acquired, they are binned into data arrays according to their detected coordinates in space. First, consider the simpler 2D case of a single slice and imaging with axial septa, in which a slice is defined by events occurring within the same crystal ring or adjacent crystal rings (Figure 1.2). Each line of coincidence connecting two crystal elements within the slice is described in terms of coordinates (R, θ), which are the distance from the center and the trans-axial angle. The histogram of all events binned in (R, θ) space is called a *sinogram* (Figure 1.8). Since the raw data from each slice produces a sinogram, a multiring PET scanner with axial septa produces a stack of 2D sinograms indexed by the slice axial coordinate z. Each sinogram is reconstructed separately, resulting in a stack of 2D tomographic images that may be displayed as a volume image. (Although the end result is a 3D volume, this mode of acquisition and reconstruction is commonly referred to as "2D imaging," since each slice is independently acquired and reconstructed.)

For a multiring PET scanner operating without axial septa, coincident events arising from detected gamma rays on nonadjacent crystal rings also are recorded. In addition to the sinogram and slice coordinates (R, θ, z), the axial angle φ (or alternatively the

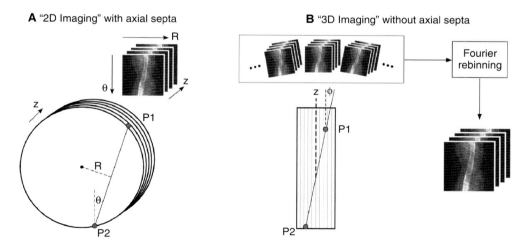

FIGURE 1.8. Binning of raw PET data into sinograms. Lines of coincidences within a trans-axial slice are represented by their distance from the origin (R) and relative angle (θ). Each coincidence event defined by the detected locations P1 and P2 is binned accordingly into a 2D histogram as a function of (R, θ), which is known as a *sinogram*. In the case of 2D imaging (A), the slices defined by the PET ring geometry are treated separately, resulting in a stack of 2D sinograms as a function of the axial coordinate z. In the case of 3D imaging (B), the relative axial angle φ presents an additional variable, which leads to multiple stacks of sinograms. Further processing (using algorithms such as Fourier rebinning) compresses the raw data into an approximate single stack of 2D sinograms, which greatly speeds image reconstruction.

ring difference) is another coordinate that must be specified, thus adding a fourth dimension to the complete description of the sinogram data (Figure 1.8B). As discussed earlier, the benefit of including multiring events is that the sensitivity of the PET scanner is greatly increased; however, the requirements for data storage and the complexity of image reconstruction also are increased. Techniques for "fully 3D reconstruction" have been well researched,[7] but many algorithms are too computationally intensive for routine clinical imaging.

Instead, rebinning methods often are used to transform the complete four-dimensional sinogram representation into an approximate stack of 2D sinograms. The commonly used Fourier rebinning algorithm has been shown to preserve the fully 3D nature of the data over a wide range of axial angles.[15] After rebinning is performed, each slice may be reconstructed independently, allowing for the use of 2D image reconstruction algorithms that are computationally much faster and more practical than fully 3D reconstruction algorithms.

Reconstruction

The typical steps involved with image reconstruction and processing are summarized in Figure 1.5. Sinogram data for the emission and transmission scans are acquired separately. Randoms correction is applied by subtracting delayed coincidence data from the prompt coincidence data. Calibration data from a prior normalization scan and dead-time loss factors are applied, as well as a decay correction factor based on the radionuclide half-life of the injected tracer. The transmission data are reconstructed first to produce attenuation correction factors, which are then applied during subsequent reconstruction of the emission data. Scatter correction is applied using both the emission and transmission images to compute and subtract the estimated scatter component. Afterward, a smoothing filter is applied to reduce high-frequency noise and produce optimal image quality.

Image reconstruction often is done using the conventional filtered backprojection (FBP) algorithm,[16] in which an apodizing filter is applied in the frequency domain to the sinogram data, followed by backprojection into image space. Since the FBP algorithm involves a single backprojection step, it is exact and requires little computational time. However, in situations with low count density or with wide variations in activity concentration, FBP is prone to artifacts and may not produce the best-quality images.

Iterative reconstruction algorithms differ from FBP in that multiple projection and backprojection steps are performed with the goal of converging toward an optimal image estimate. A common iterative algorithm is the maximum-likelihood expectation-maximization (ML-EM) method,[17] in which an image estimate first is projected and compared to the actual sinogram data, and appropriate scaling factors are computed and backprojected to produce a new and more accurate image estimate. The process is repeated for a number of iterations until a final image estimate is obtained. However, image noise is amplified with increasing number of iterations, and thus stopping criteria, regularization methods, or postfiltering, or some combination of the three, is implemented to prevent excessive noise in the final image. ML-EM assumes a Poisson statistical model and performs relatively well for low-count sinogram data. Since there are multiple projection and backprojection steps, the algorithm is more local in nature compared to FBP and is less prone to streaking and spillover artifacts. To accelerate the convergence of iterative reconstruction and to reduce computation time, the ordered-subsets expectation-maximization (OS-EM) algorithm (a modified version of ML-EM) uses ordered subsets of sinograms, such that only a fraction of the data must be processed before updating the image estimate per iteration.[18] In recent years, OS-EM iterative reconstruction has become computationally practical in clinical settings and has become the most common reconstruction algorithm used in PET oncology studies.

From the point of view of cardiac PET, the reconstruction parameters may significantly impact the quality of resultant images. Perhaps the most critical setting is the filter applied during FBP or after iterative reconstruction. The goal of proper filter selection is to minimize image noise while retaining anatomic structure.[19] Filter selection for cardiac protocols requires an understanding of the resolution performance of the PET scanner as well as consideration of the count density of the study data. FBP often performs well for cardiac PET since myocardial count density is sufficiently high in most study protocols. If OS-EM iterative reconstruction is available (as is the case on most modern PET scanners), it may be a better choice in situations in which extracardiac activity is present or in which count density is low. For dynamic PET imaging using kinetic modeling to estimate absolute perfusion values, FBP is usually considered to be the better choice because of its exact nature, even though image quality often is poorer than with OS-EM. In summary, careful selection of algorithm and associated parameters should be made based on the scanner characteristics and the imaging protocol used.

Cardiac PET—Practical Considerations

Cardiac PET is well established in clinical practice for myocardial perfusion imaging using ^{82}RbCl or ^{13}NH$_3$ and for myocardial metabolic imaging using ^{18}F-fluoro-2-deoxyglucose (FDG). General guidelines exist for patient preparation and image acquisition of cardiac PET studies.[20] However, one must keep in mind that since the designs of commercial PET scanners differ, the optimal imaging parameters may vary among scanners. A good working knowledge of the underlying physics of PET imaging is essential in establishing the cardiac PET protocol for a specific scanner. Practical considerations for cardiac PET imaging are discussed in the following sections.

Misregistration

One of the main advantages of cardiac PET over cardiac SPECT is the ability to perform accurate attenuation correction. It is important to consider, though, that the transmission data and emission data are acquired sequentially and not simultaneously. It is possible then that the two data sets may not be exactly coregistered if there is relative motion between the two acquisitions. This may occur if the patient shifts position on the table or if the heart is in a different position during stress perfusion imaging (a situation often referred to as *cardiac creep*). If motion has occurred, improper attenuation factors will be applied during image reconstruction, and the resultant images will not be quantitatively accurate. This is particularly important in cardiac PET near the lung-tissue interface, where the attenuation coefficients differ substantially (see Figure 1.7). When cardiac PET images are read, fusion images of the reconstructed emission data and the attenuation map should be viewed together routinely to assess whether relative motion has occurred.

Extracardiac Activity

Activity located nearby the heart may affect the quality of myocardial PET studies. Intense extracardiac uptake, for instance, in the bowel, may cause an artificial reduction in reconstructed activity in nearby regions. This effect is often known as *ramp filter artifact* and originates from backprojection of negative values due to the filtering step in the FBP algorithm. Conversely, spillover and streak artifacts from FBP may artificially increase the apparent uptake in nearby regions. Iterative reconstruction is affected less near regions of intense uptake and may be better suited in such cases than FBP. Extracardiac activity also may affect cardiac PET imaging by contributing scatter and random events to the myocardial regions. For example, in ^{82}Rb perfusion PET, there is significant renal uptake that may affect imaging, even though the kidneys most often are located entirely outside the axial field of view. The renal activity is effectively shielded if axial septa are used; however, if 3D imaging without septa is performed, the added scatter and random counts may degrade image quality.

Optimal Injected Activity

In addition to the typical considerations of radiation dose to the patient and the anticipated scan time, the injected dose also should account for the performance characteristics of the specific scanner. With higher activity comes a higher fraction of random events and greater dead-time losses from pulse pileup (see Figure 1.4). The optimal injected dose should be chosen with the goal of maximizing the NEC rate and the resultant image quality. The performance of the PET detectors may therefore limit the acceptable injected dose. An example is the case of ^{82}Rb imaging, in which a 60 mCi dose is commonly infused in 2D mode but would saturate most PET detectors in 3D mode. With the wide differences in detector designs and scintillation crystal properties, the scanner characteristics must be taken under consideration in the choice of injected dose for a cardiac PET scan.

2D versus 3D Imaging

Given the above discussions on extracardiac activity and injected dose, whether to use septa is an important consideration. Using septa in 2D mode will greatly reduce the contribution of random and scatter events and will reduce dead-time losses at a given injected dose, but at the expense of greatly reduced count sensitivity. Imaging in 3D mode without septa may be advantageous in situations with low injected dose, at the expense of increased background counts and with higher reliance on scatter correction accuracy. Comparisons of 2D and 3D cardiac PET have begun to appear in the literature. On modern PET scanners, 3D mode has been shown to be acceptable in comparison to 2D mode for FDG metabolic imaging of the heart.[21,22] For ^{82}Rb perfusion imaging, opinions on this topic differ depending on the PET detector hardware used in the scanner.[23,24] Research in 2D versus 3D imaging is also of interest because many PET/CT scanners in widespread use operate only in 3D mode.

Gated Imaging

Cardiac PET data acquisition may be gated using the patient's electrocardiogram signal to produce multiframe cine images. The data are acquired in multiple sinograms (typically 8), and each sinogram is reconstructed separately. (The corresponding static images are reconstructed from the total sinogram summed over the multiple gated sinograms.) The resultant gated images are displayed in a continuous loop, allowing a physician to assess wall motion and thickening in addition to regional perfusion or viability or both. Several commercial software packages allow easy display, manipulation, and segmentation of gated PET images and provide calculations of volume parameters and ejection fraction.

From a physics standpoint, the gated images are merely a set of independent images. However, the effective acquisition time per image is reduced by a factor equal to the number of frames, and thus the count density is very low. Beat rejection further reduces the acquired count density in cases with irregular heartbeat. To produce gated images of sufficient quality, more total counts must be acquired to compensate for the division of counts over multiple frames. One approach is to use a larger injected dose, provided that the PET scanner does not exhibit excessive dead-time losses and that the randoms fraction is still acceptable. More often the total scan time is lengthened to allow more counts to be acquired per frame. Longer scans can be easily done for ^{18}F-FDG PET, since its physical half-life is relatively long (110 minutes). The same holds true to some extent for ^{13}NH$_3$ PET, though its half-life is considerably shorter

(10 minutes). Gated imaging for ^{82}Rb PET is considerably more challenging, however. The half-life of ^{82}Rb is very short (76 seconds), effectively limiting the total scan time to about 5 minutes and thereby limiting the counts available for gated imaging. In all cases, the scanner performance characteristics affect the quality and feasibility of gated PET.

Summary Points

- PET imaging is based on positron annihilation and coincidence detection of paired 511 keV gamma rays.
- Electronic collimation in PET allows for higher resolution and count sensitivity compared to SPECT imaging.
- In addition to true coincidence events, background coincidence events (random, scatter) also are recorded.
- The steps of data processing and image reconstruction include corrections for attenuation, scatter, randoms, and detector normalization, resulting in quantitatively accurate PET images.
- External transmission sources are used to produce attenuation data.
- PET scanners may operate in 3D mode (without axial septa) or 2D mode (with axial septa), with a main difference being count sensitivity versus shielding of background counts.
- Scanner design and performance characteristics influence protocol selection in cardiac PET.

References

1. Valk PE, Bailey DL, Townsend DW, Maisey MN. Positron Emission Tomography: Basic Science and Clinical Practice. London: Springer; 2002.
2. Sanchez-Crespo A, Andreo P, Larsson SA. Positron flight in human tissues and its influence on PET image spatial resolution. *Eur J Nucl Med Mol Imaging.* 2004;31:44–51.
3. Levin CS, Hoffman EJ. Calculation of positron range and its effect on the fundamental limit of positron emission tomography system spatial resolution. *Phys Med Biol.* 1999;44:781–799.
4. Knoll GF. Radiation Detection and Measurement. 3rd ed. New York: John Wiley & Sons, 1999.
5. Humm JL, Rosenfeld A, Del Guerra A. From PET detectors to PET scanners. *Eur J Nucl Med Mol Imaging.* 2003;30:1574–1597.
6. van Eijk CWE. Inorganic scintillators in medical imaging. *Phys Med Biol.* 2002;47: R85–R106.
7. Bendriem B, Townsend DW. The Theory and Practice of 3D PET. Dordrecht: Kluwer Academic Publishers, 1998.
8. Strother SC, Casey ME, Hoffman EJ. Measuring PET scanner sensitivity: relating count-rates to image signal-to-noise ratios using noise equivalent counts. *IEEE Trans Nucl Sci.* 1990;37:783–788.
9. National Electrical Manufacturers Association. NEMA Standards Publication NU2; Washington, DC, 2001.
10. Daube-Witherspoon ME, Karp JS, Casey ME, et al. PET performance measurements using the NEMA NU 2–2001 standard. *J Nucl Med.* 2002;43:1398–1409.
11. Strauss LG, Conti PS. The applications of PET in clinical oncology. *J Nucl Med.* 1991;32:623–648; discussion 649–650.
12. Sugawara Y, Zasadny KR, Neuhoff AW, Wahl RL. Reevaluation of the standardized uptake value for FDG: variations with body weight and methods for correction. *Radiology.* 1999;213:521–525.
13. Watson CC. New faster, image-based scatter correction for 3D PET. *IEEE Trans Nucl Sci.* 2000;47:1587–1594.
14. Zaidi H, Koral KF. Scatter modelling and compensation in emission tomography. *Eur J Nucl Med Mol Imaging.* 2004;31:761–782.

15. Defrise M, Kinahan PE, Townsend DW, Michel C, Sibomana M, Newport DF. Exact and approximate rebinning algorithms for 3-D PET data. *IEEE Trans Med Imaging.* 1997;16:145–158.
16. Kak AC, Slaney M. Principles of Computerized Tomographic Imaging. New York: IEEE Press; 1998.
17. Lange K, Carson R. EM reconstruction algorithms for emission and transmission tomography. *J Comput Assist Tomogr.* 1984;8:306–316.
18. Hudson HM, Larkin RS. Accelerated image reconstruction using ordered subsets of projection data. *IEEE Trans Med Imaging.* 1994;13:601–609.
19. Zubal IG, Wisniewski G. Understanding Fourier space and filter selection. *J Nucl Cardiol.* 1997;4:234–243.
20. Bacharach SL, Bax JJ, Case J, et al. PET myocardial glucose metabolism and perfusion imaging: Part 1—Guidelines for data acquisition and patient preparation. *J Nucl Cardiol.* 2003;10:543–556.
21. Brink I, Schumacher T, Talazko J, et al. 3D-cardiac-PET. A recommendable clinical alternative to 2D-cardiac-PET? *Clin Positron Imaging.* 1999;2:191–196.
22. Lubberink M, Boellaard R, van der Weerdt AP, Visser FC, Lammertsma AA. Quantitative comparison of analytic and iterative reconstruction methods in 2- and 3-dimensional dynamic cardiac 18F-FDG PET. *J Nucl Med.* 2004;45:2008–2015.
23. Knesaurek K, Machac J, Krynyckyi BR, Almeida OD. Comparison of 2-dimensional and 3-dimensional 82Rb myocardial perfusion PET imaging. *J Nucl Med.* 2003;44:1350–1356.
24. Votaw JR, White M. Comparison of 2-dimensional and 3-dimensional cardiac 82Rb PET studies. *J Nucl Med.* 2001;42:701–706.

2 Instrumentation and Principles of CT

Douglas P. Boyd

The words *computed tomography* (CT) refer to a method of tomographic imaging in which a "tomographic," or cross-sectional, slice is imaged with the aid of computer processing to obtain an exact representation of the slice. Tomographic imaging is important since in conventional projection imaging, such as plane-film x-ray imaging, a small feature may be difficult to visualize because of the confusing superposition of many overlying layers of different structures. X-ray tomographic imaging was developed more than 50 years ago as an approach to cross-section slice imaging. One of the most successful commercial devices was the axial tomograph developed by Takahashi,[1] which in some ways is the precursor to modern CT scanners. The x-ray tube and a plane film positioned at a nearly perpendicular angle rotated around the body, exposing a single cross-section slice. The x-ray projections at each angle were recorded as crossing the film, and were accumulated. Today we call this a simple backprojection image. Although these images were useful, they were somewhat blurred because simple backprojection is only a first-order solution to the problem of reconstructing a cross-section image from rotational projections. This is where the computer part of the name *computed tomography* becomes critical: to provide digital processing to remove the tomographic blur. The projection data are gathered and backprojected using digital data rather than film. The resulting backprojection image is then "deblurred," or reconstructed, by applying a simple sharpening filter, which is sometimes referred to as a *convolution kernel*. You can think of this process as a kind of edge-enhancement process, and it is sometimes referred to as filtered backprojection. In the end, the marriage of computer filtering and axial tomography resulted in the new field of computed tomography.

Computed tomographic methods may be applied to many kinds of medical imaging, including x-ray CT, positron emission tomography (PET), single photon emission computed tomography (SPECT), a new kind of ultrasound imaging, ultrasound CT, and even certain forms of magnetic resonance imaging (MRI). Thus CT has revolutionized imaging by opening up the possibility of true accurate cross-section imaging and, as a side benefit, providing accurate CT numbers within each picture element of the image, thus enabling a new era of tissue characterization. As the technology continues to evolve with all the modalities, the ability to image small and subtle features deep inside the body has advanced remarkably, especially with the advent of three-dimensional (3D) volume rendering.

In this chapter we discuss the technology used in x-ray CT, including the scanner technology and applications, and a bit about the current status in the evolution of CT capabilities. Although x-ray imaging has a history of more than a century of development, x-ray CT, with only 30 years of development, is still far from its ultimate potential. Although CT is superb for soft-tissue imaging, it does not yet match conventional x-ray imaging in resolution, exposure speed, or low cost. As CT gets closer to the performance of conventional x-ray in those three categories, it will continue to replace x-ray procedures, until someday in the future, nearly all x-ray imaging will be performed by CT.

CT Development up to 1988

In 1963 and 1964 Cormack,[2,3] a physicist at Cape Town, South Africa, was working on improving the dose calculations used in radiation therapy treatment planning. Knowledge of the cross-section density distribution was required, which led him to develop the concept of reconstruction from projections. The mathematic formulas for reconstruction were then tested by Cormack on aluminum and with disks and irregularly shaped phantoms. This research was published in the *Journal of Applied Physics* and was not recognized at the time as an important solution for imaging. Many other investigators developed image reconstruction formulas for cross-sectional imaging, including solutions depending on iterative techniques. Oldendorf experimented with a rotary method for radiographic cross-sectional depiction of the brain and published his preliminary results in 1961.[4] Kuhl and Edwards reconstructed cross-sectional images from radionuclide scans.[5] Their techniques, published in 1963, constituted the basic approach that was later used in PET scanning.

Modern computed tomography (CT), however, was developed by Hounsfield working for Electronic and Musical Industries Ltd (EMI) in England.[6] His original work, with a gamma-ray source and using Perspex, produced images; however, it took more than 9 days to complete the acquisition of data. A prototype scanner using an x-ray tube was developed in 1969 and 1970, and a clinically applicable machine was installed at the Atkinson-Morely Hospital in the suburbs of London. The first clinical results were presented by Ambrose and Hounsfield in 1972 at the Congress of the British Institute of Radiology.[7] The further obvious success of the approach was due, however, to the rapid advances in small computers, making it possible to develop clinical CT scanners. Since interest for cross-sectional imaging was very intense throughout the United States, Europe, and Japan, it became apparent that such scanners had to be acquired by clinical centers and their uses further developed. The early recognition of the value of this approach was shown by the award of the Lasker Foundation in 1975 to Hounsfield, Kuhl, and Oldendorf. The Nobel Prize in Physiology and Medicine for 1979 was awarded to Cormack and Hounsfield for their discovery of computed tomography.[8]

The original EMI head scanner required long scanning time, 5 minutes, but newer machines were rapidly introduced. Working independently of Hounsfield, in 1971 Boyd and Goitein introduced the concept of a pure rotary scanner using a position-sensitive Xenon detector, a technique that later became the standard.[9] The first reconstruction of a phantom with this device required 16 hours at the UCB computer center using an iterative solution. But the first commercial whole-body scanners were destined to use a variant of Hounsfield's original translate-rotate technique and achieved scan speeds of around 20 seconds. This variation used a translating fan rather than a translating pencil beam to speed the acquisition of data. The first of these scanners was introduced by EMI in 1976 and later that year by Techniscan, followed by up to 16 other distinct manufacturers.

But it was the first rotary scanners, commercially introduced by Artronix, Varian, and later GE, that achieved the goal of 6 seconds or faster scanning,[10] to accommodate breath holding. All scanners used a full-length, position-sensitive Xenon detector to eliminate the need for translation and thereby acquire data at much faster speeds.[11]

Rotary Xenon scanners, sometimes referred to as third-generation CT, became the industry standard for more than the next 20 years, until Xenon was replaced with scintillator-photodiode arrays.

Another type of rotary scanner was developed under a grant by the National Institutes of Health. Known as the fourth generation, this instrument used a ring of stationary detectors with only the x-ray tube rotating. This approach was used by several manufacturers during the 1980s but ultimately was not competitive with rotary xenon scanners due to the added cost of a full ring of detectors. However, it was the introduction of intravenously administered iodine-containing contrast media, ionic and later nonionic, and orally administered contrast media, with rapidly improving spatial resolution, that has made abdominal computed tomography one of the preferred clinical imaging approaches.

Image Reconstruction in CT

Image reconstruction is the process that converts detector readings from hundreds of thousands of data samples into an electronic picture that represents the scanned section. The picture is composed of a matrix of picture elements (pixels), each of which has a density value represented by its CT number. Using the Hounsfield scale of CT numbers, water is 0, air is –1000, and bone is +1000. Each CT number represents a 0.1% density difference. The process of image reconstruction requires more than a billion multiplication steps to reconstruct a 512 × 512 image matrix. Since the hardware involved consists of sophisticated array processors and custom backprojection processors, the cost of the reconstruction system is significant and increases linearly with speed. Reconstruction speed can often become a limiting factor in patient throughput.

For the original scanners, iterative reconstruction methods were used. In this method the projection data are first backprojected onto the image matrix as a first-iteration image. Backprojection involves incrementing the pixels intersected by a ray with the projection value for that ray. Then projection measurements of this image are compared with the actual projection data, and the pixels are adjusted by a correction increment. This process is repeated through several iterations until the final image is obtained. Iterative reconstruction is still used today in certain situations, in which data are missing or inaccurate, to improve the image quality. For example, where there is an opaque object such as a metal prosthesis, iterative reconstruction could be used to reduce streaking. In another example, bone in the head may cause beam-hardening artifact. An iterative reconstruction can be used to first estimate the amount of bone in each projection ray and then correct for it.

Today the most popular form of image reconstruction is based on a method first described by mathematicians Ramachandran and Lakshminarayanan known as filtered backprojection.[12] This method is based on equations that describe an exact solution for reconstruction in which the projection data are first filtered using a convolution filter or kernel and then backprojected. The kernel is adjusted so that the final image is an exact representation of the scanned object. Using the Fast Fourier Transform, the number of computations required for the convolution step can be reduced from $n2$ to $n\log n$ by performing the convolution in Fourier space. The backprojection step can be speeded up by reordering and rebinning the fan projection rays into sets of parallel rays.[13] Then the backprojection process becomes a series of step-add operations. With these methods, filtered backprojection reconstruction is an order of magnitude faster than iterative reconstruction, and reconstruction speeds in the milliseconds are obtained using custom application-specific intergrated circuit (ASIC) chips that are programmed to perform the required repetitive multiplication and summing operations.

Other available reconstruction methods have been less widely used. The direct Fourier method requires fewer computations than even parallel-ray filtered backprojection. In this method the transformed projection data are placed into two-dimensional (2D) Fourier space, interpolated using a technique known as gridding,[14] and then two-dimensionally transformed back into the reconstructed image. This faster method has been used in electron beam CT (EBCT) and in baggage CT scanners.

Patient and Image Handling

The patient-handling table is usually motorized, with horizontal (axial) and vertical drives. The couch is automatically indexed in the horizontal direction under computer control to position a series of adjacent tomographic sections. Laser-produced light beams are used to localize the patient within the gantry. Selection of the scanning volume is usually based on the use of a line-scanned projection image obtained by sweeping the patient horizontally through the stationary x-ray fan beam.

Automation of the couch and integration into the scanning software enable scan planes, angles, and spacing to be selected from this image using a trackball-guided cursor at the operator's console. The scanning gantry is usually able to tilt ±20 degrees, and in some cases the couch can be tilted or angulated in the horizontal plane.

CT scanners usually come equipped with one or two display consoles. One is for the technologist's use in controlling the scanner, immediate review of images, and multiformat hardcopy production. A second console is reserved for the radiologist to read images and perform the several types of image analyses that are available. Since CT images contain quantitative information in terms of density values and contours of organs, quantitation of volumes, areas, and masses is possible. This is accomplished with region-of-interest methods, which involve the electronic outlining of the selected region of the television display monitor with a trackball-controlled cursor. In addition, various image-processing options, such as edge enhancement (for viewing fine details of edges) and smoothing filters (for enhancing the detectability of low-contrast lesions) are useful tools.

Other useful options available at the console include various software programs for off-axis reformation of images and for 3D reconstructions of surfaces. These display programs offer a great deal of flexibility in exploiting the 3D character of CT data and often enhance the interpretation of complex shapes. Recently introduced hardware options have resulted in computational speed improvements that enable many 3D display manipulations to be accomplished virtually in real time.

For many years CT images were usually photographed with multiformat cameras to produce a standard 14-in × 17-in film with 16 or 20 images on a film. Today that method is no longer practical because slices are thinner and scanning volumes larger. A CT study today may involve 1000 to 2000 slices. The solution has been to store and display CT images using a picture archiving and communications (PACS) network. The images are stored on a network server and viewed on a network workstation. The workstation is equipped with viewing software that enables the operator to scroll through large sets of images in seconds with a mouse, and to reconstruct various types of volume-rendered images in real time.

Ultrafast, Multilevel CT Using Scanning Electron Beams

During the late 1970s it seemed clear that rotary mechanical gantry systems would not become fast enough to freeze cardiac motion as required for cardiac CT, and almost every development group looked for alternative solutions. In 1978 an alternative approach to CT using a scanning electron beam tube was proposed.[15] This approach had an advantage for high-speed, multislice imaging since no mechanical

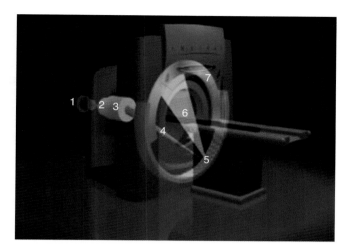

FIGURE 2.1. Artist's illustration of an electron beam ct scanner. These scanners have scan speeds as low as 33 milliseconds and, using a dual-row detector in combination with 4 target rings, can obtain 8 slices nearly simultaneously. See text for the description of the key numbered components.

motion was required. The rotating x-ray fan is produced by scanning an electron beam on semicircular tungsten rings (actually 210° arcs) below the patient. Since these large rings can be directly water cooled, the beam power can be much higher than that used in conventional x-ray tubes. Thus in the scanning electron beam system, speed is not restricted by either mechanical considerations or heat-capacity restrictions.

The principle of operation of the scanning electron beam system is illustrated in Figure 2.1. An electron gun (1) is used to produce a beam of electrons at 130 kV and 800 mA (2). After exiting the gun, the beam expands because of space-charge repulsive forces and is refocused with a series of magnetic lenses (3). Final focusing occurs near the target and is due to the self-focusing properties of an intense neutralized beam. The beam is neutralized by allowing positive ions of nitrogen gas to be captured in the beam. The beam is bent through an angle of 33 to 37 degrees by a pair of orthogonal dipole electromagnets (4). The plane of bend is rotated by applying currents to these magnets that are approximately sinusoidal and 90 degrees out of phase.

Thus, the deflected beam is caused to sweep along the circular tungsten target rings at the focus (5). Since the scanner is intended to image multiple slices, 4 target rings are provided and can be selected in sequence by varying the bend angle. An x-ray-opaque housing (collimator) defines the x-ray beam to a fan shape (6) that rotates with the motion of the electron beam spot on the water-cooled target rings. Under computer control, the focal spot is precisely steered through 210 degrees in either 50 or 100 milliseconds. The collimated x-ray beam penetrates the body and is recorded by an adjacent pair of ring-shaped detector arrays above the body (7). When installed in the hospital, this scanner looks like a conventional scanner (although the gantry aperture is larger) and requires approximately the same amount of space. Since this scanner operates completely under computer control, a wide variety of scanning sequences and operational modes are available. For dynamic studies, 2 adjacent slices are simultaneously imaged at rates of up to 17 frames per second.

Electron beam CT was first introduced commercially in 1984 as a cardiac CT scanner and was updated in 1988 as a general-purpose cardiac and radiological CT.[16] A new-model EBCT introduced in 2003 offered dual 1.5-mm slices, scan speeds as fast as 33 milliseconds, beam power of 140 kV at 1000 mA, and spatial resolution in the 14 line pairs per centimeter (lp/cm) range.

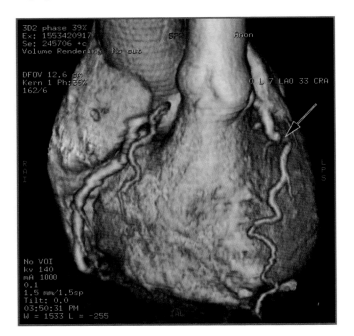

FIGURE 2.2. A volume-rendered frame from a cine sequence of the heart using ebct. This frame is at 39% of the r-r interval. In this multiphase study, 8 phases were obtained covering the first 460 milliseconds following the r-wave. The right coronary artery is shown to the left along with two of its ventricular branches. On the right side is the left anterior descending coronary artery with a proximal stenosis (arrow). Technical parameters are 50-millisecond scan speed, 140kv, 1000ma, 1.5-Mm slice thickness, and intravenous contrast media at 4ml/s.

Although approximately 300 EBCT systems were installed throughout the world, this amounted to only 1% to 2% of the entire CT market, which by 2004 became dominated by the newest version of multislice CT scanners, described below. EBCT technology at this time was more expensive to build and to develop than the competing mechanical scanners, and many of its key advantages in volume data acquisition were whittled away by continuous developments of multislice scanners. However, EBCT remains the champion in exposure speed and is still the only viable technology that has the potential to reach an exposure speed of 10 milliseconds as would be required to be fully competitive with coronary angiography (Figure 2.2).

Modern Multislice Cone-Spiral CT

Starting in the late 1980s, the concept of continuous spiral scanning was introduced in CT. This concept required the use of slip rings to transfer power and signals to and from the continuously rotating gantry. Previous to that time, scanners used long cables with a windup mechanism that limited rotation to only 360 degrees or a bit more. Some of the initial attempts with slip rings attempted to transfer high voltage (±70kV) for the x-ray tube and thus required extensive insulation and high-voltage standoff provisions. But soon, smaller high-frequency power supplies were developed that could be placed directly on the rotating gantry. With this development, only main power of 240 volts was needed.

One of the earliest continuous-rotate CT scanners was developed under a contract with the US Army and was intended for portable use at army field hospitals. This scanner, known as the Imatron FMS5000, was presented at the Radiological Society of North America exhibition in Chicago in 1988 (Figures 2.3 and 2.4). The FMS5000

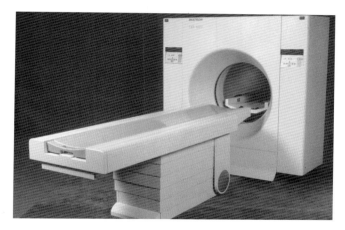

FIGURE 2.3. The Imatron FMS5000 was one of the first continuous-rotation CT scanners using low-voltage slip rings. This compact design introduced in 1998 was intended for use in army field hospitals.

components are shown in Figure 2.4. Visible are the x-ray tube (1), the compact high-voltage power supply (2, 3), the solid-state detector array (4), and the data-acquisition system (5). Later a modified version of this scanner was used to demonstrate the ability to detect explosives in airport-checked luggage (Invision CTX5000). By 2004 thousands of scanners of this type were installed at airports throughout the world.

In 2000, Willi Kalendar, using a slip-ring scanner, demonstrated the power of spiral CT.[17] In spiral CT the patient table is advanced continuously during continuous gantry rotation. Although the projection data are acquired at various z positions during the scan process (sometimes referred to as helical data), the data can be linearly interpolated back to a fixed plane by using two adjacent scans in sequence. Spiral scanning eliminated the interscan delay associated with the older step-scan methods and facilitated acquisitions of a large number of thin slices in a short interval.

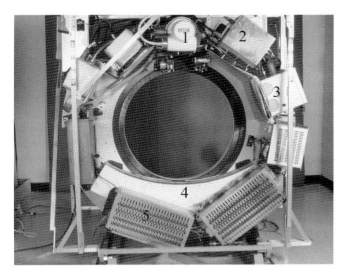

FIGURE 2.4. This photograph inside the shrouds of the Imatron FMS5000 illustrates the typical components found inside modern spiral and multislice spiral scanners. In 1998 the scan speed was 1 second. By 2005 bearings and slip rings had been improved to enable a rotation speed as fast as 350 milliseconds, and x-ray tubes increased several-fold in size and power capability. The numbered components are described in the text.

By 1999, the first multislice-spiral scanners were introduced. The first of these were called 4-slice scanners and had 4 parallel detector arrays.[18] With the acquisition of data for 4 slices simultaneously, the rate of scanning could be increased by a factor of 4, thus allowing the acquisition of volume data at a higher rate and with less tube loading. For the first time, mechanical CT could compete with many applications previously available only to electron-beam-based systems. For example, using pitch = 1 spiral scanning (advancing the table by 4 slices per revolution), a volume of 40 cm could be covered with 200 2-mm slices in only 25 seconds. Previously, this would have required 100 seconds, which is outside the x-ray-tube limitations and the limitations of patient breath holding. Slices of 2 mm are thin enough for volume rendering and maximum-intensity projection (MIP) visualization techniques to be used, especially for imaging of blood vessels, or CT angiography (CTA). These 4-slice scanners were an immediate commercial success.

Within a few years, 8-slice and then 16-slice scanners were introduced. With 16 slices, a slice thickness of 0.8 mm could be used, which enabled the concept of "isotropic resolution." This means that the resolution in the z dimension became similar to the in-plane (x,y) resolution, a useful requirement for 3D image processing. Especially with the 16-slice models, for the first time cardiac imaging became accessible with a mechanical scanner. Although the scan speed remained at 300 milliseconds for a partial scan or 500 milliseconds for a complete scan, software developers found ways to improve the performance of cardiac gating by utilizing the increased density of images. Cardiac gating with single slices had been tried and failed as early as the late 1970s, had a minor resurgence with 4-slice scanners, but became more or less viable with 16-slice scanners. Gating could be used to reduce scan speed either by a factor of 2 (from 300 milliseconds to 150 milliseconds), or by a factor of 4 (from 300 milliseconds to 75 milliseconds) by combining data from 2 or 4 heartbeats. This worked best for hearts with a consistent rate that was close to a multiple of the scanning rate. In most cases, the patient received intravenous β-blockers to slow and control the heart rate. A further advantage of the 16-slice scanners was that the slice thickness was less, and it was found that this enhanced the imaging of small-branch coronary artery vessels. For the first time cardiologists began to obtain CT scanners for the purpose of CTA of coronary arteries.

In 2005, 64-slice CT scanners became available in large numbers. The increase from 16 to 64 slices was used to reduce slice thickness an additional factor of 2, to approximately 0.5 mm, and also to increase the width of the fan from 2 cm to 4 cm, thus affording wider and faster coverage. With a 64-slice scanner it became feasible to scan a volume such as the heart or the entire chest in only a few seconds—using 0.5-mm slices. A volume of 40-cm length would now be covered with 800 slices in less than 10 seconds. At this speed, only about 40 mL of contrast media needed to be injected at 4 mL/s, a major reduction in contrast requirement. This is both a cost reduction and a benefit to the patient, who has less contrast burden on the renal system.

Although the 64-slice scanners incrementally improved the possibility of cardiac imaging with mechanical scanning, they still fall short of the speed obtainable by EBCT, and by the ideal requirement to freeze cardiac motion in the 10-millisecond range. This leaves lots of room for future development.

3D Visualization Techniques

The sheer number of slices generated by modern multislice scanners can overwhelm the viewer. Today anywhere from 1000 to 2000 slice images are routinely acquired in a study. These can be viewed with a computer-based viewer by rapid scrolling through the images using the trackball or mouse. But, increasingly, volume imaging methods are employed to visualize the scanned volume in 3D.

To start, the image slices are stacked into a 3D matrix and interpolated (if necessary) to cubic voxels (volume elements). Due to the problem of overlapping structures, processing will be necessary to see inside this cube of data. There are two fundamental approaches. One is to render the voxels as semitransparent, so the observer can look through overlying structures. The other method is to either cut away the overlying voxels or extract a slice or subvolume of voxels from within the cube. This is analogous to the procedure of exploratory surgery, where the surgeon cuts away intervening tissues to reveal what is below. Modern 3D workstations use a combination of semitransparency and cutting techniques.

One major use of volume rendering is to screen patients for colon cancer by "flying through" the air or the CO_2-inflated colon. This method is referred to as CT colonography and is rapidly replacing the more invasive method of colonoscopy using a long endoscope.

The visualization is performed by rendering the air transparent and the walls of the colon (CT values of approximately 50) semitransparent. A view is projected on the workstation screen that simulates the view from a small camera flying along a central path through the colon. The field of view of the camera is limited to just the forward direction, and the ray tracing stops a few centimeters past the wall of the colon. Thus, only a small subset of the cubic data are sampled for each image and the processing can proceed in real time. In Figure 2.5, the image is rendered as a stereo image using the Accuimage VRT program and can be viewed using blue and red stereo glasses in 3D. The stereo image is created by using 2 side-by-side stereo cameras for the blue-red images. The EBCT image shown in Figure 2.2 is also a volume-rendered image, but here parallel projection is used and the chest wall has been cut away to reveal only the surface of the heart.

For imaging of blood vessels, the MIP method usually gives the best images. In MIP imaging, the brightest pixel in a slab region of interest is projected. This will usually be a pixel within the lumen or the blood vessel. The MIP plane may be thick, thin, oblique, or even curved. For long blood vessels such as a coronary artery, it is often best to use curved reformatting by selecting points along the vessel and fitting

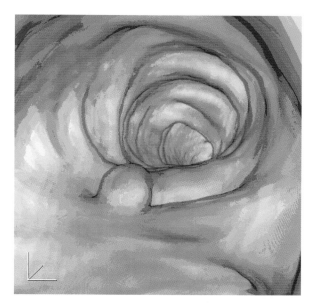

FIGURE 2.5. A volume-rendered endoscopic view inside the colon demonstrating a 4-mm polyp. Virtual colonoscopy is becoming a major application for multislice ct. This frame from the fly-through movie was rendered in stereo, and the 3d effect becomes visible when viewed with red-blue glasses.

a curved plane to those points. This then provides an image of the entire artery in a single planar image, as though the artery was straightened, and usually more closely resembles the kind of images seen in conventional angiography.

Principles of Scan Protocol Design Using Multislice CT

With the evolution of CT, the number of adjustable parameters has multiplied, causing great complexity in the design of CT protocols. Although the manufacturers provide detailed protocol books with each scanner model, these are only guidelines, intended for average clinical use. The expert radiographer can use his or her knowledge of protocol design principles to achieve superior images or less risk of radiation dose and contrast for specific problem solving. Protocol design involves a complex interplay of the parameters of slice width, scan speed, radiation dose, x-ray power, couch speed (pitch), and contrast injection technique. With multislice CT, an added complexity is that the reconstructed slice thickness may no longer correspond to the slice collimation. Thick slices can be reconstructed using multiple thin slices using the latest cone-spiral reconstruction algorithms.

In planning the protocol, the starting point is to determine the slice thickness to be used. Thick slices (4–8 mm) are preferred when low image noise is required, when dose must be minimized, for example, in screening examinations, or both. The image noise is fundamentally determined by the number of x-ray photons detected for that slice. With other parameters fixed, a 1-mm slice will acquire one eighth as many photons as an 8-mm slice. The noise in the 1-mm slice will be the square root of 8 higher than the noise of the thick slice, according to the laws of Poisson statistics. Thus, thinner slices will almost always require higher dose scanning and will be noisier than the thicker-slice alternatives. Today, slice thickness as low as 0.35 mm is available, which is 23 times less than 8 mm. In screening studies such as cardiac screening, lung screening, or virtual colonography, thicker slices are preferred to minimize radiation exposure to a healthy patient.

For diagnostic studies, the patient will normally have disease symptoms, which will justify a higher dose protocol to maximize the risk/benefit ratio. Further, in diagnostic studies, subtle distinctions of small structures or vessels or subtle contrast differences may enable an important differential determination of disease type. Therefore, these studies will generally involve higher x-ray exposure and thinner slice thickness. An exception would be for pediatric patients, who generally require lower exposure due to increased risk, and the fact that the thinner child's body may transmit 3–10 times more x-ray flux than an adult body. The attenuation distance for typical CT x-rays is approximately 5 cm, so for each additional 5 cm of body thickness, detected x-rays will be attenuated by 2.73. Thus, in contradistinction to the pediatric case, when a very obese patient is encountered, x-ray exposure must be increased greatly, and thicker slices should be considered.

To achieve optimal diagnostic quality image, consideration must be given to the signal-to-noise ratio (SNR). In the preceding paragraphs we discussed the noise part of SNR, which depends mainly on slice thickness and x-ray power and exposure time, as expressed by milliampere-seconds (mAs). But equally important is the determination of the signal. In CT the signal is represented as the contrast between adjacent tissues or structures to be imaged. CT tissue contrast varies from approximately 1000 Hounsfield units (HU) to less than 10 HU, a range of 100:1. Some typical CT contrast ranges are listed in Table 2.1.

Thus, bone and lung imaging involve a high signal, so a good SNR can be obtained with lower radiation exposure or thinner slices. On the other extreme, brain imaging requires high radiation exposure and thicker slices.

With the older single-slice spiral scanners, an important protocol design consideration involved selecting the scanning range or coverage. There were several factors

TABLE 2.1. Typical CT Contrast Ranges (Hounsfield units)

Lung tissue or vessels surrounded by air	1070 HU
Bone surrounded by soft tissue	500–3000 HU
Contrast-enhanced blood vessels	200–400 HU
Muscle and organ tissue surrounded by fat	150–170 HU
Water surrounded by soft tissue	60–70 HU
Gray matter vs white matter in brain	5–10 HU

that restricted the selection of coverage including patient breath-holding interval, contrast injection rate and maximum contrast load, slice thickness and table speed, pitch, and so on. With 16- to 64-slice scanners, the coverage issue has become less important. Tube loading is no longer a major problem and with 16 to 64 fewer revolutions required, scan times are reduced to the 5-second range for many studies. With 5-second coverage of the chest, only approximately 20 mL of contrast is needed to obtain 350 HU of enhancement using 4 mL/s of typical nonionic contrast media. This is much less than the 120 to 200 mL used by single-slice spiral scanners a few years ago. As a result, protocols involving greater coverage and thinner slices are now routinely available with modern multislice scanners.

Acquisition Versus Reconstruction Parameters

Although coverage issues are simplified, a new complication introduced by multislice CT is that the reconstruction and acquisition parameters can differ. In fact, the same scan data can be reconstructed into 2 or more reconstruction sets, for example, with thick- and thin-slice thicknesses. The thick-slice data set would be used for normal viewing and the thin slices for volume rendering. To discuss this more precisely requires the definition of certain scan parameters, as follows.

Slice Collimation

Slice collimation (SC) is the actual acquisition slice thickness. In multislice CT, the slice thickness is set by the width of adjacent detectors. Slice collimation is adjusted by summing the signals of adjacent detector channels. For example, if the minimum slice thickness is 0.5 mm, then slice collimation of 1, 1.5, and 2.0 can be obtained by summing 2, 3, or 4 adjacent channels.

Table Feed per Revolution

Table feed (TF) per revolution is the distance the table travels per 360 degrees revolution of the gantry. This defines the table speed and is an important parameter in calculating pitch.

Pitch

In single-slice spiral CT, pitch was defined as $P = SC/TF$ by analogy to the pitch of a screw. For multislice CT, pitch is now defined as $P = TF / (N \times SC)$, where N is the number of rows of multislice detectors that are active. A multislice pitch of 1 means that the table advances by the width of the active detector elements for each revolution. This definition is preferred by most physicists and adopted as an international (IEC) standard but is not uniformly adopted by manufacturers. Some manufacturers still use the older single-slice definition of pitch, which gives values that are N times larger than the convention. Pitches of up to 2 are generally useful. A pitch of less than 1 involves slice overlap and exposure would be higher depending on the amount of overlap.

Slice Width

Slice width (SW) is the actual reconstructed slice thickness, which must be equal to or larger than the slice collimation (SC).

Reconstruction Increment

Reconstruction increment (RI) is the reconstructed slice spacing. As in spiral CT, it is often advantageous to reconstruct with RI = ½SW. This gives slice overlap and is useful in determining the exact z-axis size of a lesion and can improve volume-rendered images. If the total number of slices is to be minimized, then RI = SW would be a more conventional selection.

Prospective and Restrospective Cardiac Gating

As discussed previously, gating is used to improve cardiac imaging. In the technique of prospective gating, the scan is triggered to begin at a specific delay following the R-wave (Figure 2.6). The table then moves by N slice thicknesses, and a new triggered scan is performed. This method does not actually reduce effective scan speed, but rather is used to minimize radiation exposure in coronary calcium screening studies. The prospective triggering ensures that all the slices are registered at the same cardiac interval.

In retrospective gating, a continuous multislice spiral scan with pitch of either 1 (2-way binning) or 0.5 (4-way binning) is performed and the electrocardiogram (ECG) data are recorded (Figure 2.7). This assumes an ungated pitch of 2; higher quality would be obtained with lesser pitch. Prior to reconstruction, the data are sorted into time bins representing one half or one quarter of the actual 180-degree acquisition time. For a gantry rotation of 0.4 seconds, the 180-degree acquisition time is 0.2 seconds. Under certain conditions, an effective exposure time of 0.05 seconds for 4-way binning or 0.1 seconds for 2-way binning can be achieved. The special conditions are that the heart rate must be constant and the gantry rotation speed must be adjusted so that an adjacent slice will cover the region of the prior slice with a 45-degree or 90-degree phase lag. If this condition is approximately met, then a fairly reliable gated reconstruction will be obtained. Now 64-slice scanners with gantry rotation speed of 0.35 seconds are challenging EBCT in coronary artery imaging, especially if β-blockers are used to slow the heart rate.

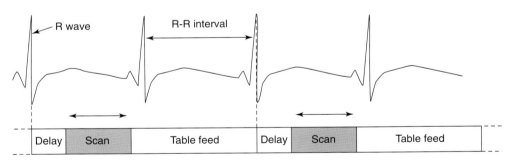

FIGURE 2.6. This figure illustrates the method of prospective gating as used for coronary calcium screening studies. As the gantry rotates continuously and the couch is stationary, a scan is triggered at a scan delay such that most of the scan occurs during the diastolic phase of the cardiac cycle. The scan uses approximately 210 degrees of gantry rotation or about 0.25 Second for modern multislice scanners. During the next heartbeat, the table is advanced by N × SC and a new scan initiated at the same delay on the third beat. Sixteen-slice scanners have a coverage of 2 cm per scan; 64-slice scanners cover 4 cm. The region of the coronary arteries covers about 10 cm and can be covered in 3 to 5 scans (6–10 heartbeats). SC, slice collimation; N, number of rows of detectors. (Diagram adapted with permission of Drs. S Edyvean and N Keat, www.impactscan.org, St George's Hospital, Tooting, London, UK.)

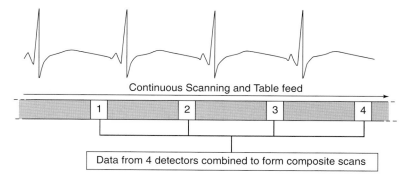

FIGURE 2.7. In retrospective gating, data are acquired continuously in spiral mode with simultaneous recording of the ECG trace. The data are sorted retrospectively into time bins representing either one half or one quarter of the scan speed. If the rotation speed is adjusted appropriately relative to the heart rate, then nearly complete data will be accumulated in each time bin. Reconstruction then provides a reduced effective scan time. (Diagram adapted with permission of Drs. S Edyvean and N Keat, www.impactscan.org, St George's Hospital, Tooting, London, UK.)

Summary Points

- Simultaneous with the development of spiral CT there have been a number of rotary scanners developed that use area detectors such as image intensifiers. These typically have from 512 to 1024 parallel slices. Image intensifiers and various flat-plate area detectors proposed for CT do not yet have the dynamic range and low-noise characteristics of the scintillator photodiode arrays used in multislice CT. In addition, flat-panel area detectors are not yet large enough for full-body scanning. However, they are becoming widely used for small-animal scanning and in dental CT.

- As flat-panel detector technology evolves, there is a trend for the area arrays to grow larger and to be modular. A tileable area detector would consist of a tiled array of detector modules stacked not only side by side as 64-slice scanners but also stacked in the z dimension, providing up to 1024 rows. It seems inevitable that multislice CT will continue to evolve in this way until coverage becomes sufficient to eliminate the need for couch translation for many studies.

- As the resolution and coverage of volume CT expands, the last remaining specification that can be improved is temporal resolution. Temporal resolution is particularly important in imaging the beating heart and especially for good-quality imaging of the coronary arteries following intravenous contrast administration.

- In 2006, the fastest commercial rotation speeds are 350 milliseconds for 360 degrees (approximately 2.5 revolutions/s). This gives the fastest possible exposure speed of about 200 milliseconds. With cardiac gating, a technique that combines data from a small number of heart cycles, the effective exposure speed can be lowered 2 to 4 times less than this in certain situations.

- As speed is increased, the x-ray intensity must be increased as well. During the first several years of spiral development, the x-ray sources grew in size and weight to accommodate higher power and higher heat capacity. Some tubes grew to a weight of more than 500 pounds, which added to the complexity of a rapidly rotating gantry. Heat capacity is important since conventional rotating anode tubes do not have a way to directly conduct heat from the anode.

- In 1993, Rand, Boyd, and Peschmann described a new concept tube in which the electron beam in the tube is fixed and the entire tube housing rotates in front of the beam.[19,20] This inverted geometry provides for direct water or oil cooling of the anode and eliminates the need for a heavy heat absorber attached to the anode. Further, the previous vacuum bearings, which were a common failure mechanism, are no longer needed.

- A similar tube known as the "Straton Tube" was introduced onto commercial multi-slice scanners in 2004; it uses a "flying spot" or "wiggler" mechanism to increase sampling in the z dimension.[21]
- The drive to faster scan speeds with cone-spiral scanners will inevitably lead to proposals for gantries with multiple x-ray tubes, resurrecting an idea first demonstrated by the Mayo Clinic's Dynamic Spatial Reconstructor (DSR) in 1977.[22] The DSR system was equipped with 14 x-ray sources and 14 corresponding area detectors, which in that case were image-intensifier systems. In principle, with such a system mechanical rotation is reduced by a factor of 14 to gather complete CT data. Using modern x-ray tubes and flat-panel detectors, it should be feasible to reach a scan speed of 30 milliseconds using approximately 6 rotating x-ray sources at 30-degree intervals.
- In a recent announcement, a 2-source, multislice CT scanner was demonstrated at the Radiological Society of North America (RSNA) in 2005; this may become the first in a series of future multisource, multislice CT scanners that will ultimately reach the full requirement for cardiac CT and compete with potential future multislice EBCT systems.[21]

References

1. Takahashi S. *Rotational Radiography*. Tokyo: Japan Society for the Promotion of Science; 1957.
2. Cormack A. Representation of function by its line integrals with some radiological applications. Part I. *J Appl Phys*. 1964;35:2722.
3. Cormack A. Representation of function by its line integrals with some radiological applications. Part II. *J Appl Phys*. 1964;35:2908.
4. Oldendorf WH. Isolated flying spot detection of radiodensity discontinuities—displaying the internal structural pattern of a complex object. *Ire Trans Biomed Electron*. 1961;8:68–72.
5. Kuhl DE, Edwards RQ. Image separation isotope scanning. *Radiology* 1963;80:653.
6. Hounsfield GN. Computerized transverse axial scanning (tomography). 1. Description of system. *Br J Radiol*. 1973;46:1016–1022.
7. Ambrose J. Computerized transverse axial scanning (tomography). 2. Clinical application. *Br J Radiol*. 1973;46:1023–1047.
8. Hounsfield GN. Nobel Award address. Computed medical imaging. *Med Phys*. 1980;7:283–290.
9. Boyd DP, Goitein M, inventors. The Board of Trustees of Leland Stanford Junior University, assignee. Fan beam X-ray or gamma-ray 3-D tomography. US patent 4,075,492, filed November 29, 1974; Issued February 21, 1978.
10. Chen ACM. Five-second fan beam CT scanner. *SPIE Appl Optical Inst Med*. 1976;96:294.
11. Boyd DP, inventor. The Board of Trustees of Leland Stanford, Jr. University, assignee. Position sensitive x-ray or gamma-ray detector and 3-D tomography using same. US patent 4,075,491, filed November 3, 1976; Issued February 21, 1978.
12. Ramachandran GN, Lakshminarayanan AV. Three-dimensional reconstruction from radiographs and electron micrographs: application of convolutions instead of Fourier transforms. *Proc Natl Acad Sci U S A*. 1971;68:2236–2240.
13. Dreike R, Boyd DP. Convolution reconstruction of fan beam projections. *Comput Graph Image Process*. 1976;5:459.
14. Penczek PA, Renka R, Schomberg H. Gridding-based direct Fourier inversion of the three-dimensional ray transform. *J Opt Soc Am A Opt Image Sci Vis*. 2004;21:499–509.
15. Boyd DP. A proposed dynamic cardiac 3-D densitometer for early detection and evaluation of heart disease. *IEEE Trans Nucl Sci*. 1979;26:2724.
16. Boyd DP, Couch JL, Napel SA, Peschmann KR, Rand RE. Ultrafast cine CT: Where have we been? What lies ahead? *Am J Card Imaging*. 1987;1:175.
17. Kalender WA, Seissler W, Klotz E, Vock P. Spiral volumetric CT with single-breath-hold technique, continuous transport, and continuous scanner rotation. *Radiology*. 1990;176:181–183.

18. Hu H. Multi-slice helical CT: scan and reconstruction. *Med Phys.* 1999;26:5–18.
19. Rand RE, Boyd DP, Peschmann KR, inventors. Imatron, Inc, assignee. Rotating X-ray tube with external bearings. US patent 4,993,005, filed November 23, 1998; Issued February 12, 1991.
20. Rand RE, Boyd DP, Peschmann KR, inventors. Imatron, Inc, assignee. High duty-cycle x-ray tube. US patent 5,104,456, filed February 1, 1991; Issued April 14, 1992.
21. Siemens. http://healthcare.siemens.com/ct_applications/dualsource/.
22. Ritman EL, Kinsey JH, Robb RA, Harris LD, Gilbert BK. Physics and technical considerations in the design of the DSR: a high temporal resolution volume scanner. *AJR Am J Roentgenol.* 1980;134:369–374.

3 Integrated PET/CT

David W. Townsend, Myrwood C. Besozzi, and Jonathan P.J. Carney

The recent development of combined positron emission tomography/computed tomography (PET/CT) instrumentation is an important evolution in imaging technology. Since the introduction of the first prototype CT scanner in the early 1970s, tomographic imaging has made significant contributions to the diagnosis and staging of disease. Rapid commercial development followed the introduction of the first CT scanner in 1972, and within 3 years of its appearance more than 12 companies were marketing, or intending to market, CT scanners; about half that number actually market CT scanners today. With the introduction of magnetic resonance imaging (MRI) in the early 1980s, CT was, at that time, predicted to last another 5 years at most before being replaced by MRI for anatomical imaging. Obviously, this did not happen, and today, with multislice detectors, spiral acquisition, and subsecond rotation times, CT continues to develop and to play a major role in clinical imaging, in particular for the assessment of cardiovascular disease. Indeed, one of the main driving forces for the current development in CT is for applications in cardiology.

Functional imaging, as a complement to anatomical imaging, has been the domain of nuclear medicine since the early 1950s. Planar imaging with the scintillation (gamma) camera, invented by Anger in 1958, was initially, and still is, the mainstay of nuclear medicine. In modern nuclear medicine, planar scintigraphy has been supplemented by tomography through the development of single photon emission computed tomography (SPECT), which can be helpful for certain clinical applications. Although early SPECT systems actually predated CT, the real growth in SPECT did not occur until after the appearance of CT, when similar reconstruction algorithms were applied to the reconstruction of parallel projections from SPECT data acquired with a rotating gamma camera.

Functional imaging with positron-emitting isotopes was first proposed in the early 1950s as an imaging technique that could offer greater sensitivity than conventional nuclear medicine techniques with single photon–emitting isotopes. The SPECT collimator is eliminated and replaced by electronic collimation—the coincident detection of 2 photons from positron annihilation—which greatly increases the sensitivity of the imaging system. However, other than some early prototypes in the 1960s, instrumentation to image positron emitters did not emerge seriously until the 1970s, and the first commercial PET scanners date from around 1980, about the time MRI also became commercially available. PET was initially perceived as a complex and expensive technology requiring both a cyclotron to produce the short-lived PET radioisotopes and a PET scanner to image the tracer distribution in the patient. Consequently, during the 1970s, PET did not experience the explosive growth of CT, or, during the 1980s, the comparable growth of MRI. However, in early 1995, the PET cardiac perfusion agent rubidium-82 (^{82}Rb), obtained from a strontium-82 (^{82}Sr)/^{82}Rb generator, was the first PET tracer to be approved by Medicare for reimbursement. Despite this, the high cost of the generator has limited the appeal of PET perfusion studies with ^{82}Rb compared to less-expensive SPECT perfusion agents.

Since the early 1970s, CT and PET have followed separate and distinct developmental paths. Both modalities have their strengths; CT scanners image anatomy with high spatial resolution, while PET can identify a functional abnormality in, for example, myocardial perfusion and metabolism. To initiate the evolution in imaging technology that was required to physically integrate CT and PET[1] in a single device, the design and development of a research prototype PET/CT scanner was undertaken with NIH support. The first combined PET/CT prototype scanner was completed in 1998,[2] and clinical evaluation began in June of that year; initial studies with the prototype focused primarily on cancer.[3–6]

While it may seem that, in many cases, it would be equally effective to view separately acquired CT and PET images for a given patient on adjacent computer displays, with[7] or without software registration, experience in the past 5 years with commercial PET/CT scanners has highlighted numerous unique advantages of the new technology. This new technology has moved to the forefront in helping physicians manage patients with cancer and, increasingly, with cardiovascular disease. However, all new ideas invite discussion and debate, and PET/CT has been called redundant and even disruptive. Debate will doubtless continue as to the role of dual-modality imaging in patient care. PET/CT is undergoing rapid evolution, and the combination of high-performance CT with high-performance PET is a powerful imaging platform that will play a major role in helping physicians manage patients with cardiovascular disease.

Cardiovascular disease claims more lives than the next leading causes of death combined, with 960,000 cardiovascular deaths annually. It kills 2600 Americans every day, and more than 58 million Americans suffer from at least one type of cardiovascular disease. It is the number one killer of women and results in the death of more women than the next 16 causes combined; myocardial infarctions kill 5.4 times more women than breast cancer does. The annual cost of diagnosing and treating patients with cardiovascular disease has been estimated at $274.2 billion. With an aging population, these figures can only increase. A cardiovascular specialist sees a wide range of pathology daily, pathologies that may have been present at birth or may have been brought on by lifestyle factors or by environmental toxins. However, irrespective of the clinical conditions under treatment, they all manifest anatomical, functional, or biochemical abnormalities, and it may often be extremely difficult to separate cause and effect. A single device that provides rapid anatomical and biochemical information in patients is obviously needed; the combined PET/CT scanner is just such a device.

The purpose of this chapter is to review the design objectives of this emerging technology and present the status of current instrumentation, including the principles and practicalities of CT-based attenuation correction. Some general protocol definitions and specific refinements for cardiac imaging are also discussed.

Initial Design Objectives

The development of the first PET/CT prototype was initiated in 1992 with the objectives to integrate CT and PET within the same device, to use the CT images for the attenuation and scatter correction of the PET emission data, and to explore the use of anatomical images to define tissue boundaries for PET reconstruction. Thus, the goal was to construct a device with both clinical CT and clinical PET capability so that a full anatomical and functional scan could be acquired in a single session, obviating the need for the patient to undergo an additional clinical CT scan. The original prototype[2] combined a single-slice spiral CT (Somatom AR.SP; Siemens Medical

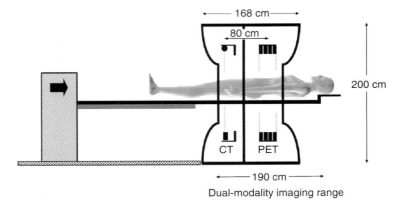

FIGURE 3.1. A schematic of a current PET-CT scanner design marketed by Siemens as the Biograph (Siemens Medical Solutions, Chicago, IL). The design incorporates a multidetector spiral CT scanner and an LSO PET scanner. The gantry is 228 cm wide, 200 cm high, and 168 cm deep. The separation of the CT and PET imaging fields is about 80 cm. The coscan range for acquiring both CT and PET is up to 190 cm. The patient port diameter is 70 cm. (Reprinted with permission from Valk P, Delbeke D, Bailey D, et al. (eds.) Positron Emission Tomography: Clinical Practice. New York: Springer, 2006.)

Solutions, Chicago, IL) with a rotating PET scanner (ECAT ART CPS Innovations, Knoxville, TN). The components for both imaging modalities were mounted on the same mechanical support and rotated together at 30 rpm. However, by the time the prototype became operational in 1998, neither the CT nor the PET components were state of the art. Nevertheless, the work convincingly demonstrated the feasibility of combining the two technologies into a single device that could acquire coregistered anatomical and functional images without the need for software realignment.

As mentioned, a number of important lessons emerged during the clinical evaluation program that followed the installation of the prototype and covered the years from 1998 to 2001.[3-6] More than 300 cancer patients were scanned, and the studies highlighted the advantages of being able to accurately localize functional abnormalities, to distinguish normal uptake from pathology, to minimize the effects of both external and internal patient movement, and to reduce scan time and increase patient throughput by using the CT images for attenuation correction of the PET data. Even during the initial evaluation, it was evident that coregistered anatomy increases the confidence of physicians reading the study.

Despite concerns over the likely cost and operational complexity of combined PET/CT technology, the major vendors of medical imaging equipment nevertheless recognized a market for PET/CT. The first commercial design comprised a CT scanner and a PET scanner enclosed within a single gantry cover and operated from separate consoles. The design involved little integration at any level and was intended primarily to be the first commercial PET/CT scanner on the market, as indeed it was. The PET scanner included retractable septa, and standard PET transmission sources were offered as an alternative to CT-based attenuation correction. Retractable septa allowed the device to acquire PET data in either two-dimensional (2D) or three-dimensional (3D) mode. Within a few months, another PET/CT design (Figure 3.1) from a different vendor appeared that had no septa and acquired data fully in 3D.[8] Since no mechanical storage was required for retractable septa and standard PET transmission sources were not offered, the design was compact; the patient port was a full 70 cm diameter throughout and the overall tunnel length was only 110 cm. Integration of the control and display software allowed the scanner to be operated from a single console. As with these and most subsequent commercial designs, both the CT and the PET were clinical state-of-the-art systems. A more open-concept PET/CT with spacing between the CT and PET scanners has since been offered by two other vendors, allowing greater access to the patient and reducing potential claustrophobic effects of the other designs.

The hardware integration of recent PET/CT designs has, therefore, remained rather minimal. The advantage is that vendors can then benefit more easily from separate advances in both CT and PET instrumentation. In the past few years, spiral CT technology has progressed from single- to dual-slice, to 4, 8, 16, and, most recently, 64 slices; in parallel, CT rotation times have deceased to less than 0.4 second, resulting in very rapid scanning protocols. Advances in PET technology have been equally dramatic, with the introduction of new, faster scintillators such as gadolinium oxyorthosilicate (GSO) and lutetium oxyorthosilicate (LSO), faster acquisition electronics, and higher resolution detectors (smaller pixels). A top-of-the-line PET/CT configuration for cardiac applications comprises a 64-slice CT scanner and an LSO-based PET scanner with 4-mm pixels.

Current Technology for PET/CT

Currently 5 vendors offer PET/CT designs: GE Healthcare, Hitachi Medical, Philips Medical Systems, Toshiba Medical Corporation, and Siemens Medical Solutions. With the exception of the SceptreP3 (Hitachi Medical; Figure 3.2E), which is based on a

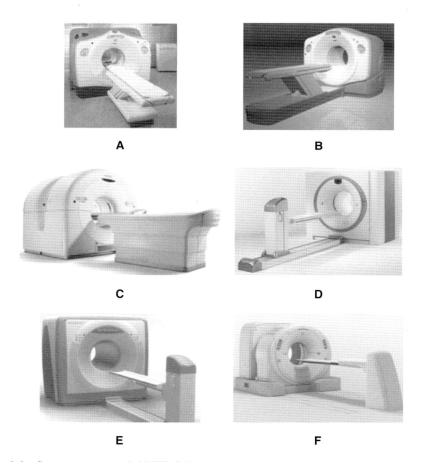

FIGURE 3.2. Current commercial PET-CT scanners from 5 major vendors of medical imaging equipment: (A) Discovery LS (GE Healthcare); (B) Discovery ST (GE Healthcare); (C) Gemini (Philips Medical Systems); (D) Biograph (Siemens Medical Solutions); (E) SeptreP3 (Hitachi Medical Systems); (F) Aquiduo (Toshiba Medical Corporation).

4-slice CT and rotating LSO detectors, all vendors offer a 16-slice CT option for higher performance, with some vendors also offering lower-priced systems with 2-, 4-, 6-, or 8-slice CT detectors. The specifications and performance of the PET components are vendor specific, with the Biograph HI-REZ (Siemens Medical Solutions; Figure 3.2D) offering the best overall spatial resolution in 3D with 4-mm × 4-mm LSO crystals; the original Biograph design was based on 6 mm × 6 mm LSO detectors. The Biograph is offered with 2, 6, 16, and now 64-slice CT scanners. The same HI-REZ PET detectors are incorporated into the Aquiduo (Toshiba Medical; Figure 3.2F) in combination with the 16-slice Aquilion CT scanner (Toshiba Medical); a unique feature of this device is that the bed is fixed and the CT and PET gantries travel on floor-mounted rails to acquire the CT and PET data. The CT and PET scanners in the Aquiduo can be moved separately, and this is the only PET/CT design in which the CT tilt option has been preserved. The Discovery LS, the original PET/CT design from GE Healthcare, combined the Advance NXi PET scanner with a 4- or 8-slice CT (Figure 3.2A); note the size difference between the smaller CT scanner in front and the larger Advance PET scanner at the rear. The more recent Discovery ST from GE Healthcare has 6-mm × 6-mm bismuth germanate (BGO) detectors in combination with a 16- or 64-slice CT scanner (Figure 3.2B); the gantry of the newly designed PET scanner now matches the dimensions of the CT scanner. The Gemini GXL (Philips Medical; Figure 3.2C) comprises 4-mm (in-plane) and 6-mm (axial) GSO detector pixels, 30 mm in depth; the Gemini is also an open design with the capability to physically separate the CT and PET scanners for access to the patient, as in the Aquiduo. Each vendor has adopted a unique design for the patient couch to eliminate vertical deflection of the pallet (Figure 3.3) as it advances into the tunnel during scanning. All designs other than the SceptreP3 and the Discovery LS offer a

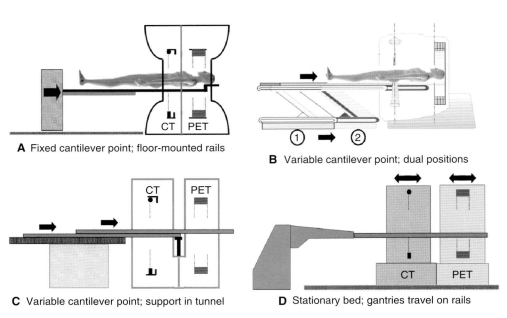

A Fixed cantilever point; floor-mounted rails

B Variable cantilever point; dual positions

C Variable cantilever point; support in tunnel

D Stationary bed; gantries travel on rails

FIGURE 3.3. Four different solutions to the patient-handling system (PHS) that eliminate variable vertical deflection of the pallet as it advances into the tunnel of the scanner. The designs include (A) a bed with a fixed cantilever point where the entire couch assembly moves on floor-mounted rails (Biograph and SeptreP3), (B) a dual-position bed with one position for CT and one for PET (Discovery LS and ST), (C) a patient couch that incorporates a support throughout the tunnel (Gemini), and (D) a fixed couch with the scanner traveling on floor-mounted rails (Aquiduo). (Reprinted with permission from Valk P, Delbeke D, Bailey D, et al. (eds.) Positron Emission Tomography: Clinical Practice. New York: Springer, 2006.)

70-cm patient port for both CT and PET, thus facilitating the scanning of radiation therapy patients in treatment position. While the Discovery and Gemini also offer standard PET transmission sources as an option, in practice most institutions use CT-based attenuation correction because of the advantage of low noise and short scan times that facilitate high patient throughput.

The Gemini, SceptreP3, Aquiduo, and Biograph designs acquire PET data in 3D mode only, whereas the Discovery incorporates retractable septa and can acquire data in both 2D and 3D mode. While the debate continues as to whether 2D or 3D acquisition yields better image quality, particularly for large patients, significant improvement in 3D image quality has undoubtedly been achieved through the use of faster scintillators and statistically based reconstruction algorithms. The scintillators GSO (Gemini) and LSO (SceptreP3, Aquiduo, and Biograph) result in lower rates of both scattered photons and random coincidences compared to BGO and offer superior performance for 3D whole-body imaging.

While there has, to date, been little actual effort to increase the level of hardware integration, there has been significant effort to reduce the complexity and increase the reliability of system operation by adopting a more integrated software approach. In early designs, CT and PET data acquisition and image reconstruction were performed on separate systems accessing a common database. Increasingly, functionality has been combined so as to reduce cost and complexity and increase reliability. Similar considerations of cost and complexity for the hardware may lead, in the future, to greater levels of integration. The likelihood is that these designs will be application specific, incorporating an 8- or 16-slice CT for oncology and a 64-slice CT specifically for cardiology.

CT-Based Attenuation Correction

The acquisition of accurately coregistered anatomical and functional images is obviously a major strength of the combined PET/CT scanner. However, an additional advantage of this approach is the possibility to use the CT images for attenuation correction of the PET emission data, eliminating the need for a separate lengthy PET transmission scan. The use of the CT scan for attenuation correction not only reduces scan times by at least 40% but also provides essentially noiseless attenuation correction factors (ACFs) compared to those from standard PET transmission measurements. Since the attenuation values are energy dependent, the correction factors derived from a CT scan at mean photon energy of 70 keV must be scaled to the PET energy of 511 keV. A requirement in performing CT-based attenuation correction is an algorithm to scale the CT Hounsfield units (HU) to the photon linear attenuation at the PET energy.

Scaling algorithms typically use a bilinear function to transform the attenuation values above and below a given threshold with different factors.[9,10] The composition of biological tissues other than bone exhibits little variation in the effective atomic number and can be well represented by a mixture of air and water. Bone tissue does not follow the same trend as soft tissue because of the calcium and phosphorus content, and thus a different scaling factor is required that reflects instead a mixture of water and cortical bone. The break point between the two mixture types has been variously set at 300 HU[9] and at 0 HU.[10] However, some tissue types, such as muscle (~60 HU) and blood (~40 HU), have Hounsfield units greater than 0 and yet are clearly not a water-bone mix. A break point around 100 HU would therefore appear to be optimal, as shown in Figure 3.4. Hounsfield units define the linear attenuation coefficients normalized to water and thus independent of the kilovolt (peak) kVp of the x-ray tube. The scale factor for the air-water mix below ~100 HU will be independent of the kVp of the tube. This does not apply to the water-bone mixing, and

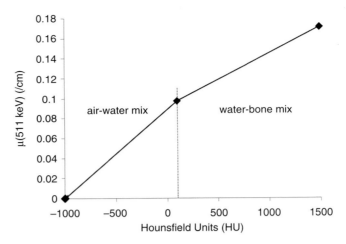

FIGURE 3.4. The bilinear scaling function used to convert CT numbers to linear attenuation values at 511 keV. The graph shows the linear attenuation coefficient at 511 keV as a function of the corresponding CT value (HU), based on measurements made with the Gammex 467 electron-density CT phantom using tissue-equivalent materials. The separation between soft tissue (air-water mixing model) and bonelike tissue (water-bone mix) is around 100 HU. (Reprinted with permission from Valk P, Delbeke D, Bailey D, et al. (eds.) Positron Emission Tomography: Clinical Practice. New York: Springer, 2006.)

therefore the scale factor for bone tissue will be kVp dependent.[11] The scaled CT images are then interpolated from CT to PET spatial resolution and the ACFs generated by reprojection of the interpolated images.

Both these algorithms perform well in transforming the CT values to 511 keV linear attenuation values; the differences between them have relatively little effect on the PET emission images. A low-dose CT scan may be performed purely for the purpose of attenuation correction, although experience in the oncology field suggests that the full benefit of the PET/CT device is obtained when both CT and PET scans are performed, as far as possible, to the individual standards of each modality. For CT, this will typically involve the administration of a CT contrast agent. Many thousands of PET/CT scans have now been performed for oncology patients in the presence of intravenous and oral CT contrast, and experience has shown that contrast administration does not generally cause a problem that could potentially interfere with the diagnostic value of PET/CT, except in well-understood instances of undiluted boluses of contrast being present.

A potentially more serious artifact in PET/CT studies arises from patient motion. The breathing protocol that is preferred for CT exams of the thorax, full-inspiration breath hold, is not suitable for performing accurate attenuation correction of the PET data. Since the duration of the PET scan extends over many breathing cycles, the PET data represent an average over the normal breathing cycle. The position of anatomical structures with breath hold at full inspiration is maximally displaced from the mean position as seen during the PET acquisition. The experience in oncological PET/CT studies has led to CT protocols that employ shallow breathing or partial-inspiration breath hold as the preferred CT protocol for PET/CT imaging. Nevertheless, there still remains the possibility of artifacts due to patient motion being introduced into the PET images in PET/CT studies using CT-based attenuation correction.

In the case of cardiac imaging, the issues in performing CT-based attenuation correction are essentially the same as for oncological studies, namely, misregistration and patient motion, and the incorrect energy scaling of foreign objects in the body including metal and CT contrast agent.[12] However, the need to perform accurate attenuation correction in cardiac PET/CT imaging is greater than in oncological PET/CT applications, since even small deviations from normal cardiac uptake patterns may have clinical significance. This has given rise, for example, to specific studies of the effect of metal artifacts in the context of cardiac imaging. This is highly relevant due to the possibility of cardiac patients presenting with pacemakers, implantable cardiac defibrillators (ICDs), and cardiac prostheses. In particular, increasing numbers of patients with ICDs in place are anticipated, due to the expanding indications for these devices[13] as the effect of their prophylactic use in reducing patient mortality continues to be established.[14]

It is well known from oncology imaging that metal objects such as dental fillings, hip prostheses, and chemotherapy ports, as well as boluses of contrast, can potentially introduce focal artifacts into the PET images.[15–17] It is therefore expected that for cardiac imaging, implanted devices may cause artifacts in the PET images.[18] DiFilippo and Brunken[19] specifically address this issue in a study of the effect of pacemaker and ICD leads, concluding that the shocking coils in ICD leads can result in artifacts at the level of a few tens of percent in myocardial uptake, depending critically on the exact placement of the leads.

Additionally, DiFilippo and Brunken[19] propose a robust protocol for CT-based attenuation correction in which a "slow CT" is acquired that averages cardiac motion over the scan duration. However, as with oncology PET/CT scans, if the CT is to be acquired for clinical purposes, such procedures as a slow CT scan do not meet the requirements of standard radiology protocols. In such protocols, the objective is to "freeze" cardiac motion rather than to average it. Thus, a standard cardiac CT protocol may not be optimal for CT-based attenuation correction. Similar considerations apply to respiratory motion. One approach to account for such movement is to acquire a CT scan that actually records respiration and cardiac motion, resulting in a sequence of time-dependent [four-dimensional (4D)] images. Existing CT reconstruction algorithms capable of generating 4D cardiac motion have been applied in the context of radiotherapy treatment planning to produce 4D CT images of respiratory motion.[20]

In the absence of gating, the PET acquisition, as a consequence of the lengthy scan duration, unavoidably averages over many cardiac and respiratory cycles. The potential to perform cardiac-gated PET is well-known, and respiratory gating of the PET acquisition for PET/CT imaging has also been studied.[21] Thus, in combination with 4D CT that maps cardiac and respiratory motion, each gated PET image could be properly attenuation corrected using the appropriate set of time-dependent CT images. This approach may be the future of cardiac PET/CT imaging.

Protocols that address motion are of particular interest for PET/CT due to the emergence of specific applications in cardiology. As previously with PET-only scanners, PET/CT may be used to evaluate myocardial perfusion and metabolism (viability), with a low-dose "slow CT" for attenuation correction. However, the true appeal of PET/CT for cardiology is as a one-stop shop for diagnosing coronary artery disease.[22,23] For such a protocol, the CT exam is performed according to current cardiac CT protocols requiring a gated CT reconstruction or a fully 4D acquisition; contrast is administered in the case of CT angiography. The objective with the CT acquisition is to obtain the best diagnostic quality and not to minimize artifacts due to the CT-based attenuation correction procedure. Conversely, the objective of the slow-CT protocol is to minimize the artifacts; thus, the use of such images for diagnostic purposes may be problematic because of mismatch of the heart wall between CT and PET.[24] A possible solution is to acquire fully gated CT and PET image sets and match the corresponding phases. In the absence of such a complete mapping of the motion, the position of the heart wall in the CT image may be shifted using the uncorrected PET image as a guide prior to performing CT-based attenuation correction.[25] Thus, for the reasons given above, the application of PET/CT technology in cardiology will likely result in more refined protocols for performing CT-based attenuation correction.

PET/CT Protocols

Data-acquisition protocols for PET/CT can, depending on the study, be relatively complex, particularly when they involve both a clinical CT and a clinical PET scan, with or without cardiac and respiratory gating. Over the past 5 years, since the technology first became commercially available, the initial rather simple and basic PET/CT protocols have been progressively refined for cardiac applications, although it will be a while before they become as well established as the corresponding protocols for cardiac CT. Issues of respiration, contrast media, operating parameters, scan time, optimal injected dose of ^{18}F-fluoro-deoxy-D-glucose (FDG), and others must be carefully addressed before definitive PET/CT protocols for specific clinical applications emerge. Nevertheless, there are certain generic features to the protocols, as shown schematically in Figure 3.5.

Depending on the specific acquisition methodology (2D or 3D), an injected dose of 10 to 20mCi of FDG is administered followed by a 60-minute uptake period. As mentioned above, the Discovery series (Figures 3.2A and 3.2B) incorporates retractable septa and can acquire PET data in either 2D or 3D mode. The remaining designs in Figure 3.2 do not incorporate septa and acquire data fully in 3D. For the Discovery PET/CT scanners, the recommended acquisition mode for PET cardiac scanning is 2D with septa extended. Following the 60-minute uptake period, the patient is positioned in the scanner with arms raised, and a topogram is acquired for 256mm starting at the sternal notch (Figure 3.5A). A field of view corresponding to a single PET bed position (around 16cm) is defined on the topogram and a spiral CT acquired for the selected field of view; a 16-slice CT scanner takes less than 10 seconds to acquire the 16-cm field of view (Figure 3.5B). Upon completion of the spiral CT scan, the patient couch is advanced into the PET scanner (Figure 3.5C); depending on the scanner design and preferred methodology, the emission data are then acquired in 2D or 3D for 10 to 15 minutes. Reconstruction of the CT images occurs in parallel with the acquisition of the PET data, allowing the calculation of scatter and attenuation correction factors to be performed during the PET acquisition. The CT-based attenuation

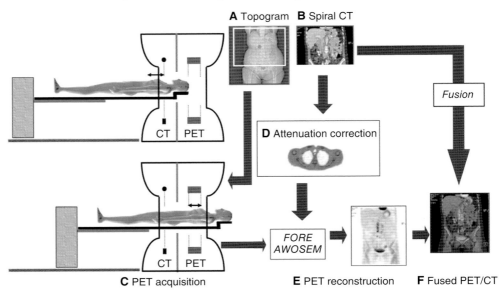

FIGURE 3.5. A typical imaging protocol for a combined PET/CT study that includes (A) a topogram, or scout, scan for positioning, (B) a spiral CT scan, (C) a PET scan over the same axial range as the CT scan, (D) the generation of CT-based ACFs, (E) reconstruction of the attenuation-corrected PET emission data using Fourier rebinning (FORE)[27] and Attenuation-Weighted Ordered-Subset Expectation Maximization (AWOSEM)[28], and (F) display of the final fused images. (Reprinted with permission from Valk P, Delbeke D, Bailey D, et al. (eds.) Positron Emission Tomography: Clinical Practice. New York: Springer, 2006.)

correction factors are calculated as described in the previous section (Figure 3.5D), and once the PET acquisition is completed, PET reconstruction commences (Figure 3.5E). PET data acquired in 2D are reconstructed with a 2D iterative reconstruction algorithm such as Order-Subset Expectation Maximization (OSEM),[26] whereas 3D data are first rebinned to 2D data sets using Fourier rebinning[27] followed by a 2D iterative reconstruction algorithm.[26] Within a few minutes of the completion of the PET acquisition, attenuation-corrected images are reconstructed and available for viewing, automatically coregistered with the CT scan by simply accounting for the axial displacement between the CT and PET imaging fields of view (Figure 3.5F). The fused image is displayed as a combination of the individual CT and PET image pixel values v_{CT} and v_{PET}, respectively. Using an α-blending approach, the fused image pixel value (v) is given by $\alpha v_{CT} + (1 - \alpha)v_{PET}$; for $\alpha = 0$, the fused image is PET, while for $\alpha = 1$ the fused image is CT. Obviously, for $0 < \alpha < 1$, the fused image represents a weighted blending of pixel values of CT and PET.

While it is not feasible with current designs to acquire the CT and PET data simultaneously, scan times have been reduced significantly by the replacement of the lengthy PET transmission scan with the CT scan. In addition, as mentioned previously, the introduction of new PET technology such as faster scintillators (LSO and GSO) can potentially reduce the emission acquisition time.

In addition to the issues related to respiration and contrast, a topic of ongoing debate is the clinical role of the CT scan. The decision to acquire a clinical gated cardiac CT scan depends on many factors, including whether such a scan was ordered by the referring physician and whether the patient has recently been subjected to a full clinical CT scan. Obviously the decision will dictate the protocol and the parameters of the CT scan. Increasingly, as PET/CT becomes established in clinical routine, the acquisition of both a clinical CT scan and a clinical PET scan should become standard practice. In addition, in the spirit of a one-stop shop, there may be complex, cardiac-specific protocols, as outlined in Chapter 16.

Finally, while there are many technical reasons to prefer the combined PET/CT approach over software image fusion, the convenience to both patient and physician should not be underestimated. For the patient, one appointment and a single scan session are required to obtain complete anatomical and functional information related to his or her disease. For the physician, the potential to have accurately registered CT and PET images available at the same time and on the same viewing screen offers unique possibilities.

Summary Points

- Even though combined PET/CT scanners have been in production for only 5 years, the technology is undergoing rapid evolution. For PET, the introduction of new scintillator materials, detector concepts, and electronics is resulting in performance improvements in count rate, spatial resolution, and signal-to-noise ratio. At the same time, the increasing number of detector rows and reduction in rotation time are transforming cardiac CT performance. The combination of high-performance CT with high-performance PET is a powerful imaging platform for the management of cardiovascular disease.
- The cardiologist may daily see a wide range of pathology. The pathology may have been present at birth or may have been brought on by lifestyle factors or environmental toxins. No matter what clinical conditions are being treated, they all have associated anatomical, functional, or biochemical abnormalities, and it may be extremely difficult to separate cause from effect. Thus, a single technology that will provide rapid anatomical and biochemical information is needed.
- Dual-modality imaging technology continues to progress at a rapid rate. The interest in this imaging technology is also increasing rapidly among physicians who are directly responsible for treating patients with cardiovascular disease. This dual

modality will permit measurements of energy substrate utilization, neuronal integrity, and markers of inflammation and cell death; high-resolution rapid CT scanners provide anatomical, angiographic, and dynamic measurements to further enhance cardiac assessment. Debates may continue, but to physicians who direct heart, lung, and vascular institutes or pain centers, PET/CT may be a breakthrough in managing cardiovascular disease.

References

1. Townsend DW, Cherry SR. Combining anatomy with function: the path to true image fusion. *Eur Radiol.* 2001;11:1968–1974.
2. Beyer T, Townsend DW, Brun T, et al. A combined PET/CT scanner for clinical oncology. *J Nucl Med.* 2000;41:1369–1379.
3. Charron M, Beyer T, Bohnen NN, et al. Image analysis in patients with cancer studied with a combined PET and CT scanner. *Clin Nucl Med.* 2000;25:905–910.
4. Meltzer CC, Martinelli MA, Beyer T, et al. Whole-body FDG PET imaging in the abdomen: value of combined PET/CT. *J Nucl Med.* 2001;42:35P.
5. Meltzer CC, Snyderman CH, Fukui MB, et al. Combined FDG PET/CT imaging in head and neck cancer: impact on patient management. *J Nucl Med.* 2001;42:36P.
6. Kluetz PG, Meltzer CC, Villemagne VL, et al. Combined PET/CT imaging in oncology: impact on patient management. *Clin Positron Imaging.* 2000;3:223–230.
7. Hawkes DJ, Hill DL, Hallpike L, Bailey DL. Coregistration of Structural and Functional Images. In: Valk P, Bailey DL, Townsend DW, Maisey MN, eds. *Positron Emission Tomography: Basic Science and Clinical Practice.* Springer, London, New York, 2003:181–197.
8. Townsend DW, Beyer T, Blodgett TM. PET/CT scanners: a hardware approach to image fusion. *Semin Nucl Med.* 2003;33:193–204.
9. Kinahan PE, Townsend DW, Beyer T, Sashin D. Attenuation correction for a combined 3D PET/CT scanner. *Med Phys.* 1998;25:2046–2053.
10. Burger C, Goerres G, Schoenes S, et al. PET attenuation coefficients from CT images: experimental evaluation of the transformation of CT into PET 511-keV attenuation coefficients. *Eur J Nucl Med Mol Imaging.* 2002;29:922–927.
11. Rappoport V, Carney JPJ, Townsend DW. X-ray tube voltage dependent attenuation correction scheme for PET/CT scanners. *IEEE Medical Imaging Conference Record.* 2004; M10–76:213.
12. Koepfli P, Hany TF, Wyss CA, et al. CT attenuation correction for myocardial perfusion quantification using a PET/CT hybrid scanner. *J Nucl Med.* 2004;45:537–542.
13. Bigger JT. Expanding indications for implantable cardiac defibrillators. *N Engl J Med.* 2002;346:931–933.
14. Moss A, Zareba W, Hall W, et al, for the Multicenter Automatic Defibrillator Implantation Trial II Investigators. Prophylactic implantation of a defibrillator in patients with myocardial infarction and reduced ejection fraction. *N Engl J Med.* 2002;346:877–883.
15. Antoch G, Freudenberg LS, Egelhof T, et al. Focal tracer uptake: a potential artifact in contrast-enhanced dual-modality PET/CT scans. *J Nucl Med.* 2002;43:1339–1342.
16. Goerres GW, Ziegler SI, Burger C, Berthold T, von Schulthess GK, Buck A. Artifacts at PET and PET/CT caused by metallic hip prosthetic material. *Radiology.* 2003;226:577–584.
17. Kamel EM, Burger C, Buck A, von Schulthess GK, Goerres GW. Impact of metallic dental implants on CT-based attenuation correction in a combined PET/CT scanner. *Eur Radiol.* 2003;13:724–728.
18. Halpern BS, Dahlbom M, Waldherr C, et al. Cardiac pacemakers and central venous lines can induce focal artifacts on CT-corrected PET images. *J Nucl Med.* 2004;45:290–293.
19. DiFilippo FP, Brunken RC. Do implanted pacemaker leads and ICD leads cause metal-related artifact in cardiac PET/CT? *J Nucl Med.* 2005;46:436–443.
20. Keall PJ, Starkschall G, Shukla H, et al. Acquiring 4D thoracic CT scans using a multislice helical method. *Phys Med Biol.* 2004;49:2053–2067.
21. Townsend DW, Yap JT, Carney JP, et al. Respiratory gating with a 16-slice LSO PET/CT scanner. *J Nucl Med.* 2004;45S:165P–166P.
22. William W. The diagnosis of coronary artery disease: in search of a one-stop shop. *J Nucl Med.* 2005;46:904–905.

23. Namdar M, Hany TF, Koepfli P, et al. Integrated PET/CT for the assessment of coronary artery disease: a feasibility study. *J Nucl Med.* 2005;46:930–935.

24. Loghin C, Sdringola S, Gould KL. Common artifacts in PET myocardial perfusion images due to attenuation-emission misregistration: clinical significance, causes, and solutions. *J Nucl Med.* 2004;45:1029–1039.

25. Wilson JW, Wong TZ, Borges-Neto F, Turkington TG. An algorithm for correction of PET/CT mismatch-induced cardiac attenuation correction artifacts. *J Nucl Med.* 2005;46S:55P.

26. Hudson H, Larkin R. Accelerated image reconstruction using ordered subsets of projection data. *IEEE Trans Med Imaging.* 1994;13:601–609.

27. Defrise M, Kinahan PE, Townsend DW, Michel C, Sibomana M, Newport DF. Exact and approximate rebinning algorithms for 3D PET data. *IEEE Trans Med Imaging.* 1997;16:145–158.

28. Comtat C, Kinahan PE, Defrise M, et al. Fast reconstruction of 3D PET data with accurate statistical modeling. *IEEE Trans Nucl Sci.* 1998;45:1083–1089.

4 Principles of Quantitation in Cardiac PET

Stephen C. Moore and Georges El Fakhri

This chapter focuses on several applications of tracer-kinetic methods to PET imaging of the heart. It will be useful, first, to review some general, basic principles of compartment analysis that have been well described by several other authors.[1-3] This review emphasizes the most important underlying assumptions and requirements for obtaining accurate quantitative measurements of myocardial perfusion or metabolism from dynamic PET image data. The review is followed by descriptions of several different tracer-kinetic techniques that have been used for imaging tissue perfusion, viability, and oxygen consumption, using a variety of radiolabeled tracers.

Basic Principles of Compartment Analysis

Review of Tracer-Kinetic Concepts

A compartment represents a unique biochemical state of a certain type of tissue, for example, myocardium that is being labeled with a tracer. The compartment is generally represented as a rectangular box, such as that shown in Figure 4.1. Arrows may be drawn to or from one or more compartments to represent active or passive transport of a given "indicator" (in our case, a radioactive tracer) from blood into a tissue compartment, or from one state of the tissue into another. As we shall see, the arrows and boxes are useful for describing mathematical models of the dynamic behavior of a radiotracer as it appears in each of the different compartments. The single tissue compartment of Figure 4.1 might provide, in some cases, a reasonable model for describing tissue blood flow (perfusion), depending on the biomolecular properties of the radiotracer. For our purposes, the box could represent myocardial tissue being perfused from the coronary arterioles.

A given radiopharmaceutical may be transported actively or passively across the capillary membranes into the myocardium with a speed characterized by a "rate constant," K_1. Once inside the myocardial tissue, the radiolabeled indicator molecules may be bound to cell-surface membranes, or even trapped within the cells, by one or more different mechanisms. These states are sometimes represented as two or more distinct compartments. It is important to realize that different tracer compartments are generally not separated spatially; that is, the tracer in a single organ—or even in a region of an organ as small as a PET voxel—can exist in several different biomolecular states simultaneously. The different states can be evaluated only through

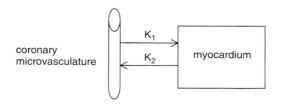

FIGURE 4.1. A single-tissue-compartment model.

careful measurements of the dynamics of tracer accumulation in and/or washout from a volume of interest (VOI). If the indicator is trapped very strongly in the tissue, the binding is essentially irreversible, which means that the tracer cannot leave the tissue and cross back into the blood. On the other hand, some tracers are bound less strongly within the tissue, in which case the binding is at least partially reversible, so the tracer can leave the tissue and return to the circulation with a rate constant, k_2. The use of a diffusible tracer, such as radiolabeled water, leads to a high value of k_2.

By convention, an uppercase symbol is used for K_1, which is defined with units of tissue perfusion, that is, milliliters of blood per minute per gram of tissue. On the other hand, k_2 and other rate constants associated with multicompartment models are written in lowercase as a reminder that they have an interpretation somewhat different from that of K_1; these are most commonly expressed simply in units of inverse time (e.g., min^{-1}). The rate, J, at which radioactivity leaves the blood to accumulate within a given mass of tissue (also called the "tissue flux" of the tracer) depends linearly on the concentration of the radiotracer in the arterial blood supply, C_A. K_1 is, in fact, the constant of proportionality in this relationship.

$$J = K_1 C_A. \tag{1}$$

J can also be shown, by the Fick principle (e.g., Lassen and Perl), to be equal to the difference between the arterial flux into the tissue and the venous flux out of the tissue,

$$J = F \cdot C_A - F \cdot C_V = F \cdot (C_A - C_V), \tag{2}$$

where F is the blood flow (in mL/min/g of tissue), C_A is the arterial blood concentration of the indicator (e.g., in Bq/mL), and C_V is the venous concentration. Clearly, then, the net tissue flux of radioactivity has units of Bq/min/g.

The unidirectional first-pass extraction, E, is defined as the fraction of tracer that moves from the capillaries to the extravascular space in the tissue of interest on a single pass through the local blood vessels. This extraction is, in turn, equivalent to the fraction of tracer disappearing from the microvasculature between the adjacent arterial and venous capillaries,

$$E = \frac{(C_A - C_V)}{C_A}. \tag{3}$$

Equations 2 and 3 may be combined to express the rate of accumulation of tracer in the tissue, as the product of flow, extraction fraction, and arterial blood tracer concentration,

$$J = K_1 C_A = (F \cdot E) C_A, \tag{4}$$

which demonstrates that the rate constant, K_1, can simply be interpreted as the product of blood flow and the unidirectional first-pass extraction fraction,

$$K_1 = F \cdot E. \qquad (5)$$

It is interesting to consider the values of K_1 expected for different kinds of tracers. With the assumption that capillaries are cylindrical in shape, Renkin[4] and Crone[5] modeled the extraction fraction in terms of capillary permeability, P, surface area, A, and blood flow, F, as

$$E = 1 - \exp\left(-\frac{PA}{F}\right) \qquad (6)$$

If the capillary permeability of a particular tracer is small, such that $PA \ll F$, then this extraction fraction may be approximated by $E \sim PA/F$. It can then be seen from equation 5 that, under such conditions, K_1 is approximately equal to the product of capillary permeability and surface area and is thus independent of flow. At the other extreme, if the permeability is very high for some other tracer, then its extraction fraction would be close to unity (i.e., 100% extraction); in this case, the rate constant, K_1, is equal to the blood flow, F, so such a tracer could be used directly to measure regional tissue perfusion.

Single-Compartment Dynamics for an Arbitrary Arterial Input Function

Consider the single-tissue-compartment model of Figure 4.1. The net flux of tracer accumulation in or washout from the myocardium, which is the time derivative of the tissue concentration, C_T, will depend on both rate constants K_1 and k_2 as well as on the values of activity concentration in the blood and myocardium:

$$J_{net} = \frac{dC_T}{dt} = K_1 C_A - k_2 C_T. \qquad (7)$$

The first term on the right side of this equation represents an increase in tracer activity moving from the blood to the tissue, while the second term represents a loss of tracer from the tissue back to the blood. If an ideal (instantaneous) bolus of blood activity with concentration C_A arrives at time t = 0, the solution to this differential equation can be shown to be

$$C_T(t) = K_1 C_A e^{-k_2 t}; \qquad (8)$$

that is, the blood activity bolus leads to an instantaneous increase in the tissue activity concentration from 0 to $K_1 C_A$, followed by an exponential decay with rate-constant k_2, representing washout of the tracer from the tissue. Because equation 8 is valid for an ideal bolus input, the system's so-called impulse response function (IRF) to the bolus of concentration, C_A, is seen to be simply

$$IRF(t) = K_1 e^{-k_2 t}. \qquad (9)$$

What if the arterial input function is more complex than a simple bolus, as it always is in clinical practice? For any compartment model, it may be shown that if the tissue activity concentration depends only linearly on the arterial blood activity concentration, then the solution of the model equation can be represented as a convolution of the arterial input function with the impulse response function. This statement can perhaps be made more intuitive if one considers that any input function can be represented as a sum of discrete boluses, each arriving at a slightly different time and characterized by a different amplitude (activity concentration). For a linear system, the net response should then be given by the sum of the time-shifted impulse response functions arising from each discrete bolus of activity, scaled by the magnitude of the arterial input function. This mathematical form is, in fact, the definition of a convolution of C_A with IRF:

$$C_t(t) = \sum_{t'} C_A(t') IRF(t-t') \equiv C_A(t) * IRF(t) \tag{10}$$

In quantitative PET studies, $C_A(t)$ is often measured by obtaining many blood samples from the radial artery during and after the injection of the radiolabeled tracer in a vein on the contralateral arm; the function $C_A(t)$ is normally completed by using a smooth mathematical interpolation between the times when arterial blood was sampled. Less invasive (and less accurate) input functions are sometimes utilized by drawing samples of arterialized venous blood from a vein in the hand.

To measure the tissue time-activity curve (TAC), PET data are acquired dynamically during and after injection of a radiolabeled tracer. The independently measured arterial input function is then used when fitting the tissue TAC to a compartment model, such as that described above by equations 9 and 10, to determine the kinetic parameters of interest, for example, K_1 and k_2. Because the kinetic parameters can vary with location, one usually defines regions or volumes of interest within the reconstructed PET slices; the tissue count data extracted from each region are then separately fitted to the model equation. Depending on the level of statistical noise in the PET images, it may also be possible to fit the dynamic data separately in each voxel to obtain high-resolution parametric images representing the detailed spatial distribution of one or more parameters of interest.

Assumptions and Requirements

Most tracer-kinetic models depend on several assumptions. First, each compartment is assumed to be well mixed and homogeneous in its tracer distribution throughout the experiment. This assumption is often satisfied only approximately, especially at earlier times, that is, shortly after the tracer is introduced to the system. At later times, activity concentration gradients are generally smaller within the compartments of interest. Second, in each compartment, the tracer concentration should be low enough that it cannot significantly perturb the system being studied. For most radiopharmaceuticals, this *tracer principle* is well satisfied, because the number of carrier molecules is generally very small in comparison with the number of cells being labeled. However, in certain receptor-imaging studies, for example, it may be possible to saturate or partially saturate the target receptors, which would violate the assumption that the underlying physiologic mechanisms behave in a steady-state fashion and would therefore require a modification of the model.

The tracer-kinetic model assumptions, when taken with some other practical considerations, allow us to define several requirements for achieving success in tracer-kinetic studies. First, an appropriate tracer should be selected for making the required measurement. For example, if one wishes to measure regional perfusion, one should not use a tracer with a very low value of capillary permeability, as discussed above. Second, the mathematical model being used to fit the time dependence of the measured data should be consistent with the underlying mechanisms of tracer delivery to and washout from the tissues of interest. As we shall see shortly, a single-tissue-compartment model may provide a very useful approximation for fitting the measured dynamic tissue data; however, if the underlying physiologic processes are better represented by a 2-compartment model, then the use of such a model should result in improved accuracy of the estimates of the tracer-kinetic parameters of interest—even though this may occur at a cost of worse precision (i.e., less reproducible estimates of the parameters) because there are additional unknown parameters to be determined in more complex compartment models. Finally, both the arterial input function and the tissue TACs should be measured with as high a degree of accuracy and precision as possible, subject to the usual constraints of scan protocols: patient comfort, scan time, and radiation dose.

For a variety of reasons, cardiac PET imaging can generally satisfy the last of these requirements very well. The heart easily fits within the axial field of view (FOV) of most modern PET scanners, which means that the entire heart can be imaged at all desired time points in a dynamic acquisition. Furthermore, because the left ventricle contains arterial blood and is relatively large—at least in comparison with the arteries supplying blood to other tissues of the body—it may be possible to reliably extract arterial input functions directly from the dynamic cardiac PET images. In fact, for myocardial imaging, the shape of an input function derived from a radial artery blood sample is degraded more by time delay and dispersion than that obtained from images of the left ventricle or atrium. Image-based determination of input functions is addressed in greater detail in the section on rubidium-82 (^{82}Rb) perfusion imaging. Finally, both the accuracy and the precision of PET images reconstructed with full corrections for scatter and attenuation are generally better than those of SPECT images, for example. Improved accuracy and precision of images translate directly into more accurate and precise estimates of all tracer-kinetic parameters of interest. SPECT is also faced with the additional serious challenge that the biodistribution of the radiotracer will be changing while the gamma camera(s) rotate to obtain a complete set of projection data for each desired acquisition time. This can lead to significant inconsistencies between projections, resulting in image artifacts, whereas dedicated PET scanners acquire all angular projection data simultaneously.

In the remainder of this chapter, we describe several existing PET techniques for the assessment of myocardial perfusion, viability, and oxygen consumption. The methods described make use of a variety of positron-emitting radionuclides and tracers, and the dynamic scan data can be represented using one or more of several different underlying compartment models and, in some cases, approximate models.

Quantitative Imaging of Myocardial Perfusion

^{15}O-Water

A positron-emitting radionuclide, oxygen-15 (^{15}O) has a half-life of 2.04 minutes. Water can be labeled with ^{15}O to form $H_2^{15}O$, a highly diffusible tracer. Soon after injection, equilibrium between the ^{15}O concentration in myocardial tissue and that in the venous blood is achieved; the ratio between the tissue concentration, C_T, and the venous blood concentration, C_V, is called the "partition coefficient" or, equivalently, the "volume of distribution." For the single-tissue-compartment model, we can use the definition of net tissue flux as the time derivative of the tracer concentration in tissue, along with the partition coefficient relation, $\lambda = C_T/C_V$, to rewrite equation 2 for the case of a highly diffusible tracer, such as ^{15}O-water:

$$\frac{dC_T}{dt} = F(C_A - C_V) = F\left(C_A - \frac{C_T}{\lambda}\right). \tag{11}$$

Although the partition coefficient, λ, is a unitless ratio, it is often referred to as the volume of distribution because it is equivalent to the volume of blood that would have the same activity as that found at equilibrium in a unit volume of tissue.

The solution to equation 11 is the following convolution:

$$C_T(t) = FC_A(t) * \exp\left(-\frac{Ft}{\lambda}\right). \tag{12}$$

It may be observed that this equation has the mathematical form expected for a single-tissue-compartment model. By comparing equation 12 with equations 9 and 10, we see that, for a highly diffusible tracer such as ^{15}O-water, $K_1 = F$, implying 100% extraction of the tracer, and $k_2 = F/\lambda$. In dog studies, Bergmann et al[6] reported a very high unidirectional first-pass extraction fraction (almost unity) for ^{15}O-water. These authors used a slightly different model, following Kety,[7] to account for observations that water does not behave like an ideal freely diffusible tracer under all conditions; that is, there are some biochemical environments that partially restrict the free diffusion of water.

In ^{15}O-water PET studies, it is difficult to separate the blood activity from the myocardial tissue images. Blood-count contamination of the tissue compartment is attributable to 2 factors: first, activity from the left ventricular blood is blurred into the myocardial wall because of the finite spatial resolution of the PET imaging system, and, second, the myocardium itself is directly perfused by arterial blood, so a fraction of the myocardial volume is occupied by arteries and arterioles. Two different approaches have been used to correct for this complication. Some investigators, for example, Bergmann[6] and Huang,[8] have subtracted labeled blood-pool images (working with either reconstructed images or sinogram projections) from the corresponding ^{15}O-water data. This can be accomplished by acquiring an initial PET image while the subject breathes C^{15}O (or carbon-11 oxygen [^{11}CO]) to perform in vivo labeling of red blood cells. When the labeled carbon monoxide has decayed away, ^{15}O-water dynamic data are acquired, after which a fraction of the C^{15}O image data is subtracted from each ^{15}O-water acquisition. The scale factor used for subtraction is computed as the ratio of the H$_2$^{15}O blood activity concentration during each dynamic acquisition to the average C^{15}O blood concentration during the blood-pool image study.

Because of possible subject motion between scans, it can be difficult to obtain high-quality ^{15}O-water images with the blood-pool contribution adequately removed. Other investigators, for instance, Iida et al,[9] proposed instead to model the measured tissue TAC as the sum of a tissue contribution from equation 12 and a blood contribution obtained from the measured arterial blood curve, $C_A(t)$, scaled by an additional unknown parameter, which corresponds to the fraction of blood-pool activity observed in the myocardium. Lammertsma et al[10] found that this approach was more accurate than the image subtraction approach based on labeled carbon monoxide imaging. A similar technique, in which a partial-volume correction was additionally included to "recover" the activity blurred outside the myocardial wall, was validated in a phantom experiment described by Herrero and colleagues.[11]

^{13}N-Ammonia

Background

Ammonia, labeled with the positron emitter nitrogen-13 (^{13}N; half-life = 10 minutes), has been extensively utilized as a perfusion indicator for PET imaging. This tracer is characterized by a high extraction fraction and is partially trapped in myocardial tissue. Schelbert et al[12] demonstrated in open-chest dog experiments that the uptake of ^{13}N-ammonia correlated nonlinearly with regional myocardial blood flow; a doubling of flow led to an ~70% increase in tracer uptake. In an isolated perfused rabbit heart model, Bergmann et al[13] studied the dependence of myocardial uptake on various metabolic factors; this and other work[14] demonstrated that the inhibition of glutamine synthetase with L-methionine diminished the metabolic trapping of ^{13}N-ammonia, indicating that the glutamic acid–glutamine reaction was primarily responsible for ammonia fixation in myocardial tissue, although other metabolic reactions also take place. In blood, NH$_3$ exists primarily in the ionic form, NH$_4$+. When NH$_4$+ enters the extravascular space, it is converted back to NH$_3$. Because of its lipid solubility, NH$_3$ diffuses across cell membranes, where it can then be metabolically trapped by conversion to ^{13}N-gluatamine.

Schelbert et al[14] also reported that their data did not agree perfectly with the Renkin-Crone model of capillary permeability; their measurement of the unidirectional first-pass extraction fraction, E', was best fitted to the functional form,

$$E' = 1 - e^{-(103+2.3F)/F},\tag{13}$$

where F, in this case, was reported in units of mL/min/100 g of tissue. By comparison with the form of equation (6), it may be seen that the surface area–permeability product for ^{13}N-ammonia appears to increase slightly with increasing flow. These authors and others have remarked that this phenomenon could be related to additional capillary recruitment that might accompany an increase in blood flow, thereby increasing the capillary surface area available for transport of the tracer to the extravascular space.

2-Compartment Model

Krivokapich et al[15] evaluated myocardial imaging of ^{13}N-ammonia in normal volunteers at rest and under exercise conditions. These authors used a model consisting of a freely diffusible ^{13}N-ammonia space (vascular plus extravascular), coupled to a metabolically trapped compartment through the forward rate constant, K_1, with a reverse rate constant, k_2. When fitting only the first 90 seconds of the blood and tissue TACs—in order to reduce possible overestimation of the true ^{13}N-ammonia input function by contamination from metabolites (^{13}N-labeled compounds other than ^{13}N-ammonia)—the researchers obtained average perfusion rates of 0.75 ± 0.43 mL/min/g at rest, and 1.50 ± 0.74 mL/min/g with exercise, and the average increase in perfusion (coronary flow reserve) was 2.2, which was considered by the authors to be reasonably representative of the coronary flow reserve expected from considerations of the average "double product" measured during exercise.

3-Compartment Model

Hutchins et al[16] proposed the use of the 3-compartment model shown in Figure 4.2. Their model was developed under the assumptions that (1) ^{13}N-ammonia behaves like a freely diffusible tracer at the capillary-myocardial tissue interface, (2) ^{13}N-ammonia is converted to ^{13}N-glutamine by glutamine synthetase and is, essentially, trapped within the myocardial tissue, (3) the extracellular and intracellular ^{13}N-ammonia concentration values rapidly equilibrate, and (4) the available glutamine synthetase level remains, essentially, unchanged throughout the study, so that the probability of converting an ammonia molecule in the tissue to glutamine remains constant.

If we define the activity concentration of the ^{13}N-ammonia in the extravascular compartment to be $C_E(t)$ and the concentration of ^{13}N-glutamine in the metabolically trapped compartment to be $C_M(t)$ then the differential equations describing the rate of change of these concentration variables (assuming correction for the physical decay of ^{13}N) are given by

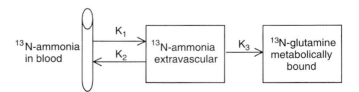

FIGURE 4.2. A 3-compartment ^{13}N-ammonia model used by Hutchins et al.[16] (Reprinted with permission from The American College of Cardiology Foundation.)

$$\frac{dC_E(t)}{dt} = K_1 C_A(t) - k_2 C_E(t) - k_3 C_E(t) \tag{14}$$

and

$$\frac{dC_M(t)}{dt} = k_3 C_E(t) \tag{15}$$

The total regional tissue activity concentration, measured at different times on the dynamic PET images, results from the sum of the values of activity concentration in the extravascular and metabolic compartments, $C_T(t) = C_E(t) + C_M(t)$. By solving differential equations (14) and (15), the total tissue activity concentration as a function of time can be shown to be given by the convolution:

$$C_T(t) = C_A(t) * \frac{K_1}{k_2 + k_3} \left[k_2 e^{-(k_2+k_3)t} + k_3 \right] \tag{16}$$

In their model equations, Hutchins et al[16] also assumed that the measured tissue TAC would contain contributions from both myocardium and blood, and they used an approach, similar to that described above for the analysis of ^{15}O-water data, to fit for the blood fraction in addition to the kinetic parameters. The resulting form used to model the measured PET activity concentration, $C_P(t)$, is

$$C_P(t) = (1 - f_A)\rho_T C_T(t) + f_A C_A(t), \tag{17}$$

where f_A is the additional fitting parameter, interpreted as the fraction of the measurement volume occupied by arterial blood (arising both from vascularized tissue and from resolution blurring of blood-pool counts into the myocardium), and ρ_T is the physical density of the tissue, needed to convert tissue concentration units, Bq/g, to Bq/mL, for consistency with the units of arterial blood concentration.

In the same paper, the researchers also evaluated the performance of this tracer-kinetic model both with and without correction for ^{13}N metabolites in the arterial input function. When fitting dynamic data acquired over 10 minutes to their 3-compartment model, they determined that the metabolite correction altered the fitted values of K_1 and k_2 by less than 10%; however, k_3 changed by more than a factor of 2 when this correction was used. Coronary flow reserve (CFR) was found to be, essentially, unchanged by metabolite correction. Myocardial blood flow, as indicated by the fitted rate-constant, K_1 (which assumes 100% extraction) averaged 88 ± 17 mL/min/100 g at rest and increased to 417 ± 112 mL/min/100 g after dipyridamole infusion (0.56 mg/kg) with handgrip exercise. The average CFR was 4.8 ± 1.3, which the authors indicated was consistent with results from other independent measurement techniques.[17,18]

Additional refinements to the quantitative imaging of ^{13}N-ammonia were reported by Kuhle et al,[19] who demonstrated that corrections for the loss of myocardial tissue counts attributable to blurring by the nonstationary PET resolution, as well as for tissue-blood spillover effects, could be improved by applying these corrections to reoriented short-axis images, rather than to the originally acquired transaxial images. Hutchins et al[20] later described a region-of-interest (ROI) strategy for minimizing the effects of resolution distortion in quantitative myocardial PET studies, demonstrating that biases in kinetic parameters could be significantly reduced by careful placement of regions of interest, as well as by fitting for a single additional parameter, which represents the fraction of the ROI that is occupied by the blood pool, as discussed above. This work was performed without any other explicit recovery-coefficient corrections for resolution blurring or blood-tissue cross-talk, and the approach was validated[21] in an open-chest dog experiment by comparison with results from microsphere-based flow measurements and with ^{15}O-water dynamic studies. A comparison of various ^{13}N-ammonia tracer models was later described by Choi et al[22] These researchers determined that myocardial blood flow (MBF) estimates from several different compartment models generally correlated well with microsphere measurements of MBF, and that MBF estimates obtained from the 4-parameter model were more variable than those from 2-parameter or modified 2-parameter model.

Rubidium

Background

Rubidium-82 (^{82}Rb) cardiac PET allows myocardial perfusion to be assessed by using a strontium-82 (^{82}Sr)/^{82}Rb column generator in clinics lacking a cyclotron to produce radionuclides such as ^{15}O-water or ^{13}N-ammonia. The short half-life of the radiotracer (76 seconds) makes possible rapid rest/stress paired studies within a very short time (~25 minutes), allowing rest and stress imaging under virtually identical conditions and decreasing the total time required to scan each patient. Rubidium is a potassium analogue that is only partially extracted by the myocardium after a single capillary pass, as is the case for cationic flow markers such as ^{13}N-ammonia or thallium-201 (^{201}Tl).[23] Therefore, extraction decreases as flow increases.[24] The extracted rubidium is taken up rapidly by myocardial cells, whose retention time is much greater than the half-life of ^{82}Rb; therefore, it falls in the category of physiologically retained tracers (e.g., ^{13}N-ammonia, ^{201}Tl), in contrast with freely diffusible tracers (e.g., ^{15}O-water). Given these characteristics, several models have been developed to describe ^{82}Rb kinetics. We present in this section the main models in order of increasing sophistication.

Extraction of ^{82}Rb in Myocardial Tissues

The extraction of ^{82}Rb by myocardial cells can be used to elucidate the functional status of myocardial tissue, and its measurement is central to the absolute quantitation of myocardial flow. As stated in the "Basic Principles of Compartment Analysis" section, the extraction is defined as the fraction of ^{82}Rb that moves from the capillaries to the extravascular space in the tissue of interest on a single pass through the local blood vessels. From equation (5), we see that flow, F, is the ratio of K_1 to extraction fraction, E. Therefore, if the extraction fraction is known, myocardial blood flow may be computed from estimates of K_1 obtained from kinetic analysis. Several authors have measured the extraction fraction in animal models. Mullani et al[25] used an open-chest dog model to measure the extraction fraction and reported the relationship between extraction fraction and flow, $E = 0.55\,e^{-0.22F}$ (Figure 4.3). Yoshida et al[26] also measured the extraction fraction in open-chest dogs and reported, $E = 1 - e^{-(0.45+0.16F)/F}$ (Figure 4.3). Marshall et al[27] performed a similar study in excised, perfused rabbit hearts and found the relationship, $E = -0.084931\,F + 0.84145$ for flow rates up to 3 mL/min/g. From Figure 4.3, it can be seen that there is a reasonable agreement among these models over a flow range of interest for patients with coronary artery disease (CAD).

Estimation of Arterial Input Functions

Arterial input functions, which are used for most quantitative tracer-kinetic techniques, can be measured invasively by arterial blood sampling, less invasively (and less accurately) by sampling arterialized venous blood, or noninvasively by drawing a VOI over the left ventricular blood pool and acquiring dynamic frames. The last approach has the advantage of being easy to perform, but it is affected by the blurring of myocardial counts into the ventricles (and vice versa) that, in turn, arise from the

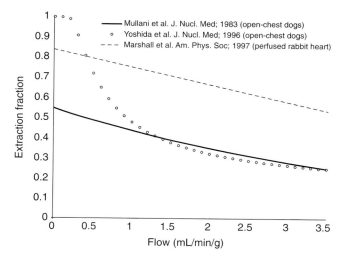

FIGURE 4.3. Parameterized extraction fraction as a function of flow from 3 different animal-model experiments.

PET camera's limited spatial resolution (~0.6cm) and from motion of the beating heart. In addition to the VOI approach, several methods have been proposed to compensate for spillover and partial volume effects based on geometrical models (e.g., References 28 and 29) using anatomic MR or CT imaging of the heart along with PET imaging. Methods like these are becoming more useful with the advent of PET/CT and the widespread use of image-registration techniques; however, they remain of limited value in the absence of anatomic data because large errors in myocardial flow estimates are associated with the use of an inaccurate estimate of myocardial wall thickness. Other approaches (e.g., Reference 30) have aimed at estimating radioactivity concentrations from sinogram (projection) data while compensating for the partial volume effect. Finally, other noninvasive methods for estimating the arterial input function, which are less sensitive to count spillover effects, include principal component analysis (PCA) and independent component analysis (ICA) (e.g., References 31–34), and generalized factor analysis of dynamic sequences (GFADS).[35] These algorithms permit estimation of left (and, in some cases, right) ventricular input functions automatically without the need to draw VOI over the ventricular cavities. Possible difficulties with the ICA and PCA approaches include the nonuniqueness of the solution and its potential lack of physiologic pertinence. These have been traditionally addressed by imposing a priori constraints on the solution. In GFADS, the nonuniqueness problem in dynamic cardiac PET is addressed by penalizing the spatial overlap of cardiac structures. After fitting the time-varying factor model to the dynamic data using a least-squares objective function, a different objective function that penalizes spatial overlap between factor images can be minimized. This process preserves the results of the least-squares fit obtained in the first step, and both steps incorporate nonnegativity constraints on the factors, as well as on the factor images.[35] The estimation of the left and right ventricular input functions should be more robust to noise than the manually drawn VOI method because all voxels in the data set are used to determine the time-activity behavior with GFADS, whereas the VOI approach utilizes a smaller number of voxels. This is illustrated in Figure 4.4, which shows the left and right ventricular input estimates from Monte Carlo simulation of a dynamic PET study obtained by drawing VOIs over the left and right cavities and by using the generalized factor analysis approach.

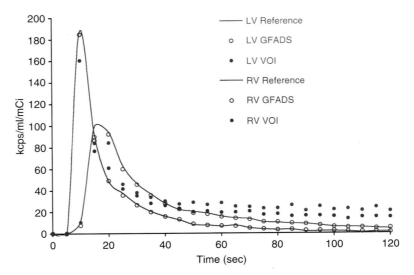

FIGURE 4.4. Left (LV) and right (RV) ventricular input functions estimated using a volume of interest (VOI) and generalized factor analysis of dynamic sequences (GFADS). (Modified by permission of the Society of Nuclear Medicine from El Fakhri G, et al., Quantitative Dynamic Cardiac 82Rb PET Using Generalized Factor and Compartment Analyses. J Nucl Med. 2005;46:1264–1271. Figure 3.)

The Single-Compartment Model

The simplest approach to model ^{82}Rb kinetics is to assume a single compartment, that is, the myocardium, with an arterial input, characterized by flow F and arterial ^{82}Rb concentration $C_A(t)$ and a venous output, characterized by flow F and arterial ^{82}Rb concentration $C_V(t)$ (Figure 4.5).

The net flux of tracer in the myocardium, J_{net} (in Bq/min/g), is, by definition, the time derivative of the ^{82}Rb concentration. From equation (2), J is also equal to the instantaneous amount of radiotracer delivered by the arterial input minus the instantaneous amount of tracer leaving through venous egress. Therefore,

$$J_{net} = \frac{dC_T(t)}{dt} = FC_A(t) - FC_V(t), \qquad (18)$$

where C_T is the ^{82}Rb concentration in Bq/g, and C_A and C_V are the arterial and venous concentrations of ^{82}Rb, respectively, in Bq/mL. The flow, F, is expressed in mL/min/g. During the passage of ^{82}Rb from the arterial to the venous capillaries, if a fraction, E, is irreversibly extracted by the myocardial cells, then the venous concentration of ^{82}Rb must be $(1 - E)$ times the arterial concentration, $C_A(t)$; this is the key assumption of the 1-compartment model. Rewriting the second term of the equation as a function of F, C_A, and the extraction fraction E yields

$$J_{net} = \frac{dC_T(t)}{dt} = EFC_A(t) \qquad (19)$$

By integrating over time, the relationship between flow and myocardial concentration of ^{82}Rb is,

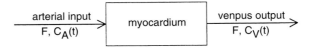

FIGURE 4.5. Single-compartment ^{82}Rb model.

$$C_T(t) = FE \int_0^t C_A(x)dx, \quad \text{or} \quad F = \frac{C_T(t)}{E \int_0^t C_A(x)dx}. \tag{20}$$

The extraction fraction can be expressed in terms of flow using any of the relations determined experimentally, such as those measured in open-chest dogs presented in the section "Extraction of ^{82}Rb in Myocardial Tissues":

$$F(0.55e^{-0.22F}) \quad \text{or} \quad F(1 - e^{-(0.45+0.16F)/F}) = \frac{C_T(t)}{\int_0^t C_A(x)dx} \tag{21}$$

Therefore, flow can be determined from measurements of the myocardial and arterial ^{82}Rb concentrations.[36]

The major advantage of the 1-compartment-model approach is its robustness to noise. Since only one parameter, flow, needs to be determined from the model, this means that flow can be determined with greater precision than it can when multiple parameters must be determined. There are also limitations to the 1-compartment model in ^{82}Rb cardiac PET. The first limitation is that, because the relation between flow and extraction (equation [21]) may not be constant with prolonged ischemia or when interventions such as reperfusion are performed, the approach must be used cautiously when estimating myocardial blood flow under these conditions.[36] Furthermore, due to the relationship between extraction and flow, the 1-compartment approach was found in dog experiments to be insensitive for flows greater than ~2.5 mL/min/g;[36] this precludes accurate estimation of coronary flow reserve during pharmacologically induced coronary hyperemia. Another limitation of the 1-compartment model is the assumption that there is no egress from myocardial cells. This is generally true for healthy myocardial cells, where the extraction and prolonged retention of rubidium indicate that it behaves as a potassium analogue; however, the assumption is probably not accurate when the cell membrane is damaged (e.g., in regions of necrosis), because rubidium can leak out of the cell. Therefore, measuring the rate of egress of rubidium from the myocardial tissue would permit assessment of the integrity of the myocardial cell membrane.[37]

The 2-Compartment Model

As explained at the end of the previous section, damage of the cell membrane, for example, in regions of necrosis, allows rubidium to leak out of myocytes. Modeling the rate of egress of rubidium from the cells can yield important physiologic information about the integrity of the myocardial cell membranes after injury; however, this requires the use of at least a 2-compartment kinetic model. As noted in the section "Extraction of ^{82}Rb in Myocardial Tissues," rubidium is partially extracted from the blood, with extraction fraction E, on its first pass through the myocardium. We present a simplified 2-compartment model of ^{82}Rb (and a similar model for ^{13}N-ammonia) first proposed by Yoshida et al,[26] and we then present the generalized 2-compartment model. The total ^{82}Rb activity concentration in the myocardium at time t, $M(t)$, which is also the measured activity in a myocardial VOI drawn on cardiac PET images, is the sum of the free rubidium in extracellular space and trapped rubidium in intracellular space:

$$M(t) = V_F C_F(t) + V_T C_T(t), \tag{22}$$

where $C_F(t)$ and $C_T(t)$ are the concentrations of rubidium in the free (extracellular) and trapped (intracellular) spaces, and V_F and V_T are the myocardial volume fractions (mL/g) occupied by free and trapped ^{82}Rb, respectively. The extraction fraction in this

2-compartment model is defined as the ratio of the amount of ^{82}Rb trapped in the intracellular space ($V_T C_T$) to the amount delivered (flow times the integrated arterial input),

$$E = \frac{V_T C_T (t)}{F \int_0^t C_F (x) dx}, \tag{23}$$

where Yoshida et al[26] approximated the integral of $C_A(t)$ in the denominator by the corresponding integral of the ^{82}Rb concentration in the free space. Replacing $V_T C_T(t)$ in Equation (22) by its expression derived from the definition of extraction fraction in Equation (23), one can express the total ^{82}Rb activity concentration in the myocardium at time t as:

$$M(t) = FE \int_0^t C_F (x) dx + V_F C_F (t), \tag{24}$$

where F is the flow, E is the extraction fraction, V_F is the free-space, or extracellular, volume, and C_F is the concentration of rubidium in the extracellular space. The concentration of rubidium in the extracellular space, $C_F(t)$, can be adequately represented for a femoral vein bolus injection by a convolution of the arterial input function with a function of the form bte^{-at}, where the parameters a and b are determined by fitting the model to the measured rubidium PET data as described by Mullani et al[25] and Goldstein et al[23] The 2-compartment model (Equation [22]) can be then rewritten as:

$$M(t) = FE \int_0^t C_A (x) * bxe^{-ax} dx + V_F C_A (t) * bte^{-at}. \tag{25}$$

The Generalized 2-Compartment Model

The 2 compartments used in rubidium kinetic modeling are the free rubidium space, or extracellular space, consisting of interstitial and vascular spaces, and the trapped rubidium, or intracellular, space.[24,26,38] Another representation of the 2-compartment model involves explicitly including the rate constants K_1 and k_2. As seen in Figure 4.6, K_1 characterizes the rate of influx of ^{82}Rb into the cells, while k_2 is the rate of egress of ^{82}Rb from the cells (in the presence of cell membrane damage).

The 2-compartment model can be generalized by modeling spillover from the right ventricle into the myocardium and by modeling a spatially distributed parameter system, where the rubidium concentration is assumed to vary from voxel to voxel. The

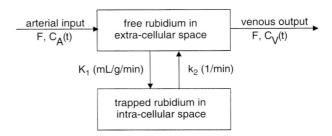

FIGURE 4.6. A 2-compartment ^{82}Rb model.

k₁ (mL/min/g)   k₂ (min⁻¹)

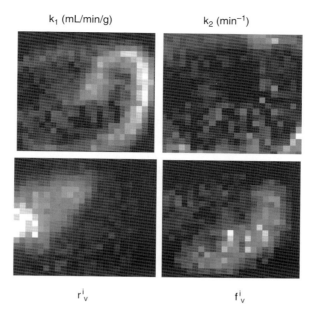

r$_v^i$ f$_v^i$

FIGURE 4.7. Parametric maps of myocardial tissue extraction (K_1) and egress (k_2) as well as right and left ventricle contributions from a dynamic resting study in 93-year-old female with known CAD but with normal myocardial perfusion. (Modified by permission of the Society of Nuclear Medicine from: El Fakhri G, et al., Quantitative Dynamic Cardiac 82Rb PET Using Generalized Factor and Compartment Analyses. J Nucl Med. 2005;46:1264–1271. Figure 4.)

amount of radioactivity measured in a myocardial volume of interest drawn on a PET cardiac study is modeled as a combination of 3 contributions: the contribution from myocardial tissue, assumed to consist of 2 compartments, along with fractional contributions from left ventricular blood and right ventricular blood.[35] As reported by El Fakhri et al,[35] modeling the right ventricle contribution yields a more stable and robust voxel-based kinetic parameter estimation. This model can be written as:

$$C_T^i(t) = L(t) \otimes K_1^i e^{-k_2^i t} + f_v^i l(t) + r_v^i R(t), \tag{26}$$

where $C_T^i(t)$ is the value of the PET-measured rubidium radioactivity in voxel i at time t, and $L(t)$ is the input function (i.e., measured LV function). K_1^i, k_2^i, f_v^i, and r_v^i are the kinetic parameters for voxel i. K_1^i (mL/min/g) characterizes myocardial tissue extraction (inflow). k_2^i (min⁻¹) characterizes myocardial tissue egress (outflow), f_v^i (dimensionless) represents the contribution to the total voxel activity from the blood input function $L(t)$, and r_v^i (dimensionless) represents the contribution from the activity in the RV, $R(t)$, which in general differs from the input function (Figure 4.4). Both $L(t)$ and $R(t)$ can be determined by the generalized factor analysis approach, as described in the section "Estimation of Arterial Input Functions."

The estimation of parametric images on a voxel-by-voxel basis yields very noisy images due to high levels of noise in TAC derived from single voxels. Use of a filtering approach reduces noise but can result in a degradation of spatial resolution of the parametric images. Another approach is to perform orthogonal grouping, that is, 3D grouping of voxels with a similar time course. The average TACs within the groups can then be used for calculation of the kinetic parameters. This approach leads to reduced levels of noise with minimal effects on spatial resolution.[35] Figure 4.7 shows an example of parametric maps of myocardial tissue extraction (K_1) and egress (k_2) as well as right and left ventricle contributions (f_v^i, r_v^i) from a dynamic resting study in a 93-year-old female with known CAD but normal myocardial perfusion.

The 3-Compartment Model

The 2-compartment model can also be generalized to a 3-compartment model in which the extracellular compartment is divided into vascular (or capillary) and interstitial spaces, since barriers for transport of rubidium are present at the level of the capillaries and the myocardial cell membrane.[39] Therefore, the 3 compartments are intracellular, interstitial, and vascular. Because of the very rapid movement of rubidium from the capillary space to the interstitial space, however, several authors (e.g., References 40, 41, 42) believe that the interstitial and vascular compartments can legitimately be grouped into a single compartment. Furthermore, Coxson et al concluded based on numerical simulations of dynamic cardiac PET data that the 1-compartment model can yield reasonably accurate estimates of myocardial blood flow and that the 2-compartment model can differentiate flow if a priori values are used for nonflow parameters.[43]

Comparison of Perfusion Measurement Techniques

This section summarizes the advantages and disadvantages of each of the perfusion tracers presented in this chapter. The reader is also referred to other comparative reviews of perfusion imaging techniques.[44] The 3 techniques we describe, based on ^{15}O-water, ^{13}N-ammonia, and ^{82}Rb, are compared by considering both physiologic properties and physical effects. The physiologic properties pertain to the extraction of the tracer and its mechanism of uptake, while physical effects include factors influencing the accuracy and precision of myocardial blood-flow estimates, such as positron range, tracer half-life, and the partial-volume effect. Both ^{13}N-ammonia and ^{82}Rb have been compared to ^{15}O-water. Nitzsche et al[45] evaluated ^{13}N-ammonia and ^{15}O-water in 15 healthy volunteers at rest and another 15 healthy volunteers at stress and showed that the values of myocardial blood flow estimated with ^{13}N-ammonia were comparable to those obtained with ^{15}O-water. Lin et al[46,47] have also shown good agreement between flow estimates obtained with ^{82}Rb and ^{15}O-water at rest and during dipyridamole stress in 11 healthy volunteers.

Physiologic Considerations

Oxygen-15 water is a metabolically inert tracer that freely diffuses across capillaries and myocardial cell membranes, yielding a rapid equilibrium between extravascular and vascular compartments. Therefore, the first-pass extraction of ^{15}O-water is close to unity and is independent of flow. However, spatial blurring of counts arising from the system spatial resolution and from motion of the beating heart makes it difficult to isolate myocardial activity from blood activity. As detailed in the section on ^{15}O-water, these limitations can be addressed by performing 2 scans and/or by additional image processing, but these approaches can be cumbersome and are affected by patient motion. As a result, it can be challenging to obtain high-quality ^{15}O-water images with the blood-pool contribution adequately removed. ^{13}N-ammonia and ^{82}Rb, on the other hand, are only partially extracted by the myocardium after a single capillary pass. The slightly greater first-pass extraction fraction of ^{13}N-ammonia (65% to 70%)[14,26] compared to ^{82}Rb (60% to 65%)[25,26] may not have a substantial clinical benefit. For both tracers, the extraction is limited by flow and decreases as flow increases, and the retention of the tracer is coupled with energy-dependent trapping mechanisms. As a consequence, mathematical models such as those described in this chapter must be used to isolate the tracer delivery and tracer retention mechanisms. The accuracy and precision of any method used to separate these effects will depend on the signal-to-noise ratio (SNR) of the data, as well as on the extraction and retention properties of the tracer, and the kinetic properties of tracer delivery.[48] Other physiologic considerations include the potential for poor contrast studies with ^{13}N-ammonia in smokers due to high lung uptake. In summary, both ^{13}N-ammonia and ^{82}Rb have useful physiologic properties that make them good candidates for routine clinical use. From an economics standpoint, ^{82}Rb, unlike ^{13}N-ammonia, does not require the presence of an on-site cyclotron for clinical use. This could prove important in the future, since a majority of nuclear medicine clinics equipped with PET and/or PET /CT scanners do not have access to on-site cyclotrons.

Physical Effects

We discuss here some factors affecting image quality, as well as the accuracy and precision of MBF estimates: positron range, the partial volume effect, and tracer half-life. The spatial resolution is affected primarily by the design of the PET scanner and by the choice of reconstruction algorithm. Although the intrinsic spatial resolution is the same for all studies, the reconstructed spatial resolution is also affected by the positron range of the radionuclide being imaged, that is, by the distance between the location of the positron decay and that of the positron's annihilation with an electron. The positron range depends on the energy of the emitted positron and varies greatly with the tissue in which the positrons are propagating. For example, the full width at half maximum (FWHM), which characterizes the loss of spatial resolution attributable to positron range, is 0.33 mm, 0.41 mm, and 0.76 mm, respectively, for ^{15}O, ^{13}N, and ^{82}Rb in soft tissues, and an even wider disparity is seen in the full-width at tenth-maximum (FWTM), that is, on the "tails" of the point-spread function. In lung tissues, the FWHM values become 0.62 mm, 0.86 mm, and 1.43 mm.[49] Clearly, ^{82}Rb is at a disadvantage in terms of loss of spatial resolution due to positron range. The greater loss of spatial resolution leads, in turn, to increased underestimation of myocardial activity attributable to increased spillover from the relatively thin myocardial wall into the cavity. This phenomenon is commonly referred to as the partial-volume effect.

The relative statistical noise (standard deviation/mean counts) in any local region of a PET image that is reconstructed by, for example, some maximum-likelihood iterative method is approximately proportional to $1/\sqrt{mean}$. Therefore, a larger number of detected counts leads to a lower degree of relative image noise; this, in turn, translates into an improved precision of estimates of myocardial flow. This can be an important consideration when performing dynamic acquisitions as short as 5–10 seconds per time frame, which might be used for ^{15}O-water and ^{82}Rb, where the mathematical models used to isolate the tracer delivery from the tracer retention depend on image SNR. Therefore, ^{15}O-water and ^{82}Rb, with half-lives of 122 seconds and 75 seconds, respectively, are at a disadvantage compared to ^{13}N-ammonia, with its half-life of 9.9 minutes, which allows longer acquisition times and, consequently, more counts, especially when an older PET scanner with slower electronics is used. Imaging performance can also be affected by dead-time and pulse pileup when high levels of activity in the field of view are imaged, as is the case following injection of 60 mCi of ^{82}Rb. Nevertheless, most new PET cameras with fast crystals and electronics can handle the high counting rates associated with a bolus injection of 60 mCi of ^{82}Rb.[35] On the other hand, the short half-lives of tracers such as ^{82}Rb allow rest and stress studies to be performed within approximately 10 minutes (8 ^{82}Rb half-lives) of each other in the same imaging session using pharmacological stress. This dramatically increases patient throughput and allows for repeated studies. A ^{13}N-ammonia rest/stress evaluation would require approximately 90 minutes compared to 25–30 minutes for a rest/stress ^{82}Rb study. Finally, given the fixed cost of a ^{82}Rb generator, the cost of each study decreases with the number of studies performed, in contrast with cyclotron-produced ^{13}N-ammonia or ^{15}O-water, where the cost of a unit dose is fixed.

PET Imaging of Myocardial Metabolism

There are several different energy sources for healthy myocardium; in the fasting, resting state, free fatty acid metabolism is by far the dominant mechanism. In fact, even after consumption of carbohydrates, it has been shown that only 30% to 50% of myocardial metabolism is glucose dependent,[50] while most of the remaining energy demands continue to be met by fatty acids. It is known that the kinetics of the radio-tracer ^{11}C-palmitate are altered in response to changes in cardiac workload[51] and ischemia.[52] Nevertheless, it has proved difficult to sort out the many metabolic pathways involved in the complex tracer-kinetic behavior of ^{11}C-palmitate. On the other hand, the behavior of fluorodeoxyglucose (FDG), a useful surrogate marker for glucose metabolism, has been studied for many years, so FDG serves as a well-characterized system that has, in fact, been exploited very effectively by nuclear medicine practitioners. The PET research community has also begun to study the utility of ^{11}C-acetate as a tracer for the assessment of oxidative metabolism. This application will be discussed following the next section on FDG imaging.

Flourine-18 Fluorodeoxyglucose

Flourine-18 (^{18}F) is widely available to clinicians and researchers today; this is primarily because its relatively long half-life (109.8 minutes) means that it can be produced by radiopharmaceutical manufacturers in a few different regional centers, and then distributed easily over a relatively wide geographic area. Production of ^{18}F fluorodeoxyglucose (FDG), in particular, has rapidly increased during the past few years, as more and more clinical indications have been approved for PET scanning. In cardiac nuclear medicine studies, FDG has been used primarily as an indicator of myocardial viability for patients with relatively severe left ventricular dysfunction, allowing clinicians to discriminate reversible from irreversible myocardial damage. For example, Di Carli et al[53] reported that if an area of mismatch between perfusion and glucose metabolism on PET images exceeded 18% of the left ventricular volume, then there was ~80% probability of improved functional outcome following revascularization.

The 3-Compartment FDG Model

From Figure 4.8, it may be seen that the standard FDG compartment model is identical in form to that shown in Figure 4.2 for ^{13}N-ammonia. Therefore, the model equations are also identical to equations (14) through (17) above, but with an obviously different interpretation. In Figure 4.2, extravascular ^{13}N-ammonia is metabolized to ^{13}N-glutamine, whereas in Figure 4.3, ^{18}F-FDG is metabolized to ^{18}F-FDG-6-phosphate, which is also largely trapped in the cells. Ultimately, however, we are more interested in quantifying the metabolism of glucose, rather than that of FDG. The metabolic pathways of glucose and FDG are virtually identical, with the important exception that glucose-6-phosphate continues to change through the glycolytic pathway. Furthermore, some of the phosphorylated glucose can revert back to the extravascular glucose pool with rate-constant k_4, whereas k_4 is, essentially, 0 for the phosphorylated FDG shown in Figure 4.8. The almost complete trapping of the

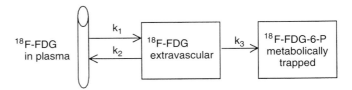

FIGURE 4.8. The standard 3-compartment ^{18}F-FDG model.

phosphorylated FDG in the second tissue compartment leads to an increase in PET signal from regions of the body characterized by a high metabolic rate, such as tumors.

Detailed analyses of the relative metabolic rates of the hexokinase-catalyzed phosphorylation of glucose versus that of FDG (e.g., References 54–56) have demonstrated that the metabolic rate for glucose can be computed after obtaining the FDG kinetic rate constants, K_1, k_2, and k_3, by fitting the TACs from dynamic PET images:

$$MRG = \frac{C_{G,P}}{L}\left(\frac{K_1 k_3}{k_2 + k_3}\right), \tag{27}$$

where MRG is the glucose metabolic rate, $C_{G,P}$ is the concentration of glucose in plasma (assumed to be constant during the experiment), and L is the so-called lumped constant, a combination of 6 different constants that arises from differences in the competing enzyme kinetics between glucose and FDG. The factor in parentheses is the product of K_1, the rate of transport of fluorine-18 (^{18}F)-FDG into the first tissue compartment, and $k_3/(k_2 + k_3)$, the fraction of irreversibly bound ^{18}F in tissue. Although it is commonly assumed that L is constant for a given tissue of interest, it has been shown that the value of the lumped "constant" in myocardium does, in fact, vary in response to changes in myocardial metabolism, which affect the kinetics of hexokinase and glucose transport.[57,58] Bøtker et al[59] later proposed a method to account for this variability, which agreed well with their measurements obtained from isolated perfused rat hearts. However, before absolute quantification of myocardial glucose uptake is possible in humans, it will be necessary to determine appropriate values for the ratio between rates of membrane transport of FDG and glucose, and for the ratio between the rates of phosphorylation of FDG and glucose. These ratios, which are assumed to be constant in the proposed approach, are not expected to be the same for rat hearts and human hearts. Wiggers et al,[60] in a study of 20 nondiabetic patients with ischemic cardiomyopathy, showed that the value of L used to calculate myocardial glucose uptake was not affected by regional differences in the metabolic state of the myocardium. Importantly, however, L did vary substantially from patient to patient in all different states of myocardial metabolism, as defined by the degree of concordance between scores used to assess regional wall motion and perfusion. These results indicate that measurements of myocardial glucose uptake obtained using a fixed value of L are likely to be strongly biased.

Patlak Analysis

If one is certain that the reverse rate constant, k_4 (representing the rate of dephosphorylation of FDG-6-P), in the tissue of interest is 0, or very small, it is possible to compute FDG utilization using a simple graphical analysis technique,[61,62] which avoids the more complicated nonlinear fitting procedure described above. The Patlak equation is

$$\frac{C_T(t)}{C_A(t)} = V_0 + K\left[\frac{\int_0^t C_A(t')dt'}{C_A(t)}\right]. \tag{28}$$

The left side of this equation is the distribution volume of FDG, and the factor in brackets on the right is defined as "stretched time." (For a continuous infusion of FDG, this factor simply reduces to conventional time, t.) K is the FDG utilization, which is equivalent to the factor in brackets in equation (27) above: $K = K_1 k_3/(k_2 + k_3)$. Equation (28) indicates that the distribution volume should be a simple linear function of stretched time, as long as the initial distribution volume, the

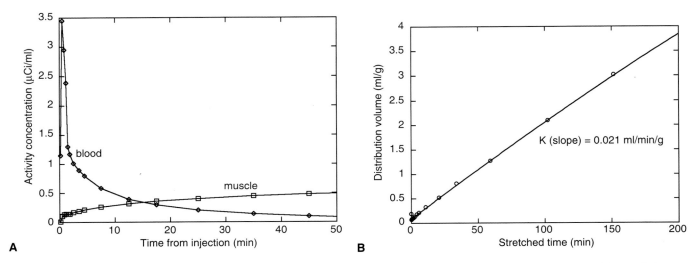

FIGURE 4.9. (A) Flourine-18 FDG TACs measured for blood and muscle and (B) corresponding Patlak plot with fitted slope, K, related to glucose utilization.

intercept V_0, and the slope of the straight line, K, (FDG utilization) are both constant. The graphical technique (e.g., Figure 4.9) consists of determining the intercept and slope of the line, for example, by straightforward linear curve fitting. If the plot is not linear over the full range of stretched time, it may indicate a violation of the assumption that there is no dephosphorylation by the tissue. While Patlak analysis is a useful technique for quickly determining FDG utilization, as well as glucose metabolic rate (if the lumped constant and the glucose blood concentration are known), it should be realized that the method does not permit the simultaneous determination of all 3 FDG rate constants. On the other hand, it is possible to fit the distribution volume to a nonlinear function of stretched time[63,64] to estimate the lumped constant; this is the basis for the approach described by Bøtker et al,[59] discussed above, to improve quantitative estimates of myocardial glucose uptake.

Single-Scan Approximate Analysis

For the case when the myocardial glucose metabolic rate must be estimated from a single FDG PET scan, obtained at time t after injection, it is possible to use an approximate, operational equation developed by Sokoloff and colleagues:[54]

$$MRG(t) = \frac{C_{G,P}}{L} = \frac{C_T(t) - K_1\left[C_A(t) * e^{-(k_2+k_3)t}\right]}{\int_0^t C_A(t')\,dt' - \left[C_A(t) * e^{-(k_2+k_3)t}\right]}. \tag{29}$$

Because no dynamic image data are available, this equation can be evaluated only using predetermined, average or "typical" values for K_1, k_2, and k_3, as well as for the lumped constant, L. The plasma blood concentration of FDG, $C_A(t)$, must be measured from multiple blood samples obtained during the interval between tracer injection and the PET scan, and the stationary glucose plasma concentration, $C_{G,P}$ can also be determined from blood sampling. $C_T(t)$ is the tissue activity concentration measured from the single PET scan acquired at time t. It is important to note that the factors in square brackets in both the numerator and denominator represent convolutions of the measured plasma blood concentration with the exponential functions.

^{11}C-Acetate Measurement of Myocardial Oxygen Consumption

Acetate in arterial blood plasma accumulates in myocardial tissue by rapid transport across a cell membrane into the mitochondrion, where it is converted by acetyl-CoA synthetase to acetyl-CoA (acetylcoenzyme-A), which enters the tricarboxylic acid (TCA) cycle, undergoing rapid transamination reactions and equilibrating with aspartate and glutamate. Acetate can be labeled with the positron emitter, carbon-11 ($T_{1/2}$ = 20.4 minutes) in the 1-position (1-^{11}C-acetate). This molecule is initially extracted to tissue in an amount approximately proportional to blood flow, where, during metabolism in the TCA cycle, ^{11}C is transferred to ^{11}CO$_2$ in accordance with oxidation rate.

Initial PET studies of ^{11}C-acetate were based mostly on its observed exponential rates of washout from tissue (e.g., References 65–67). Choi et al[68] pointed out that the numerical accuracy of indices of myocardial oxygen consumption derived from exponential fitting could depend sensitively on the choice of data points used in the analysis of TACs and by the shape of the input function. To mitigate such concerns, these authors proposed a method based on the mean transit time of tracer through tissue, determined by calculation of statistical moments of TACs.

A very thorough tracer-kinetic model incorporating 6 compartments was later developed and evaluated in experiments with isolated perfused rat hearts.[69] While this approach was accurate and comprehensive, it has generally been recognized that some simplifications would be necessary to arrive at a method that would retain good quantitative performance, while being sufficiently robust for routine use with noisy PET image data from human subjects. These considerations motivated Sun et al[70] to develop the 2-compartment model shown in Figure 4.10 for fitting PET time-activity data following injection of ^{11}C-acetate. These researchers, who validated their model in dog experiments, indicated that several simplifications could be made when using only the first 5 or 10 minutes of data after administration of the tracer. First, since the concentration of labeled glutamate was much higher than that of glutamine (in both normal and ischemic myocardium) during the first 10 minutes, 2 of the compartments (C-5 glutamine and C-1 glutamine) of the more detailed 6-compartment model could be ignored. It was also determined that the bicarbonate compartment of the 6-compartment model could similarly be dispensed with because labeled bicarbonate concentrations were relatively constant in the isolated perfused rat hearts and did not significantly influence estimates of the relevant parameters. Finally, because it was observed that labeled cellular acetate cleared rapidly and was much lower in concentration than C-5 glutamine and C-1 and C-4 aspartate, the authors decided to include cellular acetate within the same TCA compartment. With all these simplifying assumptions, the rate constant k_2 (Figure 4.10) represents the rate with which C-1 α-ketoglutarate and CO$_2$ are produced, and serves as an indicator of oxidative flux through the TCA cycle, while K_1 indicates the rate of extraction of ^{11}C-acetate into the cells. The researchers also incorporated spillover from blood to tissue, along with delay of the measured input function, into their model equations.

Given estimates of k_2, myocardial oxygen consumption (MVO$_2$) was calculated following References 69 as

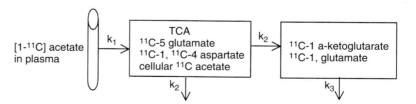

FIGURE 4.10. Simplified 2-compartment ^{11}C-acetate model of oxidative metabolism.

$$MVO_2 = 6k_2\{[Glu] + [Asp] + [TCA]\}, \tag{30}$$

where the tissue concentrations of the pools of labeled glutamate, aspartate, and other TCA intermediate compounds were assumed to be equal to those measured in previous studies of isolated perfused rat hearts. While there is no particular reason to assume that the pool sizes of these amino acids and TCA intermediaries are the same in dogs (or humans) as in rats, the researchers were, nevertheless, able to demonstrate a highly significant linear correlation between values of MVO_2 measured directly and those estimated using the simplified 2-compartment model fitting. The model was later used for fitting PET data from human subjects by Sun et al,[71] who showed that K_1 was linearly correlated with blood flow, at least in the low-flow regime, and that k_2 remained linearly correlated with MVO_2. This work indicated that, with careful calibration, both myocardial blood flow and oxygen consumption could be determined in the same resting study following administration of a single radiolabeled tracer.

Although ^{11}C-acetate imaging has several useful features, the technique also has a few limitations. First, a cyclotron on-site or very near the clinic is generally required because of the short (20.4-minute) half-life of ^{11}C and the required preparation time. Second, the tracer and model have been well validated only for the case of rest imaging; that is, the technique still needs to be extended and tested at higher flow rates under stress conditions, where, for example, the tracer extraction fraction could change significantly. Furthermore, under resting conditions, images obtained from the first 2 to 5 minutes following injection contribute mostly to the estimation of tissue perfusion, while later measurements are more affected by the rate of oxidative metabolism. Under stress conditions, the faster heart rate is likely to shorten the period of time during which the tissue flow can be reliably estimated. A shorter acquisition time would then be expected to increase the level of image noise, as discussed earlier in this chapter. In spite of these issues, ^{11}C-acetate PET imaging remains a very useful technique for assessing resting myocardial perfusion and oxygen metabolism.

Summary Points

- The unidirectional first-pass extraction fraction decreases with increasing blood flow, in a manner that is different for each different tracer of myocardial perfusion or metabolism.
- The use of more complex compartment models, characterized by a greater number of unknown kinetic parameters, may improve accuracy for the estimates of flow or metabolic rates, but this gain will generally be accompanied by a loss of precision, that is, by increased variability of the parameter estimates.
- The heart is the most convenient organ for quantitative dynamic PET imaging studies because the presence of blood pools in cross-sectional images containing the heart can greatly facilitate determination of the arterial blood input function, which is required for truly quantitative analysis.
- Oxygen-15 water, ^{13}N-ammonia, and [82]Rb are all useful for the assessment of myocardial perfusion. The first two require a cyclotron in close proximity to the PET camera; [82]Rb requires the purchase of a generator each month. The highly diffusible nature of ^{15}O-water provides, in principle, an advantage for flow imaging; however, it can be challenging to adequately separate the blood pool from the myocardium. Nitrogen-13 ammonia and [82]Rb, in contrast, are partially extracted tracers. Both exercise-stress and resting studies can be performed with ^{13}N-ammonia; however, the shorter half-life of [82]Rb restricts its use to pharmacologic-stress and resting studies. On the other hand, [82]Rb can be reinjected more frequently, which can lead to very efficient evaluation of myocardial flow and functional behavior. With the use of sophisticated compartment analysis techniques, both ^{13}N-ammonia and [82]Rb can provide information related to both myocardial perfusion and cellular viability,

although the mechanisms of transport into, trapping within, and egress from the myocytes are different for the two tracers.

- Flourine-18 FDG is a tracer of glucose metabolism, which serves as a useful indicator of myocardial viability, especially when FDG images can be directly compared to perfusion images. The half-life of ^{18}F is sufficiently long that ^{18}F-FDG can be produced regionally and distributed to many different hospitals in one area; that is, an on-site cyclotron is not required. While a detailed 3-compartment model can be applied to dynamic PET image data, the simpler Patlak method[61,62] can often be used to provide information related to the metabolic rate of FDG utilization. Unfortunately, the "lumped constant," which relates FDG utilization to the metabolic rate for glucose, is highly variable from subject to subject, although recent research suggests that useful predictors of the lumped constant in a given individual may become available in the future.

- Myocardial oxidative metabolism can be evaluated by ^{11}C-acetate imaging, using dynamic PET acquisitions with a simplified 2-compartment model. This technique requires an on-site cyclotron; however, the kinetic model permits, in principle (with careful calibration), the simultaneous determination of myocardial blood flow and oxygen consumption under resting conditions. This method has not yet been validated for use under conditions of exercise-induced or pharmacologically induced stress, which may present significant challenges.

References

1. Carson RE. Tracer kinetic modeling in PET. In: Valk PE, Bailey DL, Townsend DW, Maisey MN, eds. *Positron Emission Tomography: Basic Science and Clinical Practice.* London: Springer; 2003:147–179.
2. Morris ED, Endres CJ, Schmidt KC, Christian JT, Muzic RF, Fisher RE. Kinetic modeling in positron emission tomography. In: Wernick MN, Aarsvold JN, eds. *Emission Tomography: The Fundamentals of PET and SPECT.* Amsterdam: Elsevier; 2004:499–540.
3. Cherry SR, Sorenson JA, Phelps ME. Tracer kinetic modeling. In: *Physics in Nuclear Medicine.* Philadelphia: Saunders; 2003:377–403.
4. Renkin EM. Transport of potassium-42 from blood to tissue in isolated mammalian skeletal muscles. *Am J Physiol.* 1959;197:1205–1210.
5. Crone C. Permeability of capillaries in various organs as determined by use of the indicator diffusion method. *Acta Physiol Scand.* 1964;58:292–305.
6. Bergmann SR, Fox KAA, Rond AL, et al. Quantification of regional myocardial blood flow in vivo with $H_2^{15}O$. *Circulation.* 1984;70:724–733.
7. Kety SS. The theory and applications of the exchange of inert gas at the lungs and tissues. *Pharmacol Rev.* 1951;3:1–41.
8. Huang S-C, Schwaiger M, Carson RE, et al. Quantitative measurement of myocardial blood flow with oxygen-15 water positron computed tomography: an assessment of potential and problems. *J Nucl Med.* 1985;26:616–625.
9. Iida H, Kanno I, Takahashi A, et al. Measurement of absolute myocardial blood flow with $H_2^{15}O$ and dynamic positron-emission tomography: strategy for quantification and relation to the partial-volume effect. *Circulation.* 1988;78:104–115.
10. Lammertsma AA, DeSilva R, Araujo LI, Jones T. Measurement of regional myocardial blood flow using $C^{15}O_2$ and positron emission tomography: comparison of tracer models. *Clin Phys Physiol Meas.* 1992;13:1–20.
11. Herrero P, Markham J, Bergmann SR. Quantitation of myocardial blood flow with $H_2^{15}O$ and positron emission tomography: assessment and error analysis of a mathematical approach. *J Comp Assist Tomography.* 1989;13:862–873.
12. Schelbert HR, Phelps ME, Hoffman EJ, Huang SC, Selin CE, Kuhl DE. Regional myocardial perfusion assessed with N-13 labeled ammonia and positron emission computerized axial tomography. *Am J Cardiol.* 1979;43:209–218.
13. Bergmann SR, Hack S, Tewson T, Welch MJ, Sobel BE. The dependence of accumulation of $^{13}NH_3$ by myocardium on metabolic factors and its implications for quantitative assessment of perfusion. *Circulation.* 1980;61:34–43.

14. Schelbert HR, Phelps ME, Huang SC, et al. N-13 ammonia as an indicator of myocardial blood flow. *Circulation*. 1981;63:1259–1272.
15. Krivokapich J, Smith GT, Huang SC, et al. N-13 ammonia myocardial imaging at rest and with exercise in normal volunteers. *Circulation*. 1989;80:1328–1337.
16. Hutchins GD, Schwaiger M, Rosenspire KC, Krivokapich J, Schelbert HR, Kuhl DE. Noninvasive quantification of regional blood flow in the human heart using N-13 ammonia and dynamic positron emission tomographic imaging. *J Am Coll Cardiol*. 1990;15: 1032–1042.
17. Bergmann SR, Herrero P, Markham J, Weinheimer CJ, Walsh MN. Noninvasive quantitation of myocardial blood flow in human-subjects with oxygen-15-labeled water and positron emission tomography. *J Am Coll Cardiol*. 1989;14:639–652.
18. Araujo LI, Lammertsma AA, Rhodes CG, et al. Noninvasive quantification of regional myocardial blood flow in coronary artery disease with oxygen-15-labeled carbon dioxide inhalation and positron emission tomography. *Circulation*. 1991;83:875–885.
19. Kuhle WG, Porenta G, Huang SC, et al. Quantification of regional myocardial blood flow using ^{13}N-ammonia and reoriented dynamic positron emission tomographic imaging. *Circulation*. 1992;86:1004–1017.
20. Hutchins GD, Caraher JM, Raylman RR. A region of interest strategy for minimizing resolution distortions in quantitative myocardial PET studies. *J Nucl Med*. 1992;33: 1243–1250.
21. Muzik O, Beanlands RSB, Hutchins GD, Mangner TJ, Nguyen N, Schwaiger M. Validation of N-13 ammonia tracer kinetic model for quantification of myocardial blood flow using PET. *J Nucl Med*. 1993;34:83–91.
22. Choi Y, Huang SC, Hawkins RA, et al. Quantification of myocardial blood flow using ^{13}N-ammonia and PET: comparison of tracer models. *J Nucl Med*. 1999;40:1045–1055.
23. Goldstein RA, Mullani NA, Fisher DJ, Gould KL, O'Brien A. Myocardial perfusion with rubidium-82: II. Effects of metabolic and pharmacologic interventions. *J Nucl Med*. 1983;24:907–915.
24. Huang SC, Williams BA, Krivokapich J, Araujo L, Phelps ME, Schelbert HIR. Rabbit myocardial Rb-82 kinetics and a compartmental model for blood flow estimation. *Am J Physiol*. 1989;256:H1156–H1164.
25. Mullani NA, Goldstein RA, Gould KL, et al. Myocardial perfusion with rubidium-82: I. Measurement of extraction fraction and flow with external detectors. *J Nucl Med*. 1983;24:898–906.
26. Yoshida K, Mullani NA, Gould KL. Coronary flow and flow reserve by PET simplified for clinical application using rubidium-82 or nitrogen-13-ammonia. *J Nucl Med*. 1996;37: 1701–1712.
27. Marshall RC, Taylor SE, Powers-Risius P, et al. Kinetic analysis of rubidium and thallium as deposited myocardial blood flow tracers in isolated rabbit heart. *Am J Physiol*. 1997;272: H1480–H1490.
28. Henze E, Huang SC, Ratib O, Hoffman EJ, Phelps ME, Schelbert HR. Measurements of regional tissue and blood-pool radiotracer concentrations from serial tomographic images of the heart. *J Nucl Med*. 1983;42:987–996.
29. Herrero P, Markham J, Myears DW, Weinheimer CJ, Bergman J. Measurement of myocardial blood flow with positron emission tomography: correction for count spillover and partial volume effects. *Math Comput Model*. 1988;11:807–812.
30. Muzic RF, Chen CH, Nelson AD. A method to correct for scatter, spillover, and partial volume effects in region of interest analysis in PET. *IEEE Trans Med Imaging*. 1998;17: 202–213.
31. Wu HM, Hoh CK, Buxton DB, et al. Quantification of myocardial blood flow using dynamic nitrogen-13-ammonia PET studies and factor analysis of dynamic structures. *J Nucl Med*. 1995;36:2087–2093.
32. Sitek A, Di Bella EVR, Gullberg GT. Factor analysis with a priori knowledge- application in dynamic cardiac SPECT. *Phys Med Biol*. 2000;45:2619–2638.
33. Lee JS, Lee DS, Ahn JY, et al. Blind Separation of Cardiac Components and Extraction of Input Function from H215O Dynamic Myocardial PET Using Independent Component Analysis. *J Nucl Med*. 2001;42:938–943.
34. Fang YH, Kao T, Liu RS, Wu LC. Estimating the input function non-invasively for FDG-PET quantification with multiple linear regression analysis: simulation and verification with in vivo data. *Eur J Nucl Med Mol Imaging*. 2004;31:692–702.

35. El Fakhri G, Sitek A, Guérin B, Kijewski MF, Di Carli MF, Moore S. Quantitative dynamic cardiac 82Rb-PET imaging using generalized factor and compartment analyses. *J Nucl Med.* 2005;46:1264–1271.

36. Herrero P, Markham J, Shelton ME, Weinhelmer CJ, Bergmann SR. Noninvasive quantification of regional myocardial perfusion with rubidium-82 and positron emission tomography: exploration of a mathematical model. *Circulation.* 1990;82:1377–1386.

37. Gould KL, Yoshida D, Hess JM, Haynie M, Mullani NA, Smalling RW. Myocardial metabolism of fluorodeoxyglucose compared to cell membrane integrity for the potassium analogue rubidium-82 for assessing infarct size in man by PET. *J Nucl Med.* 1991;32:1–9.

38. Herrero P, Markham J, Shelton ME, Bergmann SR. Implementation and evaluation of a two-compartment model for quantification of myocardial perfusion with rubidium-82 and positron emission tomography. *Circ Res.* 1992;70:496–507.

39. Ziegler WH, Goresky CA. Kinetics of rubidium uptake in the working dog heart. *Circ Res.* 1971;29:208–220.

40. Bing RJ, Bennish A, Bluemchen G, Cohen A, Gallagher JP, Zaleski EJ. The determination of coronary flow equivalent with coincidence counting technic. *Circulation.* 1964;29:833–846.

41. Cohen A, Zaleski EJ, Baberon H, Stock TB, Chiba C, Bing RJ. Measurement of coronary blood flow using rubidium-84 and the coincidence counting method. *Am J Cardiol.* 1967;19:556–561.

42. Mossberg KA, Mullani NA, Gould KL, Tacgtmeyer H. Skeletal muscle blood flow in vivo: detection with rubidium-82 and effects of glucose, insulin and exercise. *J Nucl Med.* 1987;28:1155–1163.

43. Coxson PG, Huesman RH, Borland L. Consequences of using a simplified kinetic model for dynamic PET data. *J Nucl Med.* 1997;38:660–667.

44. Gould KL. Absolute myocardial perfusion and coronary flow reserve. In: *Coronary Artery Stenosis and Reversing Atherosclerosis.* New York: Oxford University Press; 1999:247–274.

45. Nitzsche EU, Choi Y, Czemin J, Hoh CK, Huang SC, Schelbert HR. Noninvasive quantification of myocardial blood flow in humans. *Circulation.* 1996;93:2000–2006.

46. Lin JW, Laine FA, Akinboboye O, Bergmann SR. Use of wavelet transforms in analysis of time–activity data from cardiac PET. *J Nucl Med.* 2001;42:194–201.

47. Lin JW, Sciacca RR, Chou RL, Laine FA, Bergmann SR. Quantification of myocardial perfusion in human subjects using 82Rb and wavelet-based noise reduction. *J Nucl Med.* 2001;42:201–208.

48. Hutchins GD. What is the best approach to quantify myocardial blood flow with PET? *J Nucl Med.* 2001;42:1183–1184.

49. Sànchez-Crespo A, Andreo P, Larsson SA. Positron flight in human tissues and its influence on PET image spatial resolution. *Eur J Nucl Med.* 2004;31:44–51.

50. Depre C, Vanoverschelde JL, Taegtmeyer H. Glucose for the heart. *Circulation.* 1999;99:578–588.

51. Schelbert HR, Henze E, Sochor H, Grossman RG, Huang SC, Barrio JR. Effects of substrate availability on myocardial C-11 palmitate kinetics by positron emission tomography in normal subjects and patients with ventricular dysfunction. *Am Heart J.* 1986;111:1055–1064.

52. Grover-McKay M, Schelbert HR, Schwaiger M, Sochor H, Guzy P, Krikokapich J. Identification of impaired metabolic reserve by atrial pacing in patients with significant coronary artery stenosis. *Circulation.* 1986;74:281–292.

53. Di Carli MF, Asgarzadie F, Schelbert HR, Brunken RC, Laks H, Phelps ME. Quantitative relation between myocardial viability and improvement in heart failure symptoms after revascularization in patients with ischemic cardiomyopathy. *Circulation.* 1995;92:3436–3444.

54. Sokoloff L, Reivich M, Kennedy C, et al. The (14C)deoxyglucose method for the measurement of local cerebral glucose utilization: Theory, procedure and normal values in the conscious and anesthetized albino rat. *J Neurochem.* 1977;28:897–916.

55. Huang S-C, Phelps ME, Hoffman EG, Sideris EJ, Selin CE, Kuhl DE. Noninvasive determination of local cerebral metabolic rate of glucose in man. *Am J Physiol.* 1980;238:E69–E82.

56. Phelps ME, Mazziotta JC, Schelbert HR. In: *Positron Emission Tomography and Autoradiography: Principles and Applications for the Brain and Heart.* New York: Raven Press; 1986:287–346.

57. Bøtker HE, Böttcher M, Schmitz O, et al. Glucose uptake and lumped constant variability in normal human hearts determined with [^{18}F]fluorodeoxyglucose. *J Nucl Cardiol.* 1997;4:125–132.

58. Harihan R, Bray M, Ganim R, Doenst T, Goodwin GW, Taegtmeyer H. Fundamental limitations of [18F]2-deoxy-2-fluoro-D-glucose for assessing myocardial glucose uptake. *Circulation.* 1995;91:2435–2444.

59. Bøtker HE, Goodwin GW, Holden JE, Doenst T, Gjedde A, Taegtmeyer H. Myocardial glucose uptake measured with fluorodeoxyglucose: a proposed method to account for variable lumped constants. *J Nucl Med.* 1999;40:1186–1196.

60. Wiggers H, Böttcher M, Nielsen TT, Gjedde A, Bøtker HE. Measurement of myocardial glucose uptake in patients with ischemic cardiomyopathy: application of a new quantitative method using regional tracer kinetic information. *J Nucl Med.* 1999;40:1292–1300.

61. Patlak CS, Blasberg RG, Fenstermacher JD. Graphical evaluation of blood-to-brain transfer constants from multiple-time uptake data. *J Cereb Blood Flow Metab.* 1983;3:1–7.

62. Patlak CS, Blasberg RG. Graphical evaluation of blood-to-brain transfer constants from multiple-time uptake data. Generalizations. *J Cereb Blood Flow Metab.* 1985;5:584–590.

63. Gjedde A. Rapid steady-state analysis of blood-brain glucose transfer in rat. *Acta Physiol Scand.* 1980;108:331–339.

64. Gjedde A. High- and low-affinity transport of D-glucose from blood to brain. *J Neurochem.* 1981;36:1463–1471.

65. Brown M, Marshall ER, Sobel BE, Bergmann SR. Delineation of myocardial oxygen utilization with carbon-11-labeled acetate. *Circulation.* 1987;76:687–696.

66. Brown MA, Myears DW, Bergmann SR. Validity of estimates of myocardial oxidative metabolism with carbon-11 acetate and positron emission tomography despite altered patterns of substrate utilization. *J Nucl Med.* 1989;30:187–193.

67. Ambrecht JJ, Buxton DB, Brunken RC, Phelps ME, Schelbert HR. Regional myocardial oxygen consumption determined noninvasively in humans with [1-^{11}C] acetate and dynamic positron emission tomography. *Circulation.* 1989;80:863–872.

68. Choi Y, Huang SC, Hawkins RA, et al. A refined method for quantification of myocardial oxygen consumption rate using mean transit time with carbon-11-acetate and dynamic PET. *J Nucl Med.* 1993;34:2038–2043.

69. Ng CK, Huang SC, Schelbert HR, Buxton DB. Validation of a model for [1-11C]acetate as a tracer of cardiac oxidative metabolism. *Am J Physiol.* 1994;266:H1304–H1315.

70. Sun KT, Chen K, Huang SC, et al. Compartment model for measuring myocardial oxygen consumption using [1-^{11}C]acetate. *J Nucl Med.* 1997;38:459–466.

71. Sun KT, Yeatman LA, Buxton DB, et al. Simultaneous measurement of myocardial oxygen consumption and blood flow using [1-carbon-11]acetate. *J Nucl Med.* 1998;39:272–280.

Part II
General Considerations for Performing PET and Integrated PET/CT

5 Radiopharmaceuticals for Clinical Cardiac PET Imaging

Josef Machac

The clinical value of cardiac positron emission tomography (PET) imaging was demonstrated more than 20 years ago,[1-3] but its clinical utilization has been low until recently. This was due to the limitation of PET imaging to research centers with a PET camera and a cyclotron, its great expense, and the lack of reimbursement for clinical PET studies. Another disincentive was lack of standardized software for cardiac PET image processing, display, or regional quantification on most PET imaging systems.

There is now an extensive infrastructure in PET imaging with an extensive network of PET and PET/CT cameras installed throughout North America. Myocardial PET perfusion imaging with rubidium-82 (^{82}Rb), reimbursed by the Centers for Medicare and Medicaid Services (CMS) since 1995, can be performed with a commercially available generator, obviating the need for a cyclotron. More recently, mobile ^{82}Rb generators have become available in some regions, allowing PET centers that are not financially able to support a 7-day-a-week ^{82}Rb service to offer PET myocardial perfusion imaging only one to several times a week. All metropolitan areas in North America now have at least one commercial F-18 fluorodeoxyglucose (FDG) supplier. FDG PET imaging is now reimbursed for myocardial viability imaging. More recently, CMS reimbursement has become available for myocardial perfusion imaging with nitrogen-13 (^{13}N) ammonia for those centers that do have a cyclotron that could until recently offer PET myocardial perfusion imaging only for patients who could afford to pay for the procedure or who participated in a funded research study.

The widespread installation of PET-CT cameras represents another leap forward. The use of CT for attenuation correction substantially shortens the acquisition time for a clinical study. The combination of PET scanners with 16-or-more-slice multidetector CT scanners offers the tantalizing possibilities of PET perfusion and viability imaging in concert with coronary calcium scoring and coronary CT angiography, which potentially represents a one-stop service. This chapter reviews the characteristics of the available radiotracers for cardiac PET imaging.

Myocardial PET Perfusion Tracers

Nitrogen-13 Ammonia

Nitrogen-13 ammonia has been used for most of the scientific investigations in cardiac PET imaging over the past two decades. Its 9.96-minute half-life (Table 5.1) requires an on-site cyclotron and radiochemistry synthesis capability. Nitrogen-13 is produced

TABLE 5.1. Characteristics of Cardiac PET Tracers

Agent	Physical Half-life[46]	Mean Positron Range (mm)[47,48,49]	Production	Extraction
N-13 NH$_3$	9.96 min	0.7	Cyclotron	80%[50]
^{82}Rb	76 s	2.6	Generator	50%–60%[51]
F-18 FDG	110 min	0.2	Cyclotron	1%–3%[52]

by bombarding O-16 water with 16.5 MeV protons via the ^{16}O $(p,\alpha)^{13}$N reaction. The target material is made of aluminum, although targets made of nickel or titanium can also be used. Two methods can be used for ^{13}N-ammonia synthesis. In the first method, the ^{13}N-labeled nitrates/nitrites formed by proton irradiation of water are reduced by either titanium (III) chloride, titanium (III) hydroxide, or Devarda's alloy in alkaline medium.[4] After distillation, trapping, and sterile filtration, ^{13}N-ammonia is ready for injection. In the second method, oxidation of ^{13}N to ^{13}N-nitrates/nitrites is prevented by the addition of ethanol as a scavenger to the target content.[5] The target content is passed through a small cation-exchange column to trap ^{13}N-ammonium ions, and ^{13}N-ammonia is then eluted with saline and filtered.

In the bloodstream, ^{13}N-ammonia consists of neutral NH$_3$ in equilibrium with its charged ammonium (NH$_4$) ion (Figure 5.1). The neutral NH$_3$ molecule readily diffuses across plasma and cell membranes, leading to virtually complete extraction from the vascular pool. Inside the myocyte, it re-equilibrates with its ammonium form, which is trapped in glutamine via the enzyme glutamine synthase.[6,7] Figures 5.2 and 5.3 show the kinetics of ^{13}N-ammonia in plasma and myocardium. Backdiffusion of ^{13}N-ammonia is proportional to blood flow and limits effective trapping.[7] Despite backdiffusion, the first-pass trapping of ^{13}N-ammonia at rest is high (Table 5.1), although, like other extractable tracers, it decreases at higher blood-flow rates (Figure 5.4). The overall trapping of ^{13}N-ammonia relies on intact metabolism, which may be impaired in ischemia and high cardiac work.

Myocardial retention of ^{13}N-ammonia may be heterogeneous; retention in the lateral wall of the left ventricle even in normal subjects is about 10% less than that of other segments. The mechanism of this finding is not known.[9] ^{13}N-ammonia images also may be degraded by occasional intense liver activity, which can interfere with the

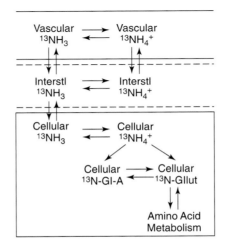

FIGURE 5.1. Schema of ^{13}N-ammonia in plasma and transport into tissue followed by metabolic trapping.

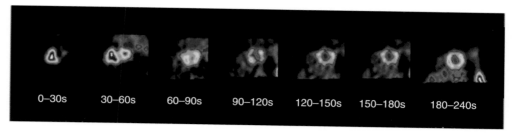

FIGURE 5.2. Serial PET images of cardiac blood clearance and uptake of ^{13}N-ammonia in a human subject. (Courtesy of Robert Gropler, MD.)

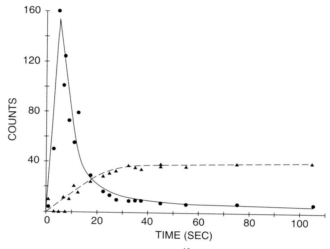

FIGURE 5.3. Plasma and myocardial kinetics of ^{13}N-ammonia in a dog, which shows faster circulation kinetics than humans. (Reproduced with permission from Schelbert HR and Schwaiger M. 1986, 581–661 (8).)

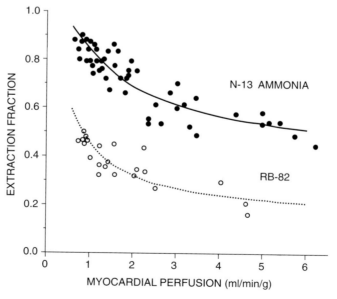

FIGURE 5.4. The relationship between uptake extraction fraction and myocardial perfusion for ^{13}N-ammonia and ^{82}Rb. As myocardial blood flow increases from 0.5 to 6.0 mL/min/g, extraction fraction decreases. (Reprinted by permission of the Society of Nuclear Medicine from: K Yoshida, N Mullani, and KL Gould. Coronary flow and flow reserve by PET simplified for clinical applications using rubidium-82 or nitrogen-13-ammonia. J Nucl Med. 1996;37:1701–1712. Figure 9.)

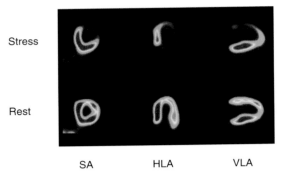

Stress

Rest

SA   HLA   VLA

FIGURE 5.5. ^{13}N-ammonia PET images demonstrating anterior and lateral defects during pharmacological stress and significant improvement at rest, consistent with ischemia. SA, short axis; HLA, horizontal long axis; VLA, vertical long axis. (Courtesy of Dr. H Schelbert.)

evaluation of the inferior wall. Although the sequestration of ^{13}N-ammonia in the lungs is usually minimal, it may be increased in patients with depressed left ventricular systolic function or chronic pulmonary disease and, occasionally, in smokers.[11] In these cases, it may be necessary to increase the time between injection and image acquisition to optimize the contrast between myocardial and background activity.

[13]N-ammonia allows the acquisition of good-quality ungated (Figure 5.5) and gated images. It takes full advantage of the superior resolution of PET relative to SPECT imaging, stemming from a sufficiently long half-life and the very short path length of the positrons emitted by [13]N (Table 5.1). Gated ^{13}N-ammonia imaging can produce accurate assessments of regional and global cardiac function.[12]

Rubidium-82

Rubidium-82 ([82]Rb) is a monovalent cationic analogue of potassium that is produced in a commercially available generator by decay from strontium-82 ([82]Sr) attached to an elution column. The [82]Sr is produced in a cyclotron by proton spallation of molybdenum with a high-energy (800 MeV) accelerator, followed by chemical purification.[13] The [82]Sr has a half-life of 25.5 days and decays to [82]Rb by electron capture. The physical half-life of [82]Rb is 76 seconds, and it decays into krypton-82, which is stable, by emitting a positron and a neutrino.

Figures 5.6 and 5.7 illustrate the generator and delivery system for [82]Rb, consisting of a cabinet, an [82]Rb generator, a pump, control electronics, and connecting tubing.

A   B

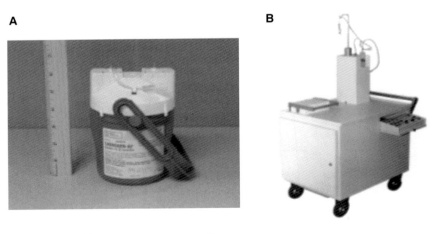

FIGURE 5.6. (A) [82]Rb generator. (B) [82]Rb delivery system. (Equipment by Bracco Diagnostics.)

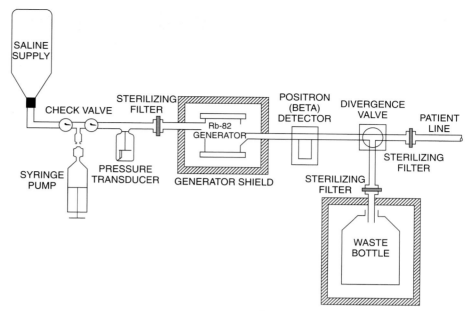

FIGURE 5.7. Schematic of an ^{82}Rb delivery system.

With a half-life of 25 days, the ^{82}Sr-containing generator is replaced every 4 weeks. Rubidium-82 is eluted with 25 to 50 cc normal saline by a computer-controlled elution pump, connected by IV tubing to the patient. The generator is fully replenished every 10 minutes; our experiments have shown that 90% of maximal available activity can be obtained within 5 minutes since the last elution.[14] Thus, serial imaging can be performed every 5 minutes. Although the short half-life of ^{82}Rb taxes the performance limits of PET scanners, it facilitates the rapid completion of a series of resting and stress myocardial perfusion studies. Rubidium-82 is a very efficient imaging agent for routine clinical usage. Because of the short half-life of ^{82}Rb and the need for the patient to lie still in the camera during the study, stress imaging of this agent is limited to pharmacological stress, although studies have obtained serviceable ^{82}Rb images with supine bicycle exercise or even treadmill exercise.[15]

Rubidium-82 is extracted from plasma with high efficiency by myocardial cells via the Na$^+$/K$^+$ ATPase pump (Figure 5.8). Myocardial extraction of ^{82}Rb is similar to that of thallium-201 (^{201}Tl)[16,17] and slightly less than ^{13}N-ammonia (Table 5.1; Figure 5.4). Figure 5.9 shows serial images of blood pool and myocardial ^{82}Rb activity in the first several minutes after injection, and Figure 5.10 shows plasma and myocardial

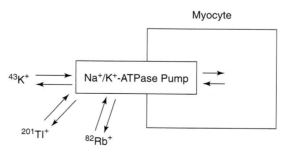

FIGURE 5.8. Diagram of myocardial uptake mechanism of monovalent cations K-43, Tl-201, and ^{82}Rb.

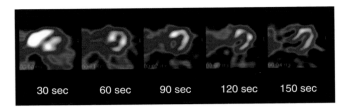

FIGURE 5.9. Serial PET images of blood pool and myocardial [82]Rb activity in the first 3 minutes after injection. (Mount Sinai School of Medicine, New York.)

[82]Rb kinetics. Extraction decreases with increasing blood flow[18,19] (Figure 5.4). In addition, [82]Rb extraction can be decreased by severe acidosis, hypoxia, and ischemia.[20–22] Thus, uptake of [82]Rb is a function of blood flow, metabolism, and myocardial cell integrity.

In spite of the short half-life of [82]Rb, modern PET gamma cameras are able to obtain good-quality images (Figure 5.11). Imaging with [82]Rb is not able to take full advantage of the superior resolution of PET because of the relatively long mean path of 2.6 mm of the energetic [82]Rb positrons and the need for filtering required to obtain optimal images with the short-lived tracer.

Oxygen-15 Water

Oxygen-15 water (^{15}O-water) is a cyclotron product with a physical half-life of 2.07 minutes. Oxygen-15 water is a freely diffusible agent with very high myocardial extraction across a wide range of myocardial blood flows.[23] The degree of extraction is independent of flow and is not affected by the metabolic state of the myocardium.[23] Because it is a freely diffusible tracer, however, imaging is challenging due to its high concentration in the blood pool. This requires subtraction of the blood pool counts from the original image to visualize the myocardium. This can be accomplished by acquiring a second set of images after a single inhalation 40 to 50 mCi of ^{15}O-carbon monoxide ([15]CO). Oxygen-15 carbon monoxide binds irreversibly to hemoglobin, forming ^{15}O-carboxyhemoglobin and thereby allowing delineation and digital subtraction of blood pool activity. The cumbersome nature of the procedure required to subtract blood pool activity of ^{15}O-water to visualize the myocardium has limited the use of this tracer in the clinical setting.

Selecting a Perfusion Tracer for Clinical Cardiac PET

Although in many ways ^{15}O-water is an ideal flow tracer, its use in the clinical setting remains limited. Besides requiring an on-site cyclotron, obtaining diagnostic

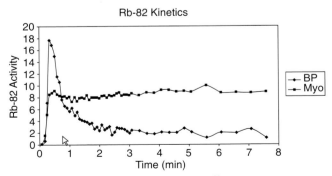

FIGURE 5.10. Kinetics of blood pool and myocardial [82]Rb activity. (Mount Sinai School of Medicine, New York.)

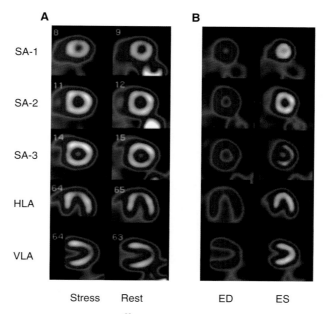

A   **B**

SA-1

SA-2

SA-3

HLA

VLA

Stress   Rest   ED   ES

FIGURE 5.11. A. Normal stress and rest ^{82}Rb PET images. B. Resting end-diastolic (ED) and end-systolic (ES) gated images, showing uniformly good contractility. (Mount Sinai School of Medicine, New York.)

images requires an impractical image subtraction procedure. The advantages of ^{13}N-ammonia are its higher first-pass tissue extraction (65% to 70%) compared to ^{82}Rb (60% to 65%)[10,19,22,24] and a longer half-life, which allows longer imaging times and better count statistics, as well as injection during treadmill exercise and subsequent imaging of the trapped radionuclide in the myocardium. However, the main disadvantage of ^{13}N-ammonia vis-à-vis ^{82}Rb is the need for an on-site cyclotron, which makes it costly and impractical. Also, the longer physical half-life of ^{13}N-ammonia makes rest-stress protocols more inefficient than with ^{82}Rb (~90 minutes vs 30 minutes, respectively). Finally, increased uptake in the liver and, occasionally, in the lungs (as in patients with heart failure and smokers) can adversely affect image quality.

Imaging of Myocardial Metabolism

Fluorine-18 Fluorodeoxyglucose

Preserved metabolism for the production of ATP is one of the critical features of myocardial viability. Flourine-18 (^{18}F) fluorodeoxyglucose (FDG) is fluorine-18-labeled 2-deoxyglucose, an analogue of glucose. Fluorine-18 is produced in a cyclotron through the (p,n) reaction, consisting of bombardment of O-18-enriched water with a proton beam with energies less than 15 MeV. High specific activity of ^{18}F fluorine is thus obtained. F-18 FDG is prepared by nucleophilic substitution on a tetraacetylmannose triflate precursor. This yields large quantities of pure D-FDG.[25]

Flourine-18 fluorine decays by the emission of a positron and a neutrino, whereby the ^{18}F fluorine decays to O-18 oxygen. The low kinetic energy of the positron, 635 keV, allows the highest special resolution among the commonly used PET radionuclides (Table 5.1). The relatively longer half-life of ^{18}F of 109.8 minutes allows sufficient time for synthesis of ^{18}F FDG, its commercial distribution in a radius of several hours from the production site, its temporary storage at the user site, the 30 to 60 minutes of

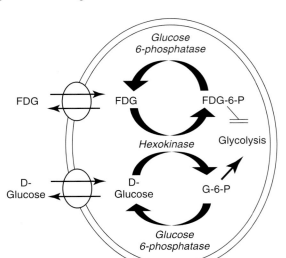

FIGURE 5.12. Schematic diagram of cellular FDG uptake and retention. (From Machac J. Gated positron emission tomography for the assessment of myocardial perfusion and function. In: Clinical gated cardiac SPECT. Germano G, Berman DS, eds, Blackwell Futura, 2006. Reprinted with permission.)

absorption time after injection, and sufficient imaging time to yield images of high quality. At the same time, it does lead to higher radiation exposure, for any given dose, compared to shorter-lived radiotracers, but at the same time similar to that of Tc-99m perfusion agents and lower than a clinical dose of [201]Tl.

Like D-glucose, FDG is transported into the myocardium by specific glucose transporters (GLUT-1 and GLUT-4) by facilitated diffusion (Figure 5.12). Inside the cell, FDG undergoes phosphorylation by the enzyme hexokinase. Because of very low levels of the enzyme glucose-6-phosphatase catalyzing the reverse reaction, FDG is essentially trapped in the cell.[26] It has been demonstrated that in a metabolic steady state, FDG uptake in the myocardium correlates linearly with uptake and utilization of exogenous glucose.[27]

Following injection, FDG is slowly taken up by body tissues, including the myocardium (Figures 5.13 and 5.14). Imaging is performed about 45 to 90 minutes after injection. As a result, the 110-minute physical half-life of ^{18}F FDG is well-suited for viability imaging (Table 5.1).

Summary Points

- There are a limited number of well-characterized PET radiopharmaceuticals for clinical imaging. Their short physical half-life allows rapid sequential imaging of

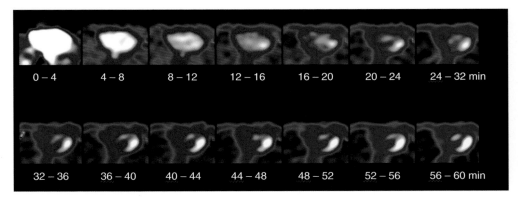

FIGURE 5.13. Serial dynamic images of plasma and myocardial ^{18}F FDG activity. (Mount Sinai School of Medicine, New York.)

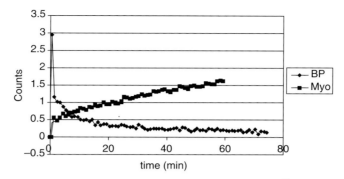

FIGURE 5.14. Kinetics of blood pool (BP) and myocardial (Myo) ^{18}F FDG activity. (Mount Sinai School of Medicine, New York.)

rest and stress perfusion imaging, which is more efficient and accurate than SPECT imaging.

- The known tracer kinetics of PET radiopharmaceuticals, coupled with the technical advantages of PET (e.g., attenuation correction, high temporal resolution), allow quantitation of myocardial blood flow that can be used to improve diagnosis of coronary artery disease (see Chapters 11 and 12).
- The main disadvantage of the available tracers is cost. As clinical PET expands its role into cardiac imaging, we will probably see significant investments in research and development of long-lived (e.g., ^{18}F) perfusion agents than could potentially be distributed by unit doses, similar to the successful model of [18]FDG.

References

1. Gould KL, Schelbert HR, Phelps ME, Hoffman EJ. Noninvasive assessment of coronary stenoses with myocardial perfusion imaging during pharmacologic coronary vasodilatation. V. Detection of 47 percent diameter coronary stenosis with intravenous nitrogen-13 ammonia and emission-computed tomography in intact dogs. *Am J Cardiol.* 1979;43: 200–208.
2. Schelbert HR, Wisenberg G, Phelps ME, et al. Noninvasive assessment of coronary stenoses by myocardial imaging during pharmacologic coronary vasodilation. VI. Detection of coronary artery disease in human beings with intravenous N-13 ammonia and positron computed tomography. *Am J Cardiol.* 1982;49:1197–1207.
3. Tillisch J, Brunken R, Marshall R, et al. Reversibility of cardiac wall-motion abnormalities predicted by positron tomography. *N Engl J Med.* 1986;314:884–888.
4. Vaalburg W, Kamphuis JA, Beerling-van der Molen HD, Rijskamp A, Woldring MG. An improved method for the cyclotron production of 13N-labelled ammonia. *Int J Appl Radiat Isot.* 1975;26:316–318.
5. Wieland B, Bida G, Padgett H, et al. In-target production of [13N]ammonia via proton irradiation of dilute aqueous ethanol and acetic acid mixtures. *Int J Rad Appl Instrum [A].* 1991;42:1095–1098.
6. Schelbert HR, Phelps ME, Hoffman EJ, Huang SC, Selin CE, Kuhl DE. Regional myocardial perfusion assessed with N-13 labeled ammonia and positron emission computerized axial tomography. *Am J Cardiol.* 1979;43:209–218.
7. Schelbert HR, Phelps ME, Huang SC, et al. N-13 ammonia as an indicator of myocardial blood flow. *Circulation.* 1981;63:1259–1272.
8. Schelbert HR, Schwaiger M. PET studies of the heart. In: Phelps ME, Mazziotta JC, Schelbert HR, eds. *Positron Emission Tomography and Autoradiography, Principles and Applications for the Brain and Heart.* New York: Raven Press; 1986:581–661.
9. Beanlands RS, Muzik O, Hutchins GD, Wolfe ER Jr, Schwaiger M. Heterogeneity of regional nitrogen 13-labeled ammonia tracer distribution in the normal human heart:

comparison with rubidium 82 and copper 62-labeled PTSM. *J Nucl Cardiol.* 1994;1: 225–235.

10. Yoshida K, Mullani N, Gould KL. Coronary flow and flow reserve by PET simplified for clinical applications using rubidium-82 or nitrogen-13-ammonia. *J Nucl Med.* 1996;37: 1701–1712.

11. Tamaki N, Ruddy TD, Dekamp R. Myocardial perfusion. In: Wahl RL, Buchanan JW, eds. *Principles and Practice of Positron Emission Tomography.* Philadelphia, PA: Lippincott Williams & Wilkins; 2002:320–333.

12. Hickey KT, Sciacca RR, Bokhari S, et al. Assessment of cardiac wall motion and ejection fraction with gated PET using N-13 ammonia. *Clin Nucl Med.* 2004;29:243–248.

13. Thomas KE. Strontium 82 production at Los Alamos National Laboratory. *Int J Appl Radiat Isot.* 1987;38:175–180.

14. Kim SH, Machac J, Almeida O. Optimization of rubidium-82 generator performance. *Clin Nucl Med.* 2004;29:135.

15. Chow BJ, Ananthasubramaniam K, dekemp RA, Dalipaj MM, Beanlands RS, Ruddy TD. Comparison of treadmill exercise versus dipyridamole stress with myocardial perfusion imaging using rubidium-82 positron emission tomography. *J Am Coll Cardiol.* 2005;45: 1227–1234.

16. Meerdink DJ, Leppo JA. Experimental studies of the physiologic properties of technetium-99m agents: myocardial transport of perfusion imaging agents. *Am J Cardiol.* 1990;66: 9E–15E.

17. Leppo JA, Meerdink DJ. Comparison of the myocardial uptake of a technetium-labeled isonitrile analogue and thallium. *Circ Res.* 1989;65:632–639.

18. Mack RE, Nolting DD, Hogancamp CE, Bing RJ. Myocardial extraction of Rb-86 in the rabbit. *Am J Physiol.* 1959;197:1175–1177.

19. Becker L, Ferreira R, Thomas M. Comparison of 86Rb and microsphere estimates of left ventricular bloodflow distribution. *J Nucl Med.* 1974;15:969–973.

20. Selwyn AP, Allan RM, L'Abbate A, et al. Relation between regional myocardial uptake of rubidium-82 and perfusion: absolute reduction of cation uptake in ischemia. *Am J Cardiol.* 1982;50:112–121.

21. Schelbert HR, Ashburn WL, Chauncey DM, Halpern SE. Comparative myocardial uptake of intravenously administered radionuclides. *J Nucl Med.* 1974;15:1092–1100.

22. Goldstein RA, Mullani NA, Marani SK, Fisher DJ, Gould KL, O'Brien HA Jr. Myocardial perfusion with rubidium-82. II. Effects of metabolic and pharmacologic interventions. *J Nucl Med.* 1983;24:907–915.

23. Schelbert HR. Evaluation of myocardial blood flow in cardiac disease. In: Skorton DJ, Schelbert HR, Wolf GL, Brundage BH, eds. *Cardiac Imaging. A Companion to Braunwald's Heart Disease.* Philadelphia: WB Saunders; 1991:1093–1112.

24. Mullani NA, Goldstein RA, Gould KL, et al. Myocardial perfusion with rubidium-82. I. Measurement of extraction fraction and flow with external detectors. *J Nucl Med.* 1983; 24:898–906.

25. Hamacher K, Coenen HH, Stocklin G. Efficient stereospecific synthesis of no-carrier-added 2-[18F]-fluoro-2-deoxy-D-glucose using aminopolyether supported nucleophilic substitution. *J Nucl Med.* 1986;27:235–238.

26. Gallagher BM, Ansari A, Atkins H, et al. Radiopharmaceuticals XXVII. 18F-labeled 2-deoxy-2-fluoro-d-glucose as a radiopharmaceutical for measuring regional myocardial glucose metabolism in vivo: tissue distribution and imaging studies in animals. *J Nucl Med.* 1977;18:990–996.

27. Ratib O, Phelps ME, Huang SC, Henze E, Selin CE, Schelbert HR. Positron tomography with deoxyglucose for estimating local myocardial glucose metabolism. *J Nucl Med.* 1982; 23:577–586.

6 Iodinated Contrast Agents for Cardiac CT

M. Raquel Oliva and Koenraad J. Mortele

Cardiac computed tomography (CT) is a noninvasive imaging test that requires the use of intravenously administered contrast material and high-resolution, high-speed CT machinery to obtain detailed volumetric images of cardiac anatomy, coronary circulation, and great vessels. Most contrast-enhanced CT examinations in the West are performed with nonionic iodinated contrast media. However, adverse events still exist and consist of allergylike contrast reactions, chemo- or osmotoxic contrast reaction, contrast media–induced nephropathy, injection-related adverse events, and complications due to various coexisting conditions. Identification of patients at risk for developing contrast media reactions is likely to prevent serious adverse events and to enhance safety. Likewise, appropriate management strategies can be adopted to reduce morbidity and mortality associated with adverse reactions of iodinated contrast media used in cardiac CT scanning.

Therefore, to enhance patient safety, during and after contrast-enhanced cardiac CT examinations, radiologists and technologists must understand risk factors that predispose to contrast media–related adverse reactions and adopt preventive and management strategies. This chapter presents risk factors, prevention, and management strategies for adverse reactions associated with the use of iodinated contrast media in cardiac CT scanning.

Classification of Iodinated Contrast Media

Since their introduction in 1928 and 1929, iodinated contrast media have been recognized as the phenomenon of present-day radiological imaging. Current iodinated contrast media differ in viscosity, osmolality, and chemotoxicity and are classified into the following categories: high, low, and iso-osmolar; ionic and nonionic; monomeric and dimeric contrast media (Table 6.1).

The ionic contrast media dissociate into ions when dissolved in water and have a higher osmolality compared to human blood. These contrast agents have high osmolality and are associated with higher incidence of adverse reactions compared to contrast media with low osmolality. The cardiovascular effects of contrast media are in part related to their osmolality and include abnormalities of conduction and contractility, although changes in hemodynamic parameters are generally not significantly different among the various nonionic contrast media.[1,2] The lower-osmolar contrast

TABLE 6.1. Classification of Iodinated Contrast Media

High Osmolar	Low Osmolar	Iso-Osmolar
Ionic Monomers	*Ionic Dimers*	*Nonionic Dimers*
Diatrizoate (Hypaque)	Ioxaglate (Hexabrix)	Iodixanol (Visipaque)
Iothalamate (Conray)		
	Nonionic Monomers	
	Iohexol (Omnipaque)	
	Iopamidol (Isovue)	
	Ioversol (Optiray)	
	Ioxilan (Oxilan)	
	Iopromide (Ultravist)	

media cause less discomfort and fewer cardiovascular and anaphylactic-type reactions.[3]

Contrast Media–Related Adverse Reactions

The precise pathogenesis of contrast reactions following intravascular administration of iodinated contrast media is not known.[4] The overall incidence of contrast reactions is 0.4% to 3% with nonionic formulations and 5% to 12% with ionic formulations.[4,5]

Classification of adverse reactions following administration of contrast media helps in documentation and formulation of appropriate management strategies in an easy and standard manner (Table 6.2). The American College of Radiology (ACR) has classified adverse reactions of iodinated contrast media used in CT scanning according to their severity and need for medication into the following categories: mild, moderate, and severe adverse reactions.[6] In addition, depending on the time of their occurrence after the administration of contrast media, adverse reactions have also been classified as acute when they occur within 1 hour after contrast media adminis-

TABLE 6.2. Classification of Adverse Reactions to Iodinated Contrast Media

Mild Reactions

Nausea, vomiting, cough, warm (heat), headache, altered taste, itching, pallor, flushing, sweats, rash, hives, nasal stuffiness, swelling (eyes and face), dizziness, shaking, chills, anxiety

Signs and symptoms appear self-limited without evidence of progression. Requires observation to confirm resolution and/or lack of progression but usually no treatment.

Moderate Reactions

Pronounced skin reactions, bradycardia, bronchospasm/wheezing, tachycardia, laryngeal edema, hypertension, dyspnea, hypotension

Clinical findings should be considered as indications for immediate treatment. These situations require close, careful observation for possible progression to a life-threatening event.

Severe Reactions

Unresponsiveness, clinical manifested arrhythmias, profound hypotension, convulsion, and cardiopulmonary arrest

Requires prompt recognition and treatment; almost always requires hospitalization.

tration and delayed when they occur after 1 hour but within 1 week of contrast injection.[7] Most life-threatening adverse reactions following administration of contrast media have an acute onset. Whereas acute contrast media–related adverse reactions vary in severity from mild to severe, the delayed adverse reactions are typically mild and usually do not require any medication.

Screening At-Risk Patients for Contrast Media–Related Adverse Reactions

Several risk factors predispose patients to adverse reactions to contrast media including active bronchospasm, previous cardiac disease, dehydration, allergy of any kind, female gender, renal diseases, and hematological and metabolic conditions.[5,8] For example, patients with a history of renal failure are 5 to 10 times more likely to develop contrast media–induced nephropathy.[9] Similarly, compared to normal population, patients with a history of acute asthma are twice as likely to have adverse allergiclike reactions. Concurrent therapy with nephrotoxic drugs such as aminoglycosides increases the likelihood of renal failure following administration of contrast media.[10] Despite common misconceptions, shellfish allergies and hay fever are not associated with increased incidence of nonrenal adverse reactions following contrast media administration. Prior identification of at-risk patients can help in planning preventive strategies to avoid occurrence or minimize severity of adverse reactions. In addition, permanent documentation and communication of each adverse reaction to contrast media in patients' medical records are critical for preventing future complications.

To identify at-risk patients for adverse reactions to contrast media, many studies have documented the usefulness of screening forms or simple questionnaires prior to contrast administration.[3,11] A sample screening form used in the Brigham and Women's Hospital is shown in Figure 6.1. In addition to basic demographic information, the screening form has 3 main sections, which include allergy and adverse event history, renal function assessment, and review of other medical conditions (Figure 6.1). Each patient is requested to complete the screening form prior to his or her contrast-enhanced CT examination. Screening forms help identify, document, and communicate risk factors in each patient prior to contrast administration so that appropriate preventive measures can be adopted.

In addition to the screening form completed by each patient undergoing contrast-enhanced CT scanning, each adverse reaction to contrast media must be recorded and communicated to the patient, to reporting radiologists, as well as to referring physicians. At our institution, a specific contrast media–related adverse reaction form is used (Figure 6.2) and incorporated into the radiology report, radiology information system, and hospital information system.

Preventive Measures for Contrast Media–Related Adverse Reactions

Several preventive measures can be adopted to avoid or minimize adverse reactions to contrast media. If possible, nephrotoxic drugs must be discontinued prior to contrast administration to minimize risk of contrast media–induced nephropathy. In addition, adequate hydration (oral or intravenous), unless contraindicated, should also be considered to prevent renal insufficiency.[3] Likewise, to prevent nonrenal adverse reactions, corticosteroids can be administered in patients with history of prior contrast reaction, in whom contrast media cannot be avoided.[6,8] The ACR guidelines recommend a premedication regimen consisting of 32 mg methylprednisolone orally, 12 hours and 2 hours before the contrast media injection.[6] Notably, this regimen does not recommend use of antihistaminic drug-based prophylaxis for nonrenal adverse reactions.

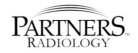

☐ BWH
☐ FH
☐ MGH
☐ NSMC
☐ NWH

PATIENT IDENTIFICATION AREA

IV CONTRAST PATIENT QUESTIONNAIRE

1. **Patient's name:** _____
2. **Medical record number:** _____   **Patient's age:** _____
3. **Date of the exam:** _____ / _____ / _____   **Gender:** ☐ Male ☐ Female
4. **Weight:** _____ **lbs**
5. Did you have something to **eat on the past 4 hours**?   ☐ Yes   ☐ No
6. Do you have any **allergy requiring medical treatment**?   ☐ Yes   ☐ No
    If yes, please list them:

    _____   _____   _____   _____

7. Have you ever had a **contrast (dye) injection**?   ☐ Yes   ☐ No
8. Have you ever had a **contrast (dye) reaction**:   ☐ Yes   ☐ No
    If yes please report:
    a) **Type of reaction** you had: ☐ Rash, hives   ☐ Nausea, vomiting
                                       ☐ Swelling: eyes, face   ☐ Shortness of breath
                                       ☐ Other: _____   _____
    b) Have you been **premedicated for today's study**?   ☐ Yes   ☐ No
9. Are you taking **Metformin** (Glucophage®, Glucovance®)?   ☐ Yes   ☐ No
10. Are you on or have you received **interleukin-2 therapy** in the past 2 years?   ☐ Yes   ☐ No
11. Are you currently taking any other **medication**?   ☐ Yes   ☐ No
    If yes please list them:

    _____   _____   _____   _____

12. **Do you have any of the following conditions?**   ☐ Yes   ☐ No
    If yes, please mark / list what do you have:
    ☐ **Kidney disease** (_____)   ☐ **Asthma**
    ☐ **Family history or kidney failure**   ☐ **Sickle cell anemia**
    ☐ **Diabetes** (For how long? _____ years) ☐ **Thyroid disease** (Has your doctor advised
    ☐ **Cardiac disease** (_____)   you not to receive iodinated contrast?)
    ☐ **Multiple myeloma**   ☐ **Pheochromocytoma**
    ☐ **Lupus**
    If none of the boxes are marked, none of the above disease conditions are present.
13. **Female** patients:
    Are you **pregnant**?   ☐ Yes   ☐ No
    Are you **breast-feeding**?   ☐ Yes   ☐ No
14. Have you received **contrast general instructions** and how to self administer **oral contrast**   ☐ Yes   ☐ No
    (Oral contrast will only be used in specific examinations and the instructions will only be given in this situation)
15. **Comments**:

_____	_____
Patient's (guardian's) Signature	Technologist / Nurse Signature (witness)
These sections are to be completed by hospital employee:	

Serum **creatinine** level: ☐ Value: _____ (Exam date: _____ / _____ / _____)   ☐ Criteria for checking not met

Estimated **creatinine** clearance: ☐ (CrCl): _____   CrCl (ml/min) = (140-age [yr]) x lean body weight [lb]/2.2
                                                           Cr [mg/dl] x (72 for men, 85 for women)

Contrast Order:
Type: ☐ Ultravist®, ☐ Omnipaque®, ☐ Opitray®   ☐ Other: _____
Concentration: ☐ 300   ☐ 370 ☐ Other: _____ (mg/ml)   **Volume:** _____ ml (1IV dose)
Ordered by: _____MD

0600865 (4/04)

FIGURE 6.1. Sample screening form for iodinated contrast media used in the Brigham and Women's Hospital, Partners HealthCare System, Department of Radiology, Boston, MA.

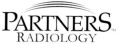

PARTNERS
RADIOLOGY

❏ BWH
❏ FH
❏ MGH
❏ NSMC
❏ NWH

PATIENT IDENTIFICATION AREA

CONTRAST: ADVERSE DRUG EVENT FORM

1. Patient's name: _____

2. Patient's medical record number: _____

3. Date: _____ / _____ / _____   Time: _____ (AM / PM)

4. **Contrast:**
   a. **Type:** ❏ Ultravist®, ❏ Omnipaque®, ❏ Opitray®   ❏ Other: _____
   b. **Lot number:** _____
   c. **Concentration:** ❏ 300   ❏ Other: _____ (mg/ml)
   d. **Amount of contrast injected:** ❏ 100ml ❏ Other _____ ml
   e. **Time administered:** _____ (AM / PM)
   f. **Ordered by:** _____ MD   **Given by:** _____ RN / RT/ MD

5. **Type of reaction:**

❏ Cutaneous (rash, hives)	❏ Cough	❏ Hypertension
❏ Itching	❏ Pallor	❏ Bradycardia
❏ Nausea/ Vomiting	❏ Flushing	❏ Dyspnea / Bronchospasm
❏ Nasal stuffiness	❏ Sweats	❏ Laryngeal edema
❏ Headache	❏ Swelling: eyes, face	❏ Convulsion
❏ Dizziness	❏ Vasovagal	❏ Arrhythmias
❏ Shaking / Chills	❏ Hypotension (with tachycardia)	❏ Cardio pulmonary arrest

   Other: _____

6. **Severity of the reaction:**
   ❏ **MILD:** Signs and symptoms appear self-limited without evidence of progression. Requires observation to confirm resolution and/or lack of progression but usually **no treatment** (includes **treatment of mild dermal reaction** with Benadryl® - diphenhydramine).
   ❏ **MODERATE:** Moderate degree of clinically evident focal or systemic signs and symptoms, which require close observation (medication treatment is required but **no hospitalization**).
   ❏ **SEVERE: Potentially life threatening signs** and symptoms which require hospitalization.

7. **Treatment given at the Radiology Department:**

❏ Observation	❏ Epinephrine - ❏ SC ❏ IV
❏ Diphenhydramine (Benadryl®) - ❏ Oral ❏ IM ❏ IV	❏ Transferred to ED or hospital ward
❏ Oxygen	❏ Code team called
❏ Steroids	❏ Other: _____

   Treatment given by: _____

8. **Recommendations for future studies** (Based on this event):
   ❏ **Routine protocol.**
   ❏ **Pre-treatment with corticosteroid** followed by nonionic contrast media.
   ❏ **Alternative exams** without iodinated contrast media should be considered in consultation with radiologist.

9. **Communication:**

❏ Contrast card given to the patient	❏ Entered in patient's medical record
❏ Dictated in both the body and impression of radiologist report.	❏ Other: _____

10. **Present:**
    Radiologist: _____ MD   Nurse _____ RN/LPN
    Technologist _____   Other _____

11. **Comments:**

This contrast adverse side effect form was filled out by: _____

0600864 (4/04)

FIGURE 6.2. Sample of contrast adverse event documentation form used in the Brigham and Women's Hospital, Partners HealthCare System, Department of Radiology, Boston, MA.

Management Strategies for Contrast Media–Related Adverse Reactions

Prompt recognition and treatment of adverse reactions to contrast media may prevent an adverse reaction from becoming severe or even life threatening (Table 6.3). Mild adverse reactions are self-limited and show no evidence of progression. Patients with

TABLE 6.3. Guidelines for Management of Patients with Contrast Media–Related Adverse Reactions

Urticaria

Discontinue injection
No treatment needed in most cases
H1-receptor blocker: Diphenhydramine PO/IM/IV 25–50 mg
If severe or widely disseminated: Epinephrine SC (1:1000) 0.1–0.3 mL (if no cardiac contraindication)

Facial or Laryngeal Edema

Epinephrine SC (1:1000) 0.1–0.3 mL
If hypotension evident: Epinephrine (1:10,000) slowly IV 1.0 mL
Repeat as needed to a maximum of 1.0 mg
Oxygen 6–10 L/min (via mask)
If not responsive to therapy or obvious acute laryngeal edema, seek assistance and consider intubation

Bronchospasm

Oxygen 6–10 L/min (via mask)
Monitor: Electrocardiogram, oxygen saturation, blood pressure
β-agonist inhalers (metaproterenol, terbutaline, or albuterol)
Epinephrine SC (1:1000) 0.1–0.3 mL
If hypotension evident: Epinephrine (1:10,000) slowly IV 1.0 mL
Repeat as needed to a maximum of 1.0 mg
Call for assistance for severe bronchospasm (or if oxygen saturation <88% persists)

Hypotension with Tachycardia

Legs elevated 60 degrees or more
Monitor: Electrocardiogram, oxygen saturation, blood pressure
Oxygen 6–10 L/min (via mask)
Rapid administration of large volumes of isotonic Ringer's Lactate or normal saline
If poorly responsive: Epinephrine (1:10,000) slowly IV 1.0 mL
Repeat as need up to a maximum of 1.0 mg
If still poorly responsive: Transfer to intensive care unit for further treatment

Hypotension with Bradycardia (Vagal Reaction)

Monitor vital signs
Legs elevated 60 degrees or more
Secure airway: give oxygen 6–10 L/min (via mask)
Secure IV access: Rapid administration of large volumes of isotonic Ringer's lactate or normal saline
Atropine 0.6–1.0 mg IV slowly
Repeat atropine up to a total dose of 0.04 mg/kg (2–3 mg)

Hypertension, Severe

Monitor: Electrocardiogram, oxygen saturation, blood pressure
Nitroglycerine 0.4 mg tablet, sublingual (may repeat 3 times) or topical 2% ointment, apply 1-in strip
Sodium nitroprussiate diluted with 5% dextrose; monitor potential hypotension; review dosage and administration
    instructions prior to use; titrate with infusion pump
Transfer to intensive care unit or emergency department
For pheochromocytoma: Phentolamine 5.0 mg IV

Seizures or Convulsions

Oxygen 6–10 L/min (via mask)
Consider diazepam 5.0 mg or midazolam 2.5 mg IV
If longer effect needed, obtain consultation; consider phenytoin infusion 15–18 mg/kg at 50 mg/min
Careful monitor of vital signs required

Pulmonary Edema

Elevate torso
Oxygen 6–10 L/min (via mask)
Diuretics-furosemide 40 mg IV, slow push
Consider morphine
Transfer to intensive care unit or emergency department

mild reactions require observation to confirm lack of progression of signs and symptoms. Generally, no treatment is necessary, except antihistaminic drugs, such as diphenhydramine, to treat pruritus.

Patients with moderate adverse reactions require monitoring and treatment to prevent further complications, which can be accomplished in the radiology department. Although treatment of moderate adverse reactions varies according to their manifestations, patients must be observed until the onset of resolution of signs and symptoms.

Patients who experience severe adverse reactions need advanced and prompt treatment according to signs and symptoms. These patients usually require hospitalization until their condition has stabilized and major complications have been ruled out. It is important to leave intravenous access lines in place for at least 20 minutes after completion of contrast-enhanced CT examinations, as most life-threatening adverse reactions occur immediately or within the first few minutes after injection of contrast medium.[6] Future use of iodinated contrast media must be avoided in patients with severe adverse reactions. However, if absolutely necessary, contrast media can be readministered for future studies following premedication with corticosteroids.

Contrast Media and Renal Toxicity

Contrast media–induced nephropathy usually refers to reduction in renal function induced by contrast media. It is defined by an increase in serum creatinine by more than 25% or 44 μmol/L within 3 days of intravenous contrast media administration.[10,12] The exact pathophysiology of contrast media–induced nephropathy is not fully understood. Predisposing factors include history of diabetes mellitus, underlying renal insufficiency, dehydration, cardiovascular disease, diuretic use, advanced age (70 years or more), multiple myeloma, hypertension, and hyperuricemia.[8,13] Screening forms can help identify patients with these predisposing factors.[14]

In most patients, contrast media–induced nephropathy is self-limited and renal function usually returns to baseline within 7 to 10 days, without progressing to chronic renal failure.[9] However, to avoid further deterioration of renal function, patients with contrast media–induced nephropathy should not be given intravenous iodinated contrast media before the renal function has returned to the baseline levels. If mandatory, contrast media should be administered following adequate hydration in order to facilitate the elimination of contrast media by the kidneys.

Estimation of serum creatinine levels prior to administration of contrast media should be performed in high-risk patients with history of renal disease, renal surgery, diabetic nephropathy, dehydration, congestive heart failure, paraproteinemia syndromes, collagen vascular disease (e.g., lupus), or concurrent administration of nephrotoxic drugs.[6,10] Special attention must be paid to patients receiving metformin, as the kidneys eliminate almost 90% of the drug. As contrast media–induced nephropathy in these patients can lead to the development of fatal lactic acidosis, metformin must be discontinued at the time of the contrast media administration and withheld for 48 hours after the injection. Renal function must be reassessed prior to reinstatement of metformin.[6,10]

Recently, creatinine clearance has been recommended for more accurate estimation of renal function to aid identification of patients with preexisting renal insufficiency.[15] Creatinine clearance levels of more then 60 mL/min indicate normal renal function; levels of 25 to 50 mL/min indicate presence of moderate renal insufficiency, whereas creatinine clearance of less than 25 mL/min indicates severe renal insufficiency. Creatinine clearance (CCr) can be estimated using the following equation based on the Cockroft and Gault formula [15]:

$$CCr(mL/min) = \frac{(140 - age\ [\text{in years}]) \times \text{Lean body weight [lb]}/2.2}{\text{Serum creatinine } (mg/dL) \times (72\ \text{for men; 85 for women})}$$

Combination of predisposing conditions and renal function allows classification of patients in different risk categories for development of contrast media–induced nephropathy. Patients with low risk have unknown or normal renal function and no predisposing conditions. These subjects can receive contrast media without estimation of serum creatinine. Patients with intermediate risk have mild renal insufficiency and diabetes mellitus. In these subjects, although contrast media can be administered in the usual dose, oral hydration and follow-up serum creatinine is recommended. On the other hand, in high-risk patients with moderate to severe renal insufficiency, either an alternate imaging study should be considered or intravenous hydration should be given with the contrast media (1mL/kg/h saline injection 12 hours before and after contrast media administration).

Recent studies have evaluated several drugs, such as acetylcysteine, fenoldapan, and theophylline, for prophylaxis of contrast media–induced nephrotoxicity with variable success.[10,12] A recent meta-analysis reported good aggregate trial evidence to suggest that patients who have an elevated serum creatinine level at baseline benefit from receiving periprocedural acetylcysteine in the prevention of contrast-induced acute renal failure.[16] Other reports described a lower incidence of nephrotoxicity with the iso-osmolar contrast agent iodixanol (Visipaque) in patients who underwent angiography.[17,18,19] Different from the low-osmolar contrast agents, the volume of iso-osmolar contrast did not affect the incidence of contrast-induced nephropathy in patients with chronic kidney disease when undergoing cardiac catheterization.[19]

For a patient on long-term dialysis, urgent dialysis after the use of nonionic contrast media is not necessary, unless there is a significant underlying cardiac dysfunction, or very large volumes of contrast media are used.[6,8] It is important, however, to limit the volume of contrast material administered in these patients.

Contrast Media Extravasation

Extravasation of contrast medium is a well-recognized complication of contrast-enhanced CT examinations.[20] Generally, even large extravasated volumes are not significant in most patients. However, in children and in patients with poor perfusion at the injection site, extravasation can lead to skin sloughing or other tissue injury. Close follow-up for several hours is essential to determine the severity and prognosis of the insult. There is no consensus regarding the best approach for the management of extravasation.[20] Immediate treatment should consist of elevation of the affected extremity to reduce edema by decreasing the hydrostatic pressure in capillaries. This can be supplemented with immediate application of warm compresses (which cause regional vasodilatation and resorption of extravasated fluid) followed by application of cold compresses (which cause vasoconstriction and limit inflammation) for 15 to 60 minutes, 3 times a day for 1 to 3 days, until symptoms resolve.[20] Patients should be followed until resolution of extravasation.

Surgical consultation is recommended if extravasated volume exceeds 30mL for high-osmolar contrast; 60mL for low-osmolar contrast media in the wrist, ankle, or dorsum of the hand; and 50mL for high-osmolar contrast or 100mL for low-osmolar contrast media at other injection sites.[6] Immediate surgical consultation is necessary in the following circumstances: increase in swelling or pain after 2 to 4 hours, altered tissue perfusion (as evidenced by decreased capillary refill following extravasation), change in sensation in the affected limb, and skin ulceration or blistering.

Iodinated Contrast Media in Patients with Coexisting Conditions

Cardiovascular Disease

In patients with underlying cardiovascular disease, iodinated contrast media may cause cardiac conduction abnormalities or alterations in myocardial contractility, which are in part related to osmolality. However, changes in cardiac hemodynamics are comparable amongst different contrast media.[1,2,21]

Pheochromocytoma

Hypertensive crisis has been reported in patients with pheochromocytoma following administration of iodinated contrast media during angiography and venography.[22] Fear of similar adverse reactions to contrast medium administration with CT scanning has led to noncontrast imaging in patients with suspected or known pheochromocytoma.[22] Although low-osmolar nonionic contrast media injection may not cause a hypertensive crisis in patients with pheochromocytoma, there is very little literature on safety of iodinated contrast medium in these patients and use of α-adrenergic blocking drugs prior to contrast administration.[23] Therefore, noncontrast CT scanning is often recommended for patients with known or suspected pheochromocytoma.[22,23]

Thyroid Disease

Administration of iodinated contrast media may cause thyrotoxicosis in patients with Graves' disease and multinodular goiter with thyroid autonomy, especially in elderly patients and patients living in areas of iodine deficiency.[24] Although patients at high risk of thyrotoxicosis should be carefully monitored by endocrinologists following contrast medium administration, prophylaxis is not generally recommended. In addition, iodinated contrast medium can compromise thyroid scintigraphy and radioiodine treatment of thyroid malignancies for 2 months after administration of contrast media.[24]

Sickle Cell Anemia

Iodinated contrast media have traditionally been contraindicated in patients with sickle cell disease because their high osmolality may induce osmotic shrinkage of red blood cells, impair blood flow through the microcirculation, and precipitate or exacerbate a sickle cell crisis.[25,26] However, recent studies have shown that low-osmolar contrast media have no effect on red cell volume and filterability of sickle cells.[25] Therefore, high-osmolar contrast media for CT scanning must be avoided in patients with sickle cell disease and replaced by an isosmolar contrast medium.

Breastfeeding

As the gastrointestinal tract of infants absorbs less than 1% of the ingested contrast medium, the expected dose absorbed by infants from the breast milk is less than 0.01% of the intravascular dose given to the mother.[27] This amount of contrast medium represents less than 1% of the recommended dose for an infant undergoing a contrast-enhanced CT study. The potential risk to the infant includes direct toxicity and allergic sensitization or reaction, which are theoretical concerns but have not been reported. Available data suggest that it is safe for the mother and infant to continue breastfeeding following administration of contrast media.[6] However, if the mother is concerned about potential negative effects to her infant, she may abstain from breastfeeding for 24 hours with active expression and discharge of milk from both breasts using a breast pump.

Pregnancy

In exceptional circumstances, when a radiographic examination is essential, iodinated contrast media may be given to the pregnant female. Following administration of iodinated agents to the mother during pregnancy, thyroid function should be checked in the neonate during the first week.[8]

Practical Recommendations for Cardiac CT

Intravenous contrast is administered using a dual-head power injector through an 18-gauge needle into an antecubital vein at a rate of 4 to 5 mL/s; the injection is followed immediately by a 40-mL saline flush. The purpose of a saline flush is to diminish beam-hardening artifact within the right ventricle that obscures the right coronary artery. It also facilitates delivery of the entire contrast volume in a short bolus.[21]

At the Brigham and Women's Hospital, scan delay is calculated based on a test bolus technique: 10 cc of iopromide (Ultravist 370, Berlex Laboratories, Wayne, NJ) is injected while scanning a fixed level in the ascending aorta. From this, a curve of the contrast density rise and fall is generated. The time to peak enhancement +3 seconds is used as the scan delay. The amount of contrast is calculated based on the scan range (the time it will take to scan from the origin of the coronary arteries to the apex of the heart), multiplied by the injection rate (typically 5 mL/s). A good technique shows the highest contrast in the left ventricle and coronary arteries with less density in the right ventricle and pulmonary arteries.[21] The use of contrast materials with higher iodine concentrations yields progressively higher levels of vascular attenuation at 16- to 64-channel CT coronary angiography.[28]

Summary Points

- Although contrast-enhanced cardiac CT scanning provides useful diagnostic information, adverse reactions following administration of contrast media can affect patient safety.
- Because cardiac CT is now performed in a high throughput environment, safety strategies for screening and preventing adverse reactions in at-risk patients and comprehensive management guidelines should be adopted.

References

1. McClennan BL, Stolberg HO. Intravascular contrast media: ionic versus nonionic—current status. *Radiol Clin North Am*. 1991;29:437–454.
2. Spencer CM, Goa KL. Iodixanol: a review of its pharmacodynamic and pharmacokinetic properties and diagnostic use as an x-ray contrast medium. *Drugs*. 1996;52:899–927.
3. Maddox TG. Adverse reactions to contrast material: recognition, prevention, and treatment. *Am Fam Physician*. 2002;66:1229–1234.
4. Cohan RH, Ellis JH. Iodinated contrast material in uroradiology. Choice of agent and management of complications. *Urol Clin North Am*. 1997;24:471–491.
5. Mortelé KJ, Oliva MR, Ondategui S, Ros PR, Silverman SG. Universal use of nonionic iodinated contrast medium for CT: evaluation of safety in a large urban teaching hospital. *AJR Am J Roentgenol*. 2005;184:31–34.
6. Cohan RH, Matsumoto JS, Quagliano PV. Committee on Drugs and Contrast Media. *Manual on Contrast Media*. 5th ed. Reston, VA: American College of Radiology; 2004.
7. Webb JA, Stacul F, Thomsen HS, Morcos SK. Members of the Contrast Media Safety Committee of the European Society of Urogenital Radiology. Late adverse reactions to intravascular iodinated contrast media. *Eur Radiol*. 2003;13:181–184.
8. ESUR—European Society of Urogenital Radiology Contrast Media Safety Committee. *Guidelines on Contrast Media*. Version 4.0. 2004.
9. Tublin ME, Murphy ME, Tessler FN. Current concepts in contrast media–induced nephropathy. *AJR Am J Roentgenol*. 1998;171:933–939.
10. Morcos SK, Thomsen HS, Webb JA. Contrast-media-induced nephrotoxicity: a consensus report. Contrast Media Safety Committee, European Society of Urogenital Radiology (ESUR). *Eur Radiol*. 1999;9:1602–1613.

11. Ashley JB, Millward SF. Contrast agent–induced nephropathy: a simple way to identify patients with preexisting renal insufficiency. *AJR Am J Roentgenol.* 2003;181:451–454.
12. Morcos SK. Contrast media–induced nephrotoxicity—questions and answers. *Br J Radiol.* 1998;71:357–365.
13. Thomsen HS. Guidelines for contrast media from the European Society of Urogenital Radiology. *AJR Am J Roentgenol.* 2003;181:1463–1471.
14. Waybill MM, Waybill PN. Contrast media–induced nephrotoxicity: identification of patients at risk and algorithms for prevention. *J Vasc Interv Radiol.* 2001;12:3–9.
15. Bostom AG, Kronenberg F, Ritz E. Predictive performance of renal function equations for patients with chronic kidney disease and normal serum creatinine levels. *J Am Soc Nephrol.* 2002;13:2140–2144.
16. Guru V, Fremes SE. The role of N-acetylcysteine in preventing radiographic contrast-induced nephropathy. *Clin Nephrol.* 2004;62:77–83. Review.
17. Sandler CM. Contrast-agent-induced acute renal dysfunction—is iodixanol the answer? *N Engl J Med.* 2003;348:551–553.
18. Erdogan A, Davidson CJ. Recent clinical trials of iodixanol. *Rev Cardiovasc Med.* 2003; 4(suppl 5):S43–S50.
19. Tadros GM, Malik JA, Manske CL, et al. Iso-osmolar radio contrast iodixanol in patients with chronic kidney disease. *J Invasive Cardiol.* 2005;17:211–215.
20. Bellin MF, Jakobsen JA, Tomassin I, et al. Contrast Media Safety Committee of the European Society of Urogenital Radiology. Contrast medium extravasation injury: guidelines for prevention and management. *Eur Radiol.* 2002;12:2807–2812.
21. Johansen JG. Assessment of a non-ionic contrast medium (Amipaque) in the gastrointestinal tract. *Investigative Radiology.* 1978;13:523–527.
22. Raisanen J, Shapiro B, Glazer GM, et al. Plasma catecholamines in pheochromocytoma: effect of urographic contrast media. *AJR Am J Roentgenol.* 1984;143:43–46.
23. Mukherjee JJ, Peppercorn PD, Reznek RH, et al. Pheochromocytoma: effect of nonionic contrast medium in CT on circulating catecholamine levels. *Radiology.* 1997;202: 227–231.
24. Van Der Molen AJ, Thomsen HS, Morcos SK. Effect of iodinated contrast media on thyroid function in adults. *Eur Radiol.* 2004;14:902–907.
25. Rao VM, Rao AK, Steiner RM, et al. The effect of ionic and nonionic contrast media on the sickling phenomenon. *Radiology.* 1982;144:291–293.
26. Losco P, Nash G, Stone P, Ventre J. Comparison of the effects of radiographic contrast media on dehydration and filterability of red blood cells from donors homozygous for hemoglobin A or hemoglobin S. *Am J Hematol.* 2001;68:149–158.
27. Cademartiri F, Mollet NR, van der Lugt A, et al. Intravenous contrast material administration at helical 16-detector row CT coronary angiography: effect of iodine concentration on vascular attenuation. *Radiology.* 2005;236:661–665.
28. Lawler LP, Pannu HK, Fishman EK. MDCT evaluation of the coronary arteries, 2004: how we do it—data acquisition, postprocessing, display, and interpretation. *AJR Am J Roentgenol.* 2005;184:1402–1412.

7 CT Anatomy of the Heart

Lawrence M. Boxt and Martin J. Lipton

The development of magnetic resonance imaging and computed tomography (CT) of the heart has provided significant advances in the diagnosis and management of patients with acquired and congenital heart disease. Certainly, the dramatic improvement in temporal resolution obtained using electrocardiogram (ECG)-gated multidetector CT scanning has set the stage for the implementation of this mature technology into the daily practice of cardiac medicine. A particular characteristic of cardiac CT scanning is acquisition of image data in the axial body plane. That is, conventional cardiac imaging has been in radiographic projection (plain films, cineangiography) and, subsequently, in tomographic section (echocardiography and nuclear imaging). However, image data was never presented to the cardiac imager in axial body section. Although the heart lies obliquely in the chest, and the axial body section therefore displays cardiac structure oblique to the intrinsic cardiac axes, image data obtained in this format provides a wealth of anatomic information. Since most cardiologists are not familiar with image data displayed in this view, the cardiac imager utilizing this exciting modality should become familiar with the appearance of the heart in axial section. Furthermore, acquisition of isotropic image voxels on higher resolution (namely, 64-detector) CT scanners provides a robust data set for the reconstruction of the heart in arbitrary or traditional cardiac-based sections. To construct these axes, one must first be able to recognize standard cardiac landmarks on the original axial data acquisition sets.

The purpose of this chapter is to describe the anatomy of the heart. We utilize thin-section axial tomographic acquisitions as obtained on a conventional 64-detector CT scanner. Our description follows the flow of blood into and out of the heart. Each particular anatomic structure is described in terms of its morphologic structure and anatomic relationships and displayed in axial section as well as in reconstruction in oblique section, normal or parallel to the intrinsic cardiac axes. The chapter is designed to serve two purposes. It is a tutorial in cardiac anatomy, as depicted in axial section on contrast-enhanced ECG-gated CT examination. It is also an atlas or reference for novice and experienced cardiac imagers to help recognize normal cardiac structures when viewed in tomographic section.

Right Atrium

The superior vena cava passes through the mediastinum to the right of the ascending aorta (Figures 7.1 and 7.2) and drains into the right atrium just posterior to the orifice of the right atrial appendage (Figures 7.3–7.6). The posterior wall of the superior vena

---

This approach to the description and evaluation of the anatomy of the heart, as depicted by ECG-gated contrast-enhanced multidetector CT, was previously presented in Boxt LM, CT Anatomy of the Heart. Int J of Cardiovasc Imag 2005;21:13–27.

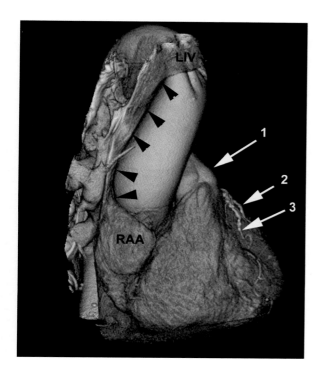

FIGURE 7.1. Surface-rendered, three-dimensional reconstruction of the heart and great arteries of a 34-year-old woman displayed in mild right anterior oblique view. The left innominate vein (LIV) drains from left to right anterior to the great arteries of the aorta, joining the unopacified right innominate vein (contrast injection was from the left upper extremity) to form the superior vena cava (arrowheads). The right atrial appendage (RAA) curves around the AoA to the anterior atrioventricular ring. The right ventricle (RV) lies anteriorly, bounded superiorly by the pulmonary valve sinuses of Valsalva (1), on the right by the atrioventricular ring, and on the left by the (moderately atherosclerotic) anterior descending coronary artery (3) and first diagonal branch (2).

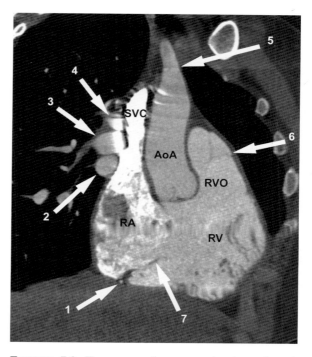

FIGURE 7.2. Tomogram from examination of patient in Figure 7.1, reconstructed in right anterior oblique (RAO) section through the origin of the innominate artery (5). The highly opacified superior vena cava (SVC) descends into the right atrium (RA) to the right of the ascending aorta (AoA). The right hilar vessels, namely the right upper-lobe pulmonary vein (2), right pulmonary artery (3), and right upper-lobe pulmonary artery (4), are labeled. Embedded in the fat of the anterior atrioventricular ring, the right coronary artery (1) is viewed in cross section. Extending from the ring, and viewed as a filling defect within the right ventricle (RV), is a tricuspid valve leaflet (7). Notice how the anterior atrioventricular ring, containing the tricuspid valve, is separated from the pulmonary valve (6). The right ventricular outflow (RVO) tract is labeled.

FIGURE 7.3. The proximal right pulmonary artery (RP) is seen extending from the medial aspect of the main pulmonary artery (MP), passing behind the ascending aorta (AoA) and superior vena cava (SVC) toward the right hilum. The right upper-lobe pulmonary vein (2) lies lateral to the SVC and anterior to the RP; the left upper-lobe pulmonary vein (5), similarly, lies anterior to the left pulmonary artery (LP). Both right (3) and left (4) internal mammary arteries lie to the right and left of the sternum (S), respectively. As the right main bronchus (RB) separates from the left main bronchus (LB), the soft tissue of the subcarinal space develops. The air-filled esophagus (1) lies behind the LB. AoD, descending aorta.

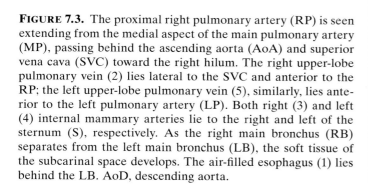

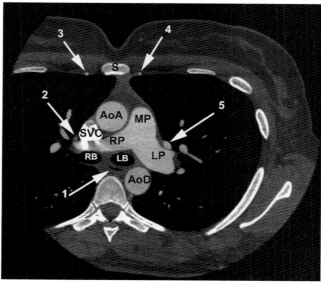

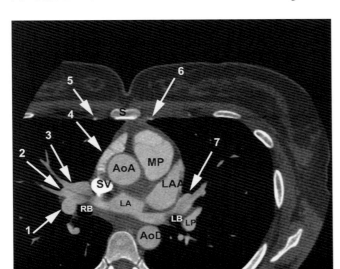

FIGURE 7.4. The left atrium (LA) lies posterior to the ascending aorta (AoA) and anterior to the descending aorta (AoD). Drainage of the right (3) and left (7) upper-lobe pulmonary veins to the LA is seen. At this level, the right upper-lobe (2) and lower-lobe (1) pulmonary arteries have separated; the lower-lobe pulmonary artery lies adjacent to the right main bronchus (RB). The left atrial appendage (LAA) lies anterior to the upper-lobe vein (7). The left lower-lobe pulmonary artery (LP) lies posterior to the LB. Notice how the right atrial appendage (4) wraps around the AoA. The right (5) and left (6) internal mammary arteries and sternum (S) are identified. MP, main pulmonary artery; SVC, superior vena cava.

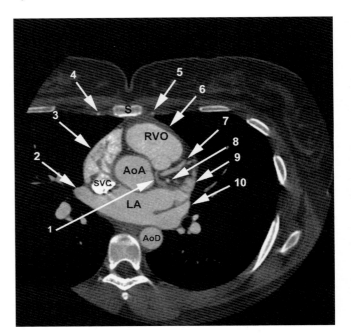

FIGURE 7.5. The anterior cardiac vein (1) has crossed over the anterior descending coronary artery (7) and is coursing toward the posterior atrioventricular ring. To the left of the vein, a portion of the proximal circumflex artery (8) is seen, immediately anterior to the left atrial appendage (9). The left upper-lobe pulmonary vein (10) lies posterior to the left atrial appendage (LAA). The right upper-lobe pulmonary vein (2) is just entering the left atrium (LA). The anterior aspect of the superior vena cava (SVC) is now nearly confluent with the right atrial appendage (3). Notice the thin right ventricular outflow tract (RVO) myocardium (6). The right (4) and left (5) internal mammary arteries and sternum (S) are labeled. AoA, ascending aorta; AoD, descending aorta.

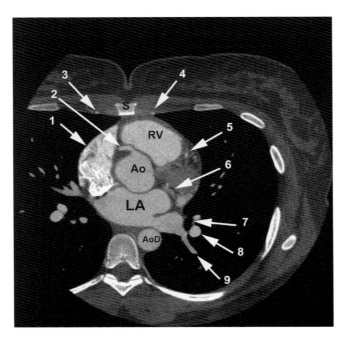

FIGURE 7.6. The right coronary artery (2) arises from the anterior aortic sinus of Valsalva and immediately turns to the right, entering the anterior atrioventricular ring between the right heart border forming the right atrium (1) and right ventricle (RV). The anterior descending coronary artery (5) runs along the top of the interventricular septum, behind the RV. The great cardiac vein (6) passes into the posterior atrioventricular ring in front of the left atrium (LA). The left lower-lobe bronchus (7), artery (8), and vein (9) are labeled. The right (3) and left (4) internal mammary arteries and sternum (S) are seen. Ao, ascending aorta; AoD, descending aorta.

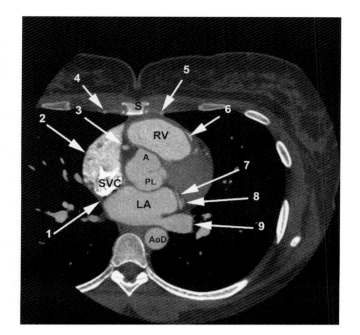

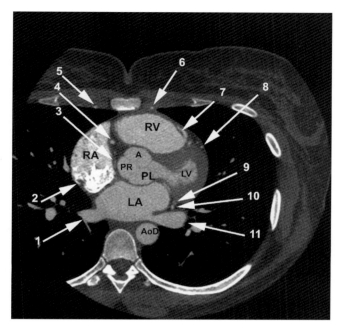

FIGURE 7.7. The right coronary artery (3) is seen in cross section, embedded within the low-attenuation fat of the anterior atrioventricular ring. The anterior (A) and posterior left (PL) aortic sinuses of Valsalva are seen. The sinus venosus interatrial septum (1) separates the posterior wall of the distal superior vena cava (SVC) from the left atrium (LA). A band of myocardium (6) extends from the interventricular septum to the right ventricular (RV) free wall. Within the fat of the posterior atrioventricular ring, the proximal circumflex coronary artery (7) and great cardiac vein (8) are seen. After passing anterior to the descending aorta (AoD), the left lower-lobe pulmonary vein (9) enters the LA. The right (4) and left (5) internal mammary arteries and sternum (S) are seen. (2), right atrium.

FIGURE 7.8. The 3 aortic sinuses of Valsalva, the anterior (A), posterior right (PR), and posterior left (PL), are seen in the center of the heart. The right coronary artery (4) is seen in cross section within the anterior atrioventricular ring. Passing between the right atrium (RA) and the PR, the sino-atrial node artery (3) heads toward the medial aspect of the superior vena cava. The crista terminalis is identified as a filling defect (2) along the lateral aspect of the RA. A muscular trabeculation (7) within the right ventricle (RV) is identified as a linear filling defect extending from the interventricular septum toward the RV free wall. At this level, the anterior descending coronary artery (8) is viewed in cross section. Passing within the posterior atrioventricular ring, the great cardiac vein (9) and circumflex coronary artery (10) are both viewed in cross section. Both the right (1) and left (11) lower-lobe pulmonary veins are identified. The right (5) and left (6) internal mammary arteries and sternum (S) are seen. AoD, descending aorta; LA, left atrium; LV, left ventricle.

cava as it enters the right atrium is the sinus venosus portion of the interatrial septum, which separates the superior vena cava from the left atrium (Figure 7.7). The cavity of the right atrium (Figures 7.8–7.13) is segregated into an anterior trabeculated portion and a posterior smooth-walled portion by the crista terminalis, the remnant of the vein of the sinus venosus. The lateral right atrium wall is very thin; the distance between the cavity of the right atrium and the outer lateral border of the heart should be no greater than 3 mm. Increased thickening usually means a pericardial effusion or pericardial thickening.

The coronary sinus extends from the confluence of the great cardiac vein, between the left atrium and left ventricle in the posterior atrioventricular ring, and then passes beneath the left atrium to the diaphragmatic surface of the heart to drain into the right atrium medial and slightly superior to the entry of the inferior vena cava (Figures 7.13 and 7.14). The eustachian valve separates these two structures.

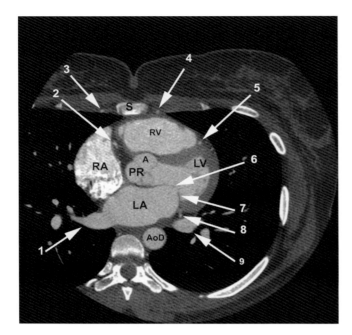

FIGURE 7.9. The anterior (6) mitral leaflet extends to the posterior right (PR) aortic sinus of Valsalva; the posterior (7) leaflet attaches on the posterior atrioventricular ring, adjacent to the circumflex coronary artery (8), viewed in cross section. At this anatomic level, the right lower-lobe pulmonary vein (1) is seen draining into the left atrium (LA); the left lower-lobe vein (9) is not yet confluent with the LA. The right (2) and left (5) coronary arteries are viewed in cross section. The right (3) and left (4) internal mammary arteries and sternum (S) are seen. A, anterior aortic sinus of Valsalva; AoD, descending aorta; LV, left ventricle; RA, right atrium; RV, right ventricle.

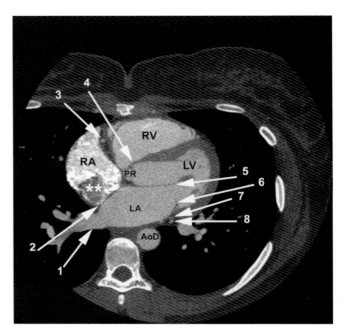

FIGURE 7.10. At this anatomic level, the secundum interatrial septum (2) separates the right atrium (RA) from the left atrium (LA). Notice the difference in thickness between the muscular and membranous (4) interventricular septum, which lies anterior and inferior to the posterior right aortic sinus of Valsalva (PR). The secundum interatrial septum separates the RA from the LA and, in this example, is visualized adjacent to the negative filling defect (**) caused by unopacified blood entering the RA from the inferior vena cava. The right coronary artery (3) is viewed in cross section in the anterior atrioventricular ring; the great cardiac vein (7) and circumflex coronary artery (8) are viewed in cross section in the posterior atrioventricular ring. The right lower-lobe pulmonary vein (1) enters the LA at the level of the secundum interatrial septum. Notice the posterior mitral leaflet (6) and the anterior leaflet (5) in continuity with the aortic annulus and PR. AoD, descending aorta; LV, left ventricle; RV, right ventricle.

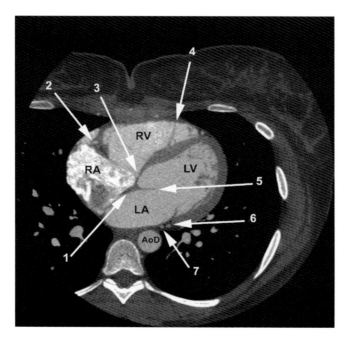

FIGURE 7.11. The membranous interventricular septum (3), anterior mitral leaflet (5), and primum interatrial septum (1) are seen in fibrous continuity. The right coronary artery (2) is seen in cross section in the anterior atrioventricular ring. A myocardial trabeculation (4) is seen within the right ventricle (RV), extending from the interventricular septum to the free wall. Within the posterior atrioventricular ring, the great cardiac vein (6) and circumflex coronary artery (7) are viewed in cross section. AoD, descending aorta; LA, left atrium; LV, left ventricle; RA, right atrium.

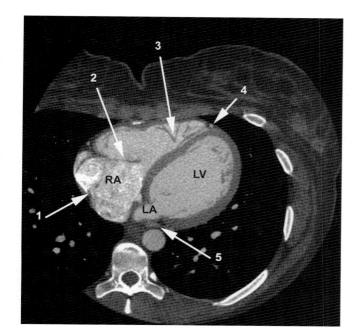

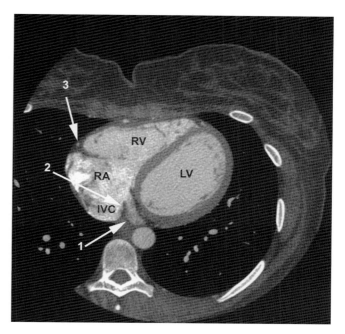

FIGURE 7.12. The crista terminalis (1) is seen as a filling defect in the lateral aspect of the right atrium (RA). The anterior tricuspid leaflet (2) extends from the anterior atrioventricular ring into the right ventricle (RV). Muscular trabeculae (3) appear as filling defects within the cavity of the RV. The anterior descending coronary artery (4) is viewed in cross section along the interventricular septum. The great cardiac vein (5) is turning in the posterior atrioventricular ring to pass beneath the left atrium (LA). LV, left ventricle.

FIGURE 7.13. The coronary sinus (1) is the continuation of the great cardiac vein beneath the left atrium in the inferior aspect of the posterior atrioventricular ring. Coronary sinus blood flow is segregated from flow in the inferior vena cava (IVC) by the eustachean valve (2). The right coronary artery (3) is viewed in cross section within the anterior atrioventricular ring. LV, left ventricle; RA, right atrium; RV, right ventricle.

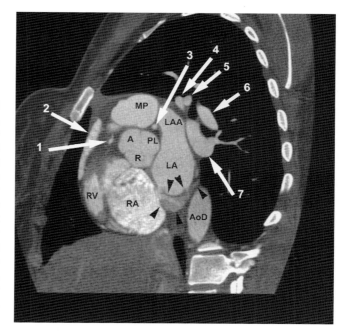

FIGURE 7.14. Tomogram reconstructed in short axis section through the aortic root, in the anterior (A), posterior left (PL), and posterior right (R) aortic sinuses of Valsalva. The coronary sinus (arrowheads) passes anterior to the descending aorta (AoD) and beneath the left atrium (LA) to enter the right atrium (RA) from behind. The RA and right ventricle (RV) are separated by the low-attenuation fat of the anterior atrioventricular ring. A portion of the right coronary artery (1) is viewed in the superior portion of the anterior atrioventricular ring. The right atrial appendage (2) lies anterior to the artery in the ring. After originating from the PL, the left main coronary artery (3) has turned behind the main pulmonary artery (MP) and begins to pass beneath the left atrial appendage (LAA). The segmental left upper-lobe pulmonary vein (4 and 5), the left pulmonary artery (6), and the left lower-lobe pulmonary vein (7) form the vessels of the left hilum.

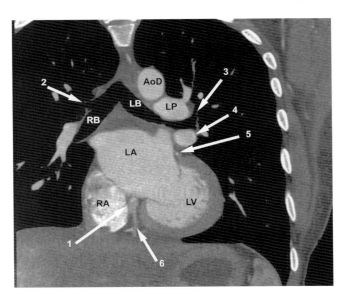

FIGURE 7.15. Coronal tomogram reconstructed through the tracheal bifurcation, demonstrating the left main bronchus (LB) and origin of the left upper-lobe bronchus (3) and the right main bronchus (RB) and origin of the right upper-lobe bronchus (2). The interatrial septum is a curvilinear low-attenuation band separating the left atrium (LA) from the right atrium (RA). The posterior cardiac vein (6) is seen draining cephalad into the coronary sinus (1), which runs along the inferior aspect of the LA. The confluence of the left pulmonary veins (4) lies beneath the hilar LB and superior to the posterior atrioventricular ring, which contains the circumflex coronary artery seen in cross section (5), and the mitral valve, which separates the LA from the left ventricle (LV). AoD, descending aorta; LP, left pulmonary artery.

The interatrial septum (Figures 7.7–7.12, 7.15, and 7.16) usually bows toward the right atrium. Normal thinning in the region of the foramen ovale may be seen. This change in septal thickness is exaggerated in individuals with extra fat deposits around the heart and elsewhere. The right atrium should appear nearly the same size as the left atrium. Measurement of right atrial size is less difficult than estimation of its volume. Nevertheless, right atrium enlargement is associated with clockwise cardiac rotation.

The right atrial appendage (Figures 7.1, 7.4, 7.5, 7.14, and 7.17) is a broad-based, triangular structure, contained within the pericardium, that extends from about the middle of the heart obliquely around the ascending aorta. The right atrial appendage is collapsed when right atrium pressure and volume are normal; the pectinate muscles

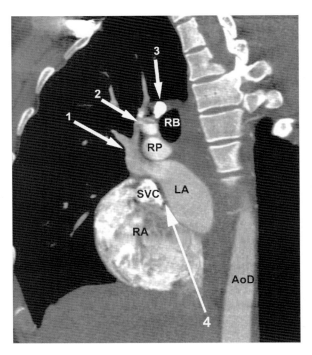

FIGURE 7.16. Left anterior oblique tomogram obtained through the right hilum. The interatrial septum is a curvilinear low-attenuation line, bowing toward the right atrium (RA), which separates the RA and the left atrium (LA). The right pulmonary artery passes along the top of the LA. At this level, the right upper-lobe pulmonary artery (2) has separated from the right pulmonary artery (RP). The right upper-lobe pulmonary veins become confluent (1), pass from anterior to inferior to the right pulmonary artery, and then posterior to the superior vena cava (SVC) to drain into the LA. The proximal superior vena cava (3) is labeled. The sinus venosus interatrial septum (4) separates the back wall of the SVC from the LA. AoD, descending aorta; RB, right main bronchus.

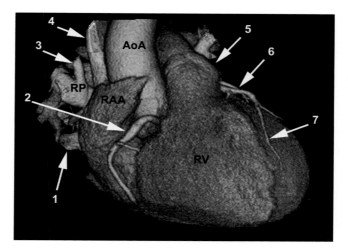

FIGURE 7.17. Surface-rendered, three-dimensional reconstruction displayed in anteroposterior view. The right atrial appendage (RAA) extends from inferior and laterally on the right, medially, anteriorly toward the anterior aspect of the ascending aorta (AoA). The right coronary artery (2) is seen passing from the aorta toward the right to enter the anterior atrioventricular ring and descend toward the diaphragmatic surface of the heart. The right ventricle (RV) is midline, bounded by the right coronary artery on the right, the pulmonary valve (5) superiorly, and the mid- (6) and distal (7) anterior descending coronary artery. The right lower-lobe pulmonary vein (1), right upper-lobe pulmonary artery (3), and superior vena cava (4) are labeled.

characteristically seen in the right atrium anterior to the crista terminalis tend to prevent its collapse. When the right atrial appendage is enlarged, its pectinate muscles appear as intracavitary filling defects, analogous to myocardial bundles in the right ventricle.

The tricuspid valve (Figures 7.2, 7.12, and 7.13) may be visualized in axial CT sections. The septal and anterior leaflets appear as long filling defects attached to the atrioventricular ring and connected to the right ventricle free wall and septum by very fine chordae, and papillary muscles of varying size.

Right Ventricle

The right ventricle resides immediately posterior to the sternum, more or less in the midline (Figures 7.1 and 7.2). Unless hypertrophied, the right ventricular free wall myocardium is only about 2 to 3 mm in thickness and at end diastole may be difficult to visualize. The shape of the right ventricle can be surmised by visualizing the ventricle as the sum of the axial sections obtained during CT examination (Figures 7.4–7.13, 7.17, and 7.18). From the level of the pulmonary valve, moving caudad, the shape of the ventricle changes. The right ventricular outflow tract is round, surrounded by the ventricular infundibulum, and lies to the patient's left. Moving in a caudad direction, the chamber increases in size, assuming a triangular shape: the base is formed by the atrioventricular ring, and the apex is at the intersection of the free wall and interventricular septum.

The tricuspid valve is separated from the pulmonary valve by the infundibulum (Figure 7.2). The right ventricular surface of the interventricular septum is irregular. Although the septomarginal trabeculation may not always be identified, papillary muscles extending from it to the tricuspid valve leaflets are commonplace. Numerous muscle bundles extend from the interventricular septum across the right ventricle

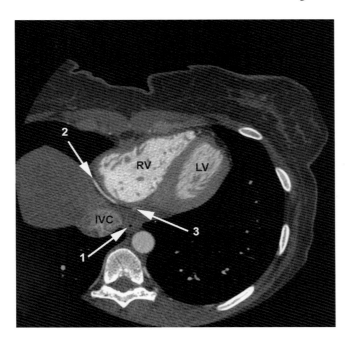

FIGURE 7.18. The right coronary artery (2) passes along the inferior aspect of the anterior atrioventricular ring toward the cardiac crux. The posterior cardiac vein (3) enters the posterior atrioventricular ring. The air-filled esophagus (1) lies between the suprahepatic inferior vena cava and descending aorta.

chamber to the free wall (Figures 7.2, 7.7, 7.8, 7.11, and 7.12). The inferior-most of these is the moderator band, which carries the conducting bundle.

The interventricular septum (Figures 7.8–7.13, 7.19–7.22) appears as intermediate attenuation muscle. The bulk of the septum appears relatively thick (never greater than 1.5 times the thickness of the free wall) and normally bows toward the right ventricle. The posterior superior aspect of the septum is embryologically derived from the endocardial cushions; this is the membranous and atrioventricular septum. It appears as a thin (not uncommonly fatty-infiltrated, low-attenuation) structure,

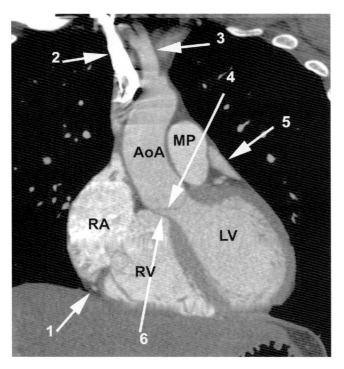

FIGURE 7.19. Tomogram reconstructed in coronal plane through the aortic valve. The membranous interventricular septum (6) extends from the crest of the muscular septum to the annulus of the aortic valve (4). The muscular interventricular septum separates the right ventricle (RV) and left ventricle (LV). The right coronary artery (1) is viewed in cross section in the anterior atrioventricular ring, which separates the right atrium (RA) from the right ventricle (RV). The left atrial appendage (5) is viewed in cross section just to the left and slightly inferior to the main pulmonary artery (MP). The right innominate vein (2, very opacified secondary to a right upper extremity injection) lies to the right of the innominate artery (3). AoA, ascending aorta.

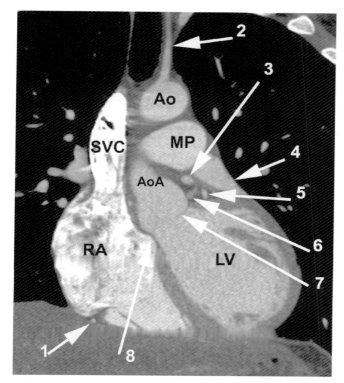

FIGURE 7.20. Image reconstructed 6 mm posterior to Figure 7.19. The atrioventricular septum (8) separates the left ventricle (LV) from the right atrium (RA) and extends from the muscular septum to the aortic annulus (7). The right coronary artery (1) is viewed in cross section. In this section, beneath the main pulmonary artery (MP) and left atrial appendage (4), the left main coronary artery (3) has left the posterior left aortic sinus. The circumflex artery (5) is viewed in cross section. Slightly inferior to and between the two arteries is the anterior cardiac vein (6) in cross section. Notice the isolated left vertebral artery (2) arising from the midaortic arch (Ao). AoA, ascending aorta; SVC, superior vena cava.

FIGURE 7.22. Tomogram reconstructed in left anterior oblique section through the aortic valve (2) and membranous interventricular septum (1). The posterior mitral leaflet (10) and circumflex coronary artery (9) are related to the posterior atrioventricular ring. The anterior mitral leaflet (11) is continuous with the aortic valve (2), which itself is continuous with the membranous interventricular septum (1). The proximal right coronary artery (3) is viewed in cross section beneath the right atrial appendage (4), within the anterior atrioventricular ring. The left main coronary artery (5) just distal to its orgin from the posterior left aortic sinus of Valsalva and proximal to the origins of the anterior descending and circumflex arteries. In this view, one may see the continuation of the main pulmonary artery (MP) as the left pulmonary artery (LP) after crossing the left bronchus (LB), and the continuation of the right pulmonary artery (RP) from the MP posterior to the ascending aorta (AoA). The origin of the innominate artery (6), proximal left common carotid artery (7), and left lower-lobe pulmonary vein (8) are labeled. LA, left atrium; RV, right ventricle.

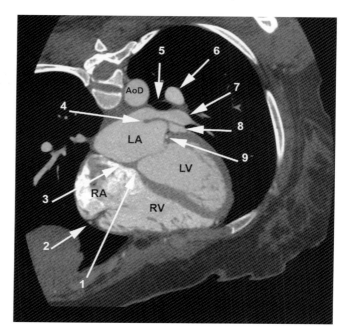

FIGURE 7.21. Tomogram reconstructed in 4-chamber view through atrioventricular (1) and primum interatrial (3) septa. The redundant endothelium (4) between the left upper-lobe pulmonary vein (7) and left atrial appendage (8) is often referred to as the "Q-tip sign." The left bronchus (5) lies medial to the left pulmonary artery (6) as the artery passes over the bronchus. The right coronary artery (2) is viewed in cross section in the anterior atrioventricular ring; the circumflex coronary artery (9) is viewed in cross section in the posterior atrioventricular ring. AoD, descending aorta; LA, left atrium; LV, left ventricle; RA, right atrium; RV, right ventricle.

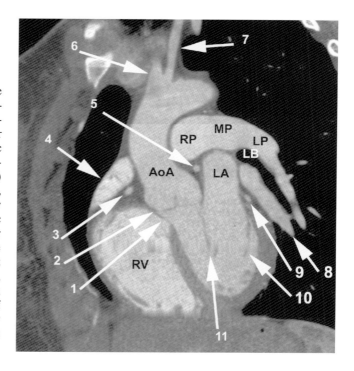

which has a characteristic anatomic relationship with the aortic valve, primum interatrial septum, and anterior mitral and septal tricuspid leaflets.

Pulmonary Artery

The pulmonary valve lies slightly out of the axial plane, so it may appear elongated in conventional axial acquisition (Figures 7.3 and 7.4). The caliber of the main pulmonary artery should be about the caliber of the ascending aorta at this anatomic level. The left pulmonary artery is the extension of the main pulmonary artery over the top of the left atrium. When the pulmonary artery crosses the left bronchus, it becomes the left pulmonary artery (Figures 7.14 and 7.15). The right pulmonary artery originates from the underside of the main pulmonary artery (Figure 7.22), passes along the roof of the left atrium, posterior to the ascending aorta and superior vena cava, to enter the right hilum (Figure 7.16). The pericardium is reflected over the top of the main pulmonary artery.

Pulmonary Veins

The upper-lobe pulmonary veins lie anterior to their respective pulmonary arteries (Figures 7.3 and 7.4). As the left upper-lobe vein courses inferiorly, it passes in front of the left pulmonary artery and enters the left atrium immediately posterior to the orifice of the left atrial appendage. The right upper-lobe vein lies anterior to the right pulmonary artery. It passes from anterior to posterior and inferiorly to enter the left atrium immediately posterior to the entrance of the superior vena cava into the right atrium (Figure 7.16). The left lower-lobe pulmonary vein (Figures 7.6–7.9) always courses in a caudad direction directly anterior to the descending thoracic aorta before entering the posterior left aspect of the left atrium. The right lower-lobe vein (Figures 7.8–7.10) drains to the right posterior inferior aspect of the left atrium.

Left Atrium

The left atrium lies posterior, superior, and toward the left with respect to the right atrium (Figures 7.4–7.16). The two atria share the interatrial septum, which forms an oblique surface between the two. The interatrial septum normally thins in the region of the foramen ovale. The left atrium is just about the same size as the right atrium. The inner surface of the left atrium is bald smooth. The confluence of the left upper-lobe pulmonary vein and orifice of the left atrial appendage is a redundant endothelium, which may appear to be thickened in its most medial aspect (Figure 7.21). The left atrial appendage is long and fingerlike (Figures 7.4 and 7.19–7.21). Analogous to the right atrial appendage, it contains pectinate musculature. However, these myocardial trabeculations are always smaller in caliber than those of the right atrial appendage, and almost never cross from one face of the appendage to the other. The left atrial appendage runs from caudad to cephalad, around the left aspect of the heart, below the level of the pulmonary valve.

The mitral valve lies within the posterior atrioventricular ring, immediately subjacent to the circumflex coronary artery. Fibrous continuity between the anterior mitral leaflet and the aortic annulus is characteristically found in morphologic left ventricles. Ordinarily, the chordae tendineae of the anterior and posterior mitral leaflets are not visualized on CT examination. However, introduction of ECG-gated 16- and 64-detector systems have improved the spatial and temporal resolution to a point where these structures are now commonly identified.

Left Ventricle

The left ventricle is generally football shaped. That is, it is symmetrical, with a long axis and two orthogonal shorter axes (Figures 7.8–7.13, 7.15, 7.18, 7.19, 7.20, and 7.22). The left ventricular papillary muscles are always seen as filling defects in the left ventricular cavity. Analogous to visualization of the chordeae, attachment of the papillary muscles to the chordeae is frequently visualized on the newer scanners.

The posterior atrioventricular ring also contains the great cardiac vein. This vein lies anterior to the circumflex artery and passes around the ring between the left atrium and left ventricle to run beneath the left atrium prior to its drainage into the right atrium. Before entering the right atrium, it receives other venous tributaries, which run along the epicardial surface of the heart.

The left ventricle lies posterior and to the left with respect to the right ventricle. The left ventricular myocardium is nearly uniform in thickness (1 cm at end diastole). However, in axial acquisition, the poster left ventricle wall may appear thicker than the septal or apical myocardium, because it has been cut obliquely with respect to its internal axis. Although some trabecular myocardial filling defects may be identified within the ventricular cavity, the left ventricle is characterized by its smooth walls and two large papillary muscles. These always originate from the posterior wall of the ventricle. The plane of the interventricular septum is directed anterior to the coronal plane and inferiorly toward the left hip. It normally bows toward the right ventricle. The aortic valve shares the fibrous trigone of the heart and is, as previously described, in continuity with the anterior mitral leaflet.

The aortic valve has three sinuses of Valsalva: the anterior, posterior left, and posterior right (Figures 7.7–7.10 and 7.14). The right coronary artery originates from the anterior sinus. The left main coronary artery arises from the posterior left sinus. The posterior right sinus is the most inferior sinus and provides no coronary artery. This so-called noncoronary sinus abuts the right and left atria.

Coronary Arteries

The right coronary artery originates from the anterior aortic sinus of Valsalva. It takes a short right turn to enter the fat within the anterior atrioventricular ring (Figures 7.6, 7.17, 7.23, and 7.24), and passes around to the intersection of the atrioventricular

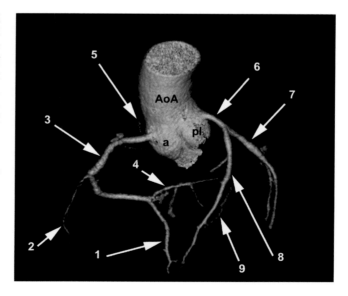

FIGURE 7.23. Surface-rendered, three-dimensional CT coronary arteriogram displayed in cranialized left anterior oblique view. The right coronary artery (3) is seen arising from the anterior aortic sinus of Valsalva (A). After taking a rightward course, it provides the conus artery (5), and then descends in the anterior atrioventricular ring. It provides a large marginal branch (2) along the anterior surface of the right ventricle not opacified, and then at the bottom of the ring (the cardiac crux), providing the posterior descending coronary artery (1). The right coronary artery continues in the inferior aspect of the ring as the posterior left ventricular branch (4). In this view, the left main (6), anterior descending (8) and circumflex (7) coronary arteries are demonstrated. Notice the segment of the anterior cardiac vein (9) running with the anterior descending artery. AoA, ascending aorta; PL, posterior left aortic sinus of Valsalva.

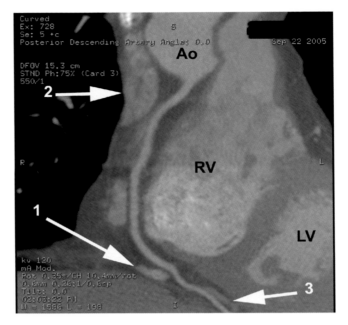

FIGURE 7.24. Multiplanar reformatted tomogram of the course of the right coronary artery. The artery originates from the anterior sinus of Valsalva of the aorta (Ao), passes in the anterior atrioventricular ring between the right atrial appendage (2) and right ventricle (RV), around the underside of the RV, over the coronary sinus (1), and along the inferior aspect of the interventricular septum as the posterior descending artery, coursing with the posterior cardiac vein (3). LV, left ventricle.

ring and the interventricular septum, the so-called crux of the heart. The posterior descending artery perfuses the inferior interventricular septum and may act as an important collateral bed in patients with atherosclerotic heart disease. In 85% of individuals, the posterior descending artery arises from the distal right coronary artery; this is called a right-dominant circulation.

The sinoatrial node artery arises from the proximal right coronary artery and passes behind the superior vena cava to the top of the interatrial septum. Marginal branches from the right coronary artery arise at a right angle from the plane of the atrioventricular ring and then course within the epicardial fat across the right ventricular free wall. The highest marginal branch from the right coronary artery is the conus artery. In right-dominant circulations, the distal right coronary artery continues in the posterior atrioventricular ring as the posterior left ventricular branches.

The left main coronary artery arises from the posterior left aortic sinus of Valsalva (Figures 7.23 and 7.25). The artery continues posteriorly and passes beneath the left atrial appendage to enter the posterior atrioventricular ring. It continues within the ring as the circumflex artery (Figures 7.5, 7.7–7.11, 7.15, 7.20, 7.23, and 7.26). Marginal branches arise from the posterior atrioventricular ring and pass along the posterior left ventricle wall. In 15% of individuals, the circumflex artery continues around the posterior atrioventricular ring, and the posterior descending artery arises from the distal left circumflex or is its continuation itself. These individuals are called left dominant.

Before the left main artery passes beneath the left atrial appendage, the anterior descending artery arises along the top of the interventricular septum (Figures 7.1, 7.23, and 7.25). Within the epicardial fat, it passes along the top of the septum in the interventricular groove (Figures 7.17 and 7.27) to the cardiac apex. As the right coronary artery defines the right margin of the right ventricle, the anterior descending artery defines the left border, and thus the position of the right ventricle, an indicator of right ventricle size. Diagonal branches of the anterior descending artery pass along the anterolateral aspect of the ventricle.

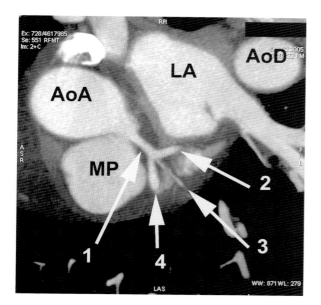

FIGURE 7.25. Multiplanar reformatted tomogram of the origin of the left coronary artery. The left main artery (1) arises from the posterior left aortic sinus of Valsalva. The circumflex artery (2) passes into the posterior atrioventricular ring, lateral to the left atrium (LA). The anterior descending artery (4) continues posterior to the main pulmonary artery (MP) over the top of the interventricular septum. Note the ramus medianus branch (3) arising from the bifurcation of the left main artery. AoA, ascending aorta; AoD, descending aorta.

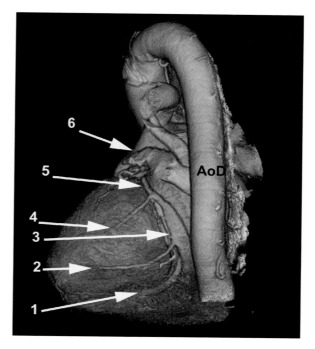

FIGURE 7.26. Surface-rendered, three-dimensional reconstruction of the heart and aorta, viewed from behind. The circumflex artery (5) passes within the posterior atrioventricular ring along with the great cardiac vein (3). The left atrial appendage (6) is seen passing from posterior to anterior just to the left of the main pulmonary artery (not demonstrated). The marginal cardiac (2 and 4) and the posterior cardiac veins (1) are seen entering the great cardiac vein prior to draining through the coronary sinus (not visualized).

FIGURE 7.27. Surface-rendered, three-dimensional reconstruction of the heart. Display in left anterior oblique view. The anterior descending artery (5) runs along the top of the interventricular septum between the right ventricle and left ventricle. Note the large first diagonal artery branch (4). A portion of the right coronary artery (1) is seen emerging from beneath the right atrial appendage (2) to enter the anterior atrioventricular ring. Notice that the main pulmonary artery lies anterior and to the left of the ascending aorta (AoA). The left atrial appendage lies lateral and slightly inferior to the main pulmonary artery, anterior to the left upper-lobe pulmonary vein (3).

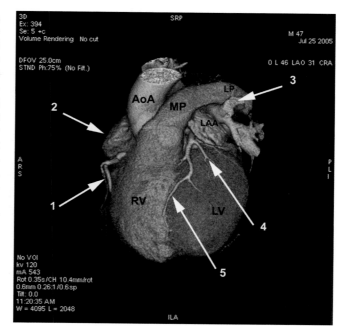

Cardiac Veins

The location, size, and course of the major cardiac veins vary considerably among patients. The venous drainage of the heart is carried by three very different sets of veins: the coronary sinus and its tributaries, the anterior cardiac veins, and the Thebesian veins. Venous return from the left ventricular myocardium is through the anterior interventricular, the middle (or marginal) cardiac, and the posterior cardiac veins (Figures 7.5–7.8, 7.10–7.13, 7.14, 7.18, and 7.26). The anterior interventricular (or anterior cardiac) vein ascends in the anterior interventricular sulcus, parallel to the anterior descending coronary artery, and passes over the base of the heart toward the posterior atrioventricular ring, to enter the great cardiac vein. The great cardiac vein spirals with the circumflex coronary artery in the posterior atrioventricular ring, receives the marginal and posterior cardiac veins, and drains into the right atrium as the coronary sinus. The marginal cardiac veins originate from the posterior or lateral aspects of the left ventricle and drain into the great cardiac vein. Not uncommonly, they drain directly into the coronary sinus.

Venous return from the right ventricular free wall is via the anterior cardiac veins. These veins travel along the anterior aspect of the heart (at nearly a right angle with respect to the right coronary artery), cross the anterior atrioventricular ring, and enter the right atrium either directly or through a small right atrial cardiac vein. The Thebesian veins are very small vessels that drain myocardial blood directly back to the cardiac chambers.

Pericardium

The heart is contained within the middle mediastinum by the pericardium. The visceral pericardium is adherent to the ventricular myocardium and cannot be visually separated from the epicardial fat. The parietal pericardium may be identified as a paper-thin high-signal-intensity surface surrounding the heart and great arteries (Figure 7.28). On the left side of the heart, it attaches over the top of the main pulmonary artery (Figure 7.29). The ascending aorta is enveloped up to about the level of the azygos vein. Recesses (potential spaces) in the pericardium are typically found anterior to the ascending aorta and medial to the main pulmonary artery (the anterior aortic recess), between the ascending aorta and transverse right pulmonary artery (the superior pericardial recess) (Figure 7.30) and around the entry of the pulmonary

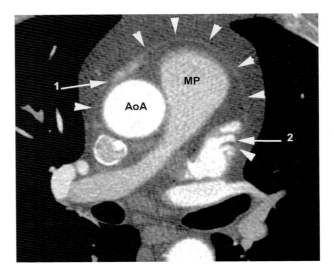

FIGURE 7.28. Axial image processed to enhance contrast and make the pericardium more obvious. The pericardium (arrowheads) surrounds the heart, containing the right (1) and left (2) atrial appendages, ascending aorta (AoA), and main pulmonary artery (MP).

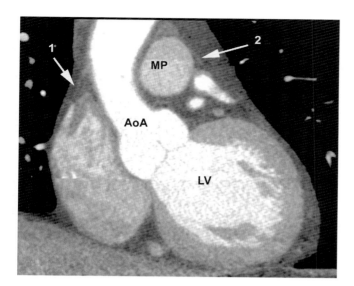

FIGURE 7.29. Tomogram reconstructed in coronal section, processed to enhance the pericardium. The reflection of the pericardium on the ascending aorta (AOA; 1) and main pulmonary artery (MP; 2) are displayed. LV, left ventricle.

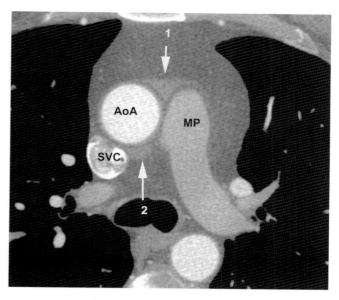

FIGURE 7.30. Axial image processed to enhance contrast and make pericardial fluid more obvious. The space (2) between the ascending aorta (AoA) and main pulmonary artery (MP) is the anterior aortic recess. Posterior to the AoA and inferior to the right pulmonary artery (not visualized) is the superior pericardial recess (2). SVC, superior vena cava.

veins to the left atrium. Visualization of the parietal pericardium depends on the presence and extent of low-density fatty deposition in the pericardial fat pad and middle mediastinum.

Summary Points

- Recognition of normal cardiac and vascular structures is critical to correct interpretation of contrast-enhanced cardiovascular CT imaging.
- Clinical interpretation requires a systematic, often time-consuming, review of axial and processed cardiac CT images.

8 Patient and Occupational Dosimetry

Frank P. Castronovo, Jr., and A. Robert Schleipman

With the introduction of dual-modality positron emission and transmission computed tomography (PET/CT) systems, concurrent acquisition and subsequent generation of coregistered functional (PET) and anatomic (CT) images have become the preferred diagnostic method.[1-4] This capability has caused concern about increased patient radiation doses and occupational exposures to healthcare personnel.[5-8] To address this concern, we need to determine the patient's optimum administered radiopharmaceutical dosage and the appropriate CT scanning parameters as well as to instruct personnel in radiation-exposure-reduction techniques. The CT component can be used to correct for tissue attenuation, which is otherwise accomplished with an external radionuclide source, or to generate diagnostically suitable CT images. In either case, there should be an attempt to minimize the radiation dose while maintaining the diagnostic efficacy of the scan.

Greater awareness about radiation doses has been heightened by the recent Biological Effects of Ionizing Radiation (BEIR VII) update on the risks of low-level radiation.[9] Specifically, the report concluded that radiation risks were somewhat higher than prior estimates, following a linear nonthreshold (LNT) relationship.

Radiation safety aspects encompass both the patient and those staff attending these procedures. The patient is exposed to ionizing radiation from both the PET and CT components of the test, whereas the occupational exposure is limited primarily to the PET portion. This chapter discusses the radiation dosimetry associated with the cardiac scanning procedures currently used in nuclear medicine. Emphasis will be placed on PET/CT and hybrid protocols that combine myocardial perfusion PET and CT coronary angiography.

Basic Concepts

The type of radiation utilized in nuclear cardiology is called ionizing radiation, meaning that the radiation has enough energy to remove an electron out of its orbital shell, producing an ion pair in its wake (the "free" electron plus the atom from which the electron came). The types of radiation of interest to our specialty that cause ionizations are either particulate (beta minus, beta plus, alpha, proton, electron) or electromagnetic (gamma, x-rays). When ionizations are produced within the body, energy is deposited within tissues. The amount of energy deposited determines the radiation dose. When undergoing a PET scan, the patient receives radiation exposure from two sources: the

TABLE 8.1. Physical Properties of Radionuclides Used in Nuclear Cardiology

Radionuclide	Physical Half-life $(T_{1/2p})$, minutes	Γ Constant, (mSv/hr)/MBq @ 1 m	Half Value Layer (HVL), cm, Pb
^{82}Rb	1.26	2.104E-4	0.70
^{15}0	2.06	1.940E-4	0.41
^{13}N	9.97	1.938E-4	0.41
^{18}F	109.74	1.879E-4	0.41
^{99m}Tc	361.2	3.317E-5	0.03
^{201}Tl	4386.00	2.372E-5	0.02

Source: Data from Ref. 20.

administered radiopharmaceutical and the attenuation correction segment of the protocol. The latter can be from either a CT or an external radionuclide source. Occupational exposure results from the handling and administration of the radiopharmaceutical and from proximity to the radioactive patient, who remains radioactive for a short period of time. Several basic radiation quantities and units are defined in Appendix A. Throughout this chapter, units are expressed in the International System of Units (SI).

Exposure of the Patient to Radiation

Internal Radiopharmaceutical Exposure

In 1948, a method was reported for determining the absorbed dose from internally administered radionuclides primarily with long half-lives and high-energy beta and gamma emissions.[10] This methodology was used until the mid-1960s, when radionuclides with shorter half-lives, lower photon energies, and much more complex decay schemes were introduced. To meet this challenge, the Society of Nuclear Medicine created the Medical Internal Radiation Dose (MIRD) Committee in 1968, which subsequently introduced the "absorbed fraction," and, in 1975, the "S" methodologies.[11–13] Computer programs eventually simplified this calculation, as did the publication of several reports from the International Commission on Radiological Protection (ICRP).[14–17]

Absorbed doses to organs from the administration of a radiopharmaceutical and the determination of the resultant effective doses are supplied in ICRP Publication 80.[18] The effective dose methodology is dependent on tissue-weighting factors, as described in ICRP Publication 60.[19] Physical properties associated with radionuclides employed in nuclear cardiology are listed in Table 8.1.[20] Specific radiopharmaceuticals utilized in nuclear cardiology with their corresponding effective doses are shown in Table 8.2.[18]

TABLE 8.2. Effective Doses for Adult Patients from Radiopharmaceuticals Used in Nuclear Cardiology

Radiopharmaceutical	Procedure	Effective dose, mSv/MBq
^{99m}Tc-sestamibi	Rest	9.0E-03
	Stress	7.9E-03
^{99m}Tc-tetrofosmin	Rest	7.6E-03
	Stress	7.0E-03
^{201}Tl-thallous chloride	Rest or stress	2.1E-02
^{18}F-fluorodeoxyglucose	Rest	1.9E-02
^{13}N-ammonia	Rest or stress	2.0E-03
^{82}Rb-rubidium chloride	Rest or stress	3.4E-03
^{15}O-water	Rest or stress	9.3E-04

Source: Data from Ref. 18.

External Radiation Exposure

Transmission Imaging

PET or single photon emission computed tomography (SPECT) procedures often include a transmission scan to correct for tissue attenuation of the image data. A gallium-68/germanium-68 (^{68}Ge/^{68}Ga) coincidence source, a gadolinium-153 (^{153}Gd) line source, or a transmission CT scanner can be used to correct for attenuation. The patient's estimated effective radiation dose from radionuclide transmission corrections is minimal (0.0013–0.0013 mSv), whereas CT attenuation is higher (0.23–5.66 mSv).[1,6,21]

CT Scan

When diagnostic-quality CT images are acquired, the effective radiation doses are higher than those obtained for attenuation correction alone. Since their introduction in 1998, multidetector scanners (MDCT) have found their way into cardiology practice. Unlike radiopharmaceuticals, where a specific radionuclide has a unique list of physical constants, CT scanners possess a number of operational variables that influence radiation dose.[22,23] These include tube potential, tube current, tube rotation time, slice thickness, pitch factor, beam filter, geometric efficiency, and focal spot to center of rotation distance. The scanner model and setup, as well as the patient's morphology, organ of interest, gender, and age, factor into the patient's radiation dose. The setup consists of a protocol supplied by the scanner manufacturer with items adjusted by the technologist as desired. For a specific scanner, patient dose is linearly related to the product of scanning time(s), tube current (milliamperage [mA], the number of x-rays produced), and tube voltage (peak kilovoltage [kVp], which determines how penetrating the x-rays are). Higher kVp is desired to create constant image noise. If a constant mA is used, the dose is then inversely related to the pitch (table travel per rotation relative to beam collimation). With a pitch <1, data acquisition occurs with overlap, whereas a pitch >1 produces gaps. Both the slice thickness and the scan volume are linearly related to dose.[22] A multidetector technique allows the scanner to acquire more slices per rotation. The most important factor for managing patient dose is the mAs, the tube current multiplied by the scan time in seconds. How these various CT parameters influence patient dose is illustrated in Table 8.3.[22,23]

The principal CT radiation dose indicator is the CT dose index (CTDI). This index integrates the radiation dose delivered both within and beyond the scan volume and corresponds to the total energy deposited in the patient (or phantom) divided by the mass of a single section.[23] A weighted CT dose.index (CTDIw) is used for contiguous

TABLE 8.3. Effect of Scan Parameters on Radiation Dose for a Spiral Chest CT

CT Parameter	Procedure A	Procedure B
Tube voltage (kVp)	140	140
Tube current (mA)	165	110
Scan volume (cm)	31	31
Slice thickness (mm)	5	5
Pitch	1	2
Radiation Dose		
Lung (mGy)	24.3	8.15
Effective dose (mSv)	7.1	2.4

Source: Data from References 22 and 23.

scanning and represents the average radiation dose across the field of view, incorporating variations in the absorbed dose from the periphery to the center of the object. These dose indicators do not represent the patient's actual radiation dose; rather, they are the standardized index of the average dose delivered for each specific scan being considered, which can then be used to determine effective dose.

Overlapping sequential scans or noncontiguous studies produce the CTDIvol, which represents the average dose within a particular scan volume. This value is multiplied by the total length (cm) to arrive at the dose-length-product (DLP). A higher radiation dose is obtained with an increased axial scan length. To minimize dose, it is therefore important to scan only the area of interest. The special dose quantities, CTDIvol and DLP, can be obtained from direct display on the scanner or by measurement of standardized phantoms. A medical physicist is best qualified to perform the latter determinations. A more direct, but more expensive, method is to estimate the radiation exposure with an anthropomorphic whole-body phantom (e.g., Alderson RANDO) distributed with thermoluminescent dosimeters (TLDs).[24] Finally, the effective dose, in mSv, is calculated by multiplying the DLP in units of mGy.cm, by a region-specific conversion factor (RSCF), in units of mSv/mGy.cm.[25]

Determination of the Patient's Effective Dose

The patient's effective dose from a nuclear cardiology procedure is made up primarily of a combination of two components: the CT scan and the administered radiopharmaceutical. The methodology associated with determining the effective dose is described above. In essence, the absorbed dose of each organ exposed is multiplied by a tissue-weighting factor. Each corrected organ dose is then summed to arrive at the dose equivalent. A sample calculation for an adult patient receiving 740 MBq of fluorine-18 fluorodeoxyglucose (^{18}F-FDG) is presented in Appendix B.[18,19] Similar methodology can be used to calculate effective dose from a conventional posteroanterior (PA) chest radiograph, as shown in Appendix C.[26]

To arrive at the CT contribution to the dose equivalent, the conversion factors for a general anatomic region are used, as described by the European Guidelines on Quality Criteria for Computed Tomography.[27] As discussed above, the effective dose is determined by multiplying DLP by RSCF. Several RSCFs have been published for various parts of the anatomy, as follows: head (0.0023 mSv/mGy.cm), chest (0.017 mSv/mGy.cm), and pelvis (0.019 mSv/mGy.cm).[25,27] A sample calculation is provided in Appendix D. Table 8.4 lists the effective doses associated with PET and integrated PET/CT procedures.

Radiation Doses to the Breast and Skin

The increased utilization of multidetector CT has resulted in a greater awareness of nontarget radiation doses. Organs often incidental to the x-ray beam include breast, thyroid, lens of the eye, gonads, and skin. Dose to the skin more often becomes a concern during CT-fluoroscopy, which has no established application as yet in cardiology. However, skin effects have occurred after interventional cardiac procedures.[28] The thyroid, lens of the eye, and gonads are outside of the anatomical region scanned during cardiac CT studies. The breasts, however, are within the primary beam of x-rays, as demonstrated by the calculated doses to this tissue from various radiological procedures in Table 8.5.[29-31] The effective dose (in mSv) is obtained by multiplying the absorbed radiation dose (in mGy) by a radiosensitivity factor, which is 0.05 for the breast.[19] The effective doses from CT procedures expose the breast to substantially higher effective doses than those determined for radiopharmaceuticals.[18,19,32] To counter this, the application of thinly layered bismuth garments has been shown to

TABLE 8.4. Patient Effective Doses from Cardiac PET and Integrated PET/CT

	Effective Dose per Procedure (mSv)	Radiopharmaceutical Dosage and Scan Parameters
Scout		
CT	0.04	120 kVp, 10 mA
Transmission		
CT (^{82}Rb stress/rest)	0.73	140 kVp, 30 mA, pitch = 1.35
CT (dynamic ^{18}F-FDG)	0.83	140 kVp, 30 mA, pitch = 1.375
CT (cardiac viability ^{18}F-FDG)	0.83	140 kVp, 30 mA, pitch = 1.375
Emission		
^{82}Rb chloride (rest + stress)	12.58	1850.0 MBq for each scan
^{13}N-ammonia (rest + stress)	5.55	925.0 MBq for each scan
^{15}O-water (rest + stress)	2.75	1480.0 MBq for each scan
Coronary artery calcium score (CAC)	3.69	120 kVp, 300 mA, pitch = 0.563 – 1.0
CT Coronary angiogram (CTA)		
Acquisition 1: localization	0.7	120 kVp, 80 mA, pitch = 1.375
Acquisition 2: bolus	0.74	120 kVp, 80 mA
Acquisition 3: "snapshot"	25.71	120 kVp, 440 mA
Total	27.21	

Source: CT dose calculations provided by Richard Nawfel, MS, Medical Physicist, Radiology, Brigham and Women's Hospital, Boston, Massachusetts, USA; Personal Communication, August, 2005.
Radiopharmaceutical dosages and scan parameters reflect those used at most institutions.

reduce the CT breast dose by 50%.[33] However, the logistics of routinely applying this type of protective device have not yet been incorporated into daily clinical practice. It is estimated that 1 in 9 women will develop breast cancer during their lifetime.[34] The probability of radiogenic fatal breast cancer is 1/250,000 per mGy of absorbed dose, or 1/2500 per mSv effective dose.[19]

Exposure of Personnel to Radiation

In contrast to the mathematical modeling, calculations, and simulations performed to determine patient or specific organ doses, measurement of radiation exposures to hospital staff is relatively straightforward. Prospectively, one can summarize ion chamber measurements obtained at variable distances from patients and other sources; retrospectively, one can review personal dosimeter findings. [7,8] The individual deep dose is calculated from personal monitors worn on the trunk. Hand (wrist or finger) badges worn during compounding and administration of radiopharmaceuticals measure extremity dose. Newer electronic personal detectors (EPDs) yield instanta-

TABLE 8.5. Breast and Skin Radiation Doses

Breast Doses: Radiopharmaceuticals

Procedure	Dosage	Effective Dose (mSv)
^{18}F-FDG	370 MBq	0.159
^{99m}Tc-MIBI (rest)	407 MBq	0.077
^{99m}Tc-MIBI (stress)	1332 MBq	0.226
^{99m}Tc-Myoview (rest)	407 MBq	0.019
^{99m}Tc-Myoview (stress)	1332 MBq	0.067
^{82}Rb-chloride	1850 MBq	0.018
^{13}N-ammonia	740 MBq	0.067
^{201}Tl-thallous chloride	93 MBq	0.180
^{15}O-water	1110 MBq	0.016

Breast and Skin Doses: X-Rays

Procedure*	Breast		Skin (C/kg)†
	mGy	mSv	
Chest x-ray: PA and lateral	0.059	0.003	1.8E-05
Mammogram	3.5	0.175	
CT-angiography	44.1	2.21	
CT-angiography: 64 slice	75.1	3.76	
CT-pulmonary embolism	54.5	2.73	
CT-chest: 4 slice	16.2	0.81	
CT-chest: 16 slice	13.5	0.68	
CT-chest: 64 slice	15.9	0.80	
Cardiac catheterization: PA-female	55.8	2.79	8.74E-02‡

Source: Data from References 16, 18, 29–32.
*As explained in the text, tube potential, mAs, and so on can vary. Average values are shown.
†2.58E-04 C/kg = 1 R
‡Assume 64 minutes of fluoroscopy, plus 4.9 minutes of cine at 9.8E-04 C/kg and 5.03E-03 C/kg, respectively.
Checking for skin changes is recommended after a radiation dose of 5.16E-02 C/kg. Skin changes were not observed with this patient.

neous dose recordings that are useful in high-dose-rate settings, though in the clinical setting of diagnostic exposures, artifactual readings and decreased radiosensitivity (relative to TLDs) have been reported.[35,36]

For all ionizing radiations, effective dose equivalent is the standard descriptor for personal dose, which is expressed in sieverts (Sv) or increments thereof, for example, μSv and mSv. The deep-dose equivalent (body) is used to estimate cancer risk. Lens dose is used to estimate risk of radiation cataractogenesis, and shallow (skin) dose to estimate probability of deterministic skin effects.

Barring lifesaving actions of emergency personnel in a radiation disaster, identical regulatory limits are imposed on all radiation workers, whether they are surgical nurses, nuclear medicine residents, or power plant operators. Authorized radiation users within the European Union and many other health ministries (following ICRP guidelines), work under a lower annual allowable effective dose limit than do those

TABLE 8.6. Maximum Occupational Annual Dose Limits

	US	ICRP
Effective Dose		
Deep	50 mSv	20 mSv
Declared pregnancy	5 mSv	2 mSv*
Radiation Weighted Dose		
Lens of the eye	150 mSv	150 mSv
Shallow (skin/extremities)	500 mSv	500 mSv

Source: Data from References 19, 37, 38.
*More recent European Commission Directive = 1.0 mSv for declared pregnancy.

in the United States (Table 8.6).[19,37] Pregnant radiation workers are further limited to not exceed 5.0 mSv in the United States, and no more than 1.0 mSv in the European Union countries, once pregnancy has been declared.[19,38] Annual limits of radionuclide intake (ALI), through ingestion or inhalation, are also codified. The actual amount varies by radionuclide, for example, ingestion of 2960 MBq of technetium-99 ([99mTc]) vs 2590 MBq of [18F], though they have the same threshold outcomes: a total effective dose equivalent of 50 mSv.[39]

Contributions to Occupational Radiation Exposure

Noninterventional CT, as in calcium scoring, PET/CT, SPECT-CT, and CTA (CT-based angiography) contributes minimal dose to staff members, as their duties are performed behind shielded consoles. However, with radionuclides a number of factors contribute to occupational exposures. These include exam volume, acuity of patients (requiring proximity of medical staff), tracer photon yield, photon energy, and decay rate. Each radionuclide possesses a unique decay constant, λ (where the physical half-life = $0.693/\lambda$), and every photon-emitting radionuclide has its own gamma constant, Γ, a descriptor of source strength based on energy and photon yield. As listed in Table 8.1, one can appreciate the steady increase in exposure, per unit dose, from thallium-201 ([201Tl]) to [99mTc], [18F], and nitrogen-13 ([13N]), and then on to rubidium-82 ([82Rb]).[20] As implied by the increasing half-value layer (HVL) gradient, increased shielding is also required to attenuate these photons. In addition to the 0.511 MeV annihilation photons common to positron emitters, [82Rb] also emits a high-energy (0.78 MeV) gamma photon.

As most cardiac imaging activities must be carried out proximal to the radiation source, occupational dose measurement generally falls into several task-based categories. These are:

- preparation, administration, and disposal of radiopharmaceuticals
- monitoring and care of the radioactive patient
- quality control of radiopharmaceuticals and imaging instruments

Reported Occupational Doses

A review of the literature yields a spectrum of dose estimates, for example, per exam, per technologist, per quarter, per year.[36,40–45] The better-designed studies further standardize results with corrections for administered dose, sensitivity of monitoring equipment, and recorded time and distance from the source or patient.

Table 8.7 summarizes the occupational exposures from PET studies as reported in the literature. Most of the published data reflect the wide use of [18F]-FDG PET, which is not necessarily cardiac specific, with the exception of its application to assess

TABLE 8.7. Occupational Effective Dose Equivalent for PET

Reference	Radiotracer	μSv per MBq administered	μSv per complete procedure	μSv per day	μSv per year
40	^{18}F-FDG	0.01–0.023	5.9–11.5	58	12400
41	^{18}F-FDG + ^{13}N-NH$_3$ + ^{11}C-methionine	0.017	5.5	14.4	3456*
36	^{18}F-FDG	0.024–0.038	10.7	46.0	7500–10000
44	^{18}F-FDG	0.01	4.1		3085
43	^{18}F-FDG	0.025	4.5	31	6665
45	^{18}F-FDG	0.009	3.13	12.5†	3000*
42	^{82}Rb chloride	0.0003	0.9 (stress + rest)	10.8‡	2592*

Source: Data from References 36, 40–45.
*Assuming 5 days/week × 4 weeks/month × 12 months/year.
†4 patients/day.
‡12 patients/day.

myocardial viability. Chiesa et al first published results comparing occupational dose from ^{18}F-FDG PET studies to other scintigraphic procedures.[40] The authors presented values for syringe preparation, escort of patients, quality assurance procedures, and scan acquisition. Benatar et al included ^{13}N-NH$_3$ and ^{11}C exams in their report on technologist exposures, though these made up only 3.4% and 5.7%, respectively, of their measured PET procedure volume.[41] Schleipman et al compared ^{82}Rb to ^{99m}Tc-MIBI in pharmacologic stress myocardial perfusion imaging.[42] Excluding the ^{82}Rb studies, the average dose per technologist approximates 6.5 μSv, ranging from 3.13 to 11.5 μSv per procedure. Despite this wide variability, when standardized to administered radioactivity, the mean occupational dose approximates 0.02 μSv/MBq.

Though ^{82}Rb has a larger gamma-ray constant, its rapid radioactive decay results in a lower dose contribution than does ^{18}F-FDG. The study by Schleipman et al demonstrated a sixfold decrease in exposure for exercise staff performing pharmacologic stress tests, when utilizing ^{82}Rb as compared to ^{99m}Tc-MIBI.[42] However, those in close proximity (0.5 m from the patient) during the first 3 minutes postinjection received high levels of exposure (approximately 15 μSv/patient); thus, from a radiation protection perspective, actual exercise testing of these patients on a routine basis is not recommended.

Radiation Protection Considerations

The universal principles of radioprotection—reduce time near the source, maintain a practical distance, use appropriate shielding, and control for contamination by frequent surveys and use of personal protective equipment—are equally relevant with positron emitters. Specific adaptations include using automated blood pressure monitors and medication pumps that decrease time spent in close contact with the radioactive patient, as well as employing PET-specific shielding, which has become more widely available.[44–46] Some syringe and vial containers contain a plastic sleeve that absorbs positrons, while others may be comprised of tungsten or tungsten-lead alloys that more efficiently absorb the 0.511 MeV annihilation photons. As with all other areas of radiological imaging, a qualified medical physicist determines facility shielding for examination areas, waiting rooms, and hot labs.[47–50] Finally, trainees should be taught to perform as many patient-centered tasks, such as obtaining consent or baseline electrocardiogram (ECG) monitoring, prior to injection of radio-tracers whenever possible.

Summary Points

- The benefits to health from diagnostic imaging are well established. Cardiology patients have benefited from the explosion of minimally invasive nuclear cardiology, CT, and fluoroscopic procedures in the past few years.
- Equally established, however, is the need to minimize the possible deleterious effects from ionizing radiation that may be overprescribed or improperly applied. Those who operate this increasingly sophisticated equipment have met this challenge by correctly and successfully performing these procedures. However, increased radiation doses, especially in the PET suite, are an unfortunate by-product of this success. It is therefore the responsibility of the authorized radiation user or clinician to maintain a program whereby the radiation dose received by patients and personnel is maintained as low as reasonably achievable. This can best be achieved by education combined with an institutional quality-management program dedicated to improving this environment.

References

1. Schwaiger M, Ziegler S, Nekolla S. PET/CT: challenge for nuclear cardiology. *J Nucl Med.* 2005;46:1664–1678.
2. Bruken RC, DiFilippo FP, Howe WC, et al. Measurement of left ventricular ejection fraction using gated cardiac PET with CT based attenuation correction [abstract]. *J Nucl Med.* 2005;46(suppl 2):173P. Abstract 499.
3. Namdar M, Hany TF, Koepfli P, et al. Integrated PET/CT for the assessment of coronary artery disease: a feasibility study. *J Nucl Med.* 2005;46:930–935.
4. Nekolla S, Souvatzoglou M, Hausleiter J, et al. Integration of function and morphology in cardiac PET/CT: a feasibility study in patients with chronic and ischemic heart disease. *J Nucl Cardiol.* 2005;2(suppl):S45.
5. Hunold P, Vogt FM, Schmermind A, et al. Radiation exposure during cardiac CT: effective doses at multi-detector row CT and electron-beam CT. *Radiology.* 2003;226:145–152.
6. Wu TH, Huang YH, Lee JJ, et al. Radiation exposure during transmission measurements: comparison between CT- and germanium-based techniques with a current PET scanner. *Eur J Nucl Med Mol Imaging.* 2004;31:38–43.
7. Gomez-Palacios M, Terron JA, Dominguez P, et al. Radiation doses in the surroundings of patients undergoing nuclear medicine diagnostic studies. *Health Phys.* 2005;89:(suppl 2):S27-S34.
8. Lundberg TM, Gray PJ, Bartlett ML. Measuring and minimizing the radiation dose to nuclear medicine technologists. *J Nucl Med.* 2002;30:25–30.
9. BIER VII, Phase 2. *Health Risks from Exposure to Low Levels of Ionizing Radiation.* Washington, DC: National Academies Press; 2005. Available at: http://www.nap.edu/catalog/11340.html. Accessed January 24, 2006.
10. Marinelli LD, Quimby EH, Hine GJ. Dosage determinations with radioactive isotopes. II. Practical considerations in therapy and protection. *AJR Am J Roentgenol.* 1948;59:260–280.
11. Society of Nuclear Medicine. Medical Internal Radiation Dose (MIRD) Publications. Suppl 1, Pamphlets 1–3. New York: Society of Nuclear Medicine; 1968.
12. Snyder WS, Ford MR, Warner GG, et al. *"S" Absorbed Dose per Unit Cumulated Activity for Selected Radionuclides and Organs.* New York: Society of Nuclear Medicine; 1975. MIRD Pamphlet 11.
13. Dillman LT, Von der Lage FP. *Radionuclide Decay Schemes and Nuclear Parameters for Use in Radiation Dose Estimation.* New York: Society of Nuclear Medicine; 1975. NM/MIRD Pamphlet 10.
14. MIRDOSE 3, Oak Ridge, TN: Oak Ridge Internal Information Center, 1994.

15. New Internal Radiation Dose and Modeling Software; FDA Approves Commercial MIRDOSE Successor. *J Nucl Med.* 2004;45:26N, 27N.

16. International Commission on Radiological Protection (ICRP). *Radiation Dose to Patients from Radiopharmaceuticals.* Oxford: Pergamon Press; 1987. ICRP Publication 53.

17. International Commission on Radiological Protection (ICRP). *Summary of the Current ICRP Principles for Protection of the Patient in Nuclear Medicine.* Oxford: Pergamon Press; 1993. A report by Committee 3.

18. International Commission on Radiological Protection (ICRP). *Radiation Dose to Patients from Radiopharmaceuticals.* Oxford: Pergamon Press; 1998. ICRP Publication 80.

19. International Commission on Radiological Protection (ICRP) *Recommendations of the International Commission of Radiological Protection.* Oxford: Pergamon Press; 1991. ICRP Publication 60.

20. Shleien B, Slaback LA, Kirky BK, eds. *The Health Physics and Radiological Health Handbook.* Baltimore: Williams & Wilkins; 1998.

21. Perisinakis K, Theocharopoules N, Korkavitsas N. Patient effective radiation dose and associated risks from transmission scans using ^{153}Gd live sources in cardiac SPECT studies. *Health Phys.* 2002;83:66–74.

22. Hamberg LM, Rhea JT, Hunter GJ, et al. Multi-detector row CT: radiation dose characteristics. *Radiology.* 2003;226:762–772.

23. International Commission on Radiological Protection (ICRP). *Managing Patient Dose in Computed Tomography.* Oxford: Pergamon Press; 2000. ICRP Publication 87.

24. Brix G, Lechel U, Veit R, et al. Assessment of a theoretical formalism for dose estimation in CT: an anthropomorphic phantom study. *Eur Radiol.* 2004;14:1275–1284.

25. McNitt-Grey M. AAPM/RSNA Physics Tutorial for Residents: Topics in CT. *Radiographics.* 2002;22:1541–1553.

26. International Commission on Radiological Protection (ICRP). *Exposure of the U.S. Population from Diagnostic Medical Radiation.* Oxford, Pergamon Press; 1989. ICRP Publication 100.

27. European Commission. *European Guidelines on Quality Criteria for Computed Tomography.* EUR 16262 EN, May 1999. Available at: http://www.drs.dk/guidelines/ct/quality/index.htm. Accessed January 24, 2006.

28. Wagner LK, Eifel PJ, Geise RA. Potential biological effects following high x-ray dose interventional procedures. *J Vasc Interv Radiol.* 1994;5:71–84.

29. Parker MS, Hui FK, Camacho MA, et al. Female breast radiation exposure during CT pulmonary angiography. *AJR Am J Roentgenol.* 2005;185:1228–1233.

30. McCollough CH, Liu HH. Breast dose during electron beam CT: measurements with film dosimetry. *Radiology.* 1995;196:1153–1157.

31. Nawfel, R, Yoshizumi T. Update on radiation CT. *AAPM News Letter.* March/April 2005:12–13.

32. Thomas SR, Stabin MG, Castronovo FP. Radiation absorbed dose from $^{(201)}$Tl-thallous chloride. *J Nucl Med.* 2005;46:502–508.

33. Hopper KD, King SH, Lobell ME, et al. The breast: in-plane x-ray protection during diagnostic thoracic CT shielding with bismuth radio-protective garments, *Radiology.* 1997;205:853–858.

34. Schnall MD. Breast imaging technology: application of magnetic resonance imaging to early detection of breast cancer. *Breast Cancer Res.* 2000;3:17–21.

35. Deji S, Nishizawa K. Abnormal responses of electronic pocket dosimeters caused by high frequency electromagnetic fields emitted from digital cellular telephones. *Health Phys.* 2004;87:539–544.

36. Biran T, Weininger J, Malchi S, et al. Measurement of occupational exposure for a technologist performing ^{18}F-FDG PET scans. *Health Phys.* 2004;87:539–544.

37. US Nuclear Regulatory Commission (NRC). *Program-Specific Guidance About Medical Use Licenses.* Washington, DC: US Nuclear Regulatory Commission; 1998. NUREG-SR 1556. Vol. 9.

38. Council of the European Union. Guideline 96/29/EURATOM laying down basic safety standards for the protection of the health of workers and the general public against the dangers arising from ionizing radiation. *J Eur Comm.* 1996;L159:0001–0114.

39. US Code of Federal Regulations. *Annual Limits on Intake (ALIs) and Derived Air Concentrations (DACs) of Radionuclides for Occupational Exposure, Effluent Concentrations for Release in Sewerage.* 10 CFR Part 20, Appendix B. Available at: http://www.nrc.gov/

reading-rm/doc-collections/cfr/part020/full-text.html#part020-appb. Accessed January 24, 2006.

40. Chiesa C, De Sanctis V, Crippa F, et al. Radiation dose to technicians per nuclear medicine procedures: comparison between technetium-99m, gallium-67, and iodine-131 radiotracers and fluorine-18 fluorodeoxyglucose. *Eur J Nucl Med.* 1997;24:1380–1389.

41. Benatar NA, Cronin BF, O'Doherty MJ. Radiation dose rates from patients undergoing PET: implications for technologists and waiting areas. *Eur J Nucl Med.* 2000;27:583–589.

42. Schleipman, AR, Castronovo FP, Di Carli, MF, et al. Occupational radiation dose associated with Rb-82 myocardial perfusion positron emission tomography imaging. *J Nucl Cardiol.* 2006;13:378–384.

43. Robinson CN, Young JG, Wallace AB, Ibbetson VJ. A study of the personal radiation dose received by nuclear medicine technologists working in a dedicated PET center. *Health Phys.* 2005;88(suppl 1):S17–S21.

44. Roberts FO, Gunawardana DH, Pathmaraj K, et al. Radiation dose to PET technologists and strategies to lower occupational exposure. *J Nucl Med Tech.* 2005;33:44–47.

45. Guillet B, Quentin P, Waultier S, et al. Technologist radiation exposure in routine clinical practice with 18F-FDG PET. *J Nucl Med Tech.* 2005;33:175–179.

46. Brown TF, Yasillo NJ. Radiation safety considerations for PET centers. *J Nucl Med Tech.* 1997;25:98–102.

47. Methé BM. Shielding design for a PET imaging suite: a case study. *Health Phys.* 2003;84(suppl 5):S83-S88.

48. Anderson JA, Matthews D. Site planning and radiation safety in the PET facility. Paper presented at: Proceedings of the 44th Annual Association of Physicists in Medicine; July 14–18, 2002; Montreal, Canada.

49. Erdman M, King S, Miller K. Recent experiences with shielding a PET/CT facility. *Health Phys.* 2004;87(suppl 1):S537-S539.

50. Cao Z, Corley JH, Allison J. ^{18}F protection issues: human and γ-camera considerations. *J Nucl Med Tech.* 2003;31:210–215.

Appendix A: Radiological Units

Exposure: Amount of ionization produced in air from photons (x-rays and/or gamma rays). The conventional unit is the Roentgen (R), which is equivalent to 2.08E+09 ion pairs/cm^3 in air at STP, or 2.58E-04 coulombs/kg air. The SI unit is coulombs/kg air. 1R = 1000 mR.

Absorbed Dose: The amount of absorbed energy per gram of material from particulate radiation. The conventional unit is the rad, and it equals 100 ergs per gram. The SI unit is the gray (Gy), which equals 1 joule/kg. 1 rad = 0.01 Gy. 1 Gy = 100 rads. 1 rad = 1000 mrad.

Dose Equivalent–Radiation Protection: A quantity that reflects the modifying effects of different types of radiation and the relative radiosensitivity of the irradiated tissue. This unit is defined as the absorbed dose times a weighting factor for radiation type, called a quality factor (QF). The conventional unit is the rem, and it equals the rad × QF. Since the radiation types in nuclear cardiology have the same weighting factor, rad and rem are equivalent. The SI unit is the sievert (Sv), which equals 100 rem. Radiation badge readings are expressed in terms of mrem or mSv.

Dose Equivalent-Radiation Risk: A double-weighted absorbed dose, using QF and a weighting factor for each tissue irradiated. The latter represents the fraction of the total fatal cancer and serious inherited disorders (stochastic risk) resulting from the irradiation of that organ or tissue, called the effective dose (ED). It is defined as a summation of the tissue equivalent doses, each multiplied by the appropriate tissue-weighting factor. ED = sum (W$_t$ × H$_t$). The conventional unit is the rem, and the SI unit is the sievert (Sv), with 1 Sv = 100 rem. The sum of fatal cancers for whole-body irradiation is 1 in 20,000 per mGy (100 mrem), with the baseline cancer mortality being 1 in 6.7 to 1 in 4.[18]

Activity: Amount of radioactivity expressed as the nuclear transformation rate. The conventional unit is the Curie (Ci), which is defined as 3.7E+10 disintegrations/s (dps). The SI unit is the Bequerel (Bq), which is defined as 1 dps. 1 mCi = 37 MBq.

Appendix B: Patient Effective Dose Calculation for ^{18}F-FDG

Organ	W_t*	mGy/MBq	mSv/MBq
Bladder	0.05	1.6E-01	8.0E-03
Bone surface	0.01	1.1E-02	1.1E-04
Breast	0.05	8.6E-03	4.3E-04
Stomach	0.12	1.1E-02	1.3E-03
Colon	0.12	1.3E-02	1.6E-03
Liver	0.05	1.1E-02	5.5E-04
Lungs	0.12	1.0E-02	1.2E-03
Esophagus	0.05	1.1E-02	5.5E-04
Red marrow	0.12	1.1E-02	1.3E-03
Skin	0.01	8.0E-03	8.0E-05
Testes	0.20	1.2E-02	2.4E-03
Thyroid	0.05	1.0E-02	5.0E-04
Remaining organs	0.05	2.0E-02	1.0E-03
Effective dose			1.9E-02

Source: Data from References 18, 19.
*W_t = Weighting factor.

Appendix C: Patient Effective Dose Calculation for a PA Chest X-Ray

Effective Dose Calculation

Organ	Absorbed Dose (mGy)	Weighting Factor	Effective Dose (mSv)
Marrow	0.021	0.12	0.003
Breast	0.059	0.05	0.003
Lung	0.124	0.12	0.015
Thyroid	0.079	0.05	0.004
Bone	0.082	0.01	0.001
Gonads	0.005	0.20	0.001
Total			0.027 (2.7 mrem)

Source: Data from The International Commission on Radiological Protection.[26]
Projection: PA (screen/film).
Skin entrance exposure: 5.7E-06 C/kg (22 mrad).

Appendix D: Patient Effective Dose Calculation for a CT of the Lung

Scan parameters:	120 kVp, 250 mAs, 5–7 mm collimation, pitch = 1
Length of scan:	25 cm
Phantom studies:	CTDI$_{100}$, center = 10 mGy
CTDI$_{100}$, periphery:	18 mGy

Calculations:

CTDIvol = [1/3 CTDI$_{100}$, center + 2/3 CTDI$_{100}$, periphery]/pitch = (3.3 + 12)/1
= 15 mGy

Dose-related product (DLP) = (CTDIvol)(length of scan) = (15)(25) = 375 mGy.cm.

ED = (DLP)(Region-specific conversion factor) = (375 mGy.cm)(0.017 mSv/mGy.cm)
= 6.4 mSv.

Data from References 23, 25.

Part III
Diagnostic Approaches to Patients with CAD

9 Patient Preparation and Stress Protocols for Cardiac PET and Integrated PET/CT Imaging

Sharon E. Crugnale and Sharmila Dorbala

In the operation of a stress test laboratory, the foremost concerns are patient safety, study quality, and efficiency. In addition to quality of care, customer service also plays a significant role in ensuring that patients have a satisfying experience and that the referring physicians continue to utilize services. Myocardial positron emission tomography (PET) and PET/computed tomography (CT) perfusion imaging are noteworthy for high efficiency, rapid throughput, and, in a high-volume setting, low operational costs. This chapter reviews the requirements regarding equipment, personnel, patient screening and preparation, and stress protocols used in a cardiac PET and integrated PET/CT imaging laboratory.

Laboratory Equipment

The stress-testing equipment (Table 9.1) includes the electrocardiogram (ECG) cart, 2 ECG modules with radiotranslucent wiring and electrode adaptors, and radiotranslucent electrodes.[1] Radiotranslucent wires, electrode grabbers, and electrodes are necessary only for cardiac PET/CT imaging and not for dedicated PET imaging. This is due to the streaking artifact that metal wires and electrodes may cause on the CT. The wires will ideally be at least 12 inches long. This will allow the attached module to remain far enough away from the chest so it does not alter the CT images.

An ECG cart with a full arrhythmia disclosure feature is highly recommended. The staff is often in the control room during the patient's rest imaging as well as during some of the stress-testing infusions to decrease radiation exposure. A full-disclosure ECG will allow all ECG information to be retained. A direct ECG monitor in the console room (as in cardiac catheterization laboratories) is optimal.

Two ECG modules are suggested to ensure efficiency of the laboratory. While one patient is having his or her exam in the PET room, the next patient can be evaluated and prepared with the second ECG module in the preparation room. This will optimize efficiency in the PET imaging room.

Of course, as in any stress-testing laboratory, emergency equipment must be readily available. This includes a code cart with a multifunction defibrillator/pacer, oxygen,

TABLE 9.1. Recommended Supplies for Cardiac PET/CT Stress Testing

1. ECG stress cart with full arrhythmia disclosure capability
2. Radiotranslucent ECG leads
3. Radiotranslucent ECG lead adapters
4. Radiotranslucent wires
5. Automated blood pressure monitoring device
6. ECG gating device
7. ECG monitoring device in console room (optional)
8. IV supplies, syringes and needles, intravenous tubing, solutions, stand, adhesive tape
9. Pharmacological stress agents
10. Normal saline bags
11. 3-way stop cock
12. Medication box
13. Emergency crash cart with defibrillator
14. Oxygen
15. Suction equipment
16. Nasal cannula, ventimask, nonrebreathing mask, O$_2$ mask

and suction. The defibrillator should be tested on a daily basis.[1] It is also helpful to have a medication box for minor incidents that do not require a full code (e.g., supraventricular tachycardia).

Laboratory Personnel

Exercise staff members may include exercise physiologists, exercise specialists, physical therapists, ECG technicians, nurses, and physician assistants.[1] Appropriate training and performance skills for exercise-testing personnel are available in published guidelines.[2] To ensure patient safety and satisfaction while maintaining efficient throughput of the laboratory and excellent study quality, 4 essential personnel are optimal. First is a staff member trained to perform exercise and pharmacological stress testing. This is usually a physician (often a fellow) or nurse, who plays a dual role preparing and giving the medication necessary for testing. Second, a certified nuclear medicine technologist who has been trained in cardiac PET or PET/CT is necessary to operate the camera as well as the rubidium-82 (^{82}Rb) generator and infusion system. Third, an exercise physiologist whose role is to prescreen and prepare each patient for testing as well as perform the tests with the covering physician and recover the patients after testing. Last, a patient coordinator is helpful in maintaining the laboratory throughput and efficiency. All staff members must have received training in basic life support.[1] Because many patients referred for cardiac PET are at higher risk than those referred for cardiac single photon emission computed tomography (SPECT), training in advanced cardiac life support is strongly encouraged.

Patient Preparation and Screening

Patient preparation and screening are key components for a successful cardiac PET or PET/CT laboratory. Patient preparation and screening begin at least 1 to 2 days prior to the study. The first step is to review the referring physician's order to correlate the procedure with history to determine whether there are any contraindications to testing and to confirm that the appropriate radiopharmaceuticals (e.g., fluorine-18 fluoro-2-deoxyglucose [^{18}F-FDG] when viability testing is required) are available for the exam. Second, the patient should be contacted (2 days prior to exam if possible) with instructions to fast (except for water) for a minimum of 6 hours prior to the exam and to refrain from caffeine-containing foods (e.g., chocolate) and beverages (e.g., tea, coffee) for a minimum of 12–24 hours prior to the exam. The patient must also discontinue theophylline-containing medications for at least 48 hours prior to the exam, and if the patient is diabetic, he or she should be instructed about insulin administration prior to the test according to institutional protocols. To perform a vasodilator stress test (adenosine or dipyridamole), oral dipyridamole, including dipyridamole-containing medications such as aggrenox, should be held for 48 hours prior to the test, if medically feasible. If not, these patients should be stressed using dobutamine. Last, patients should be given a brief overview of the exam. This helps reduce patient anxiety and also helps to identify those patients with claustrophobia prior to the exam day.

Patient preparation on the day of the exam begins on arrival. A patient's first encounter may be the most important in establishing trust and cooperation. A patient's perception concerning the quality of his or her care is formed during the first 30 seconds of the encounter. It is important to remember that patients usually have limited knowledge of nuclear medicine and that the term *nuclear* alone as well as the term *stress test* can often cause uneasiness and fear. Therefore, it is important that each individual involved with the patient be professional and courteous. Patient cooperation is essential to a quality outcome of the study.

Once the patient has arrived for the exam, he or she should be placed in a designated room for test preparation. In this room, the patient will have an intravenous (IV) line placed, ECG leads, and an ECG monitoring system placed using the modified Likar's positioning (Figure 9.1). The patient is given a standard medical screening in preparation for the stress test[3,4] (Figure 9.2). On completion of the medical screening, the patient will have a focused physical exam including vital signs and cardiopulmonary exams. Once the patient has been completely evaluated for testing, 3 essential questions should be answered:

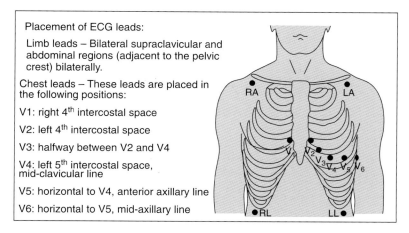

FIGURE 9.1. Recommended lead placement for stress testing (Mason-Likar modification). RA, right arm lead; LA, left arm lead; LL, left leg lead; RL, right leg lead. ("Figure 12—lead ECG System on page 286", from Bioelectromagnetism: Principles and Applications of Bioelectric and Biomagnetic Fields by Jaakko Malmivuo and Robert Plonsey, copyright © 1995 by Oxford University Press, Inc. Image adapted and reproduced by permission of Oxford University Press, Inc.)

Nuclear Cardiology Laboratory, XYZ Hospital

PATIENT
IDENTIFICATION
AREA

ID: NAME:

Date of test: __/__/__   [__] Outpatient   [__] In-patient

Test Location - Nuclear Medicine/Cardiology

DEMOGRAPHICS:

DOB: Age: Sex: ☐ Male   ☐ Female

Height (in):_____   Weight: (lbs)_____ **(kg)_____ BSA:_____

Address& Phone:_____

STAFF PHYSICIAN: _____, MD, **REFERRING PHYSICIAN:**_____, MD

FELLOW: PHYSIOLOGIST: TECHNOLOGIST:

MOST RECENT STRESS TEST:

FIGURE 9.2. Standard medical screening form.

1. Is the correct test being performed?
2. Are there contraindications for testing? (see "Stress-Testing Protocols," below)
3. What is the individualized patient risk associated with testing?

   Once the patient has had a thorough screening, a detailed explanation of the test should be given. This is of particular importance not only to alleviate the patient's anxiety but also to enhance patient cooperation. For instance, it is vital that the patient be aware of how movement and abnormal breathing will alter the exam results. The last step in the patient-screening procedures is the informed consent. At this point, the patient should have a clear understanding of the specific benefits and risks that are involved with the procedure and should provide written informed consent to proceed with the exam.

BRIEF HISTORY:

Cardiac Risk Factors	Yes
Hypertension	
Dyslipidemia	
Diabetes mellitus	
Family Hx	
Tobacco	
Obesity	
Postmenopausal	
None	

Prior Cardiac History	Date
No Cardiac Hx	
Recent MI (< 1month)	
Prior MI (>1 month)	
CABG	
PTCA	
CHF	
Valvular Dz	
Vascular Dz	

Chest Pain History		
Substernal	Yes	No
Exertional	Yes	No
Relieved by rest / NTG	Yes	No
NYHA Class		
I		
II		
III		
IV		

REASON FOR TEST	YES		YES	COMMENTS
Chest pain evaluation		Post-MI evaluation		
Dyspnea		Post-CABG		
Palpitations		Post-PCI		
Pre-op evaluation		Assess Myocardial Viability		
Pre-Transplant eval		Arrhythmias		
CHF		Other		
Allergies:				
MEDICATIONS	YES		YES	COMMENTS
Digoxin		Nitrates		
Betablockers		ACE inhibitors		
Ca Blockers		Other		

FIGURE 9.2. *Continued.*

Stress-Testing Protocols

Selection of the stress protocol for PET and PET/CT myocardial perfusion studies depends on the patient and the clinical question at hand. This section reviews the stressors and protocols, pharmacology, and contraindications.

Vasodilators

Adenosine is a direct coronary vasodilator, whereas dipyridamole blocks the cellular reuptake of adenosine, thereby increasing the plasma concentration of adenosine and causing vasodilation. Intravenous adenosine and dipyridamole cause maximal coronary vasodilation by direct relaxation of vascular smooth muscle cells at both epicardial and resistance vessels (primarily endothelium-independent mechanism). However, there is evidence that ~20% of the maximal coronary vasodilator response caused by adenosine or dipyridamole is related to the release of nitric oxide (NO) from intact endothelium due to increased shear stress on endothelial cells caused by the hyperemic response.[5] The flow increase in response to adenosine is blunted in regions of the myocardium supplied by stenotic coronary arteries, resulting in a lower radiotracer concentration in those segments compared to those supplied by normal or nondiseased coronary arteries. There is also evidence that myocardial segments that are collateral dependent may experience an actual decrease in flow below resting flow (coronary steal) because of a decrease in collateral perfusion pressure.[6] Previously, hand grip has been used in conjunction with vasodilator stress testing to improve myocardial blood flow.[7] However, isometric exercise during vasodilator stress appears to result in blunting of peak hyperemic myocardial blood flow and hence is no longer used.[8]

Adenosine

Adenosine is infused through a peripheral IV line at 140μg/kg/min (0.14mg/kg/min) over 4 or 6 minutes using a pump. It induces peak hyperemia ~1 to 2 minutes after the start of the infusion, and myocardial blood flow returns rapidly to the baseline state within 2 minutes after cessation of adenosine administration.[9] The radiotracer is injected at midpoint into the infusion. It is optimal to have 2 intravenous lines for these patients so as to avoid bolusing or holding adenosine for the duration of radiotracer infusion (especially for the somewhat large ^{82}Rb infusion, 15–30mL). Heart rate, blood pressure, and ECG should be monitored and recorded every minute during the infusion and until the patient is back to baseline (usually within 5 minutes of termination).

Dipyridamole

Dipyridamole is infused through a peripheral IV line at 142μg/kg/min (0.56mg/kg total dose) over 4 minutes, using a pump or a manual injection. The FDA-approved maximal dose is 60mg. Dipyridamole causes local irritation at the site of injection, which can be minimized by a 1:1 dilution with normal saline. Maximal hyperemia is achieved 2 to 3 minutes after termination of the 4-minute infusion, at which point radiotracer injection should be performed. Heart rate, blood pressure, and 12-lead ECG should be monitored and recorded every minute during the infusion and until the patient returns to baseline. Aminophylline is given at 1mg/kg, as a slow IV bolus over 1 minute if the patient is symptomatic or if there are signs of ischemia (ST segment depression).

Inotropic Agents

Dobutamine is a potent β-1 agonist that increases myocardial oxygen demand by increasing myocardial contractility, heart rate, and blood pressure. The presence of a coronary stenosis can limit the flow increase in that vessel, leading to an imbalance in perfusion in that region compared to myocardium supplied by normal coronary arteries. Patients who cannot exercise and who are not good candidates for dipyridamole or adenosine because of contraindications, for example, chronic obstructive pulmonary disease, asthma, or high-degree atrioventricular block, would be good candidates for dobutamine-atropine stress.[10] In addition, one of the advantages of dobutamine over the vasodilator agents is the ability to assess the ischemic threshold with dobutamine.

Dobutamine is a synthetic catecholamine with a half-life of approximately 2 minutes. It is infused using standard protocols in 2- to 3-minute increments starting at 10μg/kg/min to a maximum of 40 to 50μg/kg/min. Additional IV atropine (increments of 0.25mg to a maximum of 2mg) may be used to increase heart rate in individuals with submaximal heart-rate response (<85% age-predicted maximal heart rate). A prior history of angle closure glaucoma, myasthenia gravis, obstructive gastrointestinal tract, and prostatism are relative contraindications to atropine administration.[11] When maximal heart rate is achieved, the radiotracer is injected and dobutamine infusion continued for an additional 1 to 2 minutes. As with adenosine protocols, 2 intravenous lines are required for dobutamine protocols, so as to avoid bolusing or holding dobutamine during the duration of radiotracer infusion.

Exercise

Circulatory and hemodynamic response to exercise is complex. Briefly, in response to exercise, circulating catecholamines increase and lead to increased heart rate and myocardial contractility. This results in increased myocardial oxygen consumption and in normal hearts increased myocardial blood flow. This response is abnormal in areas of the myocardium supplied by diseased coronary arteries, due to fixed coronary stenosis, leading to reduced myocardial blood flow relative to demand and stress-induced ischemia. Exercise stress is physiological and provides clinical (chest pain), hemodynamic (blood pressure changes) and electrocardiographic (ST segment changes) information that is invaluable in the clinical management of patients with suspected or known coronary artery disease.[12] Exercise protocols can also be tailored to the patient's exercise capacity and the reason for the test. Treadmill exercise is widely used in the United States, while upright bicycle exercise is preferred in other countries. Supine bicycle exercise is more convenient to use with PET imaging,[13] but patient motion remains a consideration, especially if dynamic imaging for absolute coronary blood flow quantitation is planned. Upright bicycle exercise or treadmill exercise[14] have also been used with ^{82}Rb[14] and N-13 ammonia (^{13}N-ammonia). However, attention to occupational radiation exposure to staff personnel is required, especially in connection with the large radioactive doses required for ^{82}Rb.

Relative Efficacy of Stressors on Hyperemic Myocardial Blood Flow

In normal coronary arteries, adenosine (and dipyridamole) induces coronary vasodilatation by activation of coronary adenosine A_{2A} receptors and increases coronary blood flow to 4 to 5 times baseline levels. Theophylline and methylxanthine competitively inhibit adenosine receptors. Consequently, caffeine intake can blunt increases in peak myocardial blood flow during hyperemia, resulting in artificially low coronary flow reserve.[15] Thus, it is important to instruct patients to avoid intake of caffeinated food and beverages, including decaffeinated beverages or medications, 12 to 24 hours prior to vasodilator stress testing. The normal hyperemic myocardial blood response to vasodilator stressors[16] was initially felt to be significantly greater than that of exercise or dobutamine stress.[17] However, more recently, 20 normal volunteers were studied using oxygen-15 water (^{15}O-water), and myocardial blood flow during maximal dobutamine with atropine infusions was shown to be similar to that of dipyridamole infusion (Figure 9.3).[18] This difference of myocardial blood flow was caused partly by the increased heart rate associated with atropine infusion (mean heart rate of 110 bpm for dobutamine vs 163 bpm for dobutamine with atropine). Second, the prior study used ^{13}N-ammonia, and myocardial blood flow estimated by this tracer is lower than that obtained by using ^{15}O-water.[18]

Sympathetic stimulation caused by exercise causes an increase in heart rate and myocardial contractility, resulting in an increase in myocardial metabolism and a compensatory increase in coronary blood flow via metabolic autoregulation. This increase is not seen in diseased coronary arteries, due to baseline vasodilation resulting in lower coronary flow and reduced radiotracer delivery to myocardial segments supplied by stenosed coronary arteries.

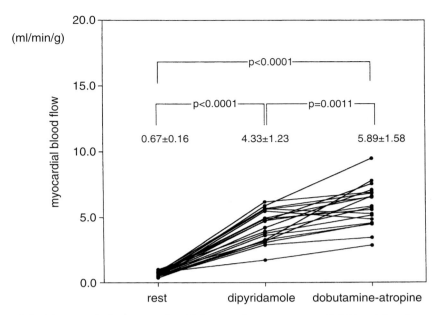

FIGURE 9.3. Line graph demonstrating higher peak stress myocardial blood flow in response to maximal dobutamine-atropine stress compared to dipyridamole. (From Tadamura E, Iida H, Matsumoto K, et al. Comparison of myocardial blood flow during butamine-atropine infusion with that after dipyridamole administration in normal men. J Amer Coll Cardiol. 2001;37:130–136. Reprinted with permission from the American College of Cardiology Foundation (18).)

Side Effects of Pharmacologic Stressors

Adenosine is known to activate all 4 known adenosine receptor subtypes (A_1, A_{2A}, A_{2B}, and A_3). Flushing and lightheadedness or dizziness may be seen due to stimulation of peripheral A_{2A} and possibly A_{2B} adenosine receptors. First- and second-degree atrioventricular (AV) block (6%) may result from stimulation of A_1 receptors in the AV node. Bronchoconstriction may be seen in subjects with bronchospastic lung disease, due to stimulation of A_{2B} and possibly A_3 receptors. Side effects from adenosine, albeit minor, are reported in a large proportion of patients (~60%–75%). However, they rarely require termination of infusion or administration of aminophylline. More serious side effects are rare and can be treated with intravenous aminophylline (1 mg/kg IV).[19] Side effects from adenosine and dipyridamole have prompted development of newer selective adenosine A_{2A} receptor agonists. Due to their selective activation of A_{2A} receptors, if approved these agents may potentially be tested in the future for patients with bronchoconstrictive diseases, in whom we currently we use dobutamine.

Side effects from dipyridamole are less intense compared to those of adenosine. Heart block is less commonly seen with dipyridamole, while headache and stinging at the site of injection are more frequent. If bothersome or serious, side effects can be treated with intravenous aminophylline as described above.[20]

Dobutamine infusion may result in nausea, vomiting, palpitations, chest pain, hypotension, and arrhythmias.[21] Since dobutamine increases myocardial oxygen demand, although uncommon, it can potentially induce true ischemia and angina. No incidence of myocardial infarction or death was reported in 2 studies.[21,22] Dobutamine is avoided in patients with aortic aneurysms (>6cm), patients immediately postmyocardial infarction, and patients with acute unstable angina.

Absolute contraindications for stress testing in general are listed below:

- Acute myocardial infarction (within 2 days)
- Unstable angina not previously stabilized by medical therapy. Appropriate timing of testing depends on level of risk of unstable angina, as defined by Agency for Healthcare Research and Quality (AHRQ) Unstable Angina Guidelines.

- Uncontrolled cardiac arrhythmias causing symptoms or hemodynamic compromise
- Symptomatic severe aortic stenosis
- Uncontrolled symptomatic heart failure
- Acute pulmonary embolus or pulmonary infarction
- Acute myocarditis or pericarditis
- Acute aortic dissection

Relative contraindications can be superseded if the benefits of exercise outweigh the risks. Relative contraindications for stress testing include the following:

- Moderate stenotic valvular heart disease
- Electrolyte abnormalities
- Severe arterial hypertension (systolic blood pressure >220 mm Hg and/or diastolic blood pressure >110 mm Hg)
- Severe arterial hypotension (systolic blood pressure <90 mm Hg)
- Tachyarrhythmias or bradyarrhythmias
- Hypertrophic cardiomyopathy and other forms of outflow tract obstruction

(Absolute contraindications and relative contraindications for stress testing adapted from Gibbons et al.[23] with permission from the American College of Cardiology Foundation.)

Specific contraindications to adenosine or dipyridamole include the following:

- Second- or third-degree AV block without a functioning artificial pacemaker
- Sinus node disease or symptomatic bradycardia without a functioning artificial pacemaker
- Bronchospastic lung disease (e.g., asthma, chronic obstructive pulmonary disease)
- Known hypersensitivity to adenosine or dipyridamole
- Intake of theophylline, oral dipyridamole, or dipyridamole-containing compounds (e.g., Aggrenox) within 48 hours of the test

Summary Points

- Cardiac PET and PET/CT will most certainly play a more significant role in the future of nuclear cardiology. Ideally, all patients referred for pharmacologic stress testing will be referred for a cardiac PET study. However, when this is not possible, specific categories of patients, including the obese, females, and those with indeterminate SPECT exams could benefit from PET myocardial perfusion imaging.
- Patient preparation plays an essential role in the efficiency and satisfaction of any stress-testing laboratory.
- Together, cardiac SPECT and cardiac PET and PET/CT have the potential to become a gold standard in cardiac testing, decreasing the amount of diagnostic invasive procedures performed.

References

1. Pina IL, Balady GJ, Hanson P, Labovitz AJ, Madonna DW, Myers J. Guidelines for clinical exercise testing laboratories. A statement for healthcare professionals from the Committee on Exercise and Cardiac Rehabilitation, American Heart Association. *Circulation*. 1995;91:912–921.
2. Franklin BA. *ACSM's Guidelines for Exercise Testing and Prescription*. 6th ed. Spiral ed. Baltimore: Lippincott Williams & Wilkins; 2000.
3. Malmivuo J, Plonsey R. *Bioelectromagnetism : Principles and Applications of Bioelectric and Biomagnetic Fields*. New York: Oxford University Press; 1995.

4. Pina IL, Chahine RA. Lead systems: sensitivity and specificity. *Cardiol Clin.* 1984;2: 329–335.

5. Buus NH, Bottcher M, Hermansen F, Sander M, Nielsen TT, Mulvany MJ. Influence of nitric oxide synthase and adrenergic inhibition on adenosine-induced myocardial hyperemia. *Circulation.* 2001;104:2305–2310.

6. Becker LC. Conditions for vasodilator-induced coronary steal in experimental myocardial ischemia. *Circulation.* 1978;57:1103–1110.

7. Brown BG, Josephson MA, Petersen RB, et al. Intravenous dipyridamole combined with isometric handgrip for near maximal acute increase in coronary flow in patients with coronary artery disease. *Am J Cardiol.* 1981;48:1077–1085.

8. Czernin J, Auerbach M, Sun KT, Phelps M, Schelbert HR. Effects of modified pharmacologic stress approaches on hyperemic myocardial blood flow. *J Nucl Med.* 1995;36: 575–580.

9. Wilson RF, Wyche K, Christensen BV, Zimmer S, Laxson DD. Effects of adenosine on human coronary arterial circulation. *Circulation.* 1990;82:1595–1606.

10. Iskandrian AS, Verani MS, Heo J. Pharmacologic stress testing: mechanism of action, hemodynamic responses, and results in detection of coronary artery disease. *J Nucl Cardiol.* 1994;1:94–111.

11. Elhendy A, van Domburg RT, Bax JJ, et al. Dobutamine-atropine stress myocardial perfusion SPECT imaging in the diagnosis of graft stenosis after coronary artery bypass grafting. *J Nucl Cardiol.* 1998;5:491–497.

12. Guidelines for exercise testing. A report of the American College of Cardiology/American Heart Association Task Force on Assessment of Cardiovascular Procedures (Subcommittee on Exercise Testing). *J Am Coll Cardiol.* 1986;8:725–738.

13. Wyss CA, Koepfli P, Mikolajczyk K, Burger C, von Schulthess GK, Kaufmann PA. Bicycle exercise stress in PET for assessment of coronary flow reserve: repeatability and comparison with adenosine stress. *J Nucl Med.* 2003;44:146–154.

14. Chow BJ, Ananthasubramaniam K, dekemp RA, Dalipaj MM, Beanlands RS, Ruddy TD. Comparison of treadmill exercise versus dipyridamole stress with myocardial perfusion imaging using rubidium-82 positron emission tomography. *J Am Coll Cardiol.* 2005;45: 1227–1234.

15. Bottcher M, Czernin J, Sun KT, Phelps ME, Schelbert HR. Effect of caffeine on myocardial blood flow at rest and during pharmacological vasodilation. *J Nucl Med.* 1995;36: 2016–2021.

16. Di Carli M, Czernin J, Hoh CK, et al. Relation among stenosis severity, myocardial blood flow, and flow reserve in patients with coronary artery disease. *Circulation.* 1995;91: 1944–1951.

17. Krivokapich J, Smith GT, Huang SC, et al. 13N ammonia myocardial imaging at rest and with exercise in normal volunteers. Quantification of absolute myocardial perfusion with dynamic positron emission tomography. *Circulation.* 1989;80:1328–1337.

18. Tadamura E, Iida H, Matsumoto K, et al. Comparison of myocardial blood flow during dobutamine-atropine infusion with that after dipyridamole administration in normal men. *J Am Coll Cardiol.* 2001;37:130–136.

19. Cerqueira MD, Verani MS, Schwaiger M, Heo J, Iskandrian AS. Safety profile of adenosine stress perfusion imaging: results from the Adenoscan Multicenter Trial Registry. *J Am Coll Cardiol.* 1994;23:384–389.

20. Lette J, Tatum JL, Fraser S, et al. Safety of dipyridamole testing in 73,806 patients: the Multicenter Dipyridamole Safety Study. *J Nucl Cardiol.* 1995;2:3–17.

21. Elhendy A, Valkema R, van Domburg RT, et al. Safety of dobutamine-atropine stress myocardial perfusion scintigraphy. *J Nucl Med.* 1998;39:1662–1666.

22. Dakik HA, Vempathy H, Verani MS. Tolerance, hemodynamic changes, and safety of dobutamine stress perfusion imaging. *J Nucl Cardiol.* 1996;3:410–414.

23. Gibbons RJ, Balady GJ, Beasley JW, et al. ACC/AHA Guidelines for Exercise Testing. A report of the American College of Cardiology/American Heart Association Task Force on Practice Guidelines (Committee on Exercise Testing). *J Am Coll Cardiol.* 1997;30: 260–311.

10 PET and Integrated PET/CT Myocardial Imaging Protocols and Quality Assurance

Sharmila Dorbala and Marcelo F. Di Carli

The primary clinical applications of positron emission tomography (PET) myocardial perfusion imaging are to diagnose, localize, and quantify the severity of coronary artery stenoses. As a result, most clinical applications of myocardial perfusion imaging are performed in conjunction with stress testing. Exercise stress testing with single photon emission computed tomography (SPECT) is widely used in the evaluation of patients with known or suspected coronary artery disease.[1-3] Although exercise stress testing offers several advantages, the short physical half-life of most PET radiotracers makes it logistically impractical for use in conjunction with PET imaging. In addition, a significant proportion of patients referred for stress imaging are unable to exercise adequately due to difficulties with ambulation related to prior stroke, peripheral vascular disease, orthopedic problems or deconditioning.[3] Submaximal exercise can reduce test sensitivity for detection of ischemic heart disease and should be avoided. Pharmacologic stress testing with dipyridamole,[4,5] adenosine[4,6,7] or dobutamine infusions[8-9] are useful to evaluate patients that are unable to exercise or have suboptimal exercise capicity.[3] Chapter 9 provides a detailed discussion of stress protocols. The aim of this chapter is to provide a review of clinically useful imaging protocols for evaluation of CAD, along with guidelines for quality control of PET and PET/CT images. For a better understanding of protocols for PET myocardial perfusion imaging, the reader should be familiar with basic principles of PET and PET/CT (discussed in Chapters 1 and 3) and PET radiopharmaceuticals (discussed in Chapter 5).

Myocardial Perfusion Imaging Protocols

Imaging protocols are tailored to the clinical question and vary depending on the radiotracer and stress protocol used. The differences in imaging protocols among the 3 PET perfusion tracers are summarized in Table 10.1.

Imaging protocols for PET and integrated PET/CT imaging using different myocardial perfusion imaging agents are shown in Figures 10.1 through 10.3. Imaging protocols using adenosine stress are shown in Figure 10.2A-E. For clinical imaging, rubidium-82 (^{82}Rb) or nitrogen-13 (^{13}N)-ammonia is used, with either single-frame (gated or nongated) or multiframe (dynamic) imaging. Single-frame gated imaging is the standard for both rest and stress components of the study. This protocol allows measurements of left ventricular (LV) function at rest and during peak stress, thereby

TABLE 10.1. Differences in Imaging Protocols for the 3 Commonly Used PET Perfusion Radiotracers

Characteristic	^{13}N-ammonia	^{82}Rb	^{15}O-water
Image acquisition	Dynamic/static/gated	Dynamic/static/gated	Dynamic
Prescan delay*	3 minutes	70–90 seconds	N/A
	4–7 minutes: longer circulation time	120 seconds: longer circulation time	
Dose-2D	15–25 mCi	40–60 mCi	40 mCi
Dose-3D	15 mCi	15–20 mCi	10 mCi
		30–40 mCi 3D LSO	
Interval between doses	50 minutes	10 minutes	7 minutes
Scan duration	~20 minutes	~6 minutes	~5 minutes
Mode of stress	Treadmill, bicycle	Treadmill, bicycle	Supine bicycle
	Adenosine, dipyridamole, or dobutamine	Adenosine, dipyridamole, or dobutamine	Adenosine, dipyridamole, or dobutamine
Laboratory throughput	Good	Excellent	N/A
Cyclotron on-site	Yes	No	Yes
Semiquantitative image interpretation	Yes	Yes	No

*Longer circulation time: if left ventricular ejection fraction <30%, severe chronic obstructive pulmonary disease, occlusion of proximal vein.

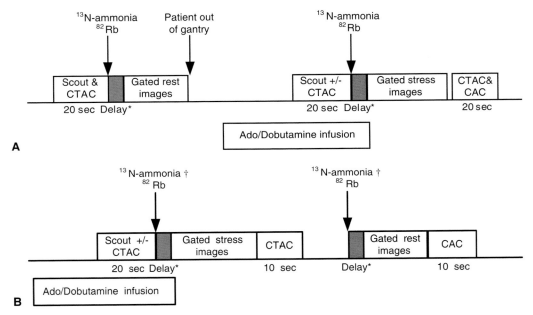

FIGURE 10.1. Schematic of protocols using PET and integrated PET/CT with different myocardial perfusion imaging agents, and adenosine or dobutamine stress. CTAC: CT attenuation correction and PET-AC: radionuclide transmission scan. Radiotracer dose: ^{82}Rb—40–60 mCi for 2D; 15–20 mCi for 3D. ^{13}N-ammonia: 15–25 mCi; recommended 50-minute delay between repeat injections or low and high dose (15 mCi for rest followed by 30 mCi for stress). *Delay: prescan delay from injection of radiotracer to beginning of image acquisition. ^{82}Rb: 70–90 seconds is standard; if longer circulation time is anticipated, 120 seconds is applied (see text); for 3D acquisition 180 seconds is standard. ^{13}N-ammonia: 3 minute is standard; if long circulation time, 4–7 minutes; for 3D acquisition, 7 minute prescan delay is used. Scout and CTAC are started at middle of adenosine infusion and 1–2 minutes prior to stopping dobutamine infusion and may be obtained after injection of radiotracer for ^{13}N-ammonia. Stress and rest image duration: ^{82}Rb—5 minutes for 2D and 3 minutes for 3D acquisition; ^{13}N-ammonia—15 minutes. CAC: calcium score, which is optional on PET/CT systems. Dynamic protocols: gated rest images recommended before stress to avoid effects of stunning. †Moving patient out of the gantry between rest and stress studies and repositioning with a repeat scout and if needed a repeat CTAC study as shown in Figures 10.1A and C, 10.2A and C, and 10.3B will improve patient tolerability of the test, particularly with ^{13}N-ammonia imaging. ‡List mode acquisition is available with the latest generation PET/CT scanners eliminating the need for a separate dynamic and gated study.

providing a powerful adjunct to perfusion imaging for diagnosing and assessing risk in CAD. Multiframe imaging is used in protocols in which measurements of coronary blood flow and flow reserve are planned. As described in Chapter 5, laboratories using ^{13}N-ammonia require a very tight coordination between the timing of imaging and delivery of the radiotracer from the cyclotron laboratory. Adenosine protocols are simple to perform and quick. They require two intravenous (IV) lines, one for the adenosine infusion and the other for the radiotracer injection. Also, the more pronounced side effects from adenosine infusion (as compared to dipyridamole) may predispose to artifacts from patient motion or breathing motion.

Imaging protocols using dipyridamole stress are shown in Figure 10.2A–E. The less intense side effects from the more gradual onset of hyperemia with dipyridamole make this protocol more acceptable to some patients. Peak hyperemia is achieved between 2 and 3 minutes after completing the dipyridamole infusion. Thus, the same IV line can be used for the radiotracer injection. In addition, this brief time delay makes it practical for technologists to sequentially complete all steps of image acquisition without time pressure.

Imaging protocols for dobutamine stress are shown in Figures 10.1A–E. As with vasodilators, gated dobutamine-stress images (especially with [82]Rb) are obtained at very close to maximal stress and may demonstrate ischemic wall motion abnormalities and effects of global stunning on LV ejection fraction (EF). Like adenosine stress, dobutamine also requires two IV lines.

Imaging protocols for exercise PET exercise myocardial perfusion imaging are shown in Figures 10.3A and B. Treadmill exercise PET is best performed in

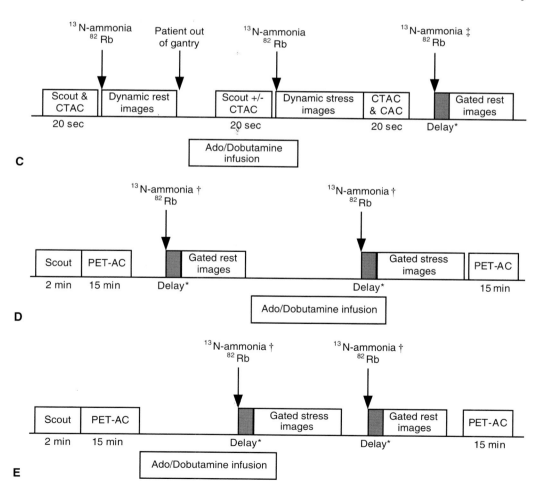

FIGURE 10.1. *Continued.*

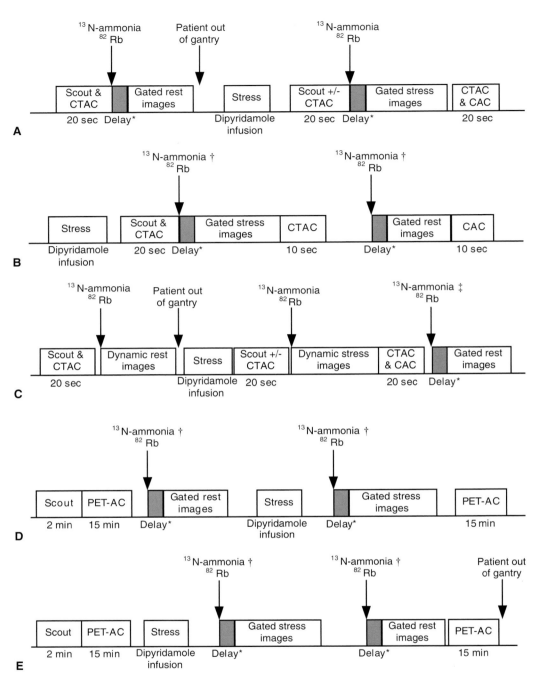

FIGURE 10.2. Schematic of protocols using PET and integrated PET/CT with different myocardial perfusion imaging agents and dipyridamole stress. Definitions are identical to those in Figure 10.1.

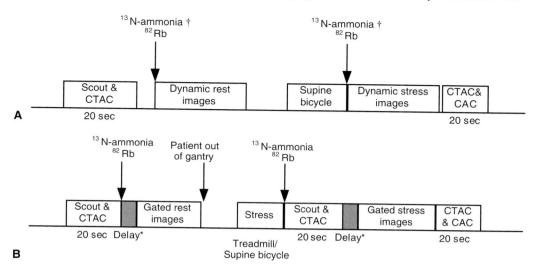

FIGURE 10.3. Schematic of protocols using PET and integrated PET/CT with different myocardial perfusion imaging agents and exercise stress.

conjunction with ^{13}N-ammonia (9.96-minute half-life) but is also feasible with ^{82}Rb imaging. The short half-life of ^{82}Rb (76 seconds) makes it technically challenging to combine it with treadmill exercise.[10–12] Supine bicycle stress imaging with single-frame or multiframe imaging is also possible for ^{13}N-ammonia imaging.[13,14] Exercise PET imaging is time inefficient compared to pharmacological stress testing. In addition, it may result in greater radiation exposure to staff personnel conducting the test. This may become the rate-limiting step as laboratory volume increases.

Performing Myocardial Perfusion Imaging

There are two important factors to consider in imaging obese individuals: the PET table weight limit and gantry diameter. Although these parameters may vary among the different manufacturers, the usual table weight limit is around 180 kg, and gantry diameter is larger for newer PET/CT systems compared to older, dedicated, PET-only systems (70 cm vs 55 cm). Other patient-related factors that may be important to consider for PET myocardial perfusion imaging are claustrophobia, ability to follow commands and to raise the arms above shoulders, and ability to lie still for the duration of the scan.

Patient Positioning

Patients are usually imaged supine with arms raised above their shoulders. This can be achieved with arm support and is usually well tolerated. In patients unable to raise their arms, imaging could be performed with arms at the side of the patient. However, it is important to maintain the same arm position during transmission and emission imaging to avoid artifacts. Arms-down imaging can be problematic when using integrated PET/CT systems because the dense bones in the arms may result in streak artifacts from beam hardening. These artifacts may adversely impact the quality of the CT transmission scan and consequently the emission images. In very large patients, arms-down imaging may result in a tight fit within the gantry and lead to truncation artifacts. Finally, with arms-down imaging, residual activity within the IV line may be seen within the field of view, resulting in difficulties with image normalization.

Scout Scan

The scout scan is a simple topographic image of the body, used to ensure appropriate patient positioning. Using dedicated PET systems, a scout scan can be obtained with a fast (~2-minute) transmission scan with an external coincidence source of germanium-68/gallium-68 (^{68}Ge/^{68}Ga). For laboratories using ^{82}Rb, the scout scan can also be obtained with an emission image following a small amount of the radiotracer (~10–20 mCi). With integrated PET/CT systems, a scout image is obtained in about 5 seconds using a low-energy CT scan (10 mA). In patients with enlarged heart size, both an anteroposterior (AP) and a lateral scout may sometimes be necessary for appropriate localization of the heart volume in the chest. The typical landmarks used for the scout are bifurcation of the trachea as the upper margin; usually the lower margin of the heart fits well within the field using this landmark (Figure 10.4). The size of the heart on the scout image in PET/CT systems can be used to estimate circulation and blood pool clearance times and to assist in selection of optimum prescan delay time (described below).

Transmission Scan

Transmission scans can be obtained using ^{68}Ge/^{68}Ga rod sources in dedicated PET systems or using a CT scan or cesium-137 (^{137}Cs) point sources in integrated PET/CT systems. As described in Chapter 1, this transmission tomogram provides anatomically specific density maps of the thorax that are used to correct PET image data for photon attenuation. Adequate coregistration between the transmission and emission data is key to obtaining artifact-free images. The clinical implications of using conventional (gamma-ray sources) versus CT-based transmission imaging are summarized in Table 10.2. The main advantages of CT-based transmission imaging are the consistent quality of transmission maps and the speed that results in greater patient tolerance and improved throughput. However, the main disadvantage relates to the relatively higher frequency of misregistration between transmission and emission images that often results in artifacts. Misregistration artifacts with CT are more frequently seen during stress due to the differences in breathing patterns during peak hyperemic stress. In our experience, postemission (stress) transmission imaging minimizes this problem.[15] Metallic implants may lead to artifacts on CT transmission images.[16] Although stents, surgical clips, and pacemaker wires do not usually pose a problem, implantable cardioverter defibrillator (ICD) wires appear to affect attenua-

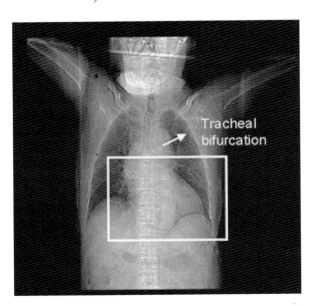

FIGURE 10.4. Scout scan obtained on a hybrid PET/CT system illustrating the selection of field of view for cardiac imaging.

TABLE 10.2. Clinical Differences Between Conventional Gamma Ray and CT-Based Transmission Imaging

Variable	CT-Transmission	Gamma Ray-Transmission
Source	X-ray	^{68}Ge/^{68}Ga rods or ^{137}Cs point source
Scan duration	10–20 seconds	4–15 minutes*
Breathing cycles	~2–3 breathing cycles	Many breathing cycles
Laboratory throughput	Excellent	Good
Misregistration from breathing	More frequent	Less frequent
Misregistration from patient motion	Less frequent	More frequent
Artifacts from metallic implants	Yes	No
Patient tolerance	Excellent	Good

*Depending on the age of sources.

tion correction and result in increased PET counts (hot spots).[17] Although it is theoretically possible that such hot spots may mask stress-induced perfusion defects, this has not been a problem in our practice. Impact of artificial heart valves on quality of transmission scans is not known, but is likely to be minimal.

Emission Scan

The duration of emission images and dose of injected radiotracer depend on a number of factors, such as the physical half-life of the radiotracer, the mode of acquisition (two-dimensional [2D] vs three-dimensional [3D]), and the type of scanner crystal (bismuth germanate [BGO] or lutetium oxyorthosilicate [LSO]/gadolinium oxyorthosilicate [GSO]), as described in Chapter 1. Typical scan durations are described in Table 10.1.

Single-Frame Gated Imaging

Single-frame imaging refers to acquisition of PET images into 1 bin (nongated or static) or to acquisitions into 8 or 16 bins with electrocardiogram (ECG) triggering (gated). Cardiac PET images can be gated to patient respiration or to the ECG. Although respiratory gating is of value in improving image resolution for oncology applications[18] and in radiation therapy planning, its value in cardiac imaging is not well established. A good ECG tracing will be necessary to ensure appropriate ECG triggering of image acquisition. Leads for gating ECG are placed with the patient's arms raised above the head to ensure secure placement without baseline sway during acquisition. An 8-frame gating is usually adequate for assessment of LV function and volumes. Higher frame gating (16 frame) may result in larger LV end diastolic volume (EDV) with higher LVEF,[19] without significant differences in detection of regional wall motion abnormalities.[20] Gating could be performed prospectively, retrospectively, combined prospectively and retrospectively, or using variable temporal resolution methods.[21] In prospective gating, the most commonly used mode, an average R-R interval, is used to set up a fixed gating interval. This mode has a fixed temporal resolution and is prone to error when there are changes in R-R cycle length during the acquisition. A fixed percentage of this R-R cycle is typically used to reject beats. Opening this gating window to accept counts within a wide range of the R-R interval may minimize count loss from gating errors, but this may result in wall-thickening errors and may adversely influence quantitative parameters, as shown with single photon emission computed tomography (SPECT) imaging.[22] Other available gating approaches include a retrospective gating with fixed temporal resolution, in which the gating is applied from the

TABLE 10.3. Differences Between Dynamic and Gated PET Myocardial Perfusion Imaging

Characteristic	Dynamic Imaging	Gated Imaging
Absolute MBF quantification	Yes	No
Frames	Multiple	Single
Estimation of LV function	No (possible with list mode acquisition)	Yes
Detection of ischemic WM abnl	No (possible with list mode acquisition)	Yes
Prescan delay	Accurate	Estimated
Image resolution	Excellent	Good
Clinical use	Uncommon	Widely used

Abbreviations: MBF, myocardial blood flow; LV, left ventricular; WM abnl, wall motion abnormality.

R wave backward and applied to data stored in memory, a combination of prospective and retrospective gating, and a variable temporal resolution method wherein an average of R-R intervals is adjusted dynamically to the last few heart beats. Gated images during pharmacological stress PET are acquired during peak stress and not poststress, as with SPECT imaging. This capability enables us to evaluate LV systolic function during peak stress, particularly with short-lived PET radiotracers such as [82]Rb. We found a decrease in LVEF from rest to peak hyperemic stress, as assessed by [82]Rb imaging, to be a useful marker of extensive stress-induced ischemia[15] and multivessel or left main CAD.[15] Although not yet studied, it is likely that this effect will be more pronounced with dynamic exercise or dobutamine imaging. Thus, gated PET imaging both at rest and during peak stress is important in evaluation of patients with suspected CAD. A more detailed discussion on the use of rest and peak stress-gating PET imaging is provided in Chapter 11.

Multiframe Imaging

With multiframe or dynamic imaging, image acquisition starts at the time of the radiotracer injection. A series of images (frames) are obtained rapidly over time to follow a dynamic process such as the change in radiotracer distribution over time. As discussed in Chapter 4, this acquisition mode is required to construct time-activity curves of radiotracer distribution for absolute measurements of myocardial blood flow.

As shown in Table 10.3, simultaneous acquisition of dynamic and gated images would be optimal for combined evaluation of quantitative myocardial blood flow and LV function. This is possible using list mode acquisition. In newer generation PET/CT scanners, list mode acquisition is either required or an option. Advances in computer and software technology now allow users to take advantage of this important option within the constraints of busy clinical workflows.

2D Versus 3D Acquisition

As discussed in Chapter 1, a 2D acquisition mode is one in which the lead septa are left in place, limiting random counts and scattered counts; in the 3D mode, the septa are left out, resulting in increased sensitivity (and also scatter) compared to 2D mode. There is a growing interest in using the 3D mode of acquisition for cardiac PET due to the increased sensitivity and the potential for using lower radiotracer doses, resulting in lower radiation exposure and possibly cost savings. However, 3D mode is not widely used for cardiac imaging. First, 3D mode requires significantly more acquisition and processing time and disc space,[23] although that may not be a limiting factor in the newer PET systems. Second, although 3D mode in principle affords significantly higher sensitivity than 2D mode, random counts and scatter may reduce its effective sensitivity. On 3D images, the noise equivalent count rate (NEC) and image quality may be improved by using lower doses of radiotracer, and the higher background noise can be minimized by prolonging the prescan delay (180 seconds for [82]Rb imaging). Despite these variations, 3D image quality may be suboptimal, particularly from PET systems with lower count-rate capabilities.[23,24] However, the effects of 3D acquisition on image quality and overall diagnosis of CAD (especially for [82]Rb) remain largely unknown.[25] Newer-generation PET systems equipped with LSO, GSO, or LYSO crystal technology (see Chapter 1) provide significantly higher count-rate capability and can potentially take full advantage of 3D imaging.

First-Pass Imaging

First-pass image acquisition has a high temporal resolution. Images are obtained in rapid succession to look at first-pass transit of radiotracer through the circulation. Since we image the radiotracer bolus as it enters the circulation, these images have very high count rates. These images are best obtained using PET systems with high count rate performance. First-pass imaging using [82]Rb has been validated to assess cardiac output and circulation times.[26,27]

Quality Assurance for PET and Integrated PET/CT Imaging

Adequate quality control of the imaging data is crucial to optimize clinical results. Quality control of the PET and PET/CT scanners is described in Chapters 1 and 3. Before the patient is allowed to leave the imaging room, images should be visually inspected to make sure that the quality is adequate. PET images are checked typically for the following features: count density, blood pool clearance, patient motion, attenuation correction, and image reconstruction artifacts.

Count Density

Both emission and transmission images (on dedicated PET systems) should be checked for adequacy of counts. Count-poor transmission images may be seen in dedicated PET systems when the radioactive sources are old or when imaging a large patient. Changing the source activity or acquiring longer transmission images could be considered. Count-poor emission images with poor signal-to-noise ratio may be seen occasionally. Some of the causes for count-poor images are listed in Table 10.4. Image count density directly influences diagnostic quality and reliability of the study. Troubleshooting count-poor studies must include checking the IV line for patency and kinking (Figure 10.5).

Blood Pool Clearance

Acquisition of emission images prior to complete clearance of radiotracer from the blood pool may potentially degrade image quality (Figure 10.6). Following

TABLE 10.4. Reasons for Count-Poor PET Images

1. High patient body mass index
2. Inadequate radiotracer dose
3. Poor scanner performance
4. Inadequate scan duration
5. Short half-life of radiotracer
6. Dietary and hormonal state in metabolic imaging

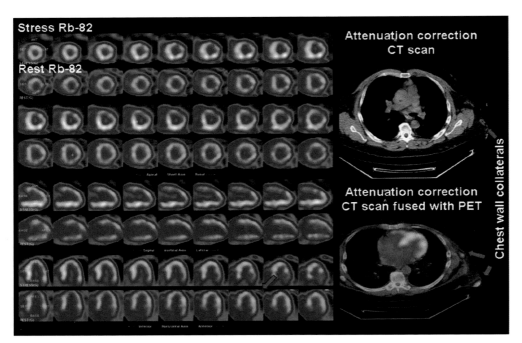

FIGURE **10.5.** Count-poor rest and stress ⁸²Rb study in a large patient studied with arms down. Fusion of the CT transmission and emission images (right panel) demonstrates intense radiotracer activity in the chest wall. This was a patient with known occlusion of the proximal veins in the right arm that led to delivery of radiotracer to the heart via well-formed chest wall collaterals (seen on the fusion image and the CT image). This resulted in increased arm-to-heart transit time and count-poor images due to decay of ⁸²Rb.

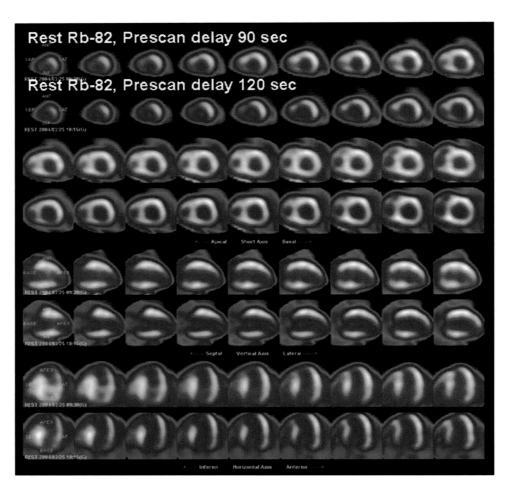

FIGURE 10.6. Sequential rest ⁸²Rb images obtained with a prescan delay of 90 seconds and 120 seconds in alternate rows, respectively. Repeat imaging with longer prescan delay improved image resolution and made the extent of the apical inferior wall defect more apparent. Images show reoriented ⁸²Rb images of the heart in short axis slices (top rows) extending from the left ventricular apex to base (from left to right), vertical long axis slices (middle rows) from the septum to the lateral wall (from left to right), and horizontal long axis slices (bottom rows) from inferior wall to anterior wall (from left to right).

intravenous injection, the radiotracer initially appears in the left ventricular blood pool and is subsequently taken up by the myocardium. Optimal image quality requires good signal-to-noise ratio, that is, good separation of blood pool activity from myocardial activity. The major determinant of time delay between radiotracer injection and optimal heart-to-blood-pool ratio is the arm-to-left-heart circulation time. The optimal prescan delay for ^{13}N-ammonia image acquisition is approximately 3 minutes and for ^{82}Rb images is between 70 and 90 seconds in normal patients. The most common factors that prolong circulation time include severe systolic dysfunction (LVEF <30%, either chronic or acute due to severe ischemia during stress) and intrinsic lung disease. A more infrequent factor includes proximal venous occlusion with flow into the chest via collaterals. Increased prescan delay (120 seconds for ^{82}Rb and 4–7 minutes for ^{13}N-ammonia) is helpful to improve image quality in cases of prolonged circulation time from any of the above factors.[28] If LVEF is not known, we may assess heart size on the scout CT image as a rough guide to LV dysfunction. As mentioned above, multiframe (i.e., dynamic) imaging can be extremely helpful in these situations for optimizing image quality.

Patient Motion

PET images are obtained by circular arrays of scintillation detectors; thus, patient movement during imaging affects all projections and can be very difficult to detect by direct inspection of the rotating projections, as assessed with SPECT imaging. Because transmission and emission imaging are sequential, patient motion during the emission images will most likely lead to misalignment between the two (Figure 10.7). The extent and direction of this misalignment will determine whether artifacts will be present on the attenuation corrected images. Images should be inspected for motion immediately upon completion. If misalignment is obvious, images should be repeated. Repeat imaging can be straightforward with generator-produced radiotracers such as ^{82}Rb but significantly more complicated for cyclotron products.

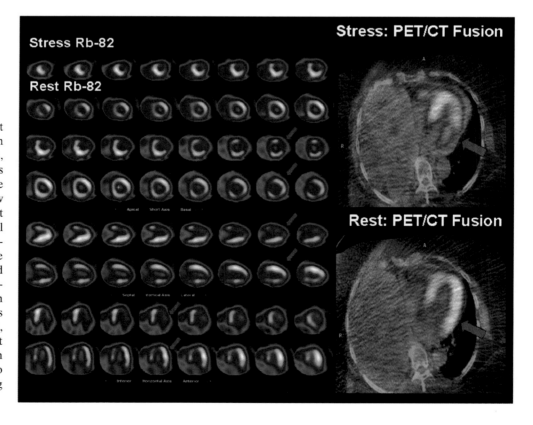

FIGURE 10.7. Stress and rest ^{82}Rb images of the heart in short axis, vertical long axis, and horizontal long axis slices as explained in Figure 10.6. The stress images show a severe perfusion defect throughout the anterolateral wall that is completely reversible at rest. Inspection of the fused transaxial emission and CT transmission images demonstrates a discontinuity in the lateral wall during stress related to patient motion, which was not seen on the rest images. The discontinuity in transmission images is also evident on the horizontal long axis images.

Attenuation Correction

Accurate attenuation correction is critical for PET images. The transmission images and attenuation map should be checked for quality. Image quality of CT transmission images may be suboptimal in heavy patients, but this has been shown not to adversely influence attenuation correction. Hence, it is not necessary to increase the CT dose in heavy patients. However, transmission images using ^{68}Ge/^{68}Ga or ^{137}Cs sources may require longer acquisition times to maintain quality as the strength of the radioactive source decreases. Because coincidence detection is the basis for PET imaging and each of the two photons is susceptible to attenuation, PET radiotracers are more prone to attenuation artifacts than SPECT radiotracers. Thus, reading of nonattenuation-corrected PET images is challenging and generally not recommended. Misregistration of transmission and emission images from respiration (Figures 10.8A and B) or from patient motion (Figure 10.7) can degrade image quality and result in false-positive scan results.[29–31] An example of misregistration of transmission and emission images is seen in Figure 10.8A, associated with a reversible anterior and anterolateral defect. Reprocessing the emission images with the CT transmission images obtained 5 minutes after completion of dipyridamole infusion (Figure 10.8B) shows resolution of the reversible defect, confirming that the previous image was an artifact from misregistration of transmission and emission images. Thus, checking for appropriate registration of transmission and emission images is crucial for interpretation of PET images.

Image Reconstruction Artifacts

Artifacts resulting from filtered backprojection reconstruction algorithms, image truncation, and beam hardening from CT transmission artifacts may be observed with cardiac PET and PET/CT imaging. As seen in SPECT myocardial perfusion imaging, excessive subdiaphragmatic activity from liver or bowel may result in decreased counts in the adjacent inferior wall myocardium when filtered backprojection is used for image reconstruction. This artifact may be particularly problematic if seen only on the stress images because it may cause an apparent reversible perfusion defect. Artifacts from filtered backprojection are not common with PET imaging since iterative methods are generally used for image reconstruction. Potential artifacts that could result from the position of the patient's arms are briefly discussed in the section on patient positioning. Image truncation artifacts appear as linear streaks through the reconstructed images. They can be seen in images of very large patients or images with a limited field-of-view reconstruction and are usually resolved by using full field-of-view reconstruction. Streak artifacts may be seen in large patients with arms-down imaging (a result of beam hardening from the large bones or metallic implants in the arm) or with metal implants in the field of view. In PET/CT systems that enable attenuation correction with either CT or an external radioactive source, a transmission scan with the radioactive source may be considered in these patients. There is preliminary evidence to suggest that a segmented reconstruction algorithm for the CT scan may help overcome artifacts from metallic implants.[32] Residual radiotracer activity in the IV line within the field of view may be an additional source of image reconstruction artifacts that can be minimized by flushing the IV tubing. A summary of the steps involved in a systematic approach to performing myocardial perfusion PET imaging is shown in Table 10.5.

Summary Points

- Widespread availability of PET/CT equipment has led to an exponential increase in the use of myocardial perfusion imaging for evaluation of patients with known or suspected CAD.

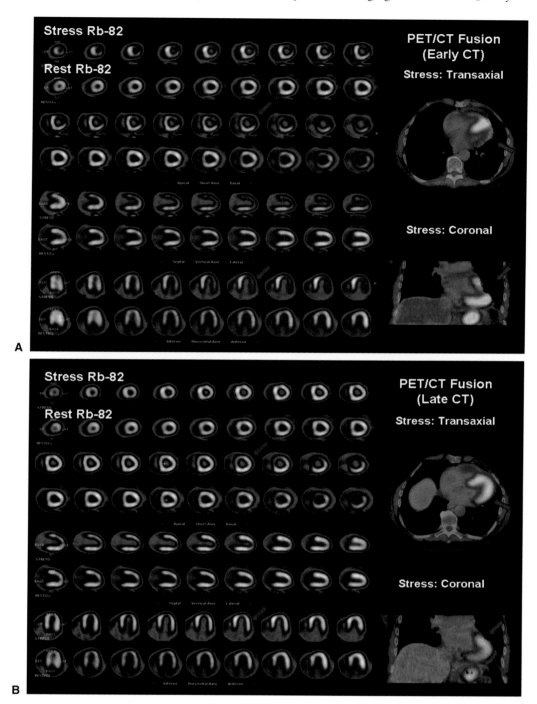

FIGURE 10.8. A and B. Stress and rest ^{82}Rb images of the heart in short axis, vertical long axis, and horizontal long axis slices as explained in Figure 10.6. The stress images show a perfusion defect of moderate intensity throughout the anterolateral wall that is completely reversible at rest. Inspection of the fused stress emission and CT transmission images show misregistration with emission image overlying the lung field, resulting in undercorrection and an apparent perfusion defect in the anterolateral wall.

TABLE 10.5. Systematic Approach to Performing PET and PET/CT Myocardial Perfusion Images

---

Before Examination

1. Check patient weight, chest circumference, claustrophobia
2. Identify contraindications to stress testing
3. Determine optimal patient positioning: supine, arms raised
4. Evaluate electrocardiogram for adequacy of gated imaging
5. Estimate prescan delay (ejection fraction, severe chronic obstructive pulmonary disease)

Examination Sequence

1. Scout for patient positioning
2. Transmission scan for attenuation correction
3. Emission scan

After Imaging

1. Quality control: count adequacy, blood pool clearance, patient motion, attenuation correction, image reconstruction artifacts
2. Image interpretation
3. Reporting

- Use of CT for localizing the heart (scout) and transmission imaging has increased laboratory throughput significantly.
- Both exercise and pharmacological stress are feasible for stress PET myocardial perfusion imaging. However, pharmacological stress protocols are simpler and more widely used.
- A single-frame 2D gated study is the most common mode of image acquisition, as 3D protocols are currently not well validated in humans.
- A rest-stress protocol with gated imaging both at rest and at peak stress is recommended. A decrease in LVEF from rest to peak hyperemic stress ^{82}Rb imaging is a useful marker of extensive stress-induced ischemia and multivessel or left main CAD.
- Absolute measurements of myocardial blood flow are feasible with multiframe or dynamic PET imaging, although they are being used primarily in the research arena.
- Quality control of PET images for adequacy of counts, adequate clearance of blood pool activity, motion artifacts, and appropriate attenuation correction and image reconstruction artifacts are critical to optimum image quality.

References

1. Ritchie JL, Trobaugh GB, Hamilton GW, et al. Myocardial imaging with thallium-201 at rest and during exercise. Comparison with coronary arteriography and resting and stress electrocardiography. *Circulation.* 1977;56:66–71.
2. Kotler TS, Diamond GA. Exercise thallium-201 scintigraphy in the diagnosis and prognosis of coronary artery disease. *Ann Intern Med.* 1990;113:684–702.
3. Tadamura E, Iida H, Matsumoto K, et al. Comparison of myocardial blood flow during dobutamine-atropine infusion with that after dipyridamole administration in normal men. *J Amer Coll Cardiol.* 2001;37:130–136.
4. Uren NG, Camici PG, Melin JA, et al. Effect of aging on myocardial perfusion reserve. *J Nucl Med.* 1995;36:2032–2036.
5. Laine H, Raitakari OT, Niinikoski H, et al. Early impairment of coronary flow reserve in young men with borderline hypertension. *J Am Coll Cardiol.* 1998;32:147–153.
6. Cerqueira MD, Verani MS, Schwaiger M, Heo J, Iskandrian AS. Safety profile of adenosine stress perfusion imaging: results from the Adenoscan Multicenter Trial Registry. *J Am Coll Cardiol.* 1994;23:384–389.

7. Kaufmann PA, Gnecchi-Ruscone T, Yap JT, Rimoldi O, Camici PG. Assessment of the reproducibility of baseline and hyperemic myocardial blood flow measurements with 15O-labeled water and PET. *J Nucl Med.* 1999;40:1848–1856.

8. Krivokapich J, Huang SC, Schelbert HR. Assessment of the effects of dobutamine on myocardial blood flow and oxidative metabolism in normal human subjects using nitrogen-13 ammonia and carbon-11 acetate. *Am J Cardiol.* 1993;71:1351–1356.

9. Hays JT, Mahmarian JJ, Cochran AJ, Verani MS. Dobutamine thallium-201 tomography for evaluating patients with suspected coronary artery disease unable to undergo exercise or vasodilator pharmacologic stress testing. *J Am Coll Cardiol.* 1993;21:1583–1590.

10. Beanlands RS, Muzik O, Melon P, et al. Noninvasive quantification of regional myocardial flow reserve in patients with coronary atherosclerosis using nitrogen-13 ammonia positron emission tomography. Determination of extent of altered vascular reactivity. *J Am Coll Cardiol.* 1995;26:1465–1475.

11. Lurie AJ, Salel AF, Berman DS, DeNardo GL, Hurley EJ, Mason DT. Determination of improved myocardial perfusion after aortocoronary bypass surgery by exercise rubidium-81 scintigraphy. *Circulation.* 1976;54:III20–III23.

12. Chow BJ, Ananthasubramaniam K, dekemp RA, Dalipaj MM, Beanlands RS, Ruddy TD. Comparison of treadmill exercise versus dipyridamole stress with myocardial perfusion imaging using rubidium-82 positron emission tomography. *J Am Coll Cardiol.* 2005;45: 1227–1234.

13. Krivokapich J, Smith GT, Huang SC, et al. 13N ammonia myocardial imaging at rest and with exercise in normal volunteers. Quantification of absolute myocardial perfusion with dynamic positron emission tomography. *Circulation.* 1989;80:1328–1337.

14. Wyss CA, Koepfli P, Mikolajczyk K, Burger C, von Schulthess GK, Kaufmann PA. Bicycle exercise stress in PET for assessment of coronary flow reserve: repeatability and comparison with adenosine stress. *J Nucl Med.* 2003;44:146–154.

15. Dorbala S, Limaye A, Crugnale S, Yang D, Fitzgerald J, Di Carli MF. Optimal timing of transmission map for rubidium 82 stress positron emission tomography (PET/CT) myocardial perfusion imaging. *J Nucl Med.* 2005;46:266p.

16. Joseph PM, Spital RD. The effects of scatter in x-ray computed tomography. *Med Phys.* 1982;9:464–472.

17. DiFilippo FP, Brunken RC. Do implanted pacemaker leads and ICD leads cause metal-related artifact in cardiac PET/CT? *J Nucl Med.* 2005;46:436–443.

18. Nehmeh SA, Erdi YE, Ling CC, et al. Effect of respiratory gating on quantifying PET images of lung cancer. *J Nucl Med.* 2002;43:876–881.

19. Navare SM, Wackers FJ, Liu YH. Comparison of 16-frame and 8-frame gated SPET imaging for determination of left ventricular volumes and ejection fraction. *Eur J Nucl Med Mol Imaging.* 2003;30:1330–1337.

20. Lalush DS, Jatko MK, Segars WP. An observer study methodology for evaluating detection of motion abnormalities in gated myocardial perfusion SPECT. *IEEE Trans Biomed Eng.* 2005;52:480–485.

21. Germano G. Digital techniques for acquisition, processing, and analysis of nuclear cardiology images. In: Sandler MP, Patton JA, Wackers FJT, Gottschalk A, eds. *Diagnostic Nuclear Medicine.* Lippincott Williams & Wilkins; 1996:207–222.

22. Nichols K, Dorbala S, DePuey EG, Yao SS, Sharma A, Rozanski A. Influence of arrhythmias on gated SPECT myocardial perfusion and function quantification. *J Nucl Med.* 1999;40:924–934.

23. Knesaurek K, Machac J, Krynyckyi BR, Almeida OD. Comparison of 2-dimensional and 3-dimensional 82Rb myocardial perfusion PET imaging. *J Nucl Med.* 2003;44: 1350–1356.

24. Votaw JR, White M. Comparison of 2-dimensional and 3-dimensional cardiac 82Rb PET studies. *J Nucl Med.* 2001;42:701–706.

25. Bacharach SL. The new generation positron emission tomography/computed tomography scanners: implications for cardiac imaging. In: Zaret BL, Beller GA, eds. *Clinical Nuclear Cardiology: State of the Art and Future Directions.* 2005:141–151.

26. Chen EQ, MacIntyre WJ, Fouad FM, et al. Measurement of cardiac output with first-pass determination during rubidium-82 PET myocardial perfusion imaging. *Eur J Nucl Med.* 1996;23:993–996.

27. Mullani NA, Gould KL. First-pass measurements of regional blood flow with external detectors. *J Nucl Med.* 1983;24:577–581.

28. Bacharach SL, Bax JJ, Case J, et al. PET myocardial glucose metabolism and perfusion imaging: Part 1—Guidelines for data acquisition and patient preparation. *J Nucl Cardiol.* 2003;10:543–556.
29. Bettinardi V, Gilardi MC, Lucignani G, et al. A procedure for patient repositioning and compensation for misalignment between transmission and emission data in PET heart studies. *J Nucl Med.* 1993;34:137–142.
30. McCord ME, Bacharach SL, Bonow RO, Dilsizian V, Cuocolo A, Freedman N. Misalignment between PET transmission and emission scans: its effect on myocardial imaging. *J Nucl Med.* 1992;33:1209–1214; discussion 1214–1215.
31. Loghin C, Sdringola S, Gould KL. Common artifacts in PET myocardial perfusion images due to attenuation-emission misregistration: clinical significance, causes, and solutions. *J Nucl Med.* 2004;45:1029–1039.
32. Mirzaei S, Guerchaft M, Bonnier C, Knoll P, Doat M, Braeutigam P. Use of segmented CT transmission map to avoid metal artifacts in PET images by a PET-CT device. *BMC Nucl Med.* 2005;5:3.

11 Myocardial Perfusion Imaging with PET

Marcelo F. Di Carli and Sharmila Dorbala

Over the past two decades, the experimental and clinical use of positron emission tomography (PET) has significantly contributed to the knowledge of cardiac physiology and metabolism. Positron tomography has emerged from the experimental arena and currently plays an important role in clinical cardiology.

Coronary stenoses may be diagnosed and located through PET myocardial perfusion imaging in patients with suspected ischemic heart disease. In addition, the physiological severity of known coronary stenoses may be precisely characterized since PET enables absolute quantification of coronary flow reserve (CFR). This chapter provides a review of myocardial perfusion assessment with PET for identification and characterization of clinical coronary artery disease (CAD), though we recognize that its clinical role continues to expand through ongoing research.

Myocardial Perfusion PET for Evaluating CAD

Chapter 10 provides a detailed discussion of the imaging protocols used in practice to evaluate myocardial perfusion with PET (Figures 10.1–10.3).

Preclinical CAD

The significant advances in our understanding of the mechanisms that initiate and facilitate the progression of coronary atherosclerosis have greatly improved our ability to target therapies aimed at preventing, halting progression, or promoting regression of atherosclerosis before it becomes clinically overt. Thus, cardiovascular medicine is witnessing a dramatic shift from the traditional paradigm of diagnosing obstructive CAD to a new paradigm in which the central goal is to detect patients who are at risk for developing CAD or who already have preclinical (albeit not obstructive) disease.

In this broader application, the traditional relative assessments of regional myocardial perfusion will likely be insensitive to identify preclinical CAD and thus will be of limited clinical value. It is now clear that endothelial dysfunction is an early event in atherosclerosis that precedes the development of structural changes in the coronary arteries; it is magnified in the presence of coronary risk factors and obstructive CAD. Consequently, endothelial dysfunction and its resulting consequences on coronary vasoreactivity are an attractive diagnostic target, especially for methods that can quantify coronary vasodilator dysfunction noninvasively, such as PET. Detection of patients at risk may offer an opportunity for early medical intervention aimed at halting the progression of atherogenesis and may ultimately lead to a reduction in cardiovascular events. In Chapter 12 the reader will find an in-depth discussion on the relationship between quantitative estimates of myocardial perfusion with PET and coronary risk factors and other measures of clinical risk.

Clinical CAD

PET has proven to be a powerful and efficient noninvasive imaging modality to evaluate regional myocardial perfusion in patients with known or suspected obstructive CAD. Several technical advantages, discussed in Chapter 1, account for the improved diagnostic power of PET. In addition, the use of short-lived radiopharmaceuticals allows fast, sequential assessment of regional myocardial perfusion (e.g., rest and stress), thereby improving laboratory efficiency and patient throughput (Figures 10.1–10.3).

Although these technical advantages have been recognized for a long time, the lack of widespread availability of PET cameras and radiotracers, its increased cost, and the sparse data supporting its use and reimbursement have all contributed to the limited clinical acceptance of this imaging technology. However, important recent developments, including changes in reimbursement and widespread availability of PET cameras due to the important role of PET in oncology, are rapidly changing the acceptance of PET in cardiology.

Diagnostic Accuracy of PET and PET/CT for Diagnosing CAD

The experience with PET for detecting obstructive CAD has been documented in 9 studies including 877 patients (Table 11.1). In these studies, regional myocardial perfusion was assessed with nitrogen-13 (^{13}N)-ammonia or rubidium-82 (^{82}Rb). The average sensitivity for detecting >50% angiographic stenosis was 91% (range, 83% to 100%), whereas the average specificity was 89% (range, 73% to 100%).

Comparative Studies of PET Versus SPECT

Three studies have performed a direct comparison of the diagnostic accuracy of ^{82}Rb PET and thallium-201 (^{201}Tl) or technetium-99 (^{99m}Tc) single photon emission

TABLE 11.1. Sensitivity and Specificity of PET for Detecting Obstructive CAD

Year	Author	Radiotracer	Prior MI (%)	Sensitivity (%)	Specificity (%)
2006	Bateman et al[4]	^{82}Rb	25	87	93
2006	Sampson et al[5]	^{82}Rb	None	93	83
1992	Marwick et al[6]	^{82}Rb	49	90	100
1992	Grover-McKay et al[7]	^{82}Rb	13	100	73
1991	Stewart et al[8]	^{82}Rb	42	83	86
1990	Go et al[9]	^{82}Rb	47	93	78
1989	Demer et al[10]	^{82}Rb/^{13}N-ammonia	34	83	95
1988	Tamaki et al[11]	^{13}N-ammonia	75	98	100
1986	Gould et al[12]	^{82}Rb/^{13}N-ammonia	NR	95	100
	Average			91	89

Source: Reprinted from Di Carli M. Advances in positron emission tomography. J Nucl Cardiol; 11:719–32, Copyright 2004, with permission from The American Society of Nuclear Cardiology.

computed tomography (SPECT) in the same or matched patient populations. Go and colleagues compared PET and SPECT in 202 patients.[9] Their results showed a higher sensitivity with PET (76% vs 93%) and no significant changes for specificity (80% vs 78% for SPECT and PET, respectively). In another study, Stewart et al compared PET and SPECT in 81 patients.[8] They observed a higher specificity for PET (53% vs 83% for SPECT and PET, respectively) and no significant differences in sensitivity (84% vs 86% for SPECT and PET, respectively). Diagnostic accuracy was higher with PET (89% vs 78%).

Bateman et al recently compared [82]Rb PET and ^{99m}Tc sestamibi SPECT with respect to image quality, reader confidence, and diagnostic accuracy in 2 matched patient cohorts undergoing clinically indicated pharmacologic-stress perfusion imaging using contemporary technology for both SPECT and PET.[4] With respect to quality, summed rest and stress PET perfusion images were more frequently rated as excellent compared to the corresponding SPECT images (79% vs 62%, respectively), but the quality of rest and stress gated images was considered comparable. Artifact-free images were more frequently observed with PET than with SPECT studies (44% vs 17%, respectively). Significant liver and/or bowel uptake affecting interpretation was more frequently observed on SPECT than on PET studies (41% vs 5%, respectively). Consequently, reader certainty as defined by a definitely normal or abnormal imaging interpretation was also higher for PET than for SPECT (96% vs 81%, respectively). Importantly, differences in image quality and reader certainty between PET and SPECT were not influenced by either patient gender or body mass index.

Overall diagnostic accuracy using either a 50% (87% vs 71%) or a 70% (89% vs 79%, respectively) angiographic threshold was higher for PET than for SPECT. Differences in diagnostic accuracy reflected primarily the increased specificity (with a marginal advantage in sensitivity) of PET versus SPECT, and applied to both men and women, and to obese and nonobese individuals.

Diagnosing Multivessel CAD with Myocardial Perfusion PET

As depicted in Table 11.1, the relative assessment of myocardial perfusion with PET remains a sensitive means for diagnosing or ruling out the presence of obstructive CAD. As with SPECT, however, PET often uncovers only that territory supplied by the most severe stenosis. This is based on the fact that in patients with CAD, coronary vasodilator reserve is often abnormal even in territories supplied by noncritical angiographic stenoses,[13,14] thereby reducing the heterogeneity of flow between "normal" and "abnormal" zones and limiting the ability to delineate the presence of multivessel CAD.

In a recent study, Bateman et al reported that PET was better than SPECT for diagnosing multivessel CAD (71% vs 48%, respectively). In this study, however, it was unclear what was the precise mix of patients with "multi-vessel CAD" (e.g., 2 vs 3 vessels vs left main disease) and whether the two groups (PET and SPECT) were equally balanced (i.e., location and severity of coronary artery stenoses). The apparent advantage of PET in this study may be related to differences in tracer kinetics between [82]Rb and ^{99m}Tc sestamibi. The relatively higher extraction of the former at relatively high flow rates could explain, at least in part, the improved ability of PET to uncover other areas supplied by stenosed coronary arteries. Nonetheless, PET still misclassifies ~30% of the patients with multivessel CAD as having single-vessel disease, or presumably misses some patients with balanced ischemia (sensitivity for detecting 70% stenosis was 86%).

As discussed in Chapter 10, one advantage of PET is its distinct ability to assess left ventricular function at rest and during peak stress (as opposed to poststress with SPECT). Recent data from our laboratory suggest that in normal subjects, LVEF increases during peak vasodilator stress.[1] In patients with CAD, however, changes in LVEF (from baseline to peak stress) are inversely related to the magnitude of perfu-

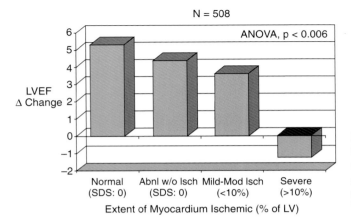

FIGURE 11.1. Bar chart illustrating the inverse relationship between the delta change in left ventricular ejection fraction (LVEF) during peak vasodilator stress and the magnitude of myocardium ischemic as assessed by perfusion imaging. SDS, summed stress score. (Data from Dorbala S, Limaye A, Sampson U, et al. [1].)

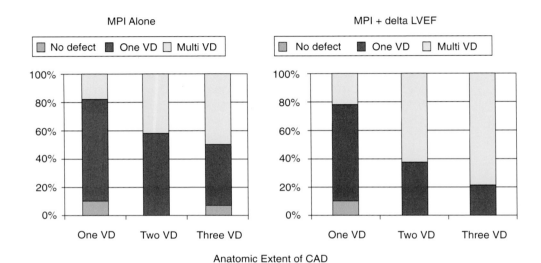

FIGURE 11.2. Bar chart illustrating the value of perfusion alone (left panel) and perfusion plus changes in left ventricular ejection fraction (LVEF) for ascertaining the anatomic extent of CAD as defined by coronary angiography. (Data from Dorbala S, Sampson U, Limaye A, et al. [2].)

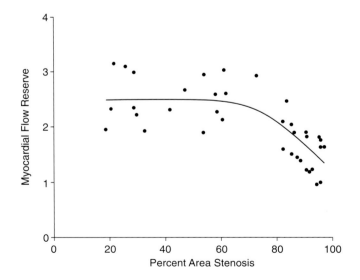

FIGURE 11.3. Scatter plot of the relation between myocardial flow reserve (peak/rest myocardial blood flow) and quantitative coronary angiographic measurements of percent area stenosis ($r = 0.78$, $p < 0.00001$). (Reproduced with permission from Di Carli M, Czernin J, Hoh CK, et al. [3].)

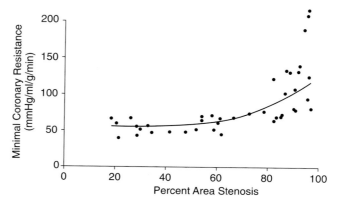

FIGURE 11.4. Scatter plot of the relation between coronary vascular resistance and quantitative coronary angiographic measurements of percent area stenosis ($r = 0.78$, $p < 0.00001$). (Reproduced with permission from Di Carli M, Czernin J, Hoh CK, et al. [3].)

sion abnormalities during stress (reflecting ischemic myocardium) (Figure 11.1). Indeed, patients with multivessel disease or left main disease show a frank drop in LVEF during peak stress even in the absence of apparent perfusion defects (see Part VI, Case 7). In contrast, patients without significant CAD or with 1-vessel disease show a normal increase in LVEF (see Part VI, Cases 1 and 2). Consequently, the diagnostic sensitivity of gated PET for correctly ascertaining the presence of multivessel disease increases from 50% to 79% (Figure 11.2).[2]

Alternatively, PET measurements of myocardial blood flow and coronary vasodilator reserve could also help improve detection of multivessel CAD. The reports evaluating the diagnostic performance of myocardial perfusion PET to detect angiographic stenoses (Table 11.1) examined imaging results in terms of sensitivity and specificity rather than as a continuous spectrum of severity. In patients with CAD, noninvasive measurements of coronary blood flow and vasodilator reserve by PET are inversely and nonlinearly related to stenosis severity, as defined by quantitative angiography (Figures 11.3 and 11.4). Importantly, coronary lesions of intermediate severity have a differential CFR that can be detected by PET, which decreases as stenosis severity increases, thereby allowing better definition of the functional importance of known coronary epicardial stenosis.[3,15,16] Figure 11.5 illustrates the potential use of measurements of myocardial blood flow and coronary vasodilator reserve to better delineate the extent of underlying CAD. In patients with so-called balanced ischemia or diffuse CAD, measurements of coronary vasodilator reserve would uncover areas of myocardium at risk that would generally be missed by performing only relative assessments of myocardial perfusion.

Two recent reports demonstrate the potential clinical value of measures of coronary vasodilator reserve as assessed by PET to delineate the extent of underlying CAD. Yoshinaga et al compared the clinical value of measures of coronary vasodilator reserve as assessed by PET to relative assessments of myocardial perfusion by SPECT in 27 patients with CAD.[14] They showed good agreement between SPECT defects and PET measures of vasodilator reserve in only 16 of 58 (28%) myocardial regions supplied by coronary stenosis >50% as assessed by quantitative angiography. The remaining 42 of 58 (72%) regions with angiographic stenoses showed no regional perfusion defects by SPECT but a definitely abnormal vasodilator reserve by PET. Similarly, Parkash et al recently reported on the value of quantification of coronary flow reserve versus the traditional relative assessment of myocardial perfusion to delineate the extent of CAD in a relatively small group of 23 patients.[17] In patients with 3-vessel CAD, they found that defect sizes were significantly larger using quantification methods as compared with the traditional method ($44 \pm 18\%$ vs $69 \pm 24\%$). In patients

Stress-Rest ^{82}Rubidium PET

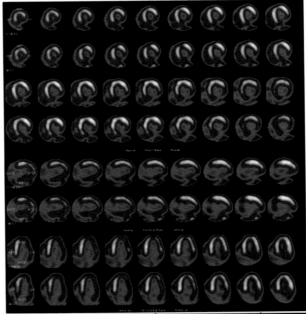

Coronary Territory	Rest MBF (mL/min/g)	Stress MBF (mL/min/g)	CFR (Stress/Rest)
LAD	0.86	0.89	1.07
LCX	0.64	0.66	1.03
RCA	0.86	1.00	1.16

FIGURE 11.5. Example of a stress and rest myocardial perfusion PET study with ^{82}Rb as the flow tracer. The images (top panel) demonstrate a medium-size and severe perfusion defect throughout the inferior and inferolateral walls, which is fixed and consistent with myocardial infarction. The quantitative data (lower panel) demonstrate impaired coronary vasodilator reserve (peak flow/baseline flow) in all 3 coronary territories. Subsequent coronary angiography demonstrated significant 3-vessel CAD. This case illustrates the potential use of blood flow quantitation to better ascertain the extent of anatomic CAD. (Reprinted from Di Carli M. Advances in positron emission tomography. J Nucl Cardiol; 11:719–32, Copyright 2004, with permission from The American Society of Nuclear Cardiology.)

with single-vessel CAD, defect sizes were smaller using quantification methods than with the traditional method (10 ± 12% vs 18 ± 17%). Thus, this is clearly an area of great clinical interest, and future studies are warranted to evaluate the added value of quantitative flow measurements for the noninvasive diagnosis of CAD.

Myocardial Perfusion PET to Monitor Progression and Regression of CAD

Lipid-lowering trials in patients with coronary atherosclerosis have demonstrated no progression or only modest regression of anatomic coronary artery stenoses compared to control patients.[18–21] Despite the lack of progression or modest regression in coronary artery stenoses, these studies have reported a proportionately greater decrease in coronary events in treated than in control patients.[18–22] This has led to the hypothesis that stabilization of atherosclerotic plaques, reduction of inducible myocardial ischemia (caused by an improvement in coronary vasodilator function), or both effects combined may be more closely related to improved clinical outcomes than the anatomic change in plaque burden. There is mounting evidence that the functional abnormalities in coronary vascular function described above can be improved by therapeutic interventions designed to improve the risk factor profile, and that these changes can be measured noninvasively with PET.

Selecting Patients for Myocardial Perfusion PET

The ACC/AHA/ASNC radionuclide guidelines from 2003[27] defined the following role for PET:

Recommendations for Diagnosis of Patients with an Intermediate Likelihood of CAD and/or Risk Stratification of Patients with an Intermediate or High Likelihood of CAD

Class I

(Conditions for which there is evidence and/or general agreement that a given procedure or treatment is useful and effective)

Adenosine or dipyridamole myocardial perfusion PET in patients in whom an appropriately indicated myocardial perfusion SPECT study has been found to be equivocal for diagnostic or risk stratification purposes. *(Level of Evidence: B, indicating that the data is derived from a single randomized trial, or from nonrandomized studies)*

Class IIa

(Conditions for which there is conflicting evidence and/or a divergence of opinion about the usefulness/efficacy of a procedure or treatment, but the weight of evidence/opinion is in favor of usefulness/efficacy)

1. Adenosine or dipyridamole myocardial perfusion PET to identify the extent, severity, and location of ischemia as the initial diagnostic test in patients who are unable to exercise. *(Level of Evidence: B)*
2. Adenosine or dipyridamole myocardial perfusion PET to identify the extent, severity, and location of ischemia as the initial diagnostic test in patients who are able to exercise but have LBBB or an electronically paced rhythm. *(Level of Evidence: B)*

(Reprinted with permission, ACC/AHA/ASNC Guidelines for the Clinical Use of Cardiac Radionuclide Imaging © 2003, American Heart Association, Inc.)

Nonetheless, the emerging data with PET and integrated PET/CT suggest that this modality could potentially expand its application in the following patient subgroups:

- *Patients requiring pharmacologic stress*: These are often the most challenging patients for SPECT, as they tend to be overweight or obese, older, and generally not able to withstand longer imaging times. Attenuation correction with SPECT, especially in the overweight and obese patients, appears to perform best in patients undergoing exercise protocols. In the setting of pharmacologic stress, the concomitant correction of areas in intense radiotracer concentration such as liver and bowel results in increased scatter into the inferior wall and degradation of SPECT image quality.[23,24] In fact, preliminary data from Bateman et al suggest that up to 50% of attenuation corrected postpharmacologic stress sestamibi SPECT images may have compromised quality and diagnostic accuracy compared to nonattenuation corrected images.[25]
- *Overweight and obese patients*: For the reasons delineated above, PET may be the first line of testing in these patient groups.
- *Women*: The improved diagnostic accuracy with PET and PET/CT may prove to be an advantage in women compared to SPECT. Indeed, data from Bateman et al discussed above and from our laboratory (Table 11.1) suggest that the diagnostic accuracy in women is probably superior with PET. This awaits confirmation by larger studies.

- *Patients with new-onset heart failure*: Integrated PET/CT, with its ability to delineate myocardial ischemia and viability and coronary anatomy, may become an important indication for PET because it can ascertain etiology of heart failure (ischemic vs nonischemic) and define management (medical therapy vs revascularization).
- *Symptomatic diabetics*: The ability of PET to more accurately delineate the presence of multivessel CAD may become very important in identifying high-risk subgroups among patients who are generally regarded as high risk, such as diabetics. The higher prevalence of obesity in this population may be another reason to select PET over SPECT.

Summary Points

- PET provides accurate diagnosis of the extent, severity, and anatomic location of coronary artery disease. A review of the current literature indicates that the sensitivity and specificity of myocardial perfusion with pharmacological stress vary from 90% to 95% in both men and women.
- An additional advantage of PET is the possibility of quantifying regional perfusion and coronary flow reserve. Experimental and clinical evidence indicates that these measurements of coronary flow reserve have a nonlinear inverse correlation with the anatomic severity of stenosis. These measurements are useful for assessing the functional implications of coronary stenoses of intermediate severity (50%–80%), especially in patients with extensive CAD.
- The high relative cost of PET requires careful selection of patients.
- The great sensitivity and, above all, the high specificity of PET for diagnosing coronary heart disease make it a particularly useful tool for the assessment of obese patients and women with a low-intermediate probability of having coronary disease. This important clinical role is expected to grow with the availability of integrated PET/CT scanners that allow a true integration (fusion) of structure and function,[26] which will allow a comprehensive examination of the heart's anatomy and function in ways never before possible.

References

1. Dorbala S, Limaye A, Sampson U, et al. Normal and abnormal responses of left ventricular ejection fraction during vasodilator stress rubidium 82 positron emission tomography (PET-CT). *J Nucl Med.* 2005;46:268P.
2. Dorbala S, Sampson U, Limaye A, et al. Diagnostic value of changes in left ventricular ejection fraction during peak vasodilator stress gated cardiac PET-CT: correlation with the extent of angiographic coronary artery disease [abstract]. *Circulation.* 2005;112: II-365.
3. Di Carli M, Czernin J, Hoh CK, et al. Relation among stenosis severity, myocardial blood flow, and flow reserve in patients with coronary artery disease. *Circulation.* 1995;91: 1944–1951.
4. Bateman TM, Heller GV, McGhie AL, et al. Diagnostic accuracy of rest/stress ECG-gated rubidium-82 myocardial perfusion PET: comparison with ECG-gated Tc-99m-sestamibi SPECT. *J Nucl Cardiol.* 2006;13:24–33.
5. Sampson UK, Limaye A, Dorbala S, et al. Diagnostic accuracy of rubidium-82 myocardial perfusion imaging with hybrid positron emission tomography-computed tomography (PET-CT) in the detection of coronary artery disease. *J Am Coll Cardiol.* 2006. In press.
6. Marwick TH, Nemec JJ, Stewart WJ, Salcedo EE. Diagnosis of coronary artery disease using exercise echocardiography and positron emission tomography: comparison and analysis of discrepant results. *J Am Soc Echocardiogr.* 1992;5:231–238.
7. Grover-McKay M, Ratib O, Schwaiger M, et al. Detection of coronary artery disease with positron emission tomography and rubidium 82. *Am Heart J.* 1992;123:646–652.

8. Stewart RE, Schwaiger M, Molina E, et al. Comparison of rubidium-82 positron emission tomography and thallium-201 SPECT imaging for detection of coronary artery disease. *Am J Cardiol.* 1991;67:1303–1310.

9. Go RT, Marwick TH, MacIntyre WJ, et al. A prospective comparison of rubidium-82 PET and thallium-201 SPECT myocardial perfusion imaging utilizing a single dipyridamole stress in the diagnosis of coronary artery disease. *J Nucl Med.* 1990;31:1899–1905.

10. Demer LL, Gould KL, Goldstein RA, et al. Assessment of coronary artery disease severity by positron emission tomography. Comparison with quantitative arteriography in 193 patients. *Circulation.* 1989;79:825–835.

11. Tamaki N, Yonekura Y, Senda M, et al. Value and limitation of stress thallium-201 single photon emission computed tomography: comparison with nitrogen-13 ammonia positron tomography. *J Nucl Med.* 1988;29:1181–1188.

12. Gould KL, Goldstein RA, Mullani NA, et al. Noninvasive assessment of coronary stenoses by myocardial perfusion imaging during pharmacologic coronary vasodilation. VIII. Clinical feasibility of positron cardiac imaging without a cyclotron using generator-produced rubidium-82. *J Am Coll Cardiol.* 1986;7:775–789.

13. Uren NG, Crake T, Lefroy DC, de Silva R, Davies GJ, Maseri A. Reduced coronary vasodilator function in infarcted and normal myocardium after myocardial infarction. *N Engl J Med.* 1994;331:222–227.

14. Yoshinaga K, Katoh C, Noriyasu K, et al. Reduction of coronary flow reserve in areas with and without ischemia on stress perfusion imaging in patients with coronary artery disease: a study using oxygen 15-labeled water PET. *J Nucl Cardiol.* 2003;10:275–283.

15. Uren NG, Melin JA, De Bruyne B, Wijns W, Baudhuin T, Camici PG. Relation between myocardial blood flow and the severity of coronary- artery stenosis. *N Engl J Med.* 1994; 330:1782–1788.

16. Beanlands RS, Muzik O, Melon P, et al. Noninvasive quantification of regional myocardial flow reserve in patients with coronary atherosclerosis using nitrogen-13 ammonia positron emission tomography. Determination of extent of altered vascular reactivity. *J Am Coll Cardiol.* 1995;26:1465–1475.

17. Parkash R, deKemp RA, Ruddy TD, et al. Potential utility of rubidium 82 PET quantification in patients with 3-vessel coronary artery disease. *J Nucl Cardiol.* 2004;11:440–449.

18. Ornish D, Brown SE, Scherwitz LW, et al. Can lifestyle changes reverse coronary heart disease? The Lifestyle Heart Trial. *Lancet.* 1990;336:129–133.

19. Brown G, Albers JJ, Fisher LD, et al. Regression of coronary artery disease as a result of intensive lipid- lowering therapy in men with high levels of apolipoprotein B [see comments]. *N Engl J Med.* 1990;323:1289–1298.

20. Kane JP, Malloy MJ, Ports TA, Phillips NR, Diehl JC, Havel RJ. Regression of coronary atherosclerosis during treatment of familial hypercholesterolemia with combined drug regimens. *JAMA.* 1990;264:3007–3012.

21. Gould KL, Ornish D, Scherwitz L, et al. Changes in myocardial perfusion abnormalities by positron emission tomography after long-term, intense risk factor modification. *JAMA.* 1995;274:894–901.

22. Watts GF, Lewis B, Brunt JN, et al. Effects on coronary artery disease of lipid-lowering diet, or diet plus cholestyramine, in the St Thomas' Atherosclerosis Regression Study (STARS). *Lancet.* 1992;339:563–569.

23. Bateman TM, Cullom SJ. Attenuation correction single-photon emission computed tomography myocardial perfusion imaging. *Semin Nucl Med.* 2005;35:37–51.

24. Nuyts J, Dupont P, Van den Maegdenbergh V, Vleugels S, Suetens P, Mortelmans L. A study of the liver-heart artifact in emission tomography. *J Nucl Med.* 1995;36:133–139.

25. Bateman T, Heller GV, McGhie AI, Friedman JD, Cullom SJ, Case JA. Attenuation-corrected Tc-99m sestamibi SPECT compared with Rb-82 myocardial perfusion PET [abstract]. *J Nucl Cardiol.* 2005;12:5118–5119.

26. Di Carli MF. Advances in positron emission tomography. *J Nucl Cardiol.* 2004;11: 719–732.

27. Klocke FJ, Baird MG, Lorell BH, et al. ACC/AHA/ASNC guidelines for the clinical use of cardiac radionuclide imaging—executive summary: a report of the American College of Cardiology/American Heart Association Task Force on Practice Guidelines. *J Am Coll Cardiol.* 2003;42:1318–1333.

12 Quantifying Myocardial Perfusion for the Assessment of Preclinical CAD

Heinrich R. Schelbert

Estimates of regional myocardial blood flow contain information on morphologic alterations of the myocardium itself but also, and importantly, on the structure and function of the upstream coronary circulation. Loss of myocytes, replacement fibrosis, and scar tissue formation are associated with regional reductions of blood flow at rest per unit mass. Conversely, regional flow at rest may also be diminished in the absence of structural alterations but in the presence of, for example, a high-grade stenosis of the epicardial conduit vessel that impinges on flow. Such flow reductions then reflect structural or functional disturbances of the upstream coronary circulation. Myocardial blood flow depends on a complex interplay between the coronary driving pressure (the pressure gradient from the aorta to the right atrium) and resistance forces that adjust the supply of blood to the energy needs of the myocardium. Besides extravascular resistive forces due to intramyocardial and intracavitary pressures and their cardiac cycle-related changes, most of the resistance to flow and its regulation resides at the level of the coronary resistance vessels. Vascular smooth muscle relaxation or constriction in the resistance vessels mediated by metabolic, neuronal, and endocrine mechanisms raises or lowers coronary and, accordingly, myocardial blood flow. The vascular-smooth-muscle-initiated changes in blood flow are modulated by endothelium-related factors that depend on flow-velocity-related shear stresses as well as on neuronal, endocrine, and paracrine factors.

Myocardial blood flow, measured in absolute units, thus serves as a measure of the functional state of the coronary circulation. This is especially true for estimates of flow responses to physiologic or pharmacologic challenges. If abnormal, these flow responses aid in identifying sites of abnormal function. Measurements of flow responses are now available noninvasively with positron emission tomography (PET) and have proved useful for identifying functional consequences of early as well as advanced stages of coronary atherosclerosis. These measurements also hold promise for exploring and defining effects of therapeutic interventions. This chapter briefly reviews methodological aspects of PET-based measurements of myocardial blood flow, examines interventions for challenging the circulatory system and for evaluating the system's responses, and then explores the potential usefulness of such measurements in individuals without but at risk for coronary artery disease.

Methodological Aspects

First, features of PET fundamental to the noninvasive quantification of myocardial blood flow include (1) its high spatial, depth-independent resolution (in the range of 8–12 mm full-width at half-maximum), (2) its quantitative imaging capability (where tissue radioactivity concentrations are determined in units of radioactivity per unit mass), and (3) its high temporal resolution capability (in the order of seconds), which affords measurements of rapidly changing radiotracer activity concentrations in arterial blood and myocardium. Second, several positron emitting tracers of myocardial blood flow are available. Foremost are nitrogen-13-labeled ammonia (^{13}N-ammonia), oxygen-15 labeled water (^{15}O-water), and, to a lesser extent, rubidium-82 chloride (^{82}Rb). The net uptake of each radiotracer as the product of its first-pass extraction fraction and myocardial blood flow correlates with myocardial blood flow (Figure 12.1) yet, with the exception of ^{15}O-water, in a nonlinear manner. Third, the tissue kinetics of the radiotracer derived from serially acquired PET images are fitted with experimentally validated tracer kinetic models for computing estimates of regional myocardial blood flow in milliliters of blood per minute per gram myocardium.

Measurements of Myocardial Blood Flow with ^{13}N-Ammonia

After a transmission image for correction of photon attenuation is recorded, acquisition of serial emission images commences while a 10-second bolus of typically 20 to 30 mCi ^{13}N-ammonia is administered intravenously. The sequence of serially acquired images typically consists of 12 frames of 10 seconds each, followed by 2 frames of 30 seconds each, followed by 1 frame of 60 seconds, and, finally, by 1 frame of 900 seconds, amounting to a total acquisition time of 19 minutes.[1–3] The final, 900-second transaxial image data set is reoriented into short and long axis slices of the left ventricular myocardium. They depict the relative distribution of myocardial blood flow and, once assembled into polar map displays, provide for semiquantitative determinations of extent and severity of perfusion defects.[4] The polar map also serves as a template for assigning regions of interest to the myocardium. The reorientation parameters applied to the late "static" image set are then applied to the serial transaxial image sets acquired during the initial 2 minutes after radiotracer injection; the reoriented short axis slices are each assembled into polar maps onto which the regions of interest assigned initially to the "static" polar map are copied. An additional 25 mm^2 region of interest is assigned to the center of the left ventricle blood pool (Figure 12.2).[3,4]

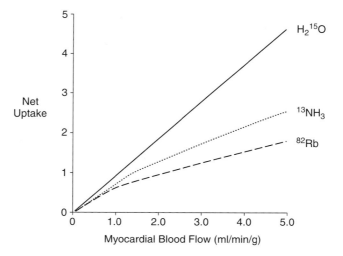

FIGURE 12.1. Net uptake of ^{13}N-ammonia, ^{15}O-water, and ^{82}Rb as a function of myocardial blood flow.

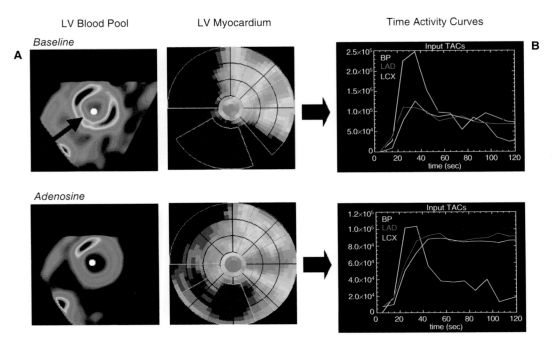

FIGURE 12.2. Determination of the arterial radiotracer input function and the myocardial response from a region of interest assigned to the left ventricular blood pool (A) and from regions of interest assigned on a polar map to the territories of the left anterior descending (LAD), left circumflex (LCX), and right coronary artery (RCA) territory for a study at baseline (upper row) and during adenosine stimulation (lower row). (B) The corresponding time-activity curves show arterial input function, LAD, and LCX and RCA myocardium. Note the markedly higher tracer uptake in myocardium in the adenosine as compared to the baseline study when related to the arterial input function.

The arterial radiotracer input function as derived from the blood pool region of interest and the myocardial tissue response derived from the myocardial regions of interest are fitted with a 2-compartment tracer kinetic model that mathematically describes the time-dependent exchange of ^{13}N-ammonia between blood and myocardium, which has been validated in animal experiments (Figure 12.3).[2,5] As shown in Figure 12.4, ^{13}N-ammonia (NH$_3$) in blood exists mostly in its ionic species of ^{13}N-ammonium (NH$_4^+$). It converts into ^{13}N-ammonia for diffusion across the capillary membrane. Because the capillary membrane exerts only a negligible barrier effect to the exchange of ^{13}N-ammonia, its first-pass extraction fraction approaches 100%. In tissue, metabolic trapping competes with flow-dependent back diffusion of the radiotracer. Once converted back to the ionic ^{13}N-ammonium, the radiotracer label becomes incorporated into glutamine via the glutamine synthase reaction and is thus effectively trapped in the myocardium.[6] Different from the rate of the glutamine synthase activity, which appears to be relatively constant over a wide range of metabolic conditions, the rate of backdiffusion of ^{13}N-ammonia from tissue into blood depends on flow. Because the fraction that diffuses back into blood increases with flow, the tracer net retention progressively declines with increasing myocardial blood flows, though in a nonlinear fashion.[6] The tracer kinetic model accounts for the flow-dependent decline of the "retention fraction" and corrects for spillover of activity from the blood pool into the myocardial region of interest (due to misplacements of registered counts), for radiotracer activity in the vascular space of the myocardium, and for partial volume-related underestimation of the true myocardial radiotracer activity concentration, and yields estimates of myocardial blood flow in milliliters per minute per gram.

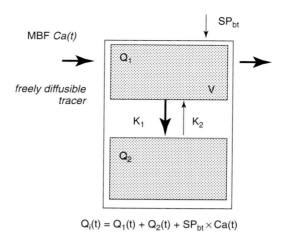

$$Q_i(t) = Q_1(t) + Q_2(t) + SP_{bt} \times Ca(t)$$

FIGURE 12.3. Three-compartment tracer kinetic models for ^{13}N-ammonia. The large box reflects the total activity present in the myocardium, and the 2 smaller compartments describe the activity present in freely diffusible form (Q_1) and in metabolically bound form (Q_2). V, volume of distribution; MBF, myocardial blood flow; SP, spillover of activity from blood into myocardium. The rate constants K_1 and k_2 describe the rates of exchange between the 2 pools.

Correction for partial volume-related underestimations of the true tissue-activity concentration (in mCi per gram myocardium) requires a "recovery coefficient." This correction factor is a function of both the spatial resolution of the imaging device and the thickness of the left ventricular myocardium.[7,8] The latter can be measured in each patient with echocardiography, gated magnetic resonance imaging, or, when hybrid PET/CT is employed, from gated contrast CT ventriculograms.[9,10] For convenience, most laboratories assume an average wall thickness of 10 mm. This value may result in over- or underestimations of true flows in patients with hypertrophic or dilated cardiomyopathies. Its use appears acceptable, however, when left ventricular dimensions are normal or for intraindividual comparisons of repeat flow measurements.

Comparison measurements of myocardial blood flow with, for example, the microsphere technique in experimental animals have confirmed the validity and accuracy of the noninvasive estimates of myocardial blood flow over a range from 0.5 to 5.0 mL/min/g.[2,5]

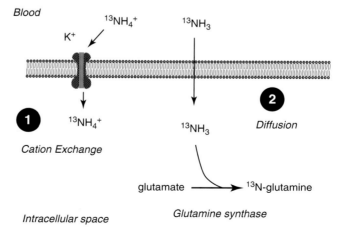

FIGURE 12.4. Tissue kinetics of ^{13}N-ammonia (see text).

Measurements of Myocardial Blood Flow with ^{15}O-Water

Flow determinations with this tracer are technically more demanding. Because of its short physical half-life of only 2.4 minutes, the radiotracer can be used only in close proximity to a cyclotron. Further, the tracer rapidly distributes into the water spaces of tissues. Accordingly, ^{15}O-water does not selectively accumulate in the myocardium. Separation of tracer activity in the myocardium from that in blood requires additional blood pool imaging with, for example, ^{15}O- or carbon-11-labeled carbon monoxide.[11–14] As an alternate and more practical approach, factor analysis has been successfully employed for discriminating between blood pool and myocardial radioactivity concentrations and their changes over time, thus obviating the need for separate blood pool imaging.[15]

After intravenous administration, ^{15}O-water rapidly distributes into and clears from the myocardium in proportion to blood flow and its concentration in blood. Using a 1-compartment tracer kinetic model, rates of myocardial blood flow are then obtained from the rate of clearance of ^{15}O-water from the myocardium.[11,16] Similar to the ^{13}N-ammonia approach, estimates of myocardial blood flow with ^{15}O-water have been found to correlate well with independent comparison measurements for example, as in animals with the microsphere technique.[13,16]

In normal human myocardium, both the ^{15}O-water and the ^{13}N-ammonia approaches yield comparable estimates of myocardial blood flows.[17] However, as an important and distinct difference, the ^{15}O-water approach selectively measures flow in myocardium capable of rapid water exchange, whereas the ^{13}N-ammonia approach measures flow across the entire myocardial wall. If normal myocardium coexists with scar tissue, then the ^{13}N-ammonia approach measures the average transmural flow, while the ^{15}O-water technique estimates flow only in the "water exchanging" myocardium or tissue.[14,18] When applied to dysfunctional myocardium with scar tissue formation, flow estimates in the hypoperfused infarct region will be diminished with ^{13}N-ammonia but may be normal or near normal with ^{15}O-water.[19] The two approaches also differ for evaluations of the relative distributions of blood flow. Because ^{15}O-water equilibrates with the water spaces of myocardium and blood, and because of rapidly changing radiotracer concentrations and its short physical half-life, "static" ^{15}O-water perfusion images are of limited value for analyzing the relative distribution of myocardial blood flow. Conversely, because ^{13}N-ammonia is selectively retained by myocardium and has a longer physical half-life, it affords perfusion images of high diagnostic quality.

Measurements of Myocardial Blood Flow with ^{82}Rb Chloride

Rubidium-82 offers distinct advantages for clinical studies of myocardial blood flow. First, it is available through a generator system with a 4- to 5-week shelf life and eliminates the need for an on-site cyclotron. Second, push-button-operated infusion systems provide for intravenous administrations of precalibrated tracer activity doses at preselected infusion rates. The ultrashort physical half-time of ^{82}Rb of only 76 seconds affords serial evaluations of myocardial perfusion at short time intervals (i.e., 10 minutes) but requires delivery of high activity doses (range, 50–60 mCi) for adequate visualization of the myocardium after 1 to 2 physical half-lives have been allowed for tracer clearance from blood. High-activity doses cause substantial dead-time-related count losses, thereby limiting accurate measurements of the radiotracer input function and the myocardial tissue response. Estimates of flow responses to pharmacological vasodilation have therefore remained "semiquantitative," where the myocardial ^{82}Rb activity concentration is normalized to the dose of activity administered.[20–22] The approach does not correct for flow-related nonlinear increases in tracer activity and thus underestimates the true flow response. Recent investigations suggest, however, the possibility of true quantification of myocardial blood flow with this radiotracer.[23–25]

Assessment of Coronary Circulatory Function

In normal individuals at low risk for coronary artery disease, average values of myocardial blood flow at rest are reported to range from 0.60 to 1.2 mL/min/g.[1,12,26–30] Some of the interstudy and interinstitutional variability relates to differences in measurement approaches including radiotracers, tracer kinetic models, and image analysis. Differences in study conditions and study populations including gender and age contribute further to the variability. Whether myocardial blood flows differ between males and females remains undetermined. Some but not all studies have observed higher flows at rest in females than in males.[27,31,32] Myocardial blood flow at rest depends on the left ventricular myocardial work and thus on the hemodynamic state.[27,32] Most investigations report statistically significant correlations between myocardial blood flow at rest and the rate pressure product (RPP; product of heart rate and systolic blood pressure) as a readily available index of cardiac work. Accordingly, increases in RPP and, thus, in myocardial work with supine bicycle exercise or with low-dose dobutamine infusion were similarly associated with proportionate increases in myocardial blood flow.[1,33,34] Differences in myocardial blood flow at rest between sedentary and trained individuals have also been reported and correspond to differences in heart rate and arterial blood pressures.[35] Moreover, age-related increases in resting myocardial blood flow as reported in several studies also depend on differences in cardiac work as reflected by an age-related increase in the RPP.[27,36,37] The dependence of blood flow on cardiac work has therefore prompted some investigators to report values of myocardial blood flow that are normalized through cardiac work (by dividing the flow estimate by the RPP).

With the exception of regional flow reductions at rest due to a critical stenosis upstream in the epicardial coronary artery or of flows that are significantly higher than predicted by the RPP, as observed, for example, in rejecting cardiac allografts,[38] measurements of myocardial blood flow at rest provide only limited information on the functional state of the coronary circulation. Fundamental to the evaluation of the coronary circulatory functions, therefore, are measurements of flow responses to physiological or pharmacological challenges, as, for example, pharmacologic stimulation of vascular smooth muscle relaxation or sympathetic stimulation with cold pressor testing. Additional information on the functional state of the epicardial conduit vessel is available through evaluation of the distribution of myocardial blood flow in the base-to-apex direction of the left ventricle.

Assessment of the Total Integrated Vasodilator Capacity

Assessment of the total integrated vasodilator capacity entails the intravenous administration of vascular smooth muscle relaxing agents, for example, adenosine, adenosine-triphosphate, dipyridamole, or specific adenosine receptor stimulating agents, and measurement of the hyperemic flow response. As illustrated in Figure 12.5, the vascular-smooth-muscle-mediated decrease in resistance at the level of the coronary microcirculation prompts an increase in coronary flow. Higher flow velocities lead to shear-stress-mediated endothelium-dependent dilation of the coronary vessels. Resistance to flow depends on its velocity, the length of the vessel and, importantly, on its diameter. The flow-related dilation can therefore be considered as a compensatory adjustment that minimizes the resistance to high-velocity flow in the conduit and resistance vessels. This adjustment is mediated through shear-stress-dependent increases in endothelial nitric oxide synthase (eNOS) activity and release of nitric oxide (NO). The flow-related vasodilation involves both the coronary conduit and the coronary resistance vessels and thus augments the total hyperemic flow initiated by selective smooth muscle relaxation. The endothelial contribution to the total hyperemic response has been confirmed in normal volunteers where pharmacologic inhibition of eNOS activity with N^G–nitro-L-arginine methyl ester (L-NAME) diminished

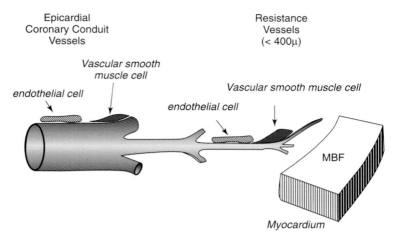

FIGURE 12.5. Schematic representation of the regulation of coronary blood flow (see text).

hyperemic flows by 21% or attenuated the adenosine-stimulated flow response by 31%.[39] Pharmacologically stimulated hyperemic flows therefore represent smooth muscle and endothelium-related vasodilator effects and thus reflect the total integrated coronary vasodilator capacity.

Sympathetic Stimulation with Cold Pressor Testing

Flow responses to sympathetic stimulation provide more direct information on endothelial function than do flow responses to pharmacological vasodilation. Exposure to cold by immersing a hand in ice water prompts a sympathetically mediated increase in heart rate and blood pressure. Thus myocardial work is normally associated with a proportionate, metabolically mediated increase in myocardial blood flow (Figure 12.6). In patients with coronary artery disease or at risk for coronary artery disease,

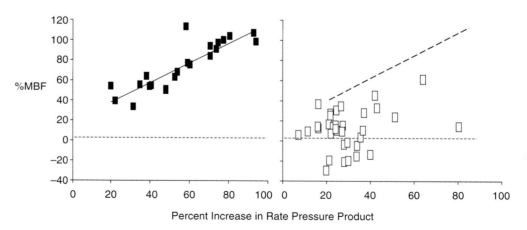

FIGURE 12.6. Responses of myocardial blood flow measured by PET and the RPP to cold pressor testing in normal individuals (panel on the left) and in individuals with risk factors for coronary artery disease (panel on the right). Note the close correlation between MBF and RPP responses in the normal volunteers but the more variable response in the at-risk individuals, where the flow changes no longer correlate with the changes in cardiac work. (Data from Zeiher AM, Drexler H, Wollshlager H, et al. [40].)

however, cold-induced flow responses may no longer correlate with changes in cardiac work. The flow response may diminished, absent, or even paradoxical; that is, flow declines rather than increases.

Several lines of evidence support the validity of the flow response to cold pressor testing as an indicator of coronary endothelial function. Cold-induced changes in coronary flow velocity were closely though inversely correlated with decreases in coronary resistance in response to endothelial stimulation with intracoronary acetyl-choline.[41] Further, acetylcholine-stimulated endothelium-dependent diameter changes corresponded to diameter changes produced by cold pressor testing.[42] Moreover, PET-measured flow responses to cold were significantly correlated with cold-induced and flow-related changes in coronary artery diameter on quantitative coronary angiography in individuals with angiographically normal coronary arteries.[40] Finally, intrave-nous administration of L-arginine, the substrate for eNOS, fully restored impaired flow responses to cold in long-term smokers,[43] suggesting that an increase in NO avail-ability accounted for the improvement of the flow response and in turn implicating diminished NO bioavailability as a determinant of the smoking-related impaired flow response.

The flow response to sympathetic stimulation reflects a delicate balance between opposing vasodilator and vasoconstrictor effects (Figure 12.7). As sympathetic stimu-lation raises heart rate and blood pressure, myocardial work increases. In response, a metabolically mediated decrease in coronary resistance initiates an increase in coro-nary flow that under normal conditions leads to a shear-stress-mediated increase in eNOS activity and release of NO. Stimulation of α-adrenergic smooth muscle recep-tors by the predominantly α-adrenergic norepinephrine causes smooth muscle con-striction. The vasoconstrictor effect is normally offset by the endothelium-related vasodilator effects so that overall flow increases. If, however, the availability of NO is diminished due to decreased synthesis or increased breakdown or both, then the vasoconstrictor effect of sympathetic stimulation may prevail so that flow increases only inappropriately or actually declines. Other endothelium-related vasoactive sub-stances are likely involved in the flow response; yet actions of NO appear to dominate. The flow response may depend further on efferent cardiac sympathetic neuronal pathways, as suggested by findings in diabetic neuropathy.[44,45] However, effects of sympathetic denervation or dysfunction await further clarification, as they probably involve both endothelium-related vasodilator and smooth-muscle-related vasocon-strictor effects.

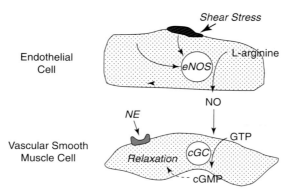

FIGURE 12.7. Highly simplified depiction of the interaction between vasoconstrictor and vasodilator forces during cold pressor testing (see text). NE, norepinephrine; eNOS, endothe-lial nitric oxide synthase; NO, nitric oxide.

Methodological Considerations of Cold Pressor Testing

The increase in heart rate and blood pressure during exposure to cold reaches a "plateau" within about 30 to 45 seconds, at which time the serial PET image acquisition commences and the radiotracer of blood flow is injected intravenously. To allow for sufficient trapping of the radiotracer in the myocardium, exposure to cold is maintained for at least another 60 seconds. Increases in heart rate and systolic blood pressure usually average about 15% to 20% and produce about a 40% to 50% increase in RPP. The increase in mean blood pressure was found to correlate with the muscle sympathetic activity during cold pressor testing[46] and thus may serve as a measure of the degree of sympathetic stimulation. Accordingly, heart rate and blood pressure should be monitored and recorded at 1-minute intervals; monitoring should continue for several minutes after termination of the cold pressor test, as posttest bradycardic hypotensive episodes may occasionally occur.

Patients should first rest comfortably and quietly on the scanner bed for at least 15 to 20 minutes to achieve a more basal hemodynamic state. Myocardial blood flow is then measured, typically first at baseline and then again during cold pressor testing. The flow response to sympathetic stimulation is defined as the flow difference between cold pressor testing and baseline and is expressed as a percentage of the baseline blood flow (% MBF) or as the flow difference between the two conditions in absolute units (ΔMBF).[47] Percent changes in flow are highly dependent on baseline flows and decline with higher baseline flows. Conversely, defined in absolute units of milliliters per minute per gram, the flow response was found to be independent of baseline flows and cardiac work.

Distribution of Myocardial Blood Flow in the Longitudinal, Base-to-Apex Direction of the Left Ventricular Myocardium

There is little resistance to flow in the normal coronary conduit vessel so that intracoronary pressures remain constant over the length of the epicardial coronary artery.[48] The resistance to high-velocity flows during hyperemia similarly remains low due to the flow-related dilation of the epicardial coronary arteries. A progressive decline in perfusion in the base-to-apex direction of the left ventricular myocardium in patients with coronary artery disease but without discrete coronary stenosis has therefore been attributed to diffuse luminal narrowing of the epicardial coronary arteries that presumably resulted in a progressive, proximal-to-distal decline in intracoronary pressure and thus in myocardial perfusion.[49] Subsequently confirmed through direct pressure measurements in coronary vessels without discrete stenosis of patients with coronary artery disease, the progressive intracoronary pressure decline was attributed to increased resistance to flow along the coronary conduit vessels.[48] Besides diffuse luminal narrowing, it is conceivable that functional alterations alone, especially at the level of the coronary endothelium, could result in a similar pressure decline. For example, attenuation or absence of the normal, flow-related dilation of the epicardial conduit vessel, as observed in endothelial dysfunction, increases the resistance to higher-velocity flows during pharmacologic vasodilation and leads to a progressive decline in intracoronary pressures. Similarly, during cold pressor testing, a decrease in conduit vessel diameter, as observed in individuals with risk factors for coronary artery disease, would also raise the resistance to flow, even though coronary flow by itself might not increase.[50] Accordingly, adenosine-stimulated increases in myocardial blood flow were noted to be attenuated in the apical relative to the basal portion of the left ventricular myocardium in individuals with risk factors for coronary artery disease.[51] Similar base-to-apex perfusion gradients have been noted during cold pressor testing.[52] This longitudinal perfusion gradient, observed during pharmacologically stimulated hyperemia as well as cold pressor testing, may thus offer additional unique information on the functional state of the epicardial conduit vessel.

Findings in Patients at Risk for Coronary Atherosclerosis

Several investigations have examined possible effects of coronary risk factors on coronary vasomotion, including long-term smoking, hypercholesteremia, estrogen withdrawal, and obesity.[3,53–55] Some but not all of these investigations observed moderate though statistically significant reductions in the total vasodilator capacity. Although hyperemic flows tended to be diminished in long-term smokers or in postmenopausal women with or without additional risk factors, these reductions in vasodilator capacity did not achieve statistical significance.[3,54] More consistent, however, were observations of an attenuated or absent flow response to sympathetic stimulation in long-term smokers, postmenopausal women, and obese individuals without other risk factors. Thus, estimates of flow responses to sympathetic stimulation appear to be more sensitive than those to pharmacological vasodilation for identifying adverse effects of risk factors on coronary function.

Most consistent have been observations in patients with hypercholesteremia.[28,53,56,57] Several studies found significant reductions in hyperemic flow responses that were correlated inversely with total or LDL cholesterol levels or with the total cholesterol to HDL cholesterol ratio.[53,57] Compared to normal controls, average reductions of hyperemic flows in hypercholesteremic patients range from 17% to 60%. Because the presence of coronary artery disease was not definitively excluded in some study populations, it remains uncertain whether the observed flow attenuations were related to hypercholesteremia alone or whether coronary artery disease contributed.

Importantly, flow measurements afford studies on the effects of risk reduction on coronary vasomotion. For example, cardiovascular conditioning including lifestyle modification, low cholesterol diet, and regular exercise for 6 weeks resulted in a 12% reduction in resting myocardial blood flows while at the same time increasing the total vasodilator capacity by about 10%.[58] Pharmacologic cholesterol lowering alone also improved hyperemic flow responses and thus enhanced the total vasodilator capacity. In hypercholesteremic but otherwise normal young volunteers with mildly reduced hyperemic blood flows in baseline, 6 months of pravastatin treatment (40 mg daily) raised hyperemic myocardial blood flows by an average of 27%.[59] Similar 31% increases in hyperemic flows were achieved in another investigation in hypercholesteremic patients with minimally diseased or normal coronary arteries.[60] Hyperemic myocardial blood flows increased from 1.82 ± 0.36 mL/min/g at baseline to 2.38 ± 0.58 mL/min/g after 6 months of cholesterol lowering with simvastatin. Of interest, the improvement of coronary vasodilator function was found to be related only indirectly to decreases in plasma cholesterol levels, as shown in another study where despite significant reductions in total and LDL plasma cholesterol levels after 2 months of fluvastatin, the hyperemic flow remained reduced initially but had improved when reexamined after 6 months of treatment.[61]

Other studies explored the effects of acute and long-term administration of vitamin C on the endothelium-dependent coronary vasomotion.[62] An acute challenge with the free radical scavenger vitamin C normalized the flow response to cold in long-term smokers but not in hypercholesteremic or hypertensive patients. After oral vitamin C administration for 2 years, the flow response to cold in smokers remained normal; there was also an improvement in the flow response in hypertensive but not in hypercholesteremic patients.

Findings in Diabetes Mellitus and in Insulin-Resistant States

Diabetes mellitus itself but also prediabetic states of insulin resistance are associated with significant increases in cardiovascular morbidity and mortality. The possibility of endothelial dysfunction as the mechanistic link between insulin resistance and cardiovascular risk has been explored in several investigations with noninvasive

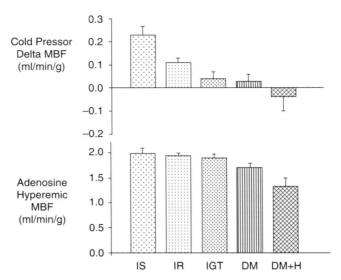

FIGURE 12.8. Flow responses to vasodilator stimulation and cold pressor testing in normal controls and in individuals with increasingly severe states of insulin resistance. IS, insulin sensitive; IR, insulin resistance; IGT, impaired glucose tolerance; DM, diabetes mellitus; HTM, hypertension. (Prior JO, et al., [47]. Adapted by permission.)

measurements of myocardial blood flow. Type 1 and type 2 diabetes mellitus patients consistently revealed an attenuation of the total vasodilator capacity that in degree paralleled the severity of the diabetic state.[45,47,63,64] For example, hyperemic flows were more severely depressed in diabetic patients with autonomic neuropathy, microangiopathy, or arterial hypertension. These investigations also observed diminished flow responses to sympathetic stimulation with cold pressor testing.[45,47,65] Again, the flow response to cold was most severely diminished in diabetic patients with evidence of microangiopathy or autonomic sympathetic neuropathy.

Prediabetic states of insulin resistance are also associated with functional alterations of the coronary circulation.[47] Compared to normal controls, flow responses to cold were significantly reduced in individuals with euglycemic insulin resistance (determined by glucose disposal rates on glucose-insulin clamping). The cold-related flow responses tended to progressively decline with more severe states of insulin resistance, while hyperemic myocardial blood flows and thus the total vasodilator capacity remained normal and declined only significantly in type 2 diabetes patients (Figure 12.8). The findings thus suggest a progressive worsening of coronary circulatory function with more severe states of insulin resistance where functional alterations are initially confined to the endothelium but subsequently also involve the total, smooth muscle, and endothelium-dependent coronary vasomotion.

Flow measurements have also been employed for evaluating responses to therapeutic interventions that, at the same time, provided information on mechanistic explanations for the functional abnormalities. For example, restoration of the flow response to cold pressor testing through intravenous administration of the iron chelator deferoxamine may implicate hydroxyl radicals as possible reasons for reductions in NO bioavailability.[66] Similarly, normalization of the flow response to cold stimulation after 3 months of treatment with the insulin-sensitizing thiazolidinediones implicates insulin resistance per se as a mechanism of endothelial dysfunction.[67]

Considerations for the Evaluation of Coronary Vasomotion

Measurements of flow responses to both sympathetic stimulation and pharmacologic vasodilation allow for a more comprehensive characterization of the functional state of the coronary circulation as compared to measurements of the vasodilator capacity only. As the estimates of hyperemic flows across the spectrum of insulin resistance demonstrated, the total vasodilator capacity may initially be fully maintained and decline only with diabetes as the most severe state of insulin resistance. Conversely, as evident from the attenuated flow responses to cold, milder forms of insulin resistance are already associated with alterations of the endothelium-related coronary vasomotion that would have remained undetected had only hyperemic flows been measured. Endothelial dysfunction might worsen with increased severity of insulin resistance, possibly due to additive effects of increased plasma cholesterol and triglyceride levels on cell signaling of eNOS activity and of free radicals on NO bioavailability or even on vascular smooth muscle function itself. Attenuation of the total vasodilator response may further reflect structural alterations of the microcirculation as findings in diabetes angiopathy suggest. Combined assessment of flow responses to cold and to vasodilation complemented by estimates of the longitudinal, base-to-apex distribution of myocardial blood flow may further allow a more definitive identification of a true impairment in coronary circulatory function, especially in view of the considerable variability of hyperemic blood flows in normal individuals.

Prognostic Value of Flow Measurements

Both the total vasodilator capacity and the flow response to cold contain predictive information on future cardiovascular events. In 51 patients with hypertrophic cardiomyopathy who were prospectively followed for a mean of 8.1 ± 2.1 years, severely reduced myocardial blood flows during dipyridamole stimulation and measured with PET were highly predictive of an unfavorable outcome including cardiac death, progression to severe congestive heart failure symptoms, or ventricular arrhythmias.[68] Another study reported on the predictive value of responses to a cold pressor stimulation. In 72 patients with angiographically normal coronary arteries, patients with attenuated or paradoxical flow responses to cold pressor testing were significantly more likely to experience, during the follow-up period of 66 ± 8 months, a cardiac event including death, acute coronary syndrome, myocardial infarction, ischemic strokes, or coronary artery bypass grafting, as compared to individuals with normal flow responses (Figure 12.9).[69]

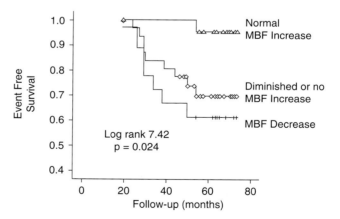

FIGURE 12.9. Flow responses to cold pressor testing and Kaplan Meier analysis of cardiovascular event-free survival. Patients are grouped according to the flow response during cold pressor testing, where, in normals, blood flow increased by at least 40%; in diminished or no response, blood flow increased by less than 40%; and in MBF decrease, blood flow paradoxical declined. (Schindler TH, et al. [69]. Adapted by permission from The American College of Cardiology Foundation.)

In the patients with hypertrophic cardiomyopathy, the reduced vasodilator capacity was attributed to functional and, more important, structural alterations of the coronary microvasculature that presumably cause myocardial ischemia. By contrast, in the study with cold pressor testing in patients with normal coronary angiograms, the PET-measured flow response appeared to identify coronary vasomotor abnormalities indicative of endothelial dysfunction, thus identifying those individuals who were at the highest risk of developing atherosclerosis. The observation of endothelial dysfunction as a predictor of future cardiovascular events in that study is consistent with those of several investigations in which invasively identified endothelial dysfunction was similarly predictive of future cardiovascular events.[70–72]

It is important to emphasize that the myocardial perfusion images at rest and during cold pressor testing or vasodilator-stimulated hyperemia were normal and were free of regional perfusion defects. This appears to be at odds with findings on stress-rest myocardial perfusion imaging with single photon emission computed tomography (SPECT) and the favorable outcome of a normal perfusion scan. Importantly, however, cardiovascular events predicted by SPECT myocardial perfusion imaging occur within 2 to 3 years, whereas cardiovascular events predicted by PET measurements of myocardial blood flow or by invasively obtained parameters of endothelial function occur after longer time periods. The PET-derived indices of abnormal coronary vasomotor function may therefore identify those patients at the greatest risk of developing coronary atherosclerosis rather than identifying the presence of coronary artery disease.

Summary Points

- Estimates of regional myocardial blood flow yield information on structural and functional disturbances of the upstream coronary circulation.
- Abnormalities in myocardial blood flow have been consistently reported in patients with coronary risk factors without clinically overt cardiovascular disease, suggesting that they could be used as a preclinical marker of atherosclerosis.
- PET-based measurements of myocardial blood flow have also been used successfully to monitor responses to therapeutic interventions.
- Both the adenosine-stimulated vasodilator capacity and the flow response to cold contain predictive information on future cardiovascular events.

References

1. Krivokapich J, Smith GT, Huang SC, et al. 13N ammonia myocardial imaging at rest and with exercise in normal volunteers. Quantification of absolute myocardial perfusion with dynamic positron emission tomography. *Circulation*. 1989;80:1328–1337.
2. Kuhle WG, Porenta G, Huang SC, et al. Quantification of regional myocardial blood flow using 13N-ammonia and reoriented dynamic positron emission tomographic imaging. *Circulation*. 1992;86:1004–1017.
3. Campisi R, Czernin J, Schoder H, et al. Effects of long-term smoking on myocardial blood flow, coronary vasomotion, and vasodilator capacity. *Circulation*. 1998;98:119–125.
4. Porenta G, Kuhle W, Czernin J, et al. Semiquantitative assessment of myocardial blood flow and viability using polar map displays of cardiac PET images. *J Nucl Med*. 1992;33:1628–1636.
5. Muzik O, Beanlands RS, Hutchins GD, Mangner TJ, Nguyen N, Schwaiger M. Validation of nitrogen-13-ammonia tracer kinetic model for quantification of myocardial blood flow using PET. *J Nucl Med*. 1993;34:83–91.
6. Schelbert HR, Phelps ME, Huang SC, et al. N-13 ammonia as an indicator of myocardial blood flow. *Circulation*. 1981;63:1259–1272.
7. Hoffman EJ, Huang SC, Phelps ME. Quantitation in positron emission computed tomography: 1. Effect of object size. *J Comput Assist Tomogr*. 1979;3:299–308.

8. Henze E, Huang SC, Ratib O, Hoffman E, Phelps ME, Schelbert HR. Measurements of regional tissue and blood-pool radiotracer concentrations from serial tomographic images of the heart. *J Nucl Med.* 1983;24:987–996.

9. Brunken RC, Perloff JK, Czernin J, et al. Myocardial perfusion reserve in adults with cyanotic congenital heart disease. *Am J Physiol Heart Circ Physiol.* 2005;289:H1798–H1806.

10. Schwaiger M, Ziegler S, Nekolla SG. PET/CT: challenge for nuclear cardiology. *J Nucl Med.* 2005;46:1664–1678.

11. Iida H, Kanno I, Takahashi A, et al. Measurement of absolute myocardial blood flow with H215O and dynamic positron-emission tomography. Strategy for quantification in relation to the partial-volume effect. *Circulation.* 1988;78:104–115.

12. Bergmann SR, Herrero P, Markham J, Weinheimer CJ, Walsh MN. Noninvasive quantitation of myocardial blood flow in human subjects with oxygen-15-labeled water and positron emission tomography. *J Am Coll Cardiol.* 1989;14:639–652.

13. Araujo LI, Lammertsma AA, Rhodes CG, et al. Noninvasive quantification of regional myocardial blood flow in coronary artery disease with oxygen-15-labeled carbon dioxide inhalation and positron emission tomography. *Circulation.* 1991;83:875–885.

14. Iida H, Rhodes CG, de Silva R, et al. Myocardial tissue fraction—correction for partial volume effects and measure of tissue viability. *J Nucl Med.* 1991;32:2169–2175.

15. Hermansen F, Ashburner J, Spinks TJ, Kooner JS, Camici PG, Lammertsma AA. Generation of myocardial factor images directly from the dynamic oxygen-15-water scan without use of an oxygen-15-carbon monoxide blood-pool scan. *J Nucl Med.* 1998;39:1696–1702.

16. Bergmann SR, Fox KA, Rand AL, et al. Quantification of regional myocardial blood flow in vivo with H215O. *Circulation.* 1984;70:724–733.

17. Nitzsche EU, Choi Y, Czernin J, Hoh CK, Huang SC, Schelbert HR. Noninvasive quantification of myocardial blood flow in humans. A direct comparison of the [13N]ammonia and the [15O]water techniques. *Circulation.* 1996;93:2000–2006.

18. Iida H, Tamura Y, Kitamura K, Bloomfield PM, Eberl S, Ono Y. Histochemical correlates of (15)O-water-perfusable tissue fraction in experimental canine studies of old myocardial infarction. *J Nucl Med.* 2000;41:1737–1745.

19. Gerber BL, Melin JA, Bol A, et al. Nitrogen-13-ammonia and oxygen-15-water estimates of absolute myocardial perfusion in left ventricular ischemic dysfunction. *J Nucl Med.* 1998;39:1655–1662.

20. Hicks K, Ganti G, Mullani N, Gould KL. Automated quantitation of three-dimensional cardiac positron emission tomography for routine clinical use. *J Nucl Med.* 1989;30:1787–1797.

21. Parkash R, deKemp RA, Ruddy TD, et al. Potential utility of rubidium 82 PET quantification in patients with 3-vessel coronary artery disease. *J Nucl Cardiol.* 2004;11:440–449.

22. Chow BJ, Ananthasubramaniam K, dekemp RA, Dalipaj MM, Beanlands RS, Ruddy TD. Comparison of treadmill exercise versus dipyridamole stress with myocardial perfusion imaging using rubidium-82 positron emission tomography. *J Am Coll Cardiol.* 2005;45:1227–1234.

23. Herrero P, Markham J, Shelton ME, Weinheimer CJ, Bergmann SR. Noninvasive quantification of regional myocardial perfusion with rubidium-82 and positron emission tomography. Exploration of a mathematical model. *Circulation.* 1990;82:1377–1386.

24. Lin JW, Sciacca RR, Chou RL, Laine AF, Bergmann SR. Quantification of myocardial perfusion in human subjects using 82Rb and wavelet-based noise reduction. *J Nucl Med.* 2001;42:201–208.

25. El Fakhri G, Sitek A, Guerin B, Kijewski MF, Di Carli MF, Moore SC. Quantitative dynamic cardiac 82Rb PET using generalized factor and compartment analyses. *J Nucl Med.* 2005;46:1264–1271.

26. Hutchins GD, Schwaiger M, Rosenspire KC, Krivokapich J, Schelbert H, Kuhl DE. Noninvasive quantification of regional blood flow in the human heart using N-13 ammonia and dynamic positron emission tomographic imaging. *J Am Coll Cardiol.* 1990;15:1032–1042.

27. Czernin J, Muller P, Chan S, et al. Influence of age and hemodynamics on myocardial blood flow and flow reserve. *Circulation.* 1993;88:62–69.

28. Pitkänen OP, Raitakari OT, Niinikoski H, et al. Coronary flow reserve is impaired in young men with familial hypercholesterolemia. *J Am Coll Cardiol.* 1996;28:1705–1711.

29. Kaufmann PA, Gnecchi-Ruscone T, Yap JT, Rimoldi O, Camici PG. Assessment of the reproducibility of baseline and hyperemic myocardial blood flow measurements with 15O-labeled water and PET. *J Nucl Med*. 1999;40:1848–1856.

30. Tadamura E, Iida H, Matsumoto K, et al. Comparison of myocardial blood flow during dobutamine-atropine infusion with that after dipyridamole administration in normal men. *J Am Coll Cardiol*. 2001;37:130–136.

31. Duvernoy CS, Meyer C, Seifert-Klauss V, et al. Gender differences in myocardial blood flow dynamics: lipid profile and hemodynamic effects. *J Am Coll Cardiol*. 1999;33: 463–470.

32. Chareonthaitawee P, Kaufmann PA, Rimoldi O, Camici PG. Heterogeneity of resting and hyperemic myocardial blood flow in healthy humans. *Cardiovasc Res*. 2001;50: 151–161.

33. Krivokapich J, Stevenson LW, Kobashigawa J, Huang SC, Schelbert HR. Quantification of absolute myocardial perfusion at rest and during exercise with positron emission tomography after human cardiac transplantation. *J Am Coll Cardiol*. 1991;18:512–517.

34. Krivokapich J, Czernin J, Schelbert HR. Dobutamine positron emission tomography: absolute quantitation of rest and dobutamine myocardial blood flow and correlation with cardiac work and percent diameter stenosis in patients with and without coronary artery disease. *J Am Coll Cardiol*. 1996;28:565–572.

35. Takala TO, Nuutila P, Katoh C, et al. Myocardial blood flow, oxygen consumption, and fatty acid uptake in endurance athletes during insulin stimulation. *Am J Physiol*. 1999;277: E585–E590.

36. Senneff MJ, Geltman EM, Bergmann SR. Noninvasive delineation of the effects of moderate aging on myocardial perfusion. *J Nucl Med*. 1991;32:2037–2042.

37. Uren NG, Camici PG, Melin JA, et al. Effect of aging on myocardial perfusion reserve. *J Nucl Med*. 1995;36:2032–2036.

38. Chan SY, Kobashigawa J, Stevenson LW, Brownfield E, Brunken RC, Schelbert HR. Myocardial blood flow at rest and during pharmacological vasodilation in cardiac transplants during and after successful treatment of rejection. *Circulation*. 1994;90:204–212.

39. Buus NH, Bottcher M, Hermansen F, Sander M, Nielsen TT, Mulvany MJ. Influence of nitric oxide synthase and adrenergic inhibition on adenosine-induced myocardial hyperemia. *Circulation*. 2001;104:2305–2310.

40. Zeiher AM, Drexler H, Wollschlager H, Just H. Endothelial dysfunction of the coronary microvasculature is associated with coronary blood flow regulation in patients with early atherosclerosis. *Circulation*. 1991;84:1984–1992.

41. Zeiher AM, Schachlinger V, Hohnloser SH, Saurbier B, Just H. Coronary atherosclerotic wall thickening and vascular reactivity in humans. Elevated high-density lipoprotein levels ameliorate abnormal vasoconstriction in early atherosclerosis. *Circulation*. 1994;89: 2525–2532.

42. Schindler TH, Nitzsche EU, Olschewski M, et al. PET-measured responses of MBF to cold pressor testing correlate with indices of coronary vasomotion on quantitative coronary angiography. *J Nucl Med*. 2004;45:419–428.

43. Campisi R, Czernin J, Schoder H, Sayre JW, Schelbert HR. L-Arginine normalizes coronary vasomotion in long-term smokers. *Circulation*. 1999;99:491–497.

44. Di Carli MF, Tobes MC, Mangner T, et al. Effects of cardiac sympathetic innervation on coronary blood flow. *N Engl J Med*. 1997;336:1208–1215.

45. Di Carli MF, Bianco-Batlles D, Landa ME, et al. Effects of autonomic neuropathy on coronary blood flow in patients with diabetes mellitus. *Circulation*. 1999;100:813–819.

46. Victor RG, Leimbach WN Jr, Seals DR, Wallin BG, Mark AL. Effects of the cold pressor test on muscle sympathetic nerve activity in humans. *Hypertension*. 1987;9:429–436.

47. Prior JO, Quinones MJ, Hernandez-Pampaloni M, et al. Coronary circulatory dysfunction in insulin resistance, impaired glucose tolerance, and type 2 diabetes mellitus. *Circulation*. 2005;111:2291–2298.

48. De Bruyne B, Hersbach F, Pijls NH, et al. Abnormal epicardial coronary resistance in patients with diffuse atherosclerosis but "normal" coronary angiography. *Circulation*. 2001;104:2401–2406.

49. Gould KL, Nakagawa Y, Nakagawa K, et al. Frequency and clinical implications of fluid dynamically significant diffuse coronary artery disease manifest as graded, longitudinal, base-to-apex myocardial perfusion abnormalities by noninvasive positron emission tomography. *Circulation*. 2000;101:1931–1939.

50. Nabel EG, Ganz P, Gordon JB, Alexander RW, Selwyn AP. Dilation of normal and constriction of atherosclerotic coronary arteries caused by the cold pressor test. *Circulation*. 1988;77:43–52.

51. Hernandez-Pampaloni M, Keng FY, Kudo T, Sayre JS, Schelbert HR. Abnormal longitudinal, base-to-apex myocardial perfusion gradient by quantitative blood flow measurements in patients with coronary risk factors. *Circulation*. 2001;104:527–532.

52. Schindler TH, Nitzsche EU, Facta AD, et al. Abnormal longitudinal, base-to-apex myocardial perfusion gradient in response to cold pressor test as assessed by PET correlates with indices of epicardial vasomotion on quantitative angiography [abstract]. *J Nucl Med*. 2004;45:4.

53. Dayanikli F, Grambow D, Muzik O, Mosca L, Rubenfire M, Schwaiger M. Early detection of abnormal coronary flow reserve in asymptomatic men at high risk for coronary artery disease using positron emission tomography. *Circulation*. 1994;90:808–817.

54. Campisi R, Nathan L, Pampaloni MH, et al. Noninvasive assessment of coronary microcirculatory function in postmenopausal women and effects of short-term and long-term estrogen administration. *Circulation*. 2002;105:425–430.

55. Schindler TH, Cardenas J, Prior JO, et al. Relationship between increasing body weight, insulin resistance, Inflammation, adipocytokine Leptin and coronary circulatory function. *J Am Coll Cardiol*. 2006;47:1188–1195.

56. Yokoyama I, Murakami T, Ohtake T, et al. Reduced coronary flow reserve in familial hypercholesterolemia. *J Nucl Med*. 1996;37:1937–1942.

57. Yokoyama I, Ohtake T, Momomura S, Nishikawa J, Sasaki Y, Omata M. Reduced coronary flow reserve in hypercholesterolemic patients without overt coronary stenosis. *Circulation*. 1996;94:3232–3238.

58. Czernin J, Barnard RJ, Sun KT, et al. Effect of short-term cardiovascular conditioning and low-fat diet on myocardial blood flow and flow reserve. *Circulation*. 1995;92:197–204.

59. Janatuinen T, Laaksonen R, Vesalainen R, et al. Effect of lipid-lowering therapy with pravastatin on myocardial blood flow in young mildly hypercholesterolemic adults. *J Cardiovasc Pharmacol*. 2001;38:561–568.

60. Baller D, Notohamiprodjo G, Gleichmann U, Holzinger J, Weise R, Lehmann J. Improvement in coronary flow reserve determined by positron emission tomography after 6 months of cholesterol-lowering therapy in patients with early stages of coronary atherosclerosis. *Circulation*. 1999;99:2871–2875.

61. Guethlin M, Kasel AM, Coppenrath K, Ziegler S, Delius W, Schwaiger M. Delayed response of myocardial flow reserve to lipid-lowering therapy with fluvastatin. *Circulation*. 1999;99:475–481.

62. Schindler TH, Nitzsche EU, Munzel T, et al. Coronary vasoregulation in patients with various risk factors in response to cold pressor testing: contrasting myocardial blood flow responses to short- and long-term vitamin C administration. *J Am Coll Cardiol*. 2003;42:814–822.

63. Yokoyama I, Momomura S, Ohtake T, et al. Reduced myocardial flow reserve in non-insulin-dependent diabetes mellitus [see comments]. *J Am Coll Cardiol*. 1997;30:1472–1477.

64. Pitkanen OP, Nuutila P, Raitakari OT, et al. Coronary flow reserve is reduced in young men with IDDM. *Diabetes*. 1998;47:248–254.

65. Pop-Busui R, Kirkwood I, Schmid H, et al. Sympathetic dysfunction in type 1 diabetes: association with impaired myocardial blood flow reserve and diastolic dysfunction. *J Am Coll Cardiol*. 2004;44:2368–2374.

66. Hattori N, Schnell O, Bengel FM, et al. Deferoxamine improves coronary vascular responses to sympathetic stimulation in patients with type 1 diabetes mellitus. *Eur J Nucl Med Mol Imaging*. 2002;29:891–898.

67. Quinones MJ, Hernandez-Pampaloni M, Schelbert H, et al. Coronary vasomotor abnormalities in insulin-resistant individuals. *Ann Intern Med*. 2004;140:700–708.

68. Cecchi F, Olivotto I, Gistri R, Lorenzoni R, Chiriatti G, Camici PG. Coronary microvascular dysfunction and prognosis in hypertrophic cardiomyopathy. *N Engl J Med*. 2003;349:1027–1035.

69. Schindler TH, Nitzsche EU, Schelbert HR, et al. Positron emission tomography-measured abnormal responses of myocardial blood flow to sympathetic stimulation are associated with the risk of developing cardiovascular events. *J Am Coll Cardiol*. 2005;45:1505–1512.

70. Schachinger V, Britten MB, Zeiher AM. Prognostic impact of coronary vasodilator dysfunction on adverse long-term outcome of coronary heart disease. *Circulation.* 2000;101: 1899–1906.
71. Suwaidi JA, Hamasaki S, Higano ST, Nishimura RA, Holmes DR Jr, Lerman A. Long-term follow-up of patients with mild coronary artery disease and endothelial dysfunction. *Circulation.* 2000;101:948–954.
72. Halcox JP, Schenke WH, Zalos G, et al. Prognostic value of coronary vascular endothelial dysfunction. *Circulation.* 2002;106:653–658.

13 Assessing Atherosclerotic Burden with CT

Javier Sanz, Santo Dellegrottaglie, and Valentin Fuster

Computed tomography (CT) has long been used for the evaluation of both normal and pathologic human anatomy. In the setting of atherosclerosis (AS) and cardiovascular disease (CVD), CT angiography has a well-established role for the detection of luminal stenoses and aneurysms in various vascular territories such as the aorta, carotid, renal, and lower-extremity arteries. Although of indisputable value in clinical practice, such findings reflect an already advanced stage of the disease. The atherosclerotic changes of the arterial wall in fact commence much earlier, as microscopic lesions progressing slowly into macroscopic plaques that often grow eccentrically without compromising the vessel lumen.[1] Reliance on changes in luminal caliber is therefore insufficient for estimating the extent and severity of atherosclerotic burden. In fact, clinical events are often caused by acute complications (rupture and thrombosis) of specific plaques that may not produce a significant luminal narrowing, particularly in the coronary tree.[2] Because AS is a systemic disorder involving multiple vascular territories, it is important not to restrict the evaluation to a single arterial system. The visualization of the coronary arteries with CT has, however, been traditionally limited by their continuous motion from both cardiac and respiratory origins.

These limitations of CT for the evaluation of CVD have been overcome to a great extent with the rapid technical improvements of ultrafast scanners during the last few years. Two modalities, described in detail in other sections of this book, are currently available for cardiac CT imaging: electron beam computed tomography (EBCT) and, more recently, multidetector-row spiral computed tomography (MDCT). Although the application of EBCT has been limited almost exclusively to the heart, MDCT offers the capability of evaluating other vascular territories. The improved volume coverage associated with MDCT enables imaging large anatomic regions in a single exam. As an example, the latest generation of 64-slice MDCT scanners can perform a whole-body angiography with submillimeter resolution in <25 seconds.[3] In addition, the increased spatial resolution achievable with newer equipment, particularly with MDCT, opens the possibility of detecting and, to a certain extent, characterizing atherosclerotic plaques at different locations, including the coronary tree. In this chapter we review the capabilities of CT imaging for the assessment of vascular calcifications (using noncontrast techniques) and noncalcified lesions (using contrast) in the coronary and extracoronary vascular systems.

Coronary Atherosclerosis

Coronary Artery Calcification

Significance

Coronary artery calcification (CAC) is absent in normal coronary arteries, and its presence is very indicative of AS,[4] although nonatherosclerotic medial dystrophic calcification has been described.[5] The prevalence of CAC increases with age, is higher in males, and is associated with traditional cardiovascular risk factors.[4] The significance of calcification in plaque biology remains incompletely understood. Once regarded as a passive phenomenon, it is known today that calcification is a complex and active process intimately related to different components of AS.[6] Calcification is most common in advanced atherosclerotic plaques, although it may be rarely observed in early type III lesions (pre-atheroma).[7] The role of calcium on plaque-surface susceptibility to shear stress and rupture is controversial. Observations of smaller amounts of calcium in patients with acute coronary syndromes versus stable disease[8] suggest that CAC occurs in the context of clinical stability and that calcification represents a healing response. However, both pathology and intravascular ultrasound (IVUS) studies have shown that culprit lesions in acute syndromes often have calcifications, which tend to be small and in a spotty pattern.[9,10] Moreover, the evidence derived from prospective studies shows that high calcium scores are associated with increased probability of events (see section Prognostic Value of CAC Scoring in Asymptomatic Subjects below). It is possible that maximal stress occurs at the areas of interface between components of different stiffness, and that small amounts of calcium result in increased vulnerability. As the calcium content progresses beyond a certain level, there could be a diminution of such areas and theoretically a reduction in stress.[6] In addition, there is a direct linear relation between the amount of CAC and total coronary plaque burden; it is estimated that for every calcified lesion there are 4 noncalcified plaques.[11]

Detection and Quantification of CAC

The high density of calcium results in pronounced x-ray attenuation. In general, most investigators use an attenuation coefficient value ≥130 Hounsfield units (HU) to define calcification with CT (Figure 13.1).[12] This threshold represents approximately

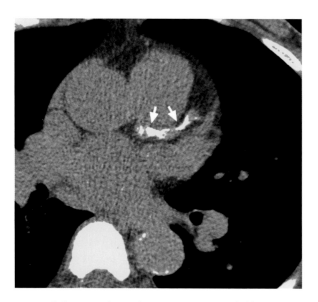

FIGURE 13.1. Coronary calcium scoring using noncontrast axial images of the thorax acquired with electrocardiographic synchronization. The pixels containing calcification (attenuation ≥130 HU) along the left main and left anterior descending arteries are highlighted in yellow.

2 standard deviations of the attenuation of blood and correlates well with histomorphometric measurements of calcified plaque.[13] Both MDCT and EBCT can be employed for CAC detection and quantification. Most of the diagnostic and prognostic data on CAC scoring have been obtained with EBCT, currently considered the standard of reference.[12] In direct comparisons, however, both modalities demonstrate excellent agreement in calcium quantification.[14] Interstudy reproducibility of calcium measurements, a factor that critically influences the interpretation of changes in CAC scores detected over a period of time, has been a matter of concern, especially for low scores. With newer scanners and optimized methodology, variability can be reduced below 10%.[15]

Three methods for calcium scoring are currently used, and reference ranges for each approach have been reported.[16] The Agatston score[17] is obtained by the summation of areas of the calcified lesions multiplied by a scaling cofactor derived from the peak attenuation in each plaque (factor of 1 for attenuation between 130 and 200 HU, 2 for attenuation between 200 and 300 HU, 3 for attenuation between 300 and 400 HU, and 4 for attenuation >400 HU). This score can be subsequently normalized for different imaging parameters such as slice thickness or reconstruction increment.[18] The Agatston score has been the most common method used in clinical and epidemiological investigations. A second approach is the volumetric method, which measures the volume of the calcified voxels and performs a continuous isotropic interpolation to avoid the nonlinearity associated with the Agatston scaling factors.[19] A third approach is the quantification of calcium mass, combining volumetric calculations with density information derived from the mean attenuation of the lesion (typically by using a calibration phantom).[18] Reproducibility is worst for the Agatston method, intermediate for the volumetric approach, and best for the mass score.[18] Interestingly, all 3 methods appear to stratify cardiovascular risk similarly.[16] A new, recently proposed approach is the analysis of calcification indexes in individual plaques rather than in the whole coronary tree.[20] Whether this method provides additional information over global scores will require further research.

Although the "normal" score is 0, there is no clear cutoff of what represents a high score. A common, simplified classification defines Agatston scores as absent (0), low (1 to 100), intermediate (101 to 400), or high (>400). However, more refined stratification in a continuous scale with age- and gender-adjusted values is recommended.[12]

Diagnostic Value of CAC Scoring

Voluminous plaques are more prone to calcification, and stenotic lesions frequently contain large amounts of calcium.[4] Therefore, quantification of CAC may be used to estimate the likelihood of significant stenoses (usually defined as luminal diameter reduction >50%). With very high sensitivity (91%), however, the practical value of this approach is limited by poor specificity (52%).[21] Nonetheless, this translates into a very low likelihood of significant luminal narrowing if the score is 0, a finding of special clinical usefulness.[12] It is important to emphasize that there is a relatively poor correlation between the site of calcification and the actual location of the stenosis, so the information provided by the calcium score is in essence an estimate of probability. In a small percentage of subjects (probably <1%), particularly at younger ages, there may still be significant stenoses caused by noncalcified plaque in the absence of CAC.[22] The global diagnostic accuracy of calcium scoring approaches 70%, similar to that of treadmill testing and slightly lower than perfusion scintigraphy or stress echocardiography.[12] Selecting the highest quartile (adjusted for age and gender) as a threshold results in less sensitivity but higher specificity and may represent a reasonable compromise.[22]

CAC scoring provides additional information to conventional risk factors in the prediction of both significant and nonsignificant luminal narrowing on angiography.[23,24] Not surprisingly, exercise testing and CT seem to reflect different aspects of the disease and offer complementary information.[24,25] As an example, one study reported a negative predictive value of 93% for the presence of significant coronary stenosis if the score was 0, even in the presence of a positive stress test, and a specificity of 100% for scores >1000.[25] CT also has been proposed as a triage method in the emergency department. A coronary origin for chest pain appears to be very unlikely in the absence of CAC,[26] although scores of 0 may be observed in the specific subset of young male smokers presenting with acute ischemic events.[27] In addition, the rate of cardiac events during subsequent midterm follow-up is very low in the subgroup of patients with chest pain and no calcification, suggesting that it is safe to discharge them from the emergency department.[28]

Evaluation of Disease Progression or Regression

Temporal variations in calcium scores may be considered surrogates of atherosclerotic disease progression or regression. In an unselected population, the mean annual progression of CAC is close to 25%, although with large interindividual variations.[29] This growth is faster in individuals with obstructive coronary disease.[30] Among the factors that drive CAC progression, the degree of baseline calcification appears to be the leading determinant, with lesser influence of age, gender, or conventional risk factors.[30,31] Notably, an accelerated increase rate may identify subjects with a higher probability of clinical events.[32,33]

In agreement with the favorable effect of statins on AS, several investigators have reported slowed progression of CAC under therapy with these drugs (5% to 10% per year).[34,35] Although net reductions were observed for subsets of patients, the degree of change is usually within the range of interstudy variability, and it is difficult to establish with certainty whether statins may actually result in "removal" of calcium from the plaque.

Prognostic Value of CAC Scoring in Asymptomatic Subjects

It is well known that the likelihood of both hard (death and myocardial infarction) and soft (revascularization or stroke) cardiovascular events increases as CAC rises. A meta-analysis of 5 prospective studies calculated risk ratios of 4.2 and 8.7 for hard events alone or in combination with revascularization, respectively, when the calcium scores were elevated above a certain threshold (variable among studies).[36] Interestingly, the risk is particularly increased for very large scores,[37] challenging the notion that calcified coronary disease represents a scenario of clinical stability. Very high absolute scores are, however, relatively uncommon in the population, with the majority of events taking place in those individuals with scores >75th percentile, adjusted for their age and gender.[38]

Current approaches for risk stratification in CVD are based on the presence of the so-called traditional risk factors (i.e., the Framingham risk score). Such scales possess demonstrated predictive value, but they are too gross to accurately identify the minority of individuals who will actually develop clinical events. CAC quantification may help place intermediate-risk individuals in a higher or lower category (Table 13.1);[33,39] however, this approach is not currently recommended for systematic use.[12] In the setting of high baseline risk (i.e., diabetes mellitus), there is some controversy on the prognostic utility of CAC measurement, whose relative "weight" might be diluted by the stronger influence of traditional risk factors.[40,41] Nonetheless, the recently published St. Francis Heart Study has demonstrated additive value for calcium scoring in the setting of low, intermediate, and high risk as defined by the Framingham index, at least for Caucasian individuals.[33] Interestingly, among low-risk individuals, only those with elevated calcium score (in the third tertile) experienced events.[33] These findings agree with a meta-analysis of those studies in which calcium scores were adjusted for traditional risk factors and where calcification levels were still able to predict increased risk (Figure 13.2).[33,42] Comparable results can be applied to the

TABLE 13.1. Probability of Coronary Events (in percent) Within 10 Years, Based on Traditional Risk Factors Before and After Coronary Calcium Scoring

Pretest Probability (Framingham Score)	Posttest Probability (CAC Score)	
	CAC Score ≥80	CAC Score <80
1.0	3.0	0.2
2.0	6.5	0.4
3.0	9.5	0.6
4.0	12.5	0.9
5.0	15.0	1.0
6.0	18.0	1.2
7.0	20.0	1.4
10.0	**27.0**	**2.2**
15.0	38.0	3.4
20.0	46.0	4.8

Source: Data from Greenland and Gaziano.[39]

aging population.[43] Moreover, CAC may be superior to conventional risk assessment and C-reactive protein for the prediction of cardiovascular events.[33] Although both CAC scoring and C-reactive protein refine risk stratification beyond the Framingham index, they provide independent and complementary information, suggesting that they reflect different physiopathologic aspects of the disease (inflammatory activity versus anatomic burden of AS).[33,44]

Prognostic Value of CAC Scoring in Symptomatic Patients

There is a paucity of evidence on the implications of CAC in the setting of symptomatic ischemic heart disease or secondary prevention. Nonetheless, available reports suggest that the prognostic value is maintained in this context. In subjects with chest pain, detectable calcification is associated with significantly increased likelihood of coronary hard events.[4] The prognostic ability may be similar or superior to the number of vessels with significant disease or a prior history of coronary events.[45]

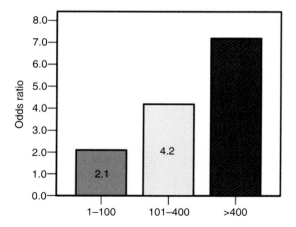

FIGURE 13.2. Incremental prognostic value of coronary calcium scoring after adjustment for conventional risk factors. The columns represent the odds ratios of cardiovascular events for different Agatston scores in relation to the patients with zero calcification, after an average follow-up of 3.5 years. (Data from Pletcher et al.[42])

Coronary Noncalcified Plaque

Plaque Detection and Quantification

The improvements in both spatial and temporal resolution in newer MDCT scanners have enabled the visualization of changes in the vessel wall when intravenous iodinated contrast agents are administered. MDCT can also provide some insights into the composition of the plaque, opening the possibility of noninvasive characterization of coronary atherosclerosis. There are virtually no data on the application of EBCT for this purpose, probably in relation to its inferior spatial resolution. In healthy subjects, the coronary arterial wall is very thin (<1 mm) and cannot be discerned from perivascular structures. However, when wall thickening occurs in the presence of atherosclerotic disease, it is possible to visualize plaques even in the absence of calcium or luminal narrowing.[46] Plaques are seen as areas of thickening of the arterial wall and exhibit attenuation properties of soft tissue (lower than the contrast–enhanced lumen but higher then the surrounding fat), as demonstrated in Figure 13.3. Atherosclerotic lesion types I and II are usually not identified due to their small size, and the sensitivities to detect types III, IV, and V_{a-c} range from 56% to 100% ex vivo.[47,48] In an in vivo comparison with IVUS, the reported sensitivity and specificity were 82% and 88%, respectively, for the detection of any coronary plaque, which in turn became 78% and 87% when only noncalcified lesions were considered.[49] Similar results were communicated in a subsequent investigation with a sensitivity of 78% and specificity of 92%.[50] Not surprisingly, the technique has limited ability to detect small plaques that may be beyond its spatial resolution.[50,51] The accuracy for the quantification of lumen or vessel wall cross-sectional areas is nonetheless satisfactory when plaques are actually visualized.[51,52] It is therefore possible to obtain indexes of global coronary disease burden by quantifying the volume of visualized plaque at multiple segments. As expected from the still-limited spatial resolution of MDCT, total plaque volume is underestimated,[49] but such measurements correlate with the extent of coronary calcification and the severity of disease.[53]

Plaque Characterization

Several features of plaque morphology, such as eccentricity and disruption, are detected with MDCT.[54] Preliminary reports confirmed the feasibility of differentiating various carotid plaque components based on their distinct x-ray attenuation prop-

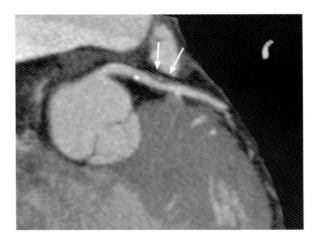

FIGURE 13.3. Contrast-enhanced coronary angiography demonstrating an eccentric plaque (arrows) that does not cause significant luminal narrowing. The plaque is mostly noncalcified, with a small central area of calcification.

TABLE 13.2. Differences in Attenuation Coefficients Between Predominantly Lipid-Rich and Fibrous Atherosclerotic Plaques

Reference Source	Attenuation (HU)		Methods		
	Lipid-rich	Fibrous	Territory	Reference Test	Other
Estes et al[55]	39 ± 12	90 ± 24	Carotid	Pathology	In vivo (EA)
Schroeder et al[57]	14 ± 26	91 ± 21	Coronary	IVUS	In vivo
Becker et al[47]	49 ± 22	91 ± 22	Coronary	Pathology	In vivo
Nikolaou et al[48]	47 ± 13	87 ± 29	Coronary	Pathology	Ex vivo
Schroeder et al[58]	42 ± 22	70 ± 21	Coronary	Pathology	Ex vivo
Viles-Gonzalez et al[51]	51 ± 25	116 ± 27	Aortic	Pathology, MRI	In vivo (rabbit)
Leber et al[50]	49 ± 22	91 ± 22	Coronary	IVUS	In vivo

Abbreviations: HU, Hounsfield units; EA, endarterectomy; IVUS, intravascular ultrasound; MRI, magnetic resonance imaging. Attenuation values expressed as mean ± standard deviation.

erties.[55] These observations were soon translated to the field of cardiac imaging once MDCT scanners became available.[56] So far, investigations have demonstrated the possibility to differentiate "soft" (lipid-rich) from fibrous lesions in ex vivo human hearts and also in vivo, in both animal models and humans. Areas rich in lipid components within the plaque, often associated with increased plaque vulnerability, have lower attenuation coefficients than fibrotic tissue (see Table 13.2).

Extracoronary Atherosclerosis

Many of the aforementioned implications of CT findings in the coronary tree can be extrapolated to other arterial systems. It is important to recognize, however, that there are territorial variations in the frequency of involvement, clinical significance, and histopathologic features of lesions. As an example, vulnerable plaques in the carotids or the lower extremities tend to be more stenotic and fibrotic than those in the aorta or coronaries.[2]

Association with CAC

When calcification is present in the coronary arteries, simultaneous although heterogeneous atherosclerotic involvement (including calcification) can be identified in other vascular territories.[59] Calcium in extracoronary locations is detected in approximately 60% of individuals above middle age.[60] Again age appears to be the main determinant for calcification (particularly in the aorta), although gender and traditional risk factors do exert some influence.[60,61] In subjects above 70 years old, the prevalence approaches 100% and affects all vascular beds in more than two thirds of cases.[60] Calcification in men appears to initiate more often in the coronaries, whereas in women the abdominal aorta and iliac arteries are also affected early.[60]

Aortic Atherosclerosis

In general, the aorta is the artery with a higher prevalence of calcification, a finding that indicates advanced atherosclerotic disease.[60] Aortic calcification is associated with CAC and with increased Framingham risk scores regardless of the level of coronary calcium.[61] Whether aortic calcification per se provides information regarding cardiovascular risk is less established than in the case of CAC, although there also appears to be a direct relation between risk and aortic calcium.[43] Two studies (which employed plain x-ray for the detection of calcification) demonstrated increased risk for stroke in particular or cardiovascular diseases in general even after controlling for traditional risk factors.[62,63] Determination of the degree of aortic calcification may also play a role in the diagnosis of obstructive coronary disease. In a comparison with invasive angiography, the presence of calcium thoracic descending aorta improved the diagnostic performance (specificity) of CAC scoring for the prediction of significant coronary stenoses.[64] Interestingly, the amount of both calcified and noncalcified plaque after the administration of contrast may represent a better predictor for this purpose (Figure 13.4).[65] It is likely that the amount of atherosclerosis detected by this method correlates with traditional risk factors and allows for estimation of the subject's burden of disease, as already demonstrated with magnetic resonance imaging (MRI).[66] Further investigation will need to concentrate on the possible additional prognostic value of such indexes of disease in overall risk assessment. Contrast-enhanced CT may also serve as a roadmap that will delineate the presence and extent of both calcified and noncalcified atherosclerotic lesions. Once lesions are detected, further characterization can be performed with targeted, high-resolution MRI, which currently shows superior capabilities for discrimination of plaque composition.[51]

Carotid Atherosclerosis

Carotid calcification is readily detected using CT techniques and is also associated with CAC.[67] Again, there is less evidence on its significance than in the case of CAC, but it appears to be more common in asymptomatic lesions.[68,69] In addition, there is a negative correlation between the degree of plaque inflammation and calcium extent.[69] Contrast-enhanced CT has similarly been used to evaluate the presence, size, morphology, and composition of noncalcified atherosclerotic lesions in the carotid arteries.[55,70,71]

Other Territories

The capability of MDCT to evaluate plaque characteristics in human popliteal arteries was recently reported in an ex vivo investigation,[72] with findings comparable to

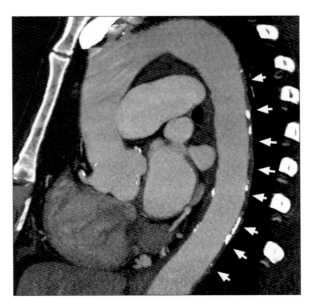

FIGURE 13.4. Maximum-intensity projection of the thoracic aorta as imaged during a contrast-enhanced coronary study. Diffuse thickening with both calcified and noncalcified plaques is clearly visible along the descending thoracic aorta (arrows).

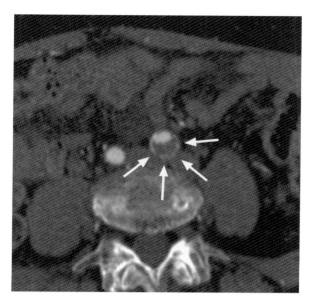

FIGURE 13.5. Axial image below the level of the aortic bifurcation. A large plaque (arrows) with extensive wall remodeling can be noted in the left common iliac artery. A normal appearance can be observed in the contralateral vessel.

those in other vascular territories (Figure 13.5). A special case may be that of valvular calcification. Both mitral annular calcification and especially calcified aortic valve disease show associations with cardiovascular risk factors, are linked to AS, and have been identified as predictors of cardiovascular events.[73,74] CT may play a role in detecting and quantifying valvular calcium, providing useful information in these patients.

Current and Future Perspectives

Noncontrast CT has demonstrated ability to detect and quantify the amount of calcification in the coronary arteries and other vascular territories. From a diagnostic perspective, this modality depicts the presence and extent of AS and, in the coronary tree, has a high negative predictive value in ruling out significant stenoses, providing a reasonable alternative to conventional stress testing. Particularly useful is the prognostic information derived from calcium scoring, which is of incremental value over traditional risk factors and newer biomarkers. These features of CT will probably result in growing interest in the technique during the next years. The issues of accessibility, radiation exposure, and cost-effectiveness may, however, preclude its systematic application in the general population. In addition, the calcium score does not provide important additional information for the evaluation of CVD, such as degree of stenosis, ventricular function, functional class or site, and extent of ischemia. The increasing availability of MDCT and fusion technologies (such as PET/CT or, perhaps in the future, MRI/CT) may overcome some of these limitations and further promote the use of this imaging modality.

In the context of noncalcified plaque, although it is feasible to visualize, measure, and characterize such lesions in humans, several existing limitations must be accounted for before application in clinical practice. In the coronary arteries, this approach is currently limited to proximal and midcoronary segments with sufficient image quality. Accurate delineation of plaque boundaries (particularly the outer limit) can be challenging and, although interobserver agreement appears to be good,[8,49] data on interstudy reproducibility are lacking. Determination of plaque composition is still rudimentary, as evidenced by the overlap in attenuation coefficients in Table 13.2, and density values are also influenced by scanning or image analysis methods.[51,75] In the next few years, it will be necessary to optimize and standardize acquisition and analysis methods before comparing results from different studies or centers. Some of the current challenges also may be overcome in part with improved spatial resolution (64-slice MDCT scanners and beyond) or quantitative approaches for plaque composition determination.[76] Today, concomitant evaluation with high-resolution MRI can provide a practical and noninvasive combination for rapid lesion detection (with CT) and plaque characterization (with MRI), resulting in a more detailed evaluation of AS and probably more refined assessment of individual risk. In the future, as some of the limitations are addressed, MDCT-determined assessment of noncalcified plaque may become a useful tool in the evaluation of the natural history of disease or of the effects of different therapeutic interventions, and provide supplementary prognostic information over current risk stratification approaches.

Summary Points

- Imaging modalities for noninvasive assessment of atherosclerosis must be able to evaluate multiple vascular territories, including the coronary tree. EBCT and MDCT currently offer such potential.
- CT imaging without the use of contrast agents accurately detects the presence of arterial calcification, a specific marker of atherosclerosis. When calcium is detected in one vascular system, atherosclerotic involvement is often present in other territories. Contrast-enhanced CT can also be employed to visualize noncalcified plaques.
- The presence of coronary calcification has high sensitivity (and negative predictive value) for the detection of significant coronary stenoses, although its use in clinical practice is limited by poor specificity.
- Serial quantification of coronary calcium can estimate the rate of progression of atherosclerotic disease in different patient groups or under specific therapeutic interventions.
- The likelihood of both hard and soft cardiovascular events increases with coronary calcium scores. This predictive value is additive to traditional cardiovascular risk stratification.
- Contrast-enhanced CT can detect the presence and quantify the extent of noncalcified lesions both in the coronary arteries and in extracoronary locations. Preliminary results suggest a potential role of CT in noninvasive plaque characterization.
- CT offers the potential to provide an overall assessment of the presence, location, and extent of atherosclerotic disease at multiple levels. These estimates of burden of disease may prove useful in the early detection of subclinical disease or the identification of those subjects with increased cardiovascular risk.

References

1. Corti R, Fuster V. New understanding, diagnosis, and prognosis of atherothrombosis and the role of imaging. *Am J Cardiol.* 2003;91:17–26.
2. Viles-Gonzalez JF, Fuster V, Badimon JJ. Atherothrombosis: a widespread disease with unpredictable and life-threatening consequences. *Eur Heart J.* 2004;25:1197–1207.
3. Flohr T, Stierstorfer K, Raupach R, Ulzheimer S, Bruder H. Performance evaluation of a 64-slice CT system with z-flying focal spot. *Rofo.* 2004;176:1803–1810.
4. Wexler L, Brundage B, Crouse J, et al. Coronary artery calcification: pathophysiology, epidemiology, imaging methods, and clinical implications. A statement for health professionals from the American Heart Association. Writing Group. *Circulation.* 1996;94:1175–1192.

5. Qiao JH, Doherty TM, Fishbein MC, et al. Calcification of the coronary arteries in the absence of atherosclerotic plaque. *Mayo Clin Proc.* 2005;80:807–809.

6. Abedin M, Tintut Y, Demer LL. Vascular calcification: mechanisms and clinical ramifications. *Arterioscler Thromb Vasc Biol.* 2004;24:1161–1170.

7. Stary HC. The development of calcium deposits in atherosclerotic lesions and their persistence after lipid regression. *Am J Cardiol.* 2001;88:16–19.

8. Leber AW, Knez A, White CW, et al. Composition of coronary atherosclerotic plaques in patients with acute myocardial infarction and stable angina pectoris determined by contrast-enhanced multislice computed tomography. *Am J Cardiol.* 2003;91:714–718.

9. Burke AP, Weber DK, Kolodgie FD, Farb A, Taylor AJ, Virmani R. Pathophysiology of calcium deposition in coronary arteries. *Herz.* 2001;26:239–244.

10. Ehara S, Kobayashi Y, Yoshiyama M, et al. Spotty calcification typifies the culprit plaque in patients with acute myocardial infarction: an intravascular ultrasound study. *Circulation.* 2004;110:3424–3429.

11. Sangiorgi G, Rumberger JA, Severson A, et al. Arterial calcification and not lumen stenosis is highly correlated with atherosclerotic plaque burden in humans: a histologic study of 723 coronary artery segments using nondecalcifying methodology. *J Am Coll Cardiol.* 1998;31:126–133.

12. O'Rourke RA, Brundage BH, Froelicher VF, et al. American College of Cardiology/ American Heart Association Expert Consensus document on electron-beam computed tomography for the diagnosis and prognosis of coronary artery disease. *Circulation.* 2000;102:126–140.

13. Rumberger JA, Simons DB, Fitzpatrick LA, Sheedy PF, Schwartz RS. Coronary artery calcium area by electron-beam computed tomography and coronary atherosclerotic plaque area. A histopathologic correlative study. *Circulation.* 1995;92:2157–2162.

14. Horiguchi J, Yamamoto H, Akiyama Y, Marukawa K, Hirai N, Ito K. Coronary artery calcium scoring using 16-MDCT and a retrospective ECG-gating reconstruction algorithm. *AJR Am J Roentgenol.* 2004;183:103–108.

15. Kopp AF, Ohnesorge B, Becker C, et al. reproducibility and accuracy of coronary calcium measurements with multi-detector row versus electron-beam CT. *Radiology.* 2002;225:113–119.

16. Rumberger JA, Kaufman L. A Rosetta stone for coronary calcium risk stratification: agatston, volume, and mass scores in 11,490 individuals. *AJR Am J Roentgenol.* 2003;181:743–748.

17. Agatston AS, Janowitz WR, Hildner FJ, Zusmer NR, Viamonte M Jr, Detrano R. Quantification of coronary artery calcium using ultrafast computed tomography. *J Am Coll Cardiol.* 1990;15:827–832.

18. Ohnesorge B, Flohr T, Fischbach R, et al. Reproducibility of coronary calcium quantification in repeat examinations with retrospectively ECG-gated multisection spiral CT. *Eur Radiol.* 2002;12:1532–1540.

19. Callister TQ, Cooil B, Raya SP, Lippolis NJ, Russo DJ, Raggi P. Coronary artery disease: improved reproducibility of calcium scoring with an electron-beam CT volumetric method. *Radiology.* 1998;208:807–814.

20. Moselewski F, O'Donnell C J, Achenbach S, et al. Calcium concentration of individual coronary calcified plaques as measured by multidetector row computed tomography. *Circulation.* 2005;111:3236–3241.

21. Nallamothu BK, Saint S, Bielak LF, et al. Electron-beam computed tomography in the diagnosis of coronary artery disease: a meta-analysis. *Arch Intern Med.* 2001;161:833–838.

22. Knez A, Becker A, Leber A, et al. Relation of coronary calcium scores by electron beam tomography to obstructive disease in 2,115 symptomatic patients. *Am J Cardiol.* 2004;93:1150–1152.

23. Brown BG, Morse J, Zhao XQ, Cheung M, Marino E, Albers JJ. Electron-beam tomography coronary calcium scores are superior to Framingham risk variables for predicting the measured proximal stenosis burden. *Am J Cardiol.* 2001;88:23E–26E.

24. Lamont DH, Budoff MJ, Shavelle DM, Shavelle R, Brundage BH, Hagar JM. Coronary calcium scanning adds incremental value to patients with positive stress tests. *Am Heart J.* 2002;143:861–867.

25. Schmermund A, Baumgart D, Sack S, et al. Assessment of coronary calcification by electron-beam computed tomography in symptomatic patients with normal, abnormal or equivocal exercise stress test. *Eur Heart J.* 2000;21:1674–1682.

26. McLaughlin VV, Balogh T, Rich S. Utility of electron beam computed tomography to stratify patients presenting to the emergency room with chest pain. *Am J Cardiol.* 1999;84:327–328, A8.

27. Raggi P, Callister TQ, Cooil B, et al. Identification of patients at increased risk of first unheralded acute myocardial infarction by electron-beam computed tomography. *Circulation.* 2000;101:850–855.

28. Georgiou D, Budoff MJ, Kaufer E, Kennedy JM, Lu B, Brundage BH. Screening patients with chest pain in the emergency department using electron beam tomography: a follow-up study. *J Am Coll Cardiol.* 2001;38:105–110.

29. Maher JE, Bielak LF, Raz JA, Sheedy PF 2nd, Schwartz RS, Peyser PA. Progression of coronary artery calcification: a pilot study. *Mayo Clin Proc.* 1999;74:347–355.

30. Shemesh J, Koren-Morag N, Apter S, et al. Accelerated progression of coronary calcification: four-year follow-up in patients with stable coronary artery disease. *Radiology.* 2004;233:201–209.

31. Yoon HC, Emerick AM, Hill JA, Gjertson DW, Goldin JG. Calcium begets calcium: progression of coronary artery calcification in asymptomatic subjects. *Radiology.* 2002;224: 236–241.

32. Raggi P, Cooil B, Shaw LJ, et al. Progression of coronary calcium on serial electron beam tomographic scanning is greater in patients with future myocardial infarction. *Am J Cardiol.* 2003;92:827–829.

33. Arad Y, Goodman KJ, Roth M, Newstein D, Guerci AD. Coronary calcification, coronary disease risk factors, C-reactive protein, and atherosclerotic cardiovascular disease events: the St. Francis Heart Study. *J Am Coll Cardiol.* 2005;46:158–165.

34. Callister TQ, Raggi P, Cooil B, Lippolis NJ, Russo DJ. Effect of HMG-CoA reductase inhibitors on coronary artery disease as assessed by electron-beam computed tomography. *N Engl J Med.* 1998;339:1972–1978.

35. Achenbach S, Ropers D, Pohle K, et al. Influence of lipid-lowering therapy on the progression of coronary artery calcification: a prospective evaluation. *Circulation.* 2002;106: 1077–1082.

36. O'Malley PG, Taylor AJ, Jackson JL, Doherty TM, Detrano RC. Prognostic value of coronary electron-beam computed tomography for coronary heart disease events in asymptomatic populations. *Am J Cardiol.* 2000;85:945–948.

37. Wayhs R, Zelinger A, Raggi P. High coronary artery calcium scores pose an extremely elevated risk for hard events. *J Am Coll Cardiol.* 2002;39:225–230.

38. Kondos GT, Hoff JA, Sevrukov A, et al. Electron-beam tomography coronary artery calcium and cardiac events: a 37-month follow-up of 5635 initially asymptomatic low- to intermediate-risk adults. *Circulation.* 2003;107:2571–2576.

39. Greenland P, Gaziano JM. Clinical practice. Selecting asymptomatic patients for coronary computed tomography or electrocardiographic exercise testing. *N Engl J Med.* 2003;349: 465–473.

40. Greenland P, LaBree L, Azen SP, Doherty TM, Detrano RC. Coronary artery calcium score combined with Framingham score for risk prediction in asymptomatic individuals. *JAMA.* 2004;291:210–215.

41. Detrano RC, Wong ND, Doherty TM, et al. Coronary calcium does not accurately predict near-term future coronary events in high-risk adults. *Circulation.* 1999;99:2633–2638.

42. Pletcher MJ, Tice JA, Pignone M, Browner WS. Using the coronary artery calcium score to predict coronary heart disease events: a systematic review and meta-analysis. *Arch Intern Med.* 2004;164:1285–1292.

43. Vliegenthart R, Oudkerk M, Hofman A, et al. Coronary calcification improves cardiovascular risk prediction in the elderly. Circulation. 2005;112:572–577.

44. Park R, Detrano R, Xiang M, et al. Combined use of computed tomography coronary calcium scores and C-reactive protein levels in predicting cardiovascular events in nondiabetic individuals. *Circulation.* 2002;106:2073–2077.

45. Keelan PC, Bielak LF, Ashai K, et al. Long-term prognostic value of coronary calcification detected by electron-beam computed tomography in patients undergoing coronary angiography. *Circulation.* 2001;104:412–417.

46. Caussin C, Ohanessian A, Lancelin B, et al. Coronary plaque burden detected by multislice computed tomography after acute myocardial infarction with near-normal coronary arteries by angiography. *Am J Cardiol.* 2003;92:849–852.

47. Becker CR, Nikolaou K, Muders M, et al. Ex vivo coronary atherosclerotic plaque characterization with multi-detector-row CT. *Eur Radiol.* 2003;13:2094–2098.
48. Nikolaou K, Becker CR, Muders M, et al. Multidetector-row computed tomography and magnetic resonance imaging of atherosclerotic lesions in human ex vivo coronary arteries. *Atherosclerosis.* 2004;174:243–252.
49. Achenbach S, Moselewski F, Ropers D, et al. Detection of calcified and noncalcified coronary atherosclerotic plaque by contrast-enhanced, submillimeter multidetector spiral computed tomography: a segment-based comparison with intravascular ultrasound. *Circulation.* 2004;109:14–17.
50. Leber AW, Knez A, Becker A, et al. Accuracy of multidetector spiral computed tomography in identifying and differentiating the composition of coronary atherosclerotic plaques: a comparative study with intracoronary ultrasound. *J Am Coll Cardiol.* 2004;43:1241–1247.
51. Viles-Gonzalez JF, Poon M, Sanz J, et al. In vivo 16-slice, multidetector-row computed tomography for the assessment of experimental atherosclerosis: comparison with magnetic resonance imaging and histopathology. *Circulation.* 2004;110:1467–1472.
52. Leber AW, Knez A, von Ziegler F, et al. Quantification of obstructive and nonobstructive coronary lesions by 64-slice computed tomography: a comparative study with quantitative coronary angiography and intravascular ultrasound. *J Am Coll Cardiol.* 2005;46:147–154.
53. Nikolaou K, Sagmeister S, Knez A, et al. Multidetector-row computed tomography of the coronary arteries: predictive value and quantitative assessment of non-calcified vessel-wall changes. *Eur Radiol.* 2003;13:2505–2512.
54. Caussin C, Ohanessian A, Ghostine S, et al. Characterization of vulnerable nonstenotic plaque with 16-slice computed tomography compared with intravascular ultrasound. *Am J Cardiol.* 2004;94:99–104.
55. Estes JM, Quist WC, Lo Gerfo FW, Costello P. Noninvasive characterization of plaque morphology using helical computed tomography. *J Cardiovasc Surg (Torino).* 1998;39:527–534.
56. Kopp AF, Schroeder S, Baumbach A, et al. Non-invasive characterisation of coronary lesion morphology and composition by multislice CT: first results in comparison with intracoronary ultrasound. *Eur Radiol.* 2001;11:1607–1611.
57. Schroeder S, Kopp AF, Baumbach A, et al. Noninvasive detection and evaluation of atherosclerotic coronary plaques with multislice computed tomography. *J Am Coll Cardiol.* 2001;37:1430–1435.
58. Schroeder S, Kuettner A, Leitritz M, et al. Reliability of differentiating human coronary plaque morphology using contrast-enhanced multislice spiral computed tomography: a comparison with histology. *J Comput Assist Tomogr.* 2004;28:449–454.
59. Davis PH, Dawson JD, Mahoney LT, Lauer RM. increased carotid intimal-medial thickness and coronary calcification are related in young and middle-aged adults: the Muscatine Study. *Circulation.* 1999;100:838–842.
60. Allison MA, Criqui MH, Wright CM. Patterns and risk factors for systemic calcified atherosclerosis. *Arterioscler Thromb Vasc Biol.* 2004;24:331–336.
61. Wong ND, Sciammarella M, Arad Y, et al. Relation of thoracic aortic and aortic valve calcium to coronary artery calcium and risk assessment. *Am J Cardiol.* 2003;92:951–955.
62. Hollander M, Hak AE, Koudstaal PJ, et al. Comparison between measures of atherosclerosis and risk of stroke: the Rotterdam Study. *Stroke.* 2003;34:2367–2372.
63. Iribarren C, Sidney S, Sternfeld B, Browner WS. Calcification of the aortic arch: risk factors and association with coronary heart disease, stroke, and peripheral vascular disease. *JAMA.* 2000;283:2810–2815.
64. Yamamoto H, Shavelle D, Takasu J, et al. Valvular and thoracic aortic calcium as a marker of the extent and severity of angiographic coronary artery disease. *Am Heart J.* 2003;146:153–159.
65. Takasu J, Mao S, Budoff MJ. Aortic atherosclerosis detected with electron-beam CT as a predictor of obstructive coronary artery disease. *Acad Radiol.* 2003;10:631–637.
66. Taniguchi H, Momiyama Y, Fayad ZA, et al. In vivo magnetic resonance evaluation of associations between aortic atherosclerosis and both risk factors and coronary artery disease in patients referred for coronary angiography. *Am Heart J.* 2004;148:137–143.

67. Wagenknecht LE, Langefeld CD, Carr JJ, et al. Race-specific relationships between coronary and carotid artery calcification and carotid intimal medial thickness. *Stroke*. 2004;35: e97–e99.
68. Hunt JL, Fairman R, Mitchell ME, et al. Bone formation in carotid plaques: a clinicopathological study. *Stroke*. 2002;33:1214–1219.
69. Shaalan WE, Cheng H, Gewertz B, et al. Degree of carotid plaque calcification in relation to symptomatic outcome and plaque inflammation. *J Vasc Surg*. 2004;40:262–269.
70. Oliver TB, Lammie GA, Wright AR, et al. Atherosclerotic plaque at the carotid bifurcation: CT angiographic appearance with histopathologic correlation. *AJNR Am J Neuroradiol*. 1999;20:897–901.
71. Walker LJ, Ismail A, McMeekin W, Lambert D, Mendelow AD, Birchall D. Computed tomography angiography for the evaluation of carotid atherosclerotic plaque: correlation with histopathology of endarterectomy specimens. *Stroke*. 2002;33:977–981.
72. Schroeder S, Kuettner A, Wojak T, et al. Non-invasive evaluation of atherosclerosis with contrast enhanced 16 slice spiral computed tomography: results of ex vivo investigations. *Heart*. 2004;90:1471–1475.
73. Fox CS, Vasan RS, Parise H, et al. Mitral annular calcification predicts cardiovascular morbidity and mortality: the Framingham Heart Study. *Circulation*. 2003;107:1492–1496.
74. Freeman RV, Otto CM. Spectrum of calcific aortic valve disease: pathogenesis, disease progression, and treatment strategies. *Circulation*. 2005;111:3316–3326.
75. Schroeder S, Flohr T, Kopp AF, et al. Accuracy of density measurements within plaques located in artificial coronary arteries by X-ray multislice CT: results of a phantom study. *J Comput Assist Tomogr*. 2001;25:900–906.
76. Komatsu S, Hirayama A, Omori Y, et al. Detection of coronary plaque by computed tomography with a novel plaque analysis system, "Plaque Map," and comparison with intravascular ultrasound and angioscopy. *Circ J*. 2005;69:72–77.

14 CT Coronary Angiography

John A. Rumberger

Direct visualization of the epicardial coronary arteries is currently the reference standard to confirm the presence or focal severity of coronary luminal disease, or both. For more than 50 years[1] the coronary angiogram has been used to define epicardial coronary disease. While conventional coronary arteriography provides exceptional spatial resolution and a general road map of the coronary system for catheter-based or surgical intervention to the heart, its chambers, and the individual arteries, it is expensive, has a small but definite risk of complications, and requires either a brief hospitalization or a period of observation for several hours after the procedure in a specialized monitored unit. When it is used for diagnosis of coronary disease, a mechanical intervention is required only about half the time.

Over the past 20 years, stress testing coupled most commonly with direct cardiac imaging (two-dimensional [2D] echocardiography or perfusion mapping) often has become the de facto arbitrator of decisions to forgo or proceed with direct, catheter-based angiography. The tacit assumptions are that stress testing with imaging is a viable substitute for determining whether a given patient does or does not have sufficient evidence for a flow-limiting (e.g., 50% to 70%) coronary stenosis. However, even in the best of hands, these tests have an accuracy of generally <90%, with, in some series, combined false-positive and false-negative rates up to 20%,[2-4] depending on the pretest likelihood ratio.[5]

For a great number of symptomatic patients with known or suspected luminal coronary disease, a convenient, noninvasive, and safe means to visualize the coronary arteries directly would be of significant clinical and economic benefit. The following discussion examines the current and future role of modern cardiac computed tomography (CT) as a viable alternative to direct coronary angiography as well as for stress testing for the diagnosis of obstructive coronary disease in selected patients.

Methods

The evolution of CT instrumentation for cardiac imaging is discussed in detail in Chapter 2, which also provides basic concepts on how to construct CT protocols for cardiac imaging. This section provides a detailed, yet practical description of how to apply the basic concepts described in Chapter 2 to clinically relevant protocols for cardiac CT imaging.

TABLE 14.1. Technical Statistics for Currently Available CT Angiography Scanners

Parameter	EBCT		MDCT	
	C-150, C-300	e-Speed	16-slice	32-64-slice
Spatial resolution (line pairs/cm)	6	9	12	14
Spatial resolution (mm)	1.5–2.0	1.0–1.5	0.75	0.4–0.6
Image acquisition time (rotation speed, msec)	100	100	450	330–350
True temporal resolution (msec)*	100	50 and 100	~250	~210
Radiation dose (mSv)†	1.5–3.0	1.5–3.0	8–12	12–25
ECG-based display	Prospective	Prospective	Retrospective	Retrospective
Slice thickness (mm)	3.0	1.5	0.75	0.4–0.6
Overlap (mm)	1	0–1.0	0	0

Abbreviations: EBCT, electron beam computed tomography; MDCT, multidetector computed tomography.

*True temporal resolution is not the same as rotational speed. Imaging requires that at least 180 degrees of data be acquired plus the width of the fan or x-ray beam (30 degrees for EBCT; 50 degrees for MDCT). So true temporal resolution is related to individual sweep (EBCT) or rotational (MDCT) speed, and the time required to acquire data from 180 + 30 = 210 degrees of arc (EBCT) or 180 + 50 = 230 degrees of arc (MDCT).

†This range is for various imaging protocols; radiation dose for CT depends on x-ray energy (kV), tube current (mA), exposure time, and, nominally, slice thickness. The numbers given are for CT angiography studies only and not for coronary artery calcium assessment in noncontrast studies.

Scan Acquisition

The following is a short synopsis of CT coronary angiography data acquisition using either electron beam computed tomography (EBCT; e-Speed) or multidetector computed tomography (MDCT) (Table 14.1).

Preprocedure

1. Load the single-barreled powered contrast injector (200-cc syringe) with 100 cc of nonionic contrast media (choose contrast with iodine concentrations of 350 to 370 mg/cc) layered with 50 to 100 cc saline. When using a dual-barreled powered contrast injector, load one 100-cc syringe with nonionic contrast media in one barrel and 100 cc of saline in the other barrel.

2. Place an 18- to 20-gauge intravenous (IV) cannula in the right arm.

3. For MDCT: Most clinicians feel at the present time that a heart rate <60 to 65 beats per minute produces the best, motion-free images. Although some vendors offer "partial-scan" reconstruction algorithms so that imaging can be done at higher heart rates, this reduces the potential to perform simultaneous multiphase ventricular function analysis and increases the radiation exposure by about 1.5-fold. The usual protocol is to administer β-blockers (be sure there is no contraindication) orally (50 mg metoprolol the night before and 50 mg 1 hour prior to the procedure) and/or intravenously (metoprolol 5 mg), with continuous electrocardiogram (ECG) monitoring, checking blood pressure every 2 minutes; if the heart rate remains above 65 to 70 beats per minute without hypotension, 5 mg to a total of 10 mg additionally of intravenous metoprolol can be administered every 5 to 15 minutes, as needed to maintain heart rate steady.

4. For EBCT—Heart rate is less of an issue and no premedications are generally given. Using the C-150/C-300 scanners (but not for the e-Speed), a heart rate faster than 70 beats per minute is desirable and sometimes 0.6 mg up to 3 mg of intravenous atropine may be given during continuous monitoring. The e-Speed scanner shortens the entire EBCT angiogram breath-hold time by 50% by acquiring dual 1.5–mm-thick slices at each scan time.

5. Determine the starting (most cephalad/superior) and ending (most caudad/distal) scan positions. Generally for CT angiography of the native coronary arteries, the average scan range is approximately 120 mm. Be sure to account for the midleft anterior descending artery often to be 10 to 15 mm cephalad to the origin of the left main artery. For CT angiography of bypass grafts, the average scan range is approximately 200 mm; imaging must include the origins of the saphenous veins from the aorta, noting that in most instances the graft to the region of the left circumflex is often the most cephalad (this is also sufficient to include superior portions of any internal mammary grafts). It is advisable to plan the scanning range to be 10 mm above the superior image selected and 10 mm below the inferior image selected in case the patient's breath holding is inconsistent.

6. Adjust the exposure to the patient's body size and weight. Larger patients can be problematic in imaging. For the older EBCT scanners (C-150/C-300), the kV is fixed at 130 and the mA is also fixed at 750. For the e-Speed, the kV operates at either 130 or 140 and the mA at 750 or 1000. For MDCT, the kV is generally at 120 and the mA is variable and should be increased from 300 in a patient weighing <60 kg up to 450–500 in a patient weighing >100 kg.

7. Access the "circulation time," that is, the time for intravenous contrast to travel from the injection site (peripheral vein) to produce maximum opacification in the systemic circulation. For EBCT, this requires injecting about 10 cc of contrast at a rate of 3.5 cc/s and acquiring a "flow mode" set of images. This image set can then define a contrast clearance curve for the ascending aorta, which then determines the "circulation time." For most MDCT, this step is not necessary, as "bolus-tracking" software is in place to start image acquisition for the CT angiogram at a point when the CT number in the aorta generally exceeds 200 Hounsfield units (HU). All CT scanners will provide feedback on the time required to complete the CT angiogram imaging prior to actually performing the study, once the scan parameters are set. Generally, contrast (layered or followed with saline) should be administered throughout the scan time. Nominal infusion rates of 3.5 cc/s have been used in most published studies. This time can be reduced to 2.5 cc/s in some individuals and may need to be increased to 5.0 cc/s in larger patients. As a quick rule of thumb, the total injection time (contrast and saline included) should be approximately 15 seconds longer than the scan time. This allows for contrast to reach maximum or adequate opacification in the systemic circulation prior to commencing scanning, because in the average person the "circulation time" is about 12 to 15 seconds. However, note that the circulation time can be as long as 50 seconds in a patient with congestive heart failure.

8. Approximately 2 to 3 minutes before commencing the actual scan examination, the patient can be given one sublingual standard nitroglycerine tablet or nitroglycerine spray (0.2 to 0.4 mg). It is the opinion and experience of the author that this dilates the coronary arteries, reduces the chances of any coronary spasm, and improves the diagnostic accuracy of the study.

9. As with all CT contrast studies, breath holding should be practiced with the patient prior to contrast injection. For EBCT, the scan acquisition time for the C-150/C-300 can be as long as 50 to 60 seconds; for the e-Speed, this is cut in half. MDCT using the 32–64-slice scanners can accomplish the entire CT angiogram in as little as 5 to 10 seconds.

Image Viewing and 3D Reconstruction

The ability to have cubic or nearly cubic image voxel dimensions extends the potential array of image displays from standard 2D images to a variety of three-dimensional (3D) representations (in virtually any imaging plane) while allowing for preservation of linear dimensions. Although there are a number of image presentations that can be accomplished, this author uses almost exclusively the maximum-intensity projection (MIP) and the volume-rendering technique (VRT). Alternating between both image presentation types while viewing a coronary segment or a larger portion of the cardiac anatomy is a valuable ability that can be found on most modern computer workstations. It is beyond the scope of the present discussion to individually discuss the attributes and liabilities of the workstations offered by various CT vendors as well as the various independent CT/MR workstations offered. However, it is this author's experience that not all workstations are created equal. When my laboratory at the Mayo Clinic first began to look at electron beam (coronary) angiography (EBA) nearly a decade ago, it would take on the order of 15 minutes or longer to "generate" one 3D view, and navigational tools for MIP imaging were crude and cumbersome. This is primarily the reason for the number of "nonevaluable" segments in the early EBCT studies (noted later). Using current workstation technology, these images are now generated on the fly with instant feedback and superlative editing and display tools. In the catheterization laboratory, a 3D feel for the overall spatial localization of the vessels and luminal disease becomes second nature, although this is usually garnered by viewing orthogonal projection-type images. However, it is often disorienting even for senior angiographers to be presented with a data set that can be viewed from any possible angle and displayed using a variety of presentation styles.

MIP is one of the most powerful 3D techniques available. Using MIP, a "slab" can be defined and oriented in the data set such that an appropriate thickness is combined into one image. A MIP image can have a thickness that is variable by the interpreter; both thick and thin MIP images are useful for diagnostic purposes. These types of data manipulation also are the closest to the presentation that might be found in the catheterization laboratory, because the subsequent image appears to be a projection of a single plane (i.e. a 2D image) at one time. A technique similar to MIP is multiplanar reconstruction (MPR). This technique allows the interpreter to place an oblique slice through the data set and view the resulting cut. The workstation software allows one to manipulate this oblique slice by rotating or translating. This allows investigation of the data set from any angle. Combinations of all 3D methods are helpful to display the anatomy, although the author recommends using only the MIP (or MRP) images for "diagnostic" purposes defining luminal abnormalities.

Many of the presentations of 3D images using EBCT and other CT methods as well as MRI are presented as a shaded surface display (SSD) in publications. However, although they provide a dramatic view of overall anatomy, they are not considered sufficient for diagnostic purposes of lumen topology. Where an SSD image provides a "hard" surface of the selected densities, VRT uses a "blending" approach to create a 3D image, such that rather than a particular surface, a combination of information from some depth around that surface contributes to the image. In this way, the image of the contrasted blood in a vessel is generated by a blend of information from and around the boundary of the lumen.

The VRT method allows for a general 3D view of the anatomy under concern; there are a variety of predesigned density ranges provided as templates on most workstations for almost any particular section of the vascular or body anatomy. MIP images can be thin or thick but represent basically a "sliding slab" view through any region. Specific coronary segments can then be brought into view during navigation, while other segments fade over the "horizon" (using a globe analogy). A MIP image is generated by knowledge that the maximum value encountered by each ray can be encoded in a 2D projection display. MIP grayscale thus reflects relative x-ray attenuation. The absence of a thresholding step, as is the case for VRT, ensures that no information is lost and subtle variations in attenuation can be appreciated. This has tremendous importance in the differentiation of calcified atheromata versus intraluminal contrast. An interactive tool, MIP can provide valuable information about the condition of a vessel by enabling the reading physician to present the CT angiographic data in an appropriate context. A disadvantage of the MIP is that a single projection image does not encode depth relationships; thus, there is value in using both MIP and VRT.

Results of Published Studies

The goal of CT angiography is to have the look and feel of standard invasive angiography (albeit with the ability to look not only at the lumen but also at the arterial mural surfaces). Thus, interpretation should proceed along established guidelines and in a systematic fashion. The author recommends using the standardized American Heart Association 15-segment model (Figure 14.1) for interpretation of the native coronary arteries. A variety of MIP and VRT images of the native coronary arteries and bypass grafts are shown in Figures 14.1 through 14.8.

The author's procedure is to start reading the left main (LM) and then proceed down the left anterior descending (LAD). Once review of the LAD is accomplished, the author returns to the LM and proceeds down the left circumflex (LCX) and its branches. Finally, the author returns to the right coronary artery (RCA) ostium and then proceeds distally to the most inferior segments. Coronary bypass grafts are best interpreted with knowledge of the operative note. Surgical clips, especially for in situ left and right internal mammary artery grafts, can be problematic in viewing the entire vessel, but patency can almost always be determined. Special attention is paid to the origin, body, and anastomotic site of all bypass grafts.

Both EBCT and 16-slice or greater MDCT have been validated against the reference standard of invasive coronary angiography for native coronary arteries and for bypass grafts. Using a 50% or greater stenosis as the definition of obstructive

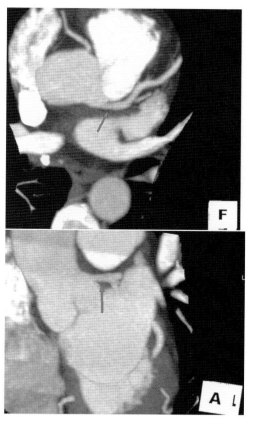

FIGURE 14.2. MIP images of the left main coronary artery (LM). LM (arrow) in standard transaxial (superior) view (top); LM (arrow) as viewed from an anterior view (bottom).

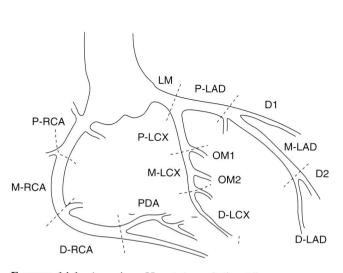

FIGURE 14.1. American Heart Association 15-segment coronary artery anatomy denotation.

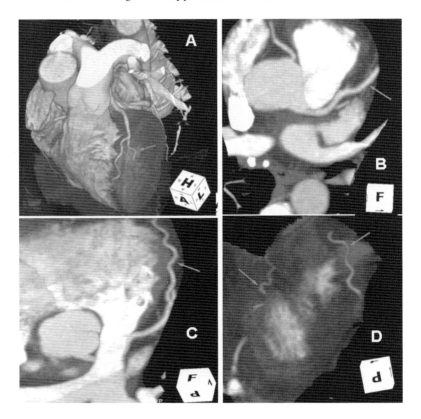

FIGURE 14.3. Images of the left anterior descending (LAD). (A) VRT anterior image showing the LAD (left arrow) and first diagonal (D1) branch (right arrow); (B) MIP view from superior angle of proximal LAD (arrow); (C) MIP view from a superior angle of the proximal and mid-LAD (arrow); (D) MIP view from an inferior angle of the distal LAD (right arrow); note the position of a portion of the posterior descending artery (PDA; left arrow).

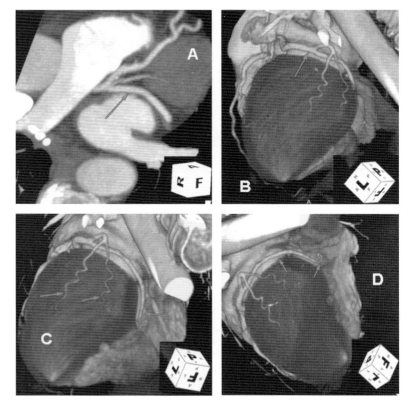

FIGURE 14.4. Images of the left circumflex (LCX). (A) MIP image of the proximal LCX from a superior view; (B) VRT image of the proximal LCX from an anterior view; (C) VRT image of two marginal branches of the LCX (arrows) and the mid-LCX from a shallow lateral view; (D) VRT image of the distal LCX from a lateral view.

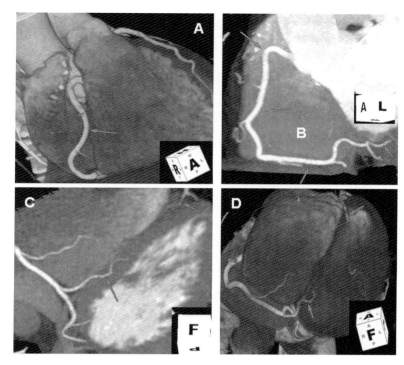

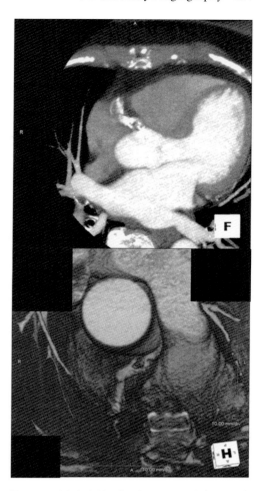

FIGURE 14.5. Images of a dominant right coronary artery (RCA). (A) VRT image from the proximal and mid-RCA segments from an anterior view; (B) thick section MIP of the entire RCA showing the proximal segment, midsegment, distal segment, and PDA (arrows); (C) MIP image of the distal RCA from an inferior view (arrow shows PDA); (D) VRT image of the distal RCA and the PDA (bottom arrow) from an inferior view, not the distal LAD (top arrow).

FIGURE 14.6. MIP (top) and VRT (bottom) images of a patient with a complex proximal RCA lesion.

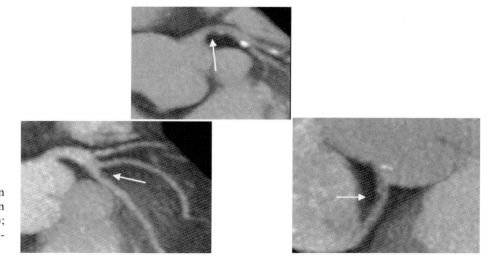

FIGURE 14.7. Images from electron beam angiography of "soft" plaque in three separate patients. LM (top); proximal LAD (bottom left); proximal RCA (bottom right).

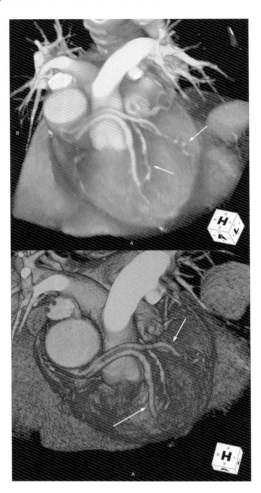

FIGURE 14.8. MIP (top) and VRT (bottom) images from electron beam angiography of target vessels and saphenous vein bypass grafts. Arrows in the top panel point to target vessels (first diagonal [right] and LAD [middle]). Arrows in the bottom panel point to saphenous bypass grafts (first diagonal [right] and LAD [middle]).

coronary/bypass disease, the overall accuracy for EBCT is now on the order of 92% to 93%; for MDCT the accuracy is on the order of 94% to 95%. The negative predictive value for both approaches is 100% in multiple studies. Table 14.2 lists summary statistics for published studies. Note that the number of "nonevaluable" segments was greater in the earlier studies than in the more recent ones. This is due to improvements in scanner technology, thinner CT slice thicknesses, improvements in CT angiography contrast and acquisition protocols, and, most of all, newer workstations. The changes to thinner CT scanning for all current systems have allowed visualization in nearly all studies to include the proximal and distal portions of the LCX and distal branches of the RCA. Views of the LCX and to some extent the posterior descending artery (PDA) were hindered for some time in the original studies by 3D rendering tools that did not allow sufficient navigation to facilitate "unveiling" of the anterior cardiac vein/coronary sinus or the middle cardiac veins that course across and often parallel to these vessels, respectively. As with all things in digital imaging, CT angiography methods have improved and the 3D rendering and workstation tools have advanced considerably.

Currently, definition of coronary in-stent stenosis remains problematic, although stent patency is straightforward in nearly all cases. Although there have been individual case reports of performing very thin CT sectioning through coronary stents, demonstrating in-stent narrowing, these methods remain currently clinically impractical. In addition, extensive coronary mural calcification can also confound focal stenosis definition. Although there are no set rules for when there is too much coronary calcification to provide global native coronary accuracy with CT angiography, a good rule of thumb is that the value of the test decreases as the coronary scores (Agatston scale) become >400. Additionally, in a symptomatic patient, data have shown that high coronary calcium scores have specificity for significant coronary obstructive disease above 90%, even in the absence of a companion CT angiography study.

CT (EBCT and MDCT) provide information on calcified plaque that specifically applies to prediction of coronary artery plaque burden and extent. Histologic,[24,25] ultrasonic,[26] and angiographic[27] studies have confirmed that coronary calcium quantified by x-ray CT is related to the extent of atherosclerotic plaque disease in a direct fashion, regardless of age or gender, although it is not a substitute for actual angiographic stenosis severity.[28] Furthermore, these measures have been shown to provide cardiac prognostic information that is separate and incremental to conventionally based risk factor analysis.[29-31]

A common issue of discussion in coronary artery calcium (CAC) quantitation by CT has been the general misunderstanding of what it actually measures; that is, it only defines "hard" plaque and provides no information on "soft" (and potentially

TABLE 14.2. Correlations of CT Angiography with Conventional Angiography for Detection of Luminal Coronary Stenoses >50% (EBCT and MDCT)

Reference	Year Published	No. of Subjects	Se (%)	Sp (%)	NE (%)
EBCT					
Nakanishi[6]	1997	37	74	91	—
Schmermund[7]	1998	28	82	88	12
Reddy[8]	1998	23	88	79	8
Rensing[9]	1998	37	77	94	19
Achenbach[10]	1998	125	92	94	25
Budoff[11]	1999	52	78	71	11
Achenbach[12]	2000	36	92	93	20
Leber[13]	2001	87	78	93	24
Ropers[14]	2002	118	90	82	24
Nikolau[15]	2002	20	85	77	11
Rasouli[16]	2003	10	94	88	8
MDCT					
Nieman[17]	2003	59	95	86	—
Ropers[18]	2003	77	92	93	12
Mollet[19]	2004	128	94	91	0
Bypass Grafts—EBCT					
Achenbach[20]	1999 (occlusion)	56	100	100	0
	1999 (stenosis)		100	97	16
Bypass Grafts—MDCT					
Ropers[21]	2002 (occlusion)	65	97	98	0
	2002 (stenosis)		75	92	—
Schlosser[22]	2004 (occlusion and stenosis)	51	96	95	6
Martuscelli[23]	2004 (occlusion and stenosis)	84	97	100	9

Abbreviations: Se, sensitivity; Sp, specificity; NE, nonevaluable coronary segments; –, not published.

vulnerable) plaque. Rumberger[32] initially studied autopsy hearts defining the use of CAC as an estimate of coronary atherosclerotic plaque burden, when looking at the coronary arteries as a whole. In nondecalcified coronary artery segments using contact microradiography, the relationship between coronary artery calcium and total atherosclerotic plaque area on a segment-by-segment basis, however, is variable; at times the tracking is intimate and at other times somewhat dissociated.[33]

Contrast-enhanced CT using both EBCT and MDCT has been shown to have the potential to define noncalcified (so-called soft) plaque on a segmental basis (Figure 14.7). Two studies have been published to support this finding. Achenbach and colleagues[34] compared intravascular ultrasound (IVUS) obtained during cardiac catheterization with noninvasive contrast-enhanced coronary studies using MDCT. They found that CT had a sensitivity of about 82% to detect coronary segments with atherosclerotic plaque but had only a 53% sensitivity of defining segments with noncalcified atherosclerotic plaque. Thus, combining CAC and contrast-enhanced segmental definition of "soft" plaque still resulted in significant underestimation of true total atherosclerotic plaque burden.

Leber et al[35] also performed a comparison between IVUS and contrast-enhanced CT. They reported a sensitivity for "soft" plaque at about 78%, a sensitivity for fibrous plaque at about 78%, while maintaining a sensitivity for "calcified" plaque (as had been shown in prior EBCT noncontrast-enhanced studies) of about 95%. Thus in about 80% of the cases, contrast-enhanced CT can be used to provide additional information about noncalcified plaque, but the total "atherosclerotic plaque burden" remains underdefined. Such studies are possible using both EBCT and MDCT, but both have specific deficiencies. EBCT is limited currently by spatial resolution on the order of 1 to 1.5 mm, as compared with submillimeter definition by MDCT. Conversely, EBCT can be used for heart rates from 50 to 120 beats/min without the need for β-blockade to lower resting heart rate because of its superior temporal resolution, which is 2 to 3 times greater than that of MDCT. All published studies using MDCT have required resting heart rates <65 beats/min for adequate image resolution.

Contrast-enhanced CT, although possessing great potential as a diagnostic catheterization for defining the absence or presence of "significant" coronary stenotic lesions, is still somewhat limited in defining "noncalcified" plaque and has not yet been shown to provide incremental value in predicting the potential for preventing heart attack.

Applications in Clinical Practice

Nobody would have imagined 30 years ago the current wide applicability of echocardiography in clinical practice, and, likewise, we may not have yet begun to fully comprehend the place of cardiac CT in patient care. Already in some sites the workup of "chest pain" in the emergency department can be supplanted with contrast-enhanced EBCT and 16+-slice MDCT. In a single test one can examine the pericardium; define global and regional left ventricular function; quantify the presence or absence of coronary calcification; examine the lumen of the major epicardial coronary arteries; obtain qualitative information about the atria, pulmonary arteries, and pulmonary veins; and examine portions of the ascending and descending aorta to rule out dissection. Following is a list of current clinical applications for CT angiography that are now possible:[36]

- Defining the origin and anatomic course of anomalous coronary artery anatomy[37]
- Serving as an alternative to conventional stress testing in a patient with atypical chest pain
- Functioning as an alternative to diagnostic catheterization in a patient with a prior equivocal stress test

- Functioning as an alternative to stress testing or diagnostic catheterization in a symptomatic patient with a mild to moderate coronary calcium score
- Serving as an alternative to stress testing or diagnostic catheterization in a patient with a newly diagnosed cardiomyopathy
- Functioning as a direct method to follow-up in a patient for coronary artery stent patency or evaluation of nonstented segments
- Functioning as a follow-up in a patient with atypical symptoms who has had prior coronary artery bypass surgery
- Functioning as an alternative to stress testing or diagnostic catheterization for preoperative noncardiac surgical clearance in an intermediate coronary risk patient

Summary Points

- Cardiac CT has been studied and validated in patients for over 20 years. Initially, it was used to define cardiac size and function and as an estimator of myocardial perfusion.
- In the 1990s, research turned to noncontrast CT and quantification of coronary artery calcium, now recognized as the most powerful means to define risk for untoward cardiac events, above and incremental to conventional risk factors.
- Within the last decade, studies have turned to CT as a means to define luminal coronary anatomy. This has been a maturation process that has been the result of improvements in scanner technology and, not inconsequently, in cardiac computer workstation technology.
- The American College of Radiology and the American College of Cardiology[38] have both now provided accreditation guidelines for radiologists and cardiologists in performing cardiac CT, especially in performing CT coronary angiography.

References

1. Ryan TJ. The coronary angiogram and its seminal contributions to cardiovascular medicine over five decades. *Circulation.* 2002;106:752–756.
2. McArthur D, Froelicher V. Exercise-induced ST depression in the diagnosis of coronary artery disease—a meta-analysis. *Circulation.* 1989;80:87–98.
3. Roger VL, Pellikka PA, Oh JK, Miller FA, Seward JB, Tajik AJ. Stress echocardiography. Part I. Exercice echocardiography: techniques, implementation, clinical applications, and correlations. *Mayo Clin Proc.* 1995;70:5–15.
4. Maddahi J, Rodrigues E, Berman DS, Kiat H. State-of-the-art myocardial perfusion imaging. *Cardiol Clin.* 1994;12:199–222.
5. Morise AP, Diamond GA. Comparison of the sensitivity and specificity of exercise electrocardiography in biased and unbiased populations of men and women. *Am Heart J.* 1995;130:741–747.
6. Nakinishi T, Ito K, Imazu M, Yamakido M. Evaluation of coronary artery stenoses using electron-beam CT and mutiplanar reformation. *J Comp Assist.* 1997;21:121–127.
7. Schmermund A, Rensing BJ, Sheedy PF, Bell MR, Rumberger JA. Intravenous electron-beam CT coronary angiography for segmental analysis of coronary artery stenoses. *J Am Coll Cardiol.* 1998;31:1547–1554.
8. Reddy GP, Chernoff DM, Adams JR, Higgins CB. Coronary artery stenoses: assessment with contrast-enhanced electron-beam CT and axial reconstructions. *Radiology.* 1998;208:167–172.
9. Rensing BJ, Bongaerts A, van Geuns RJ, van Ooijen P, Oudkerk M, de Feyter PJ. Intravenous coronary angiography by electron beam computed tomography: a clinical evaluation. *Circulation.* 1998;98:2509–2512.
10. Achenbach S, Moshage W, Ropers D, Nossen J, Daniel WG. Value of electron beam computed tomography for the noninvasive detection of high-grade coronary artery stenoses and occlusions. *N Engl J Med.* 1998;339:1964–1971.

11. Budoff MJ, Oudiz RJ, Zalace CP, et al. Intravenous three-dimensional coronary angiography using contrast enhanced electron beam computed tomography. *Am J Cardiol.* 1999;83:840–845.

12. Achenbach S, Ropers D, Regenfus M, et al. Contrast enhanced electron beam computed tomography to analyze the coronary arteries in patients after acute myocardial infarction. *Heart.* 2000;84:489–493.

13. Leber AW, Knez A, Mukherjee R, et al. Usefulness of calcium scoring using electron beam computed tomography and noninvasive coronary angiography in patients with suspected coronary artery disease. *Am J Cardiol.* 2001;88:219–223.

14. Ropers D, Regenfus M, Stilanakis N, et al. A direct comparison of noninvasive coronary angiography by electron beam tomography and navigator-echobased magnetic resonance imaging for detection of restenosis following coronary angioplasty. *Invest Radiol.* 2002;37:386–392.

15. Nikolaou K, Huber A, Knez A, Breuning R, Reiser M. Intraindividual comparison of contrast-enhanced electron-beam computed tomography and navigator echo-based magnetic resonance imaging for noninvasive coronary artery angiography. *Eur Radiol.* 2002; 12:1663–1671.

16. Rasouli ML, Budoff M, Mao S, et al. Detection of coronary stenosis using e-Speed electron beam tomography [abstract]. *Circulation.* 2003;108:IV-527.

17. Nieman K, Cademartiri F, Lemos P, Raaijmakers R, Pattynama P, de Feyter P. Reliable non-invasive coronary angiography with fast sub-millimetre multislice spiral CT. *Circulation.* 2002;106:2051–2054.

18. Ropers D, Baum U, Pohle K, et al. Detection of coronary artery stenoses with thin-slice multi-detector row spiral computed tomography and multiplanar reconstruction. *Circulation.* 2003;107:664–666.

19. Mollet NR, Cademartiri F, Nieman K, et al. MSCT coronary angiography in stable angina. *J Am Coll Cardiol.* 2004;43:2265–2270.

20. Achenbach S, Giesler A, Moshage W, Ropers D, Nossen J, Bachmann K. Noninvasive three-dimensional visualization of coronary artery bypass grafts by electron beam tomography. *Am J Cardiol.* 1997;88:792–795.

21. Ropers D, Ulzheimer S, Wenkel E, et al. Investigation of aortocoronary artery bypass grafts by multislice spiral computed tomography with electrocardiographic-gated image reconstruction. *Am J Cardiol.* 2001;88:792–795.

22. Schlosser T, Konorza T, Hunold P, Huhl H. Schmermund A, Barkhausen J. Noninvasive visualization of coronary artery bypass grafts using 16-detector row computed tomography. *J Am Coll Cardiol.* 2004;44:1224–1229.

23. Martuscelli E, Romagnoli A, D'Eliseo A, et al. Evaluation of venous and arterial conduit patency by 16-slice spiral computed tomography. *Circulation.* 2004;110:3234–3228.

24. Simons DB, Schwartz RS, Edwards WD, Sheedy PF, Breen JF, Rumberger JA. Non-invasive definition of anatomic coronary artery disease by ultrafast CT: a quantitative pathologic study. *J Am Coll Cardiol.* 1992;20:1118–1126.

25. Rumberger JA, Simons DB, Fitzpatrick LA, Sheedy PF, Schwartz RS. Coronary artery calcium areas by electron beam computed tomography and coronary atherosclerotic plaque area: a histopathologic correlative study. *Circulation.* 1995;92:2157–2162.

26. Baumgart D, Schmermund A, Goerge G, et al. Comparison of electron beam computed tomography with intracoronary ultrasound and coronary angiography for detection of coronary atherosclerosis. *J Am Coll Cardiol.* 1997;30:57–64.

27. Rumberger JA, Sheedy PF, Breen JR, Schwartz RS. Coronary calcium as determined by electron beam computed tomography, and coronary disease on arteriogram: effect of patient's sex on diagnosis. *Circulation.* 1995;91:1363–1367.

28. Rumberger JA, Sheedy PF, Breen JF, Schwartz RS. Electron beam CT coronary calcium score cutpoints and severity of associated angiography luminal stenosis. *J Am Coll Cardiol.* 1997;29:1542–1548.

29. Wong ND, Hsu JC, Detrano RC, et al. Coronary artery calcium evaluation by electron beam computed tomography and its relation to new cardiovascular events. *Am J Cardiol.* 2000;86:495–498.

30. Kondos GT, Hoff JA, Sevrukov A, et al. Coronary artery calcium and cardiac events electron-beam tomography coronary artery calcium and cardiac events: a 37-month follow-up of 5,635 initially asymptomatic low to intermediate risk adults. *Circulation.* 2003; 107:2571–2576.

31. Arad Y, Goodman KJ, Roth M, et al. Coronary calcification, coronary disease risk factors, C-reactive protein, and atherosclerotic cardiovascular disease events: The St. Francis Heart Study. *J Am Coll Cardiol.* 2005;46:158–165.

32. Rumberger JA, Simons DB, Fitzpatrick LA, Sheedy PF, Schwartz RS. Coronary artery calcium areas by electron beam computed tomography and coronary atherosclerotic plaque area: a histopathologic correlative study. *Circulation.* 1995;92:2157–2162.

33. Sangiorgi G, Rumberger JA, Severson A, et al. Arterial calcification and not lumen stenosis is highly correlated with atherosclerotic plaque burden in humans: a histologic study of 723 coronary artery segments using non-decalcifying methodology. *J Am Coll Cardiol.* 1998;31:126–133.

34. Achenbach S, Moselewski F, Ropers D, et al. Detection of calcified and noncalcified coronary atherosclerotic plaque by contrast-enhanced submillimeter multidetector spiral computed tomography. *Circulation.* 2004;109:14–17.

35. Leber AW, Knez A, Becker A, et al. Accuracy of multidetector spiral computed tomography in identifying and differentiating the composition of coronary atherosclerotic plaques. *J Am Coll Cardiol.* 2004;43:1241–1247.

36. Rumberger JA. Noninvasive coronary angiography using computed tomography: ready to kick it up another notch? *Circulation.* 2002;106:2036–2038.

37. Ropers D, Moshage W, Daniel WG, et al. Visualization of coronary artery anomalies and their anatomic course by contrast-enhanced electron-beam tomography and 3-dimensional reconstruction. *Am J Cardiol.* 2001;87:193–197.

38. Budoff MJ (Chair). ACCF/AHA Clinical Competence Statement on Cardiac Imaging with Computed Tomography and Magnetic Resonance: A Report of the American College of Cardiology Foundation/American Heart Association/American College of Physicians Task Force on Clinical Competence and Training. *J Am Coll Cardiol.* 2005;46:383–402.

15 Relative Merits of Coronary CTA and Coronary MRI

Martin J. Lipton and Warren J. Manning

Computed tomography angiography (CTA) and magnetic resonance imaging (MRI) and angiography (MRA) have now replaced x-ray angiography for many vascular beds, but only recently has the technology advanced sufficiently for these modalities to interrogate and display coronary artery morphology.

Technical obstacles to noninvasive coronary artery imaging are similar for both CTA and MRI, but their approaches to overcoming these obstacles differ. The coronary arteries are relatively small in caliber (2–5 mm), demonstrate a tortuous course, and display near-constant motion with the cardiac cycle and superimposed respiration. Thus, an imaging modality with high temporal and spatial resolution is required with respiratory motion compensation. The arteries are also surrounded by epicardial fat and underlying myocardium, necessitating methods to enhance contrast-to-noise ratio (CNR) of the coronary lumen.

Both CTA and MRI have much in common, including the ability to display the arterial lumen and its wall in cross section in any three-dimensional (3D) plane by postprocessing of the originally acquired scan data sets. Furthermore, there is no need for a prolonged hospital stay or arterial access. This chapter discusses the state-of-the-art, clinical indications and current limitations of these two minimally invasive techniques, as well as their potential role in the future.

Relative Strengths and Weaknesses of Noninvasive Coronary Artery Imaging with CT and MR

Multidetector CT (MDCT) is rapidly becoming widely available and is the primary modality for diagnosing patients with a wide spectrum of diseases other than coronary artery atherosclerosis. Electrocardiogram (ECG) gating is essential for cardiac CT applications, and it is generally agreed that 16-slice (at the minimum) and preferably 64-slice scanners can be expected to display the coronary arteries consistently and adequately.[1,2]

As discussed in Chapter 14, major limitations of CT include motion artifacts with heart rates of over 70 beats per minute related to gantry rotation speed; hence, β-blockade is commonly employed prior to scanning. However, β-blockade may be contraindicated in patients with pulmonary disease and in those with prolonged atrioventricular conduction abnormalities. Because it requires ECG gating and a regular rhythm, patients with atrial fibrillation and other irregular arrhythmias are not ideal candidates for CTA. Retrospective gating allows postscan ECG editing to improve image quality by manually excluding abnormal beats and their associated CT data. This acquisition is also necessary to obtain left ventricular data for useful analysis by providing multiphasic reconstruction of the ECG-gated CT data.[3] However, the radiation dose is several times greater than that of a conventional x-ray coronary arteriogram and considerably greater than prospective ECG-gated CT acquisition. Nevertheless, coronary angiography with MDCT may be performed in a single 10- to 20-second breath hold with total examination time less than 15 minutes. The field of view includes the whole chest if necessary for evaluating chest pain, for example, in the emergency room, or to evaluate bypass grafts including internal mammary grafts artery. In cooperative patients with appropriate heart rate and rhythm, the technique provides high-resolution images of the heart, lungs, and mediastinum as well as the bony thorax with one acquisition sequence.

A significant issue is the presence of dense, extensive epicardial calcification, which makes evaluation of arterial stenosis very difficult. Contrast-media allergy and nephrotoxicity are relative contraindications to CTA, just as they are for invasive coronary angiography. Patients with a creatinine >2.0 mg/dL are excluded unless they are receiving renal dialysis. Radiation is always a concern, particularly in younger patients, and has implications when repeat CT scans are necessary.

Coronary MRI must overcome technical hurdles similar to those of coronary CTA. Though two-dimensional (2D) coronary MRI acquisitions predominated in the 1990s,[4] targeted 3D[5] and "whole heart"[6] coronary MRI methods now predominate, using either ECG-triggered "bright blood" segmented gradient echo or steady-state free precession imaging methods.

To suppress motion related to respiration, prolonged breath holding or free breathing with MRI navigators (monitoring of diaphragmatic motion) is employed while prospective ECG triggering is used to acquire data during diastasis period (usually mid-diastole). No β-blockade is needed, as the coronary MRI acquisition period can be adjusted (lengthened or shortened) to be tailored to the patient's heart rate and diastasis period. No exogenous contrast or intravenous access is needed. For coronary lumen contrast, specific prepulses suppress signal from surrounding epicardial fat and myocardium.[7] Since no ionizing radiation or iodinated contrast is used, concerns regarding repeated examinations and studies in patients with renal dysfunction are not applicable. In addition, coronary MRI images appear to be less sensitive to the confounding impact of epicardial calcium. Another advantage of MRI is the ability to combine coronary artery imaging with assessments of LV function, myocardial perfusion, and viability in a single examination;[8,9] however, discussion of this feature is beyond the scope of this chapter.

Disadvantages of coronary MRI (vs coronary CTA) include an inferior spatial resolution with nonisotropic voxels and a greater technical burden on both the operator and the patient, as coronary MRI acquisitions often exceed 20 to 30 minutes. MRI studies also remain relatively contraindicated in the presence of pacemakers, retained pacemaker leads, and implanted cardiodefibrillators. Current free breathing methods are dependent on a regular respiratory pattern.

Relative Accuracy of CTA and Coronary MRI for Diagnosing CAD

As the number of detectors has increased, the number of coronary artery segments that can be evaluated has progressively increased, along with the precision and accuracy of CTA. Problems in assessing the degree of luminal stenosis by MDCT can be expected when compared with selective coronary angiography based on the combination of higher temporal resolution of invasive catheterization without ECG-gating motion artifacts, projection imaging, and high-contrast enhancement of the arterial

TABLE 15.1. Multicenter Coronary MRI Data for Coronary MRI Identification of a <50% Diameter Angiographic Stenosis by Quantitative X-Ray Coronary Angiography

	Patient	Vessel	LM/Multivessel
Sensitivity	93%	83%	100%
Specificity	42%	73%	85%
Prevalence	59%	25%	17%
Positive predictive value	70%	51%	54%
Negative predictive value	81%	93%	100%

Abbreviation: LM, left main.

lumen due to selective arterial injection. A major limitation of CT is in its capability to determine luminal size in regions of heavy calcified plaque, which are particularly time-consuming to interpret when calcification is extensive.

The feasibility of 2D coronary MRI for identifying stenoses in the proximal and midcoronary segments has been demonstrated in several single-center studies.[4,10] Subsequently, 3D free-breathing segmented k-space gradient echo sequences have predominated due to their more favorable postprocessing capabilities and improved signal-to-noise ration (SNR). These have generally demonstrated sensitivities and specificities of 85% to 90%.[11,12] A multicenter trial of more than 100 patients from 7 international sites demonstrated high sensitivity but only modest specificity for identifying focal stenoses (Table 15.1), with very high accuracy for discriminating between patients with multivessel disease and no disease,[14] and preliminary data suggest it to be superior to delayed-enhancement MRI.[15] Data from "whole-heart" steady-state free precession (SSFP) methodology somewhat analogous to MDCT acquisitions (though inferior in spatial resolution) have shown longer vessel segments identified, with improved SNR and CNR[6] but similar diagnostic results of 82% and 91%, respectively (Figures 15.1 and 15.2).[16] Preliminary data suggest similar overall results with 3T coronary MRI.[17]

Few studies have directly compared coronary CTA and coronary MRI for evaluating the coronary arteries in the same patient (Figure 15.3). Gerber et al in Belgium reported that coronary MRI was superior to 4-slice MDCT.[18] Subsequently, these authors studied 56 patients comparing 16-slice MDCT with navigator-gated coronary MRI in the same patients.[19] Accuracy was similar, but MDCT showed better diagnos-

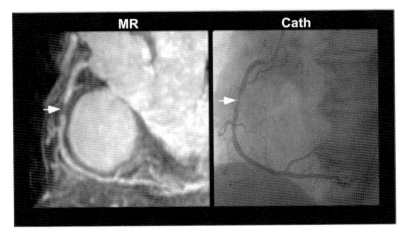

FIGURE 15.1. Whole-heart coronary MRI and corresponding x-ray angiogram in a 56-year-old man with a proximal right coronary artery stenosis (arrows).

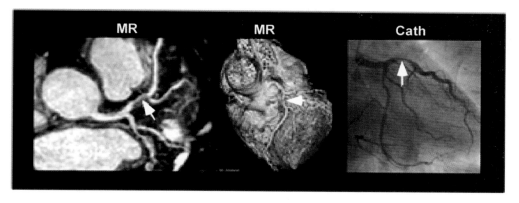

FIGURE 15.2. Whole-heart coronary MRI (left panel) with 3D software reconstruction (middle panel) and x-ray angiogram (right panel) in a patient with a proximal left anterior descending stenosis (arrows).

tic accuracy when quantitative assessment of stenosis was applied. This was true for segmental (Figure 15.4) and per-vessel analysis (Figure 15.5). Measurements of plaque and lumen areas derived by CT correlated well with intravascular ultrasound.

While the technologies of both coronary CTA and coronary MRI continue to advance, neither technology is currently ready to replace invasive x-ray arteriography, because the positive predictive value of both techniques falls short of near 100%[19] and neither has been studied as a screening test for low- to moderate-risk patients.

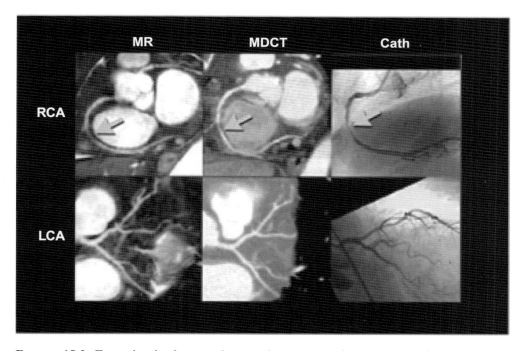

FIGURE 15.3. Example of reformatted magnetic resonance (MR; left panels), multidetector row computed tomography (MDCT; center panels), and corresponding coronary angiography images (right panels) of the right (RCA; top) and left coronary artery (LCA; bottom). The mid-RCA stenosis (arrows) was evaluated at 40% diameter stenosis using MR, 58% using MDCT, and 86% by quantitative coronary angiography. The LCA was normal.

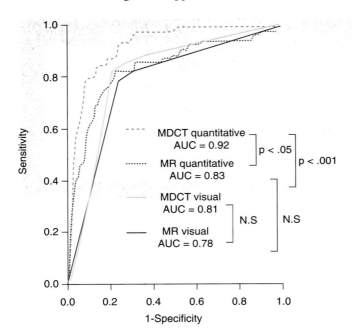

FIGURE 15.4. Receiver-operator characteristic curves demonstrating the diagnostic accuracy of visual and quantitative measurements of coronary diameter stenosis severity by MR and MDCT on a segment-by-segment analysis. Quantitative analysis of stenosis severity (>50%) significantly improved the diagnostic accuracy of MDCT but not MR. (Kefer J, et al. [19]. Reprinted with permission from The American College of Cardiology Foundation.)

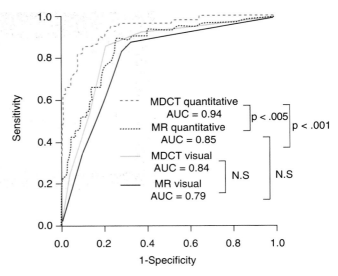

FIGURE 15.5. Receiver-operator characteristic curves demonstrating the diagnostic accuracy of visual and quantitative measurements of coronary diameter stenosis severity by MR and MDCT on a patient-by-patient analysis. Quantitative analysis of stenosis severity (>50%) significantly improved the diagnostic accuracy of MDCT but not MR. N.S., not significant. (Kefer J, et al. [19]. Reprinted with permission from The American College of Cardiology Foundation.)

Evaluation of Congenital Anomalies

There is considerable variation in coronary artery anatomy.[13,20] Both CT and MRI techniques can demonstrate congenital anomalies of the coronary arteries.[21–26] Congenital heart disease, most notably tetralogy of Fallot and transposition of the great arteries, is commonly associated with abnormal coronary artery anatomy, which may be difficult to demonstrate precisely by conventional projection x-ray coronary arteriography but may be readily identified by MR.[27] These variants may be of critical importance to the surgeon, depending on the anatomical relationships of the coronary arteries to the sternum.

Patients with anomalous coronary arteries may have no other associated congenital heart disease.[20] The incidence of coronary artery anomalies in the general population is shown in Table 15.2. Figures 15.6, 15.7, and 15.8 show examples of anomalies on

TABLE 15.2. Congenital Anomalies of the Coronary Arteries

Separate origins of LAD and CX (1 in 2000)
Separate origin of conus artery (up to 60%)
Origin of CX from RCA (<0.67%)—50% have other cardiac anomalies
Origin of LAD from RCA or right sinus, associated with sudden death
Origin of LCA from right sinus, associated with sudden death
Origin of LCA from a main pulmonary artery, associated with neonatal cardiac failure
Single coronary artery frequency is 0.024
Coronary artery fistulae, congenital stenosis, and atresia also occur

Abbreviations: LAD, left anterior descending artery; CX, circumflex artery; RCA, right coronary artery; LCA, left coronary artery.

FIGURE 15.6. Axial (left) and coronal (right) cardiac CT study demonstrating a myocardial bridge over the left anterior descending (LAD) artery entering the interventricular septum. LA, left atrium; LV, left ventricle; RV, right ventricle. (Courtesy of Lawrence Boxt, MD, Northshore University Hospital, NY.)

CTA. Despite all these anomalies, only 3 are usually life threatening. The first is a large coronary artery fistula. The second is the origin of a left main coronary artery from a pulmonary artery. The third is when a left main coronary artery or a single coronary artery passes between the two great vessels.[28,29]

Coronary MRI for identification and characterization of anomalous coronary arteries is widely accepted as a clinical tool (Figures 15.9 and 15.10). Several studies have now reported on the value of MRI in this condition,[24,25,27] including the finding of initial misinterpretation by conventional x-ray angiography.[25] Coronary anomalies are more of a concern in younger patients, which makes the absence of radiation or need for intravenous contrast a particular advantage for coronary MRI. Though coronary MRI data for anomalous disease are quite extensive, in the absence of a strong suspicion, data are insufficient to support routine coronary MRI screening among children or young adults.

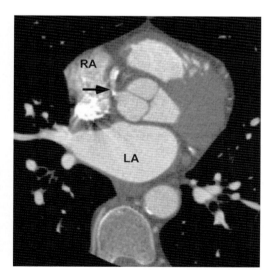

FIGURE 15.7. An axial image from an MDCT study illustrating the RCA (arrow) arising anomalously from the noncoronary aortic sinus and coursing anteriorly into the right atrioventricular groove, where it normally lies. RA, right atrial appendage; LA, left atrium.

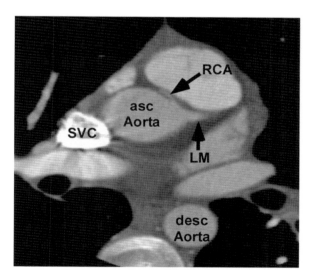

FIGURE 15.8. CTA image showing the origins of a large normal left main (LM) coronary artery and the separate origin of a small anomalous right coronary artery (RCA), both arising from the left aortic sinus. The RCA courses anteriorly between the great vessels, which can be associated with sudden death syndrome. SVC, superior vena cava; asc Aorta, ascending aorta; desc Aorta, descending aorta.

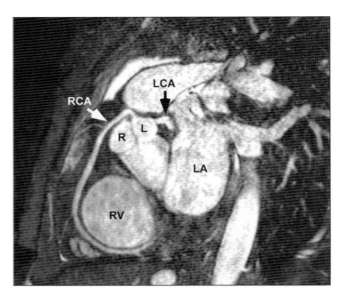

FIGURE 15.9. Coronary MRI in a patient with anomalous right coronary artery (RCA) arising from the left sinus of Valsalva (L). The left coronary artery (LCA) is also seen. LA, left atrium; R, right sinus of Valsalva; RV, right ventricle.

Evaluation of Coronary Artery Aneurysms

Although coronary artery aneurysms are relatively uncommon, data indicate an important role for coronary MRI for assessment of this condition.[30] The vast majority of acquired coronary aneurysms in children and younger adults are due to muco-cutaneous lymph node syndrome (Kawasaki disease), a generalized vasculitis of unknown etiology usually occurring in children under 5 years old. Infants and children with this syndrome may show evidence of myocarditis, pericarditis, or both, and

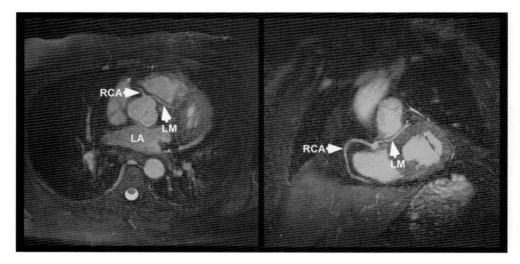

FIGURE 15.10. Coronary MRI in the axial (left panel) and oblique coronal imaging (right panel) planes in a patient with anomalous left main (LM) coronary artery originating from the right sinus of Valsalva and traversing between the pulmonary artery anteriorly and the aorta posteriorly. LA, left atrium; RCA, right coronary artery.

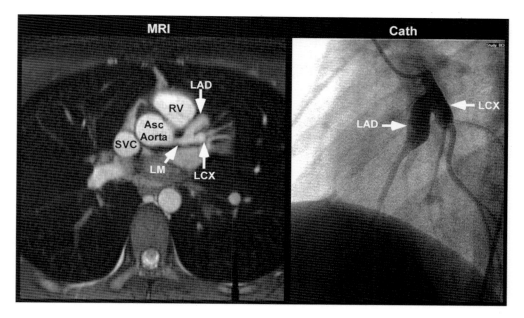

FIGURE 15.11. Coronary MRI and corresponding x-ray coronary angiogram in a patient with Kawasaki disease and left coronary artery aneurysms involving the proximal left anterior descending (LAD) and left circumflex (LCX) arteries. SVC, superior vena cava; Asc Aorta, ascending aorta; RV, right ventricle; LM, left main coronary artery.

nearly 20% will develop coronary artery aneurysms. These aneurysms are the source of both short- and long-term morbidity and mortality. For afflicted young children, transthoracic echocardiography is usually adequate for diagnosing and following these aneurysms, but echocardiography is often inadequate after adolescence and in obese children. These patients are therefore often referred for serial x-ray coronary angiography. Data from a series of adolescents and young adults with coronary artery aneurysms (Figure 15.11) defined on x-ray angiography have confirmed the high accuracy of coronary MRI for both the identification and the characterization (diameter and length) of these aneurysms.[31,32] Good correlation between coronary MRI and x-ray coronary angiography has also been reported for ectatic coronary arteries (distinct from Kawaski disease) among adults.[31,32]

Evaluation After Revascularization

The patency of bypass grafts has been extensively studied and may present diagnostic difficulty for the cardiologist.[33] The anatomy of both saphenous vein and internal mammary artery grafts is readily displayed with MDCT. The procedure has the advantage of requiring as little actual scan time as 20 to 30 seconds; usually the total procedure can be completed within 15 minutes. Further advantages of CT include the large field of view, which can be tailored to a specific area or can include the whole chest, allowing appraisal in 3D not only of graft locations, calcifications, graft and native coronary artery patency and quality but also of the position of these vessels relative to the sternum, which may be critical when repeat surgery is being considered (Figure 15.12). Furthermore, the spatial resolution is uniformly excellent and allows precise measurements to guide the surgeon.[34] Feasibility studies measuring relative graft flow by CT have also been reported.[35]

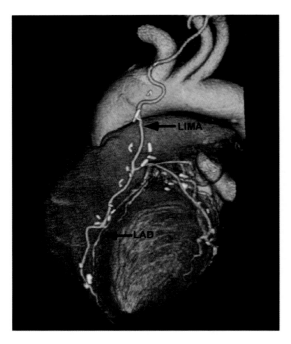

FIGURE 15.12. Cardiac MDCT study with 3D reconstruction showing patent left internal mammary artery (LIMA) graft and left anterior descending (LAD) artery.

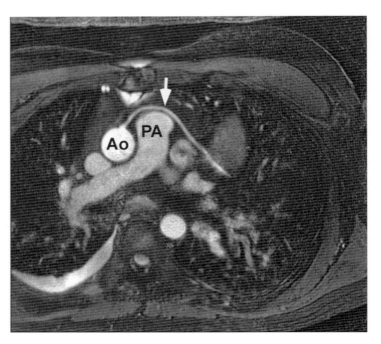

FIGURE 15.13. Coronary MRI gradient-echo image in a patient with a widely patent reverse saphenous vein graft (arrow). Ao, aorta, PA, main pulmonary artery. (Courtesy of Albert de Roos, MD, Leiden University.)

In comparison with the native coronary arteries imaging, coronary MRI of reverse saphenous vein and internal mammary artery grafts is relatively easy (in the absence of adjacent vascular clips) due to their relatively stationary position during the cardiac and respiratory cycle and their larger lumen.

If information regarding graft patency versus occlusion data are desired, conventional free-breathing ECG-gated 2D spin-echo[33,34,36] and 2D gradient-echo MRI in the transverse plane have both been reliably utilized to assess bypass graft patency (Figure 15.13). Patency is generally determined by visualizing a patent graft lumen in at least two contiguous transverse levels along its expected course (presence of flow appearing as signal void for spin-echo techniques and bright signal for gradient-echo approaches). If signal consistent with flow is identified in the area of the graft lumen on two levels, it is likely to be patent. If a patent graft lumen is not seen at any level, the graft is considered occluded. Combining spin-echo and gradient-echo imaging in the same patient does not appear to improve accuracy.[37] Both 3D noncontrast and contrast-enhanced coronary MRI have also been described for the assessment of graft patency, with slightly improved results.

A practical limitation of coronary MRI bypass graft assessment is related to local signal loss or artifacts due to nearby metallic objects (hemostatic clips, ostial stainless steel graft markers, sternal wires, coexistent prosthetic valves and supporting struts or rings, and graft stents). The inability to identify severely diseased yet patent grafts is also a hindrance to clinical utility and acceptance.

Summary Points

- Both CTA and coronary MRI are still in their adolescence compared with established cardiac imaging modalities such as echocardiography and radionuclide methods.

- Considerable potential exists for further improvements in coronary CTA and coronary MRI methods.
- CTA and MRI are useful for coronary anomalies, aneurysms, and graft patency.
- The interest in cardiac CT and MR by radiologists, cardiologists, and surgeons continues to increase. Further developments and clinical trials are under way, and the results of these are awaited with great interest.

References

1. Achenbach S, Daniel WG. Computed tomography of the coronary arteries: more than meets the (angiographic) eye. *J Am Coll Cardiol.* 2005;46:155–157.
2. Achenbach S, Ropers D, Pohle FK, et al. Detection of coronary artery stenoses using multi-detector CT with 16×0.75 collimation and 375 ms rotation. *Eur Heart J.* 2005;26: 1978–1986.
3. Juergens KU, Grude M, Fallenberg EM, et al. Using ECG-gated multidetector CT to evaluate global left ventricular myocardial function in patients with coronary artery disease. *AJR Am J Roentgenol.* 2002;179:1545–1550.
4. Manning WJ, Li W, Edelman RR. A preliminary report comparing magnetic resonance coronary angiography with conventional angiography. *N Engl J Med.* 1993;328:828–832.
5. Stuber M, Botnar RM, Danias PG, et al. Double-oblique free-breathing high resolution three-dimensional coronary magnetic resonance angiography. *J Am Coll Cardiol.* 1999; 34:524–531.
6. Weber OM, Martin AJ, Higgins CB. Whole-heart steady-state free precession coronary artery magnetic resonance angiography. *Magn Reson Med.* 2003;50:1223–1228.
7. Botnar RM, Stuber M, Danias PG, Kissinger KV, Manning WJ. Improved coronary artery definition with T2-weighted, free-breathing, three-dimensional coronary MRA. *Circulation.* 1999;99:3139–3148.
8. Plein S, Ridgway JP, Jones TR, Bloomer TN, Sivananthan MU. Coronary artery disease: assessment with a comprehensive MR imaging protocol—initial results. *Radiology.* 2002; 225:300–307.
9. Foo TK, Ho VB, Saranathan M, et al. Feasibility of integrating high-spatial-resolution 3D breath-hold coronary MR angiography with myocardial perfusion and viability examinations. *Radiology.* 2005;235:1025–1030.
10. Pennell DJ, Bogren HG, Keegan J, Firmin DN, Underwood SR. Assessment of coronary artery stenosis by magnetic resonance imaging. *Heart.* 1996;75:127–133.
11. Bogaert J, Kuzo R, Dymarkowski S, Beckers R, Piessens J, Rademakers FE. Coronary artery imaging with real-time navigator three-dimensional turbo-field-echo MR coronary angiography: initial experience. *Radiology.* 2003;226:707–716.
12. Sommer THM, Hofer U, Meyer C, Flacke S, Schild H. Submillimeter 3D coronary MR angiography with real-time navigator correction in 112 patients with suspected coronary artery disease [abstract]. *J Cardiovasc Magn Reson.* 2001;4:28.
13. Angelini P VS, Chan AV. Normal and anomalous coronary arteries in humans. In: Angeli PE, ed. *Coronary Artery Anomalies: A Comprehensive Approach.* Philadelphia: Lippincott Williams & Wilkins; 1999.
14. Kim WY, Danias PG, Stuber M, et al. Coronary magnetic resonance angiography for the detection of coronary stenoses. *N Engl J Med.* 2001;345:1863–1869.
15. Hauser TH, Yeon SB, Appelbaum E. Discrimination of ischemic vs. non-ischemic cardiomyopathy among patients with heart failure using combined coronary MRI and delayed enhancement CMR [abstract]. *J Cardiovasc Magn Reson.* 2005;7:94.
16. Sakuma H, Ichikawa Y, Suzawa N, et al. Assessment of coronary arteries with total study time of less than 30 minutes by using whole-heart coronary MR angiography. *Radiology.* 2005;237:316–321.
17. Sommer T, Hackenbroch M, Hofer U, et al. Coronary MR angiography at 3.0 T versus that at 1.5 T: initial results in patients suspected of having coronary artery disease. *Radiology.* 2005;234:718–725.
18. Gerber BL, Coche E, Pasquet A, et al. Coronary artery stenosis: direct comparison of four-section multi-detector row CT and 3D navigator MR imaging for detection—initial results. *Radiology.* 2005;234:98–108.

19. Kefer J, Coche E, Legros G, et al. Head-to-head comparison of three-dimensional navigator-gated magnetic resonance imaging and 16-slice computed tomography to detect coronary artery stenosis in patients. *J Am Coll Cardiol.* 2005;46:92–100.
20. Engel HJ, Torres C, Page HL Jr. Major variations in anatomical origin of the coronary arteries: angiographic observations in 4,250 patients without associated congenital heart disease. *Cathet Cardiovasc Diagn.* 1975;1:157–169.
21. Datta J, White CS, Gilkeson RC, et al. Anomalous coronary arteries in adults: depiction at multi-detector row CT angiography. *Radiology.* 2005;235:812–818.
22. Kim SY, Seo JB, Do KH, et al. Coronary artery anomalies: classification and ECG-gated multi-detector row CT findings with angiographic correlation. *Radiographics.* 2006;26:317–333; discussion 333–334.
23. Lipton M. In response to the article of M.A. Bekedam et al. Diagnosis and management of anomalous origin of the right coronary artery from the left coronary sinus [editorial comment]. *Int J Card Imaging.* 1999;15:253–258.
24. McConnell MV, Ganz P, Selwyn AP, Li W, Edelman RR, Manning WJ. Identification of anomalous coronary arteries and their anatomic course by magnetic resonance coronary angiography. *Circulation.* 1995;92:3158–3162.
25. Post JC, van Rossum AC, Bronzwaer JG, et al. Magnetic resonance angiography of anomalous coronary arteries. A new gold standard for delineating the proximal course? *Circulation.* 1995;92:3163–3171.
26. Schmid M, Achenbach S, Ludwig J, et al. Visualization of coronary artery anomalies by contrast-enhanced multi-detector row spiral computed tomography. *Int J Cardiol.* 2006;111:430–435.
27. Taylor AM, Thorne SA, Rubens MB, et al. Coronary artery imaging in grown up congenital heart disease: complementary role of magnetic resonance and x-ray coronary angiography. *Circulation.* 2000;101:1670–1678.
28. Cheitlin MD, De Castro CM, McAllister HA. Sudden death as a complication of anomalous left coronary origin from the anterior sinus of Valsalva. A not-so-minor congenital anomaly. *Circulation.* 1974;50:780–787.
29. Lipton MJ, Barry WH, Obrez I, Silverman JF, Wexler L. Isolated single coronary artery: diagnosis, angiographic classification, and clinical significance. *Radiology.* 1979;130:39–47.
30. Lipton MJ, Pfeifer JF, Lopes MG, Hultgren HN. Aneurysms of the coronary arteries in the adult. Clinical and angiographic features. *Radiology.* 1975;117:11–18.
31. Greil GF, Stuber M, Botnar RM, et al. Coronary magnetic resonance angiography in adolescents and young adults with Kawasaki disease. *Circulation.* 2002;105:908–911.
32. Mavrogeni S, Papadopoulos G, Douskou M, et al. Magnetic resonance angiography is equivalent to X-ray coronary angiography for the evaluation of coronary arteries in Kawasaki disease. *J Am Coll Cardiol.* 2004;43:649–652.
33. Fitzgibbon GM, Kafka HP, Leach AJ, Keon WJ, Hooper GD, Burton JR. Coronary bypass fate and patient outcome: angiographic follow-up of 5,065 grafts related to survival and reoperation in 1,388 patients during 25 years. *J Am Coll Cardiol.* 1996;28:616–626.
34. White RD, Caputo GR, Mark AS, Modin GW, Higgins CB. Coronary artery bypass patency: noninvasive evaluation with MR imaging. *Radiology.* 1987;164:681–686.
35. Rumberger JA, Feiring AJ, Hiratzka LF, et al. Quantification of coronary artery bypass flow reserve in dogs using cine-computed tomography. *Circ Res.* 1987;61:II117–II123.
36. van Geuns RJ, Wielopolski PA, de Bruin HG, et al. Magnetic resonance imaging of the coronary arteries: techniques and results. *Prog Cardiovasc Dis.* 1999;42:157–166.
37. Mavrogeni SI, Manginas A, Papadakis E, et al. Correlation between magnetic resonance angiography (MRA) and quantitative coronary angiography (QCA) in ectatic coronary vessels. *J Cardiovasc Magn Reson.* 2004;6:17–23.

16 Integrated Assessment of Myocardial Perfusion and Coronary Angiography with PET/CT

Marcelo F. Di Carli

The integration of positron emission tomography (PET) and multidetector CT (PET/CT) technology provides a potential opportunity to delineate the anatomic extent and physiologic severity of coronary atherosclerosis and obstructive disease in a single setting. It allows detection and quantification of the burden of the extent of calcified and noncalcified plaques, quantification of vascular reactivity and endothelial health, and identification of flow-limiting coronary stenoses. PET/CT also has the potential to identify high-risk plaques in the coronary and other arterial beds. Together, by revealing the degree and location of anatomic stenoses and their physiologic significance, and the plaque burden and its composition, integrated PET/CT can provide unique information that may improve noninvasive diagnosis of coronary artery disease (CAD) and the prediction of cardiovascular risk. In addition, this approach expands the diagnostic capability of nuclear cardiology to include atherosclerosis and may facilitate further study of atherothrombosis progression and its response to therapy, thus allowing assessment of subclinical disease.

Imaging Protocols

Figure 16.1 illustrates the protocol used in our laboratory for the integrated assessment of myocardial perfusion and coronary anatomy with PET/CT. The details of the myocardial perfusion protocols used are discussed in Chapter 10. Immediately after myocardial perfusion imaging, the tomograph's table is moved back into the CT position for coronary angiography. Heart-rate control is achieved by a combination of oral and IV β-blockers. Sublingual nitroglycerin is routinely used prior to contrast administration. The integrated protocol is completed in approximately 45 minutes.

Portions of the text are reproduced from Di Carli M, et al. Integrated cardiac PET-CT for diagnosis and management of CAD. J Nucl Cardiol 2006;13:139–44, with permission from The American Society of Nuclear Cardiology.

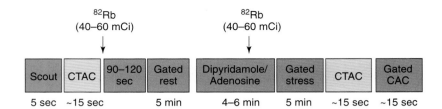

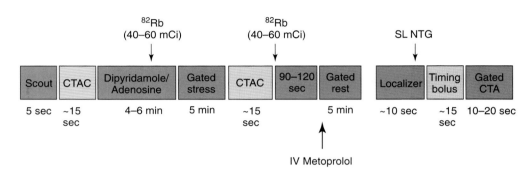

FIGURE 16.1. Integrated PET/CT imaging protocols. The top panel illustrates protocols combining myocardial perfusion and coronary artery calcium scoring. The lower panel illustrates protocols combining myocardial perfusion and CT coronary angiography. [82]Rb, rubidium-82; CTAC, CT attenuation correction; CAC, coronary artery calcium scoring.

Limitations of Single-Modality Approaches to Routine Diagnosis and Management of CAD

Computed Tomography

Lack of Access to Functional Significance

In general, decisions regarding revascularization are governed by the severity of patient symptoms and the magnitude of inducible myocardial ischemia.[1,2] This approach is based on the fact that revascularization procedures are very effective for symptomatic relief and for reducing risk of cardiac death among those with extensive inducible ischemia.[3] However, they are not effective at reducing future risk of myocardial infarction. While in general the anatomic severity of epicardial coronary stenosis is a predictor of the degree of downstream myocardial ischemia, there is great individual variability.[4,5] This is based on the fact that isolated angiographic measures of stenosis severity (i.e., diameter stenosis) are relatively modest indicators of coronary resistance, a key determinant of myocardial blood flow. Numerous other anatomic and physiologic factors that are important determinants of coronary blood flow are not accounted for by measures of stenosis severity, including factors related to plaque (shape, eccentricity), cardiac hemodynamics (left ventricular end-diastolic pressure and contractility), arterial physiology (vasomotor tone, endothelial function), stenosis characteristics (composition, stenoses in series) and collateral blood flow.[4] The effectiveness of stress perfusion imaging is based on the fact that it offers an integrated measure of the consequence of anatomic and physiologic parameters on myocardial perfusion.

Difficulties with Coronary Calcium and Stents

As described in Chapter 14, high-density objects such as calcified coronary plaques and stent struts limit the ability to accurately delineate the degree of coronary luminal narrowing. The bright (blooming) signal from such high-density objects extends beyond their true size into neighboring volume voxels, thereby leading to overestimation of stenosis severity. In addition, photon flux through such high-density areas occasionally leads to a signal void adjacent to calcified plaques or within stents that can be interpreted as "soft" (noncalcified) plaque, which could cause overestimation of plaque burden in individual patients. Although improvements in spatial resolution would decrease the impact of high-density objects, with current technology this would significantly increase radiation exposure. Thus, coronary calcifications would limit the role of multidetector computed tomography (MDCT) in some patient groups, including the elderly (>70 years)[6] and those with end-stage renal disease and diabetes in whom the prevalence of coronary calcium is increased.[7]

Limited Temporal Resolution

Clinical data show that the standard currently available temporal resolution is inadequate to cover the normal range of resting heart rates.[8] Although administration of β-blockers prior to testing seems to overcome this problem in most patients, it still remains a cause of image degradation and blurring that could lead to false-positive or false-negative results in some patients (as one tries to read "through" motion artifacts) or simply to nondiagnostic studies.

Irregular Heart Rhythm

Because of the need to acquire a gated scan, patients with atrial fibrillation and other forms of irregular heart rhythm are not candidates for CT coronary angiography. This effectively excludes CT as a diagnostic option in a significant number of patients over the age of 65.[9]

Incorporating CT Angiography into Testing Strategies

Establishing or ruling out the presence of CAD is an important goal of testing. However, this information alone is insufficient for identifying optimal patient management. Ideally, the results of noninvasive testing should also provide information regarding the risk of adverse outcomes (i.e., death and myocardial infarction) and, if possible, the risk associated with multiple potential treatment strategies.

While stress myocardial perfusion imaging has been shown to have the capability to achieve this goal,[2] this may be the most challenging limitation of CT. For example, data from the Coronary Artery Surgery Study (CASS) registry suggest that measures of ischemia and exercise performance were more useful indicators of treatment benefit than anatomic indices of CAD extent.[3] Patients with *low-risk* stress electrocardiogram (ECG) results (<1 mm ST segment depression able to exercise for >6 minutes) showed no survival advantage from revascularization over medical therapy, regardless of the angiographic extent of CAD.[1] Furthermore, even among those with *high-risk* stress electrocardiogram (ECG) results (>1 mm ST segment depression able to exercise for <6 minutes), revascularization showed improved survival over medical therapy only in patients with three-vessel CAD.[1] In keeping with these findings, more recent data in a large cohort of patients with suspected CAD who were undergoing stress single photon emission computed tomography (SPECT) imaging suggest that revascularization improves survival over medical therapy only in patients with moderate to severe ischemia.[10] Together, these findings would suggest that management decisions based solely on the extent of angiographic CAD by CT may lead to inappropriate revascularization in a considerable number of patients with stable CAD.

TABLE 16.1. Diagnostic Accuracy of CTA

	MDCT	Patients	Vessel Size (mm)	Sensitivity (%)	Specificity (%)
Nieman et al[11]	16	59	2.0	95	86
Ropers et al[12]	16	77	1.5	93	92
Martuscelli et al[13]	16	64	1.5	89	98
Mollet et al[14]	16	128	2.0	92	95
Hoffman U et al[15]	16	33	2.0	89	95
Kuettner et al[16]	16	72	**All**	**82**	98
Mollet et al[17]	16	51	2.0	95	98
Morgan-Hughes et al[18]	16	57	**All**	**83**	97
Achenbach et al[19]	16	50	1.5	93	95
Hoffman et al[20]	16	103	1.5	97	96
Leschka et al[21]	64	67	1.5	94	97
Leber et al[22]	64	59	**All**	**73**	97

Abbreviation: MDCT, multidetector computed tomography.

Positron Emission Tomography

Underestimation of the Extent of Anatomic CAD

As shown in Table 16.1, the relative assessment of myocardial perfusion with PET remains a sensitive means for diagnosing CAD. As with SPECT, however, PET often uncovers only that territory supplied by the most severe stenosis. This is based on the fact that, in patients with CAD, coronary vasodilator reserve is often abnormal even in territories supplied by noncritical angiographic stenoses,[23,24] thereby reducing the heterogeneity of flow between "normal" and "abnormal" zones and limiting the ability to delineate the presence of multivessel CAD.

Detection of CAD Versus Identification of Subclinical Atherosclerosis

While conventional stress perfusion imaging excels at the identification of CAD, its extent and severity, and the associated risks of adverse events, it fails to describe the presence and extent of atherosclerosis. The incorporation of CT technology with PET permits routine evaluation for the presence of subclinical coronary atherosclerosis in patients presenting for stress perfusion imaging. Whether incremental information can be gained by the combination of these two distinct physiologic phenomena is as yet unknown.

Value Added of Integrated PET/CT and Clinical Applications

Assessing Subclinical Atherosclerosis

Stress perfusion imaging alone fails to uncover the presence and extent of atherosclerosis. Integrated PET/CT offers an opportunity to assess the presence and magnitude of subclinical atherosclerotic disease burden (Figure 16.2) and to measure myocardial blood flow (in milliliters per minute per gram of myocardium) as a marker of endothelial health and atherosclerotic disease activity, as described in Chapters 11 and 12. As discussed in Chapter 23, image fusion with integrated PET/CT may also allow identification of so-called vulnerable plaques by enabling image fusion of structure and function (biology) (Figure 16.3). Such imaging tools would provide mechanistic insights into atherothrombotic processes, better risk stratification, optimal selection of therapeutic targets, and the means for monitoring therapeutic responses.

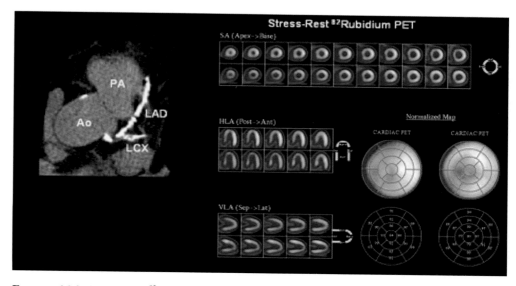

FIGURE 16.2. Integrated [82]Rb myocardial perfusion and noncontrast gated CT scan to evaluate coronary calcium content. The images demonstrate extensive (albeit nonflow limiting) coronary atherosclerosis in a patient with risk factors. Integrated PET/CT offers a more complete approach to diagnosis, risk stratification, and management than either modality alone.

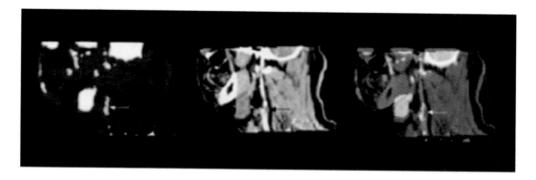

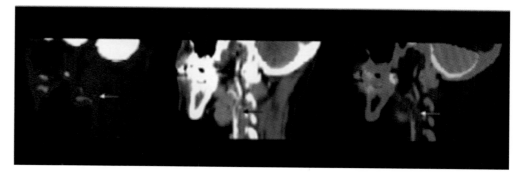

FIGURE 16.3. The upper row (from left to right) shows PET, contrast CT, and coregistered PET/CT images in the sagittal plane, from a 63-year-old man who had experienced 2 episodes of left-sided hemiparesis. Angiography demonstrated stenosis of the proximal right internal carotid artery; this was confirmed on the CT image (black arrow). The white arrows show fluorine-18 fluorodeoxyglucose (^{18}F-FDG) uptake at the level of the plaque in the carotid artery. As expected, there was high [18]FDG uptake in the brain, jaw muscles, and facial soft tissues. The lower row (from left to right) demonstrates a low level of [18]FDG uptake in an asymptomatic carotid stenosis. The black arrow highlights the stenosis on the CT angiogram, and the white arrows demonstrate minimal [18]FDG accumulation at this site on the [18]FDG PET and coregistered PET/CT images. (Reproduced from Rudd JHF, Warburton EA, Fryer TD, et al. [25]. with permission of The American Heart Association.)

Detecting Clinical CAD

One advantage of the integrated approach to the diagnosis of CAD is the added sensitivity of PET and CTA, which potentially could provide correct diagnosis in virtually all patients.[26] CT coronary angiography provides excellent diagnostic sensitivity for stenoses in the proximal and mid segments (>2 mm in diameter) of the main coronary arteries. The sensitivity of this approach is reduced substantially in more distal coronary segments and side branches (Table 16.1). This limitation may be offset by the perfusion information from PET that is rarely affected by the location of coronary stenoses. It may be argued that only stenoses in large vessels (>2 mm) are of practical interest because they can be revascularized with stents. However, diagnosing obstructive disease in more distal coronary arteries or side branches is equally important to guide medical management.

Stress perfusion PET also provides excellent sensitivity to identify patients with obstructive CAD. As described above, however, PET often uncovers only that territory supplied by the most severe stenosis and often underestimates the extent of anatomic CAD. With integrated PET/CT, this limitation can be overcome by the CT coronary angiographic information (Part VI, Case 11).

Guiding Management of CAD

Because not all coronary stenoses detected by CT coronary angiography are flow limiting, the stress myocardial perfusion PET data complement the CT anatomic information by providing instant readings about the clinical significance (i.e., ischemic burden) of such stenoses (Part VI, Case 14). Preliminary data from our laboratory suggest that the positive predictive value of CT angiography for identifying coronary stenoses producing objective evidence of stress-induced ischemia is suboptimal (~50%).[27] This finding, if confirmed, would suggest that additional noninvasive testing would be required after CT angiography before consideration for invasive catheterization. Further, the use of CT angiography as a replacement for myocardial perfusion imaging would potentially result in an enormous increase in costs of care and resource utilization due to unnecessary downstream catheterization and revascularization procedures.[28]

This apparent discrepancy between anatomic and physiologic measurements of stenosis severity is probably multifactorial. First, while CTA is an excellent method to exclude CAD, its ability to accurately assess the degree of luminal narrowing is only modest. Indeed, recent studies with 64-MDCT indicate that quantitative estimates of stenosis severity by CT correlate only modestly with quantitative coronary angiography, the former explaining only 29% of variability in the latter (Figure 16.4).[22] Image

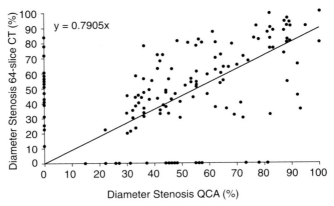

FIGURE 16.4. Scatter plot demonstrating the relationship between the severity of angiographic stenosis by quantitative CTA and quantitative coronary angiography. (From Leber AW, Knez A, von Ziegler F, et al. (22). Reproduced with permission from The American College of Cardiology Foundation.)

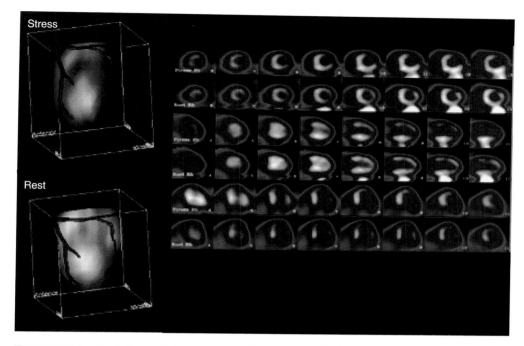

FIGURE 16.5. The left panel shows stress and rest myocardial perfusion images obtained with ^{82}Rb demonstrating a severe and reversible perfusion defect throughout the anterolateral and lateral left ventricle walls. The right panel demonstrates the fusion of three-dimensional volume rendered perfusion information with the patient's coronary artery tree derived from the contrast-enhanced MDCT coronary angiographic images (not shown). The fused images demonstrate that the culprit vessel corresponds to a marginal branch from the left circumflex artery. (Images are courtesy of Dr. Ernest Garcia from Emory University, Atlanta, GA.)

degradation by motion and calcium may lead to both under- and overestimation of luminal narrowing by CTA. Owing to similar effects, metal objects such as stents, surgical clips, and sternal wires can also interfere with the evaluation of underlying coronary stenoses. Second, as described above, isolated angiographic measures of stenosis severity (i.e., diameter stenosis) are relatively modest indicators of coronary resistance, a key determinant of myocardial blood flow.[29] Third, CTA does not provide adequate information regarding collateral flow or vasomotor tone, both of which are known to affect myocardial perfusion. In contrast, myocardial perfusion imaging provides a simple integrated measure of the effect of all these parameters on coronary resistance and tissue perfusion, thereby allowing more appropriate selection of patients who may ultimately benefit from revascularization. Finally, image fusion of the stress perfusion PET data with the coronary CT information can also help identify the culprit stenosis in a patient presenting with chest pain (Figure 16.5).

An integrated approach with PET/CT also facilitates identification of patients without flow-limiting disease (i.e., normal perfusion) who have extensive, albeit subclinical, coronary artery disease. Preliminary data from our laboratory suggest that as many as 50% of patients with normal stress perfusion PET may show extensive (non–flow limiting) coronary atherosclerosis (both calcified and noncalcified plaques) (Figure 16.2).[27] While these patients do not require revascularization, due to the absence of ischemia, they probably warrant more aggressive medical therapy.

Summary Points

- The clinical evidence suggests that integrated PET/CT is a powerful, noninvasive modality for diagnosing and managing CAD.

- The need for gated scans, the use of nephrotoxic contrast, and the potential limitations imposed by the presence of calcium call into question the generalizability of CT alone for all patients with known or suspected CAD.
- Beyond diagnosis of CAD, the most important challenge for CT coronary angiography may be in guiding management after the diagnosis of CAD.
- The greatest strength of integrated PET/CT imaging is its ability to establish the diagnosis, define risk, and guide management with a single study.

References

1. Weiner DA, Ryan TJ, McCabe CH, et al. The role of exercise testing in identifying patients with improved survival after coronary artery bypass surgery. *J Am Coll Cardiol.* 1986;8: 741–748.
2. Hachamovitch R, Hayes SW, Friedman JD, Cohen I, Berman DS. Identification of a threshold of inducible ischemia associated with a short-term survival benefit with revascularization compared to medical therapy in patients with no prior CAD undergoing stress myocardial perfusion SPECT. *Circulation.* 2003;107:2899–2906.
3. Yusuf S, Zucker D, Peduzzi P, et al. Effect of coronary artery bypass graft surgery on survival: overview of 10-year results from randomised trials by the Coronary Artery Bypass Graft Surgery Trialists Collaboration. *Lancet.* 1994;344:563–570.
4. Di Carli M, Czernin J, Hoh CK, et al. Relation among stenosis severity, myocardial blood flow, and flow reserve in patients with coronary artery disease. *Circulation.* 1995;91: 1944–1951.
5. Uren NG, Melin JA, De Bruyne B, Wijns W, Baudhuin T, Camici PG. Relation between myocardial blood flow and the severity of coronary- artery stenosis. *N Engl J Med.* 1994; 330:1782–1788.
6. Hoff JA, Chomka EV, Krainik AJ, Daviglus M, Rich S, Kondos GT. Age and gender distributions of coronary artery calcium detected by electron beam tomography in 35,246 adults. *Am J Cardiol.* 2001;87:1335–1339.
7. Hoff JA, Quinn L, Sevrukov A, et al. The prevalence of coronary artery calcium among diabetic individuals without known coronary artery disease. *J Am Coll Cardiol.* 2003;41: 1008–1012.
8. Nieman K, Rensing BJ, van Geuns RJ, et al. Non-invasive coronary angiography with multislice spiral computed tomography: impact of heart rate. *Heart.* 2002;88:470–474.
9. American Heart Association. Heart Disease and Stroke Statistics—2005 Update. American Heart Association Web site. Available at: http://www.americanheart.org/downloadable/heart/1105390918119HDSStats2005Update.pdf.
10. Hachamovitch R, Hayes SW, Friedman JD, Cohen I, Berman DS. Comparison of the short-term survival benefit associated with revascularization compared with medical therapy in patients with no prior coronary artery disease undergoing stress myocardial perfusion single photon emission computed tomography. *Circulation.* 2003;107:2900–2907.
11. Nieman K, Cademartiri F, Lemos PA, Raaijmakers R, Pattynama PM, de Feyter PJ. Reliable noninvasive coronary angiography with fast submillimeter multislice spiral computed tomography. *Circulation.* 2002;106:2051–2054.
12. Ropers D, Baum U, Pohle K, et al. Detection of coronary artery stenoses with thin-slice multi-detector row spiral computed tomography and multiplanar reconstruction. *Circulation.* 2003;107:664–666.
13. Martuscelli E, Romagnoli A, D'Eliseo A, et al. Accuracy of thin-slice computed tomography in the detection of coronary stenoses. *Eur Heart J.* 2004;25:1043–1048.
14. Mollet NR, Cademartiri F, Nieman K, et al. Multislice spiral computed tomography coronary angiography in patients with stable angina pectoris. *J Am Coll Cardiol.* 2004;43: 2265–2270.
15. Hoffmann U, Moselewski F, Cury RC, et al. Predictive value of 16-slice multidetector spiral computed tomography to detect significant obstructive coronary artery disease in patients at high risk for coronary artery disease: patient- versus segment-based analysis. *Circulation.* 2004;110:2638–2643.

16. Kuettner A, Beck T, Drosch T, et al. Diagnostic accuracy of noninvasive coronary imaging using 16-detector slice spiral computed tomography with 188 ms temporal resolution. *J Am Coll Cardiol.* 2005;45:123–127.

17. Mollet NR, Cademartiri F, Krestin GP, et al. Improved diagnostic accuracy with 16-row multi-slice computed tomography coronary angiography. *J Am Coll Cardiol.* 2005;45: 128–132.

18. Morgan-Hughes GJ, Roobottom CA, Owens PE, Marshall AJ. Highly accurate coronary angiography with submillimetre, 16 slice computed tomography. *Heart.* 2005;91:308–313.

19. Achenbach S, Ropers D, Pohle FK, et al. Detection of coronary artery stenoses using multi-detector CT with 16 × 0.75 collimation and 375 ms rotation. *Eur Heart J.* 2005; 26:1978–1986.

20. Hoffmann MH, Shi H, Schmitz BL, et al. Noninvasive coronary angiography with multislice computed tomography. *JAMA.* 2005;293:2471–2478.

21. Leschka S, Alkadhi H, Plass A, et al. Accuracy of MSCT coronary angiography with 64-slice technology: first experience. *Eur Heart J.* 2005;26:1482–1487.

22. Leber AW, Knez A, von Ziegler F, et al. Quantification of obstructive and nonobstructive coronary lesions by 64-slice computed tomography: a comparative study with quantitative coronary angiography and intravascular ultrasound. *J Am Coll Cardiol.* 2005;46: 147–154.

23. Uren NG, Crake T, Lefroy DC, de Silva R, Davies GJ, Maseri A. Reduced coronary vasodilator function in infarcted and normal myocardium after myocardial infarction. *N Engl J Med.* 1994;331:222–227.

24. Yoshinaga K, Katoh C, Noriyasu K, et al. Reduction of coronary flow reserve in areas with and without ischemia on stress perfusion imaging in patients with coronary artery disease: a study using oxygen 15-labeled water PET. *J Nucl Cardiol.* 2003;10:275–283.

25. Rudd JH, Warburton EA, Fryer TD, et al. Imaging atherosclerotic plaque inflammation with [18F]-fluorodeoxyglucose positron emission tomography. *Circulation.* 2002;105: 2708–2711.

26. Namdar M, Hany TF, Koepfli P, et al. Integrated PET/CT for the assessment of coronary artery disease: a feasibility study. *J Nucl Med.* 2005;46:930–935.

27. Di Carli MF, Dorbala S, Limaye A, et al. Clinical value of hybrid PET/CT cardiac imaging: complementary roles of multi-detector CT coronary angiography and stress PET perfusion imaging [abstract]. *J Am Coll Cardiol.* 2006;47:115A.

28. Shaw LJ, Hachamovitch R, Berman DS, et al. The economic consequences of available diagnostic and prognostic strategies for the evaluation of stable angina patients: an observational assessment of the value of precatheterization ischemia. Economics of Noninvasive Diagnosis (END) Multicenter Study Group. *J Am Coll Cardiol.* 1999;33:661–669.

29. Gould KL, Kirkeeide RL, Buchi M. Coronary flow reserve as a physiologic measure of stenosis severity. *J Am Coll Cardiol.* 1990;15:459–474.

Part IV
Diagnostic Approaches to the Patient with Heart Failure

17 PET Measurement of Myocardial Metabolism

Robert J. Gropler

There is growing evidence that perturbations in myocardial substrate use play a key role in a variety of normal and abnormal cardiac states. A decline in myocardial fatty acid metabolism and a preference for glucose as an energy substrate characterize pressure-overload left ventricular hypertrophy. Conversely, an overdependence on myocardial fatty acid metabolism with a parallel decline in carbohydrate use is characteristic of the myocardial metabolic adaptation in diabetes mellitus. What is unclear is the extent to which these metabolic switches are adaptive and to what extent they have the propensity to become maladaptive.

Accelerating our understanding of the role of alterations in myocardial substrate metabolism in these various cardiac processes is the development of transgenic models targeting key aspects of myocardial substrate use. A top priority is determining the relevance of the metabolic phenotype in these models to the human condition. In addition, applied genomics have identified numerous gene variants intimately involved in the regulation of myocardial substrate use. However, determination of the clinically significant genetic variants remains elusive. Finally, the importance of these various metabolic switches in the pathogenesis of cardiac disease can be exemplified by the current efforts to develop novel therapeutics designed to modify myocardial substrate metabolism in various diseases such as the partial fatty acid oxidation inhibitors for the treatment of ischemic heart disease. For all these reasons, the demand for accurate noninvasive imaging in myocardial substrate metabolism that can be performed in small animals and humans is increasing rapidly. Cardiac positron emission tomography (PET) is the most useful tool to meet this demand. This chapter highlights the current and future capabilities of PET metabolic imaging to furthering our understanding of cardiac disease.

Overview of Myocardial Metabolism

The myocardium is an omnivore using a variety of substrates, predominantly fatty acids, glucose, and lactate as energy sources (Figure 17.1). Under normal aerobic conditions, 50% to 70% of the total energy is obtained from the oxidation of fatty acids, the rest being obtained primarily from carbohydrates (glucose and lactate).[1,2] The proportional contribution of these various substrates to myocardial energy metabolism is exquisitely sensitive to the substrate environment, hormonal milieu, level of myocardial work, and level of myocardial blood flow. For example, under fasting conditions, myocardial fatty acid metabolism is the predominant energy source.

Low plasma insulin levels result in increased lipolysis in peripheral adipose tissue and thus in increased plasma fatty acid levels. The increased fatty acid delivery to the myocardium increases myocardial fatty acid levels, a ligand for the peroxisome proliferator-activated receptor α (PPARα) gene regulatory pathway.[3,4] PPARα is a nuclear receptor that regulates the transcription of an array of genes responsible for cellular fatty acid utilization pathways, including fatty acid uptake and oxidation. The increase in myocardial fatty acid metabolism decreases the transport of glucose into the myocytes as well as glucose oxidation, resulting in a decline in overall glucose metabolism. Under postprandial conditions, increased plasma insulin levels stimulate translocation of several glucose transporters to external sarcolemmal sites, increasing glucose uptake. Under normoxic conditions, glucose is converted to pyruvate, which is then oxidized via the tricarboxylic acid cycle. In addition, the rise in plasma insulin levels inhibits lipolysis within adipose tissue. Plasma fatty acid levels fall, which in turn decreases myocardial fatty acid metabolism. As a consequence, glucose becomes the primary substrate for oxidative metabolism. Other factors that can increase glucose uptake include an increase in cardiac work and direct catecholamine stimulation.[5,6] Under conditions of mild to moderate myocardial ischemia, myocardial fatty acid oxidation ceases and anaerobic metabolism supervenes. Glucose becomes the primary substrate for both increased anaerobic glycolysis and continued, albeit diminished, oxidative metabolism.[7,8] With successful reperfusion of ischemic myocardium, oxidative metabolism increases, frequently returning to levels comparable to those observed before the onset of ischemia.[9–11] The use of free fatty acids increases, and, with time, overall myocardial glucose use then declines.

In summary, myocardial health depends on plasticity in its substrate use to respond to a variety of stresses (e.g, changes in myocardial blood flow, work, substrate availability, or catecholamine levels). It is this loss of plasticity that characterizes the myocardial metabolic response to a variety of normal processes (i.e., normal aging)

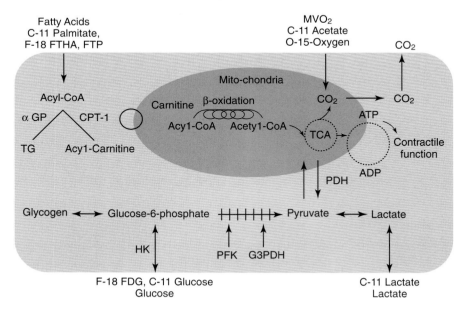

FIGURE 17.1. Summary of the various PET radiopharmaceuticals to assess myocardial substrate metabolism. FTHA, ^{18}F-fluoro-6-thia-heptadecanoic acid; FDG, ^{18}F-fluorodexoyglucose. (Reproduced and adapted by permission of the Society of Nuclear Medicine from M Schwaiger and R Hicks. The clinical role of metabolic imaging of the heart by positron emission tomography. J Nucl Med. 1991;32:565–578. Figure 1.)

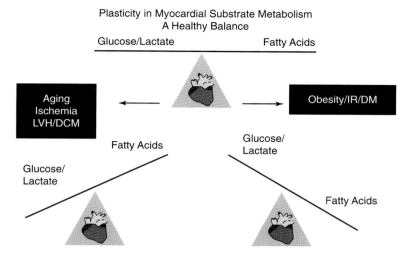

FIGURE 17.2. Summary of myocardial substrate metabolism demonstrating the need for flexibility in myocardial substrate use to maintain myocardial health. LVH, left ventricular hypertrophy; DCM, dilated cardiomyopathy; IR, insulin resistance; DM, diabetes mellitus. (Reprinted from Herrero P, Gropler RJ. *J Nucl Cardiol.* 2005;12:345–358 with permission from The American Society of Nuclear Cardiology.)

and pathological processes (pressure-overload left ventricular hypertrophy, dilated cardiomyopathy, obesity, and diabetes mellitus) (Figure 17.2). This loss of flexibility initiates a cascade of events that can have detrimental effects on myocardial mechanical function.

Challenges of Imaging Myocardial Metabolism

Accurate interpretation of a metabolic response to a pathologic state or following the institution of a therapy requires that the various determinants of myocardial substrate be taken into account. For example, therapies that decrease peripheral lipolysis will decrease fatty acid delivery to the heart, shifting myocardial substrate use from fatty acids to glucose even though there is no "direct" effect of the therapy on myocardial substrate metabolism. Moreover, the metabolic response will be different whether the changes are acute or chronic in nature. In the first instance, acute adaptation is regulated by the activation and inactivation of pathways switching metabolic fuels to the most efficient pathway of energy production for a given environment. The response of the heart to an acute increase in workload by oxidizing glycogen, lactate, and glucose is one example.[5] In the chronic setting, metabolic regulation occurs at a transcriptional level, resulting in adaptation and, in the extreme case, maladaptation of the heart. For example, the hypertrophied and failing heart switches its genetic profile to a more "fetal" pattern that favors glucose over fatty acids as an energy source.[12,13] Thus, very different metabolic patterns are present based on the time course of the stimulus. Localizing the metabolic effects of a disease process or the response to a new therapy will require that the most relevant pathways involved can be measured. For example, determining the relative potency of different partial myocardial fatty acid oxidation antagonists requires the measurement of myocardial fatty acid oxidation, not uptake or overall utilization.[14] Finally, whatever approach is used to measure myocardial substrate use, it should be possible in both rodents and in humans. In that way the potential clinical applicability of observations obtained in these experimental models of disease can be determined.

PET Tracers of Overall Oxidative Metabolism

Oxygen-15 Oxygen

Because oxygen is the final electron acceptor in all pathways of aerobic myocardial metabolism, PET with oxygen-15 oxygen (^{15}O-oxygen) has also been used to measure myocardial oxygen consumption (MVO_2). Administration of ^{15}O-oxygen is generally performed by inhalation of the gas, which results in marked spillover of radioactivity from the lungs to the heart.[15] Interpretation of tracer kinetics is complicated by the need to account for the conversion of ^{15}O-oxygen to ^{15}O-water and by blood-to-myocardial spillover. Consequently, four different scans have to be performed: a transmission scan to calculate lung volume, a ^{15}O-carbon monoxide scan to measure blood volume, a scan using a PET perfusion tracer to quantify myocardial blood flow, and the ^{15}O-oxygen scan. However, despite these complexities, a compartmental modeling approach has been devised that quantifies the myocardial oxygen extraction fraction. Thus, with the knowledge of the arterial oxygen content and myocardial blood flow, MVO_2 can be accurately calculated.[15,16] The major advantage of the approach is that it provides a measure of myocardial oxygen extraction and measures MVO_2 directly. Due to the short half-life of this tracer, ^{15}O-oxygen is readily applicable in studies requiring repetitive assessments, such as those with an acute pharmacologic intervention. Its major disadvantage is the need for a multiple-tracer study and fairly complex compartmental modeling to obtain the measurements. Despite these limitations, the ^{15}O-oxygen method has provided unique insights into the changes in MVO_2 that occur in a variety of abnormal cardiac conditions.[17,18]

Carbon-11 Acetate

Currently PET using carbon-11 acetate (^{11}C-acetate) is the most accurate and commonly used method of measuring MVO_2 noninvasively. Once taken up by the heart, acetate, a 2-carbon-chain free fatty acid, is rapidly converted to acetyl-coenzyme A (acetyl-CoA). The primary metabolic fate of acetyl-CoA is metabolism through the tricarboxylic acid cycle. Because of the tight coupling of the tricarboxylic acid cycle and oxidative phosphorylation, the myocardial turnover of ^{11}C-acetate reflects overall flux in the tricarboxylic acid cycle and, thus, overall oxidative metabolism or MVO_2. When biexponential curve fitting is used to measure the myocardial kinetics of the tracer, the rate constant k_1, which describes the myocardial clearance of ^{11}C activity (in the form of $^{11}CO_2$), correlates closely and directly with MVO_2 over a wide range of conditions.[19–21] This method has been simplified further to measure the clearance from the linear portion of the myocardial time-activity curve (k_{mono}).[19] Because of the relative simplicity of curve fitting, it is the most commonly used method to measure the myocardial kinetics of ^{11}C-acetate.

Exponential curve fitting of myocardial ^{11}C-acetate to estimate MVO_2 is susceptible to errors due to several factors. The curve fitting is sensitive to the shape of the time-activity curve in the blood. Thus, the accuracy of this method is affected not only by the injection technique but also by cardiac output and the amount of tracer recirculation.[22,23] The sensitivity of exponential curve fitting to this effect is more pronounced with the monoexponential. as opposed to the biexponential, fitting method.[23] A second potential disadvantage is that curve fitting may be sensitive to spillover effects from either the blood or the lungs. If significant, this would lead to an underestimation of the myocardial clearance of tracer and, again, an underestimation of MVO_2. Although it is not typically a problem in normal hearts, spillover may become a problem in situations in which recirculation of tracer may be significant or in which lung activity is increased, as may be seen in patients with marked left ventricular dysfunction. Finally, the curve-fitting method provides only an estimate of MVO_2. Absolute values of MVO_2 (in $\mu mol/g^{-1}/min^{-1}$) are obtained from k_{mono} based on the relationship between these two values measured directly in either dogs or humans. However, this relationship has usually been measured under normal physiologic conditions. It is unknown whether the relationship between k_{mono} and MVO_2 is altered under abnormal conditions, in which marked alterations could occur in the shape of the blood curve.

To circumvent many of these problems, compartmental modeling of myocardial ^{11}C-acetate kinetics has been developed. Compartmental modeling takes into account the effects of variability on the blood curve and spillover from the blood pool and lung fields and usually estimates MVO_2 directly, rather than converting rate constants to MVO_2 using a previously measured relationship. Indeed, measurements of MVO_2 have been shown to be more accurate when the compartmental modeling method is used as opposed to exponential curve fitting.[23] However, this method is more complex and time-consuming. The blood curve must be corrected for [11]CO_2 so that an accurate measurement of ^{11}C-acetate blood activity is obtained. Other physical factors, such as underestimation of true tissue activity due to partial volume effects, can significantly degrade the accuracy of the estimates obtained with compartmental modeling. Finally, because of the number of parameters being estimated, the need for high-quality dynamic data is greater with compartmental modeling than with exponential curve fitting. Despite these complexities, numerous groups have used compartmental modeling of myocardial ^{11}C-acetate kinetics to measure MVO_2 in a variety of normal and abnormal cardiac states.[24–26]

Hypoxic Agents

Fluoromisonidazole is a nitroimidazole, a class of compounds with high electron efficiency that serve as radiosensitizers of tissue hypoxia. It is believed that after passive diffusion into the myocyte, the nitroimidazole undergoes nitro-reduction in the cytoplasm. If adequate oxygen tension is present intracellularly, the process is reversible and the nitromidazole diffuses out of the cell. If there is an oxygen deficit, the nitro-reduction continues with subsequent irreversible binding of the products of this process to intracellular macromolecules. Consequently, the tracer will accumulate in hypoxic but still viable tissue. In contrast, tracer accumulation will not occur in normal tissue (because of normal oxygen tension) or in necrotic tissue (because it lacks the necessary enzymes to complete the nitro-reductive process). Results of experimental and clinical studies show differences that can be imaged between normal and hypoxic tissues using the PET agent ^{18}F-fluoromisonidazole.[27–30] Unfortunately, nitroimidazole-based agents suffer from two disadvantages, low cellular uptake and slow normal-tissue clearance, requiring long periods between injection and imaging.[27,30,31] Copper(II)-diacetyl-*bis*(N^4-methylthiosemicarbazone) (Cu-ATSM) is in a class of copper *bis*(thiosemicarbazones) that have been evaluated in vitro and display uptake that is hypoxia selective.[32–34] Studies using an acute myocardial infarction rat heart model, in which oxygen concentration can be controlled, showed that specific retention of ^{64}Cu-ATSM is due to oxygen depletion.[33] In intact dog hearts, Cu-ATSM has shown selective quantitative uptake in myocardium subjected to hypoxia from diverse etiologies such as reduced blood flow, excessive myocardial work, or reduced arterial oxygen tension.[35]

PET Tracers of Fatty Acid Metabolism

Carbon-11 Palmitate

Palmitate is a fatty acid that represents approximately 25% of the long-chain fatty acids circulating in the blood. It can be readily labeled with ^{11}C in the 1-carbon position and has been used extensively in experimental and clinical studies.[36] Carbon-11 palmitate (^{11}C-palmitate) is extracted rapidly by normal myocardium.[37] There is an initial vascular transit phase followed by the biexponential clearance of the tracer from the myocardium. The initial clearance rate reflects primarily β-oxidation, whereas the slower rate reflects primarily incorporation of the tracer into slow-turnover triglyceride pools.[37,38] However, the reliability of the relationship between the initial clearance rate and β-oxidation is reduced under conditions of ischemia due to enhanced backdiffusion out of the cytoplasm of nonmetabolized substrate.[39] To circumvent this problem, a compartmental model for the quantification of myocardial fatty acid metabolism has been developed and validated. In this model, palmitate enters the cytosol from the vascular pool and can proceed either into the mitochondria for β-oxidation or into a slow-turnover pool, which represents incorporation of fatty acid into triglycerides, phospholipids, or amino acids. Quantification of myocardial fatty acid oxidation with this technique requires determination of plasma fatty acid levels, myocardial perfusion, and the rate of conversion of palmitate to $^{11}CO_2$. This model has been validated in an animal model under a wide range of metabolic conditions and workloads; rates of fatty acid utilization correlated well with those measured with arterial-coronary sinus sampling.[40]

Fatty Acid Analogues

Due to the complexity of myocardial ^{11}C-palmitate kinetics, a number of fatty acid analogues with less complex metabolic fates have been developed. The 6-thia fatty acid analog 14(R,S)-[^{18}F]fluoro-6-thia-heptadecanoic acid (FTHA) was developed as a metabolically trapped tracer of β-oxidation for the myocardium.[41,42] In addition to incorporating a tracer with a more practical half-life than ^{11}C, FTHA demonstrates prolonged retention, allowing for quantitative determinations of myocardial fatty acid oxidation by the Patlak graphical analysis method.[43] Initial studies with FTHA have demonstrated that it is metabolically retained in the myocardium and that excellent image quality can be obtained both in normal humans and in those with coronary artery disease.[43-45] Experimental validation has demonstrated that FTHA trapping corresponds to fatty acid oxidation under a variety of conditions; however, this technique does not demonstrate the expected decrease in β-oxidation due to hypoxic conditions.[46] A newer 4-thia fatty acid analog, 16-[^{18}F]fluoro-4-thia-hexadecanoic acid (FTP), shows metabolic trapping similar to that of FTHA, with excellent sensitivity to the reduction in β-oxidation rates seen with hypoxia.[47] Though results with experimental models are promising, human studies are still pending.

PET Tracers of Carbohydrate Metabolism

Fluorine-18 FDG

Most studies of myocardial glucose metabolism with PET have used the glucose analogue fluorodeoxyglucose labeled with fluorine-18 FDG (^{18}F-FDG). Fluorine-18 FDG competes with glucose for facilitated transport into the sarcolemma, then with hexokinase for phosphorylation. The resultant ^{18}F-FDG-6-phosphate is trapped in the cytosol; its phosphorylation is assumed to be nonreversible because it is a poor substrate for further metabolism by either glycolytic or glycogen-synthetic pathways. The myocardial uptake of ^{18}F-FDG activity is thought to reflect overall anaerobic and aerobic myocardial glycolytic flux.[48,49] However, it should be noted that the concept that ^{18}F-FDG retention in myocardium is irreversible has been recently challenged. In dog hearts studied under conditions of high myocardial glucose use, ^{18}F-FDG egress was demonstrated as early as 9 minutes after tracer injection.[50] These results provided in vivo confirmation of observations obtained in perfused rabbit septa nearly 20 years earlier.[51] The reversible trapping resulted in nonlinear Patlak plots and significant decreases in the accuracy of the estimates of myocardial glucose utilization. In addition, acidic ^{18}F-FDG metabolites were noted in the blood, although their presence had little effect on the accuracy of the Patlak measurements of myocardial glucose use. As is the case with ^{11}C-palmitate, myocardial uptake of ^{18}F-FDG depends on the pattern of substrates presented to the myocardium as well as the hormonal milieu.[52] The preferred dietary state of patients to be studied depends on the metabolic question being addressed. For example, glucose loading is preferred to identify viable myocardium in zones of mechanical dysfunction because ischemic but viable tissue will accumulate ^{18}F-FDG, whereas necrotic tissue or scar will not take up this tracer. Conversely, to detect the metabolic sequelae of ischemia in myocardium with normal contractile function (for example, after exercise induction of ischemia), the fasted state is preferred to accentuate the difference between ischemic tissue with increased accumulation of ^{18}F-FDG and normal tissue with less uptake. The substrate environment can be further standardized by performing such studies under conditions of hyperinsulinemic-euglycemic clamp, which minimizes changes in the plasma levels of free fatty acids, insulin, and glucose during myocardial ^{18}F-FDG imaging.[53] Despite fastidious attention being paid to optimizing the substrate environment for myocardial ^{18}F-FDG imaging, uninterpretable images may still be obtained in 10% to 15% of cases.

Regional myocardial glucose utilization can be assessed in either relative or absolute terms (i.e., in $nmol/g^{-1}/min^{-1}$). To obtain images of relative myocardial ^{18}F-FDG uptake, image acquisition typically occurs ~45 to 60 minutes after the administration of ^{18}F-FDG to allow adequate time for uptake and phosphorylation of the tracer. When quantification of the rate of myocardial glucose metabolism is necessary, dynamic scanning is initiated concurrent with the administration of the tracer and continued for ~1 hour. Quantification can then be performed by either a compartmental modeling approach or by Patlak graphic analysis of myocardial ^{18}F-FDG kinetics.[54-56] Quantitative assessment of myocardial glucose uptake with PET demonstrates heterogeneity in glucose uptake: glucose uptake is higher in the posterolateral than it is in the septum and anterior wall. This disparity is most pronounced under conditions of low myocardial glucose use. These findings are independent of the level of perfusion or oxidative metabolism, suggesting that the proportional contributions of substrates to overall oxidative metabolism may differ in various parts of the left ventricular myocardium (Figure 17.3).[52,57,58]

Because ^{18}F-FDG is an analog of glucose, its initial uptake and phosphorylation differ from those of glucose. As such, a correction factor that accounts for these differences, called the lumped constant, must be known to accurately quantify myocardial glucose utilization with ^{18}F-FDG. However, the lumped constant can vary with the availability of insulin and fatty acids in plasma and with the level of perfusion.[59-63] An approach has been devised to correct for these factors, but the accuracy of this method has been validated only in isolated perfused hearts.[64] Other disadvantages of ^{18}F-FDG include the limited metabolic fate of ^{18}F-FDG in tissue, precluding determination of the metabolic fate (i.e., glycogen formation vs glycolysis) of the extracted tracer and glucose, and limitations on the performance of serial measurements of myocardial glucose utilization because of the relatively long physical half-life of [18]F. On the other hand, the myocardial kinetics of ^{18}F-FDG have been well characterized, the acquisitions scheme is relatively straightforward, and its production has become routine owing in part to the rapid growth of its clinical use in oncology; as such, it remains the most widely used tracer for determination of myocardial glucose metabolism.

Carbon-11 Glucose

More recently, quantification of myocardial glucose utilization has been performed with PET using glucose radiolabeled in the 1-carbon position with [11]C (^{11}C-glucose). PET with ^{11}C-glucose offers several advantages over PET with ^{18}F-FDG for quantifying glucose use: (1) as glucose has been labeled with ^{11}C, its metabolic fate is identical to that of glucose, obviating the need for the lumped constant correction factor and potentially assessing the metabolic fate of extracted glucose; (2) a compartmental

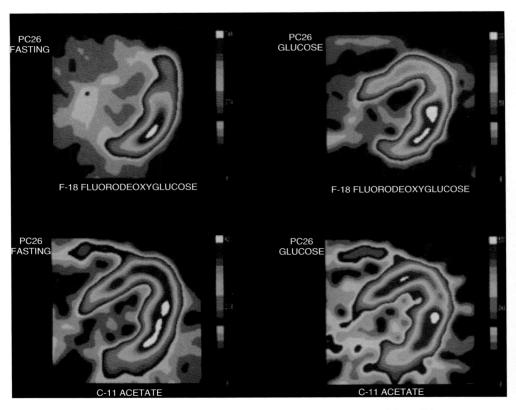

FIGURE 17.3. Midventricular PET reconstructions from a normal subject. The tomograms depicted in the upper panels were obtained after the intravenous administration of ^{18}F-FDG. Those in the bottom panels were obtained after the intravenous administration of ^{11}C-acetate. The left-side panel images were acquired after a 5- to 8-hour fast; those in the right-side panels were acquired after administration of glucose. The subject's left is represented by the right side in the image. In the fasting state, marked heterogeneity of the accumulation of ^{18}F-FDG is evident. It was attenuated markedly after administration of glucose. Accumulation and clearance of ^{11}C-acetate are homogenous with both fasting and feeding. (Reprinted by permission of the Society of Nuclear Medicine from RJ Gropler, BA Siegel, KJ Lee, SM Moerlein, DJ Perry, SR Bergmann, and EM Geltman. Nonuniformity in myocardial accumulation of fluorine-18-fluorodeoxyglucose in normal fasted humans. J Nucl Med. 1990;31:1749–1756. Figure 2.)

model to accurately characterize the kinetics of this tracer has been developed and; (3) its relatively short physical half-life allows for serial measurements of myocardial glucose utilization.[65] It has been demonstrated that, over a wide range of plasma substrate and insulin availability and levels of cardiac work, myocardial uptake of ^{11}C-glucose more closely paralleled glucose uptake by arterial-coronary sinus sampling than did uptake measured with ^{18}F-FDG (Figure 17.4).[66] As a consequence, measurements of myocardial glucose utilization were more accurate with ^{11}C-glucose than with ^{18}F-FDG. Results of preliminary studies suggest that this model can be modified to determine the fraction of extracted glucose that enters slow-turnover pools such as glycogen and the fraction that is metabolized via glycolytic/oxidative pathways.[67] However, compartmental modeling is more demanding with ^{11}C-glucose than it is with ^{18}F-FDG. The arterial input function must be corrected for the production of [11]CO_2 and ^{11}C-lactate, the synthesis of this tracer is fairly complex, and the short physical half-life of ^{11}C requires an on-site cyclotron.

Carbon-11 Lactate and Pyruvate

Both ^{11}C-labeled lactate and pyruvate have been used to assess myocardial intermediary metabolism; however, the metabolic fates of these tracers are quite complex.[68]

FIGURE 17.4. Correlation in dog hearts between Fick-derived (x-axis) measurements of the rate of myocardial glucose utilization (rMGU) and PET-derived (y-axis) rMGU using (A) 1–^{11}C-glucose, (B)^{18}F-FDG before correcting PET values for the lumped constant (LC), (C) ^{18}F-FDG after correcting PET values by the LC, and (D) ^{18}F-FDG after correcting PET values by a variable LC (LC$_v$) that accounts for varying substrate, hormonal, and work environments. Correlation with Fick-derived values was significantly close when 1–^{11}C-glucose (A), as opposed to ^{18}F-FDG was used, regardless of whether an LC was used or the type of LC used (B-D). (Reprinted by permission of the Society of Nuclear Medicine from Pilar Herrero, Terry L. Sharp, Carmen Dence, Brendan M. Harden, and Robert J. Gropler. Comparison of 1-11C-Glucose and 18F-FDG for Quantifying Myocardial Glucose Use with PET. J Nucl Med. 2002;43:1530–1541. Figure 4.)

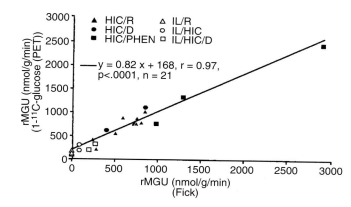

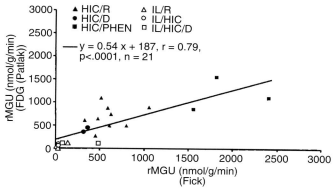

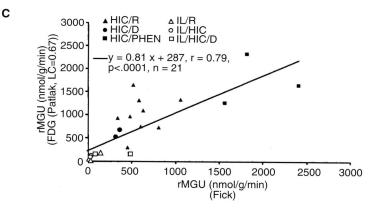

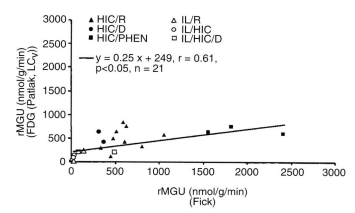

Lactate metabolism in the heart correlates with serum lactate level at rest, but this relationship may vary with exercise or ischemia. Recently, a multicompartment model was developed for the assessment of myocardial lactate metabolism using PET and L-3[^{11}C] lactic acid. Under a wide variety of conditions, PET-derived extraction of lactate correlated well with lactate oxidation measured by arterial and coronary sinus sampling.[69] This model may help delineate the clinical role of lactate metabolism in a variety of pathological conditions such as diabetes mellitus and myocardial ischemia.

Research Contributions

"Healthy" Aging

Aging has several deleterious effects on the heart: with senescence, there is impairment in diastolic filling and in systolic reserve capacity as well as blunted inotropic and chronotropic responses to certain β-adrenergic agonists. In both mouse and rat experimental models of aging, the contribution of fatty acid oxidation to overall myocardial substrate metabolism declines with age.[70,71] It appears that the cause for the decrease in fatty acid oxidation is multifactorial, including changes in mitochondrial lipid content, lipid composition and protein interactions as well as oxygen free radical injury, a decline in carnitine palmitoyltransferase-1 activity (CPT-1), the rate-limiting enzyme for mitochondrial long-chain fatty acid uptake, and age-related decline in myocardial PPARα transcript and protein levels.[72,73] Using PET, an age-related decrease in fatty acid metabolism and a relative increase in glucose utilization have been demonstrated (Figure 17.5).[74] Moreover, older individuals are not able to increase glucose utilization in response to β-adrenergic stimulation with dobutamine to the same extent as younger individuals. This impaired metabolic response may represent a stress-related energy deprivation state in the aging heart or potentially indicate that the heart is more susceptible to injury during periods of ischemia.[75]

Effects of Estrogen

Ovarian hormones have also been implicated in regulation of myocardial substrate metabolism. Estrogen supplementation in isolated working hearts from ovariecto-

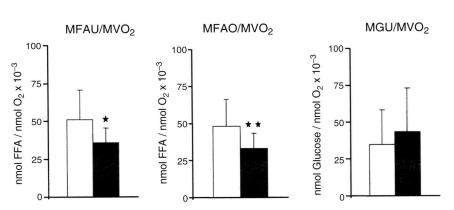

FIGURE 17.5. Values for myocardial fatty acid utilization (MFAU) and oxidation (MFAO) and myocardial glucose utilization (MGU), all corrected for myocardial oxygen consumption (MVO$_2$). Both MFAU/MVO$_2$ and MFAO/MVO$_2$ were lower in the older subjects compared with younger subjects. The MGU/MVO$_2$ did not differ between the groups. *p < 0.005; **p < 0.004. FFA, free fatty acids;. open bar, younger subjects; solid bar, older subjects. (From Kates AM, et al. (71). Reprinted with permission from The American College of Cardiology Foundation.)

mized rats demonstrates increased myocardial fatty acid oxidation that parallels impaired postischemic recovery.[76] Abnormalities in cardiac lipid metabolism in male mice deficient in PPARα were improved by the chronic administration of estrogen.[77] Myocardial blood flow, MVO$_2$, as well as glucose and fatty acid metabolism, were examined retrospectively using PET in postmenopausal women taking estrogen, estrogen and progesterone, or no hormone replacement and in age-matched men. Postmenopausal women on hormone replacement therapy containing estrogen demonstrated higher levels of myocardial fatty acid utilization and oxidation when compared to age-matched men and showed a trend toward higher fatty acid metabolism when compared to women not on hormone replacement. The increase in myocardial fatty acid utilization due to estrogen was likely secondary to a combined peripheral effect and direct myocardial effect. Moreover, the results of the study suggested that progestins attenuate the metabolic effects of estrogen.[78] Further studies are needed to verify these preliminary results and determine their clinical significance.

Hypertension and LV Hypertrophy

Several lines of evidence suggest a linkage between abnormalities in myocardial fatty acid metabolism and left ventricular hypertrophy. Initial observations obtained in children in whom genetic defects in the enzymatic pathways critical for myocardial fatty acid oxidation caused left ventricular hypertrophy.[79] More recently, a mutation in the gene encoding a regulatory subunit of adenosine monophosphate–activated protein kinase (AMPK) was found to be associated with hypertrophic cardiomyopathy.[80] Given that AMPK is another key regulator of β-oxidation, this provided further evidence for linkage between reduced myocardial fatty acid oxidation and left ventricular hypertrophy. Interventions in animals that involve inhibition of mitochondrial fatty acid β-oxidation result in cardiac hypertrophy.[81] In addition, numerous animal models of pressure-overload left ventricular hypertrophy have shown a reduction in the expression of β-oxidation enzymes, leading to a fall in myocardial fatty acid oxidation and an increase in glucose use.[12,82,83] Finally, a recent study in humans linked an Intron 7 G/C PPARα gene polymorphism to alterations in the hypertrophic phenotype. Hypertensive male patients with the PPARα CC polymorphism had a hypertrophic response significantly greater than those with the more common GG or GC genotypes, a finding that was independent of blood pressure control.[84]

PET with ^{11}C-palmitate in humans has shown that myocardial fatty acid oxidation is an independent predictor of left ventricular mass in hypertension.[85] That is, as left ventricular mass increases, there is a decline in myocardial fatty acid metabolism. This is the first confirmation in humans that the same downregulation in myocardial fatty acid metabolism occurs with hypertrophy. Another unique application of PET metabolic imaging has been in the measurement of energy transduction in normal and diseased myocardium. By combining measurements of left ventricular myocardial external work (either by echocardiography or right heart catheterization) with measurements of MVO$_2$ performed by PET with ^{11}C-acetate or ^{15}O-oxygen, it is possible to estimate cardiac efficiency.[86] Using this approach in patients with hypertension-induced left ventricular hypertrophy has shown that the transition from hypertension alone, where MVO$_2$ per gram of tissue is elevated, to hypertension with hypertrophy is associated with normalization in MVO$_2$ per gram of tissue. However, this adaptation is at the expense of reduced myocardial efficiency, which may increase the potential for the development of heart failure.[17]

Nonischemic Cardiomyopathy

In addition to left ventricular hypertrophy, alterations in myocardial substrate metabolism have been implicated in the pathogenesis of contractile dysfunction and heart failure. Animal models of heart failure have shown that in the progression from cardiac hypertrophy to ventricular dysfunction, the expression of genes encoding for enzymes regulating α-oxidation is coordinately decreased, resulting in a shift in myocardial substrate metabolism to primarily glucose use, similar to that seen in the fetal heart.[13,82,83,87-89] These metabolic changes are paralleled by reexpression of fetal isoforms in a variety of contractile and calcium regulatory proteins program.[13,90-92] The reactivation of the metabolic fetal gene program may have detrimental consequences on myocardial contractile function. The decline in myocardial fatty acid oxidation is paralleled by increased myocardial utilization of oxygen-sparing glycolytic pathways for the production of high-energy phosphates. Although this allows for reduced oxygen demands in the failing heart, the reliance of the myocardium on glucose may produce a relatively energy-deficient state that over a long time may result in decreased contractile performance.[93-95] Theoretically, the inability to metabolize fatty acids in the presence of increased fatty acid delivery may be associated with accumulation of nonoxidized toxic fatty acid derivatives, resulting in lipotoxicity and left ventricular dysfunction.[96] It should be noted that alterations in myocardial substrate use are now becoming attractive targets for novel treatments for heart failure. For example, it has been proposed that the presence of insulin resistance in heart failure patients further exacerbates the myocardial metabolic derangements because of the myocardial preference for glucose as an energy substrate. This in turn can limit adenosine triphosphate (ATP) production and lead to an energy-deficient state. Recently it has been shown that administration of glucagonlike peptide-1, an insulin sensitizer, results in increased myocardial insulin sensitivity and glucose uptake in an animal pacing model of heart failure.[97] Moreover, these metabolic changes were paralleled by dramatic improvement in left ventricular mechanical function. Similarly, the administration of pyruvate improved the contractile performance of failing human myocardial muscle strips by increasing intracellular Ca^{2+} transients as well as myofilament Ca^{2+} sensitivity.[98] The proposed mechanism for this improvement was to stimulate glucose oxidation via the activation of pyruvate dehydrogenase complex.

Early studies of myocardial metabolism assessed patients with heart failure by using PET to estimate the clearance rates of long-chain fatty acid tracers such as ^{11}C-palmitate.[99-101] Decreased rates of β-oxidation were shown in patients with myocardial long-chain acyl-CoA dehydrogenase genetic defects.[101] Furthermore, the extent of impaired clearance of ^{11}C-palmitate was shown to correlate with clinical severity. Studies using compartmental modeling of myocardial ^{11}C-palmitate and ^{11}C-glucose kinetics have shown that myocardial fatty acid uptake and oxidation are lower in patients with nonischemic dilated cardiomyopathy when compared with age-matched controls (Figure 17.6). In contrast, myocardial glucose utilization was higher in the cardiomyopathic patients. The metabolic findings cannot be explained by differences in plasma substrates or insulin, blood flow, or MVO_2.[102] Others have used PET with FTHA and ^{18}F-FDG to show that patients with heart failure exhibit increased rates of myocardial fatty acid uptake and lower rates of myocardial glucose uptake.[103,104] These results are in contradiction to those listed above. The differences likely reflected the inclusion of patients with ischemic cardiomyopathy and the lack of a control group in this study.

Combining PET measurements of MVO_2 with echocardiographic measurements of myocardial work has demonstrated that myocardial efficiency is improved in patients with heart failure with both exercise training and cardiac resynchronization therapy, implicating improved myocardial energetics as a potential mechanism.[105,106] A study with PET and ^{18}F-FDG in patients with dilated cardiomyopathy and left bundle branch block demonstrated a septal reduction in glucose uptake that is not matched by a regional reduction in perfusion. Moreover, treatment with resynchronization therapy resulted in homogenization of this unbalanced glucose metabolism.[107] Treatment with the selective β-blocker metoprolol also leads to a reduction in oxidative metabolism and an improvement in cardiac efficiency in patients with left ventricular dysfunction.[108] In patients with dilated cardiomyopathy, the percentage of glucose uptake, as measured by ^{18}F-FDG PET, can be used as a predictor for the effectiveness

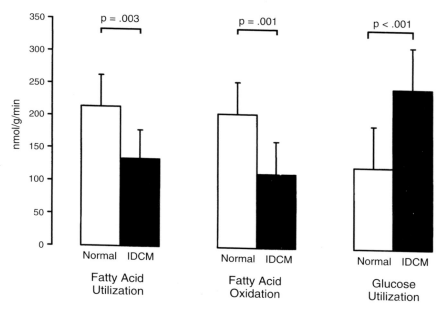

FIGURE 17.6. Myocardial fatty acid and glucose metabolism in idiopathic dilated cardiomyopathy (IDCM). Patients with IDCM exhibited significantly lower rates of myocardial fatty acid utilization and myocardial fatty acid oxidation and significantly higher rates of myocardial glucose utilization compared with normal subjects. (From Davila-Roman VG, et al. (22). Reprinted with permission from The American College of Cardiology Foundation.)

of β-blocker therapy.[109] Thus, cardiac PET can be used to study both the mechanism and the effectiveness of treatment in cardiomyopathy.

Diabetes

Diabetes mellitus is associated with increased cardiac morbidity and mortality.[110] Additionally, cardiomyopathy occurs commonly in diabetics independent of known risk factors such as coronary artery disease or hypertension.[111] Evidence is emerging that diabetic cardiomyopathy may be related to derangements in myocardial energy metabolism.[112,113] In diabetes, glucose utilization is markedly reduced and fatty acids account for 90% to 99% of MVO_2, as opposed to 50% to 70% as observed in nondiabetics.[113,114] Furthermore, the heart's capacity to switch energy substrates becomes constrained.[112,113] This dependence on fatty acid metabolism can be attributed to multiple mechanisms, including (1) The presence of high plasma levels of fatty acid enhancing both myocardial fatty acid utilization and triacylglycerol formation; (2) the presence of hypoinsulinemia causing subcellular (microsomal) localization of the glucose transporter GLUT-4 and decreased acetyl-CoA carboxylase activity; and (3) the combined effects of high cytosolic fatty acids and hypoinsulinemia reducing the activity of pyruvate dehydrogenase complex.[115,116] With the increase in myocardial fatty acid metabolism, there is an overall decline in glucose metabolism. Both insulin-mediated glucose transport and glucose transporter expression decline in diabetes mellitus.[117,118] However, rates of myocardial glucose uptake are frequently normal due to the presence of hyperglycemia.[119] Further metabolism of extracted glucose declines. The increase in fatty acid uptake results in increased citrate levels that inhibit phosphofructokinase. Glucose oxidation is inhibited at the level of pyruvate dehydrogenase complex due to increased mitochondrial acetyl-CoA levels and the phosphorylation of pyruvate dehydrogenase kinase 4 by PPARα activation.[120,121] Consequently, the maintenance of myocardial glucose uptake but a decrease in downstream metabolism results in an accumulation of glucose metabolites.[122,123] Potential detrimental effects associated with this shift in

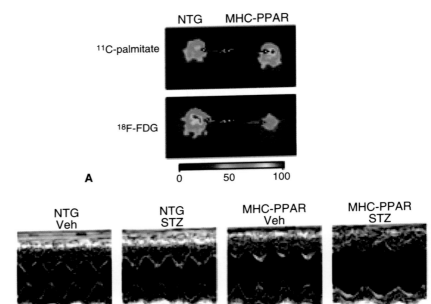

FIGURE 17.7. Metabolic characterization of the MHC-PPAR heart. Representative images of ^{11}C-palmitate and ^{18}F-FDG uptake into myocardium as assessed by small animal PET in non-transgenic (NTG) and MHC-PPAR mice. The relative amount of tracer uptake is indicated by the color scale (0–100). Arrows indicate the cardiac field. The heart field is increased into the red scale in MHC-PPAR mice infused with ^{11}C-palmitate, indicative of enhanced uptake of fatty acid. Conversely, uptake of FDG is substantially lower in hearts of MHC-PPAR mice. Representative two-dimensional-guided M-mode images of the LV obtained from control and diabetic NTG and MHC-PPAR mice. Ventricular dysfunction is present in MHC-PPAR mice and is further worsened by diabetes caused by streptozotocin (STZ) administration. (From Finck BN, Lehman JJ, Leone TC, et al. The cardiac phenotype induced by PPARα over-expression mimics that caused by diabetes mellitus. J Clin Invest 2002;109(1):121–136. Reprinted with permission from The American Society for Clinical Investigation, Inc.)

metabolism include impaired mechanical function due to the inability to increase glucose metabolism in response to increased myocardial work, myocardial lipid accumulation or lipotoxicity leading to disruption of cell membranes, electrical instability and apoptosis, and a greater sensitivity to myocardial ischemia.[124–126]

The potential mechanisms underlying diabetic cardiomyopathy have been studied in transgenic mice. Mice with cardiac-restricted overexpression of PPARα (MHC-PPAR) demonstrate a metabolic phenotype that is similar to diabetic hearts. Small animal PET studies with ^{11}C-palmitate and ^{18}F-FDG in these mice demonstrate an increase in the rates of fatty acid uptake and oxidation and an abnormal suppression of glucose uptake and oxidation (Figure 17.7). These changes occurred in tandem with activated gene expression of the myocardial fatty acid utilization pathway and reciprocal myocardial glucose transport and oxidation. Moreover, the MHC-PPAR hearts with the highest level of transgene expression developed left ventricular chamber dilation and systolic ventricular dysfunction. These data suggest that the metabolic shifts in the diabetic heart are maladaptive and contribute to cardiac dysfunction.[127]

Myocardial glucose uptake and fatty acid uptake and β-oxidation have been characterized in patients with type 1 diabetes mellitus by PET with ^{11}C-glucose and ^{11}C-palmitate, respectively. When compared to normal controls, individuals with insulin-dependent diabetes mellitus demonstrate decreased glucose uptake and a reciprocal increase in fatty acid uptake and oxidation.[128] In the setting of euglycemia and physiological plasma insulin levels, the percentage of extracted fatty acid that is oxidized is increased when compared to normoglycemic controls.[128,129] However, myocardial glucose utilization, as measured by PET with ^{18}F-FDG, can be normalized by instituting a hyperinsulinemic-euglycemic clamp.[130,131] Potential explanations for this discrepancy include differences in the levels of plasma insulin achieved (higher with the hyperinsulinemic-euglycemic clamp), different duration and severity of type 1 diabetes mellitus in the patients studied, or differences in the accuracy of PET measurements of myocardial glucose utilization with ^{18}F-FDG compared with 1–^{11}C-glucose.[66] Of note, clinical studies with PET and ^{18}F-FDG have shown that individuals with type 2 diabetes also demonstrate a reduced glucose uptake that is further exacerbated by hypertriglyceridemia.[132,133]

The increased plasma fatty acid and triglyceride levels are attractive targets to reduce the overdependence of the myocardium on fatty acid metabolism and perhaps to improve energetics and function of the left ventricle. For example, PET and ^{18}F-FDG studies in patients with type 2 diabetes mellitus before and 26 weeks after treatment with the PPARγ-agonist rosiglitazone demonstrated nearly a 40% increase in myocardial glucose utilization, which was attributed in large part to suppression of plasma fatty acid levels.[134] Thus, PET metabolic imaging can potentially be used to follow the effects of therapies designed to alter myocardial substrate metabolism in patients with diabetes mellitus.

Obesity-Insulin Resistance

There is compelling evidence obtained in experimental literature on obesity to suggest that significant increases in body mass index (BMI) induce marked increases in myocardial fatty acid metabolism. In either dietary-induced or transgenic models of obesity, myocardial fatty acid uptake and oxidation are significantly increased.[135–138] This increase, at least initially, reflects the increase in fatty acid delivery to the heart due to increased lipolysis from both visceral/abdominal and subcutaneous fat stores. Similar to diabetes mellitus, the increased delivery of fatty acids likely initiates a cascade of events that lead to increased fatty acid metabolism. Ultimately, fatty acid uptake may exceed oxidation, leading to extracted fatty acids entering nonoxidative pathways and most likely initially forming triglycerides. Moreover, the progression from insulin resistance to glucose intolerance to frank diabetes mellitus could also increase the likelihood of fatty acids entering nonoxidative pathways. The accumulation of the neutral fats or triglycerides may ultimately become detrimental.[135]

Imaging of obese young women with PET and ^{11}C-acetate and ^{11}C-palmitate has demonstrated that an increase in BMI is associated with a shift in myocardial substrate metabolism toward greater fatty acid use. Moreover, this dependence on myocardial fatty acid metabolism increased with worsening insulin resistance.[139] Paralleling the preferential use of fatty acids was an increase in MVO_2 and a decrease in energy transduction. These findings suggest that metabolic changes in obesity may play a role in the pathogenesis of cardiac dysfunction.

Coronary Artery Disease

As mentioned previously, under conditions of mild to moderate myocardial ischemia, oxidation of fatty acids ceases and glucose becomes the primary substrate for both increased anaerobic glycolysis and continued, albeit diminished, oxidative metabolism. The energetic advantage of incremental glucose utilization arises from the fact that although fatty acid oxidation yields more ATP than glycolysis under aerobic conditions, it does so at the expense of greater oxygen consumption.[140] Therapeutic interventions aimed at a shift of myocardial substrate utilization toward glucose metabolism may therefore be expected to offer benefit in those with coronary artery disease. PET has been used to study some of these "metabolic" agents that are currently available. For example, trimetazidine is a substituted piperazine that has been shown in several clinical trials to reduce angina and increase exercise capacity and systolic thickening in patients with ischemic heart disease. Although the exact mechanism has not been delineated, isolated heart models indicate that it exerts its antianginal effect by reducing the rate of fatty acid oxidation and increasing glucose oxidation.[140] An in vivo study using PET and ^{18}F-FDG demonstrated that trimetazidine further increases glucose utilization in ischemic myocardium without altering overall oxidative metabolism, suggesting a similar decrease in fatty acid oxidation.[141]

In myocardial infarction, PET has been shown to accurately identify, localize, and quantify the extent of infarction by measurements of either myocardial fatty acid or glucose or oxidative metabolism.[142–146] For example, the size of infarction quantified by PET and ^{11}C-palmitate correlated closely with enzymatic estimates of infarct size both in experimental animals and in humans.[142,146] The salutary effects on myocardial metabolism of timely reperfusion have been demonstrated with this method.[147,148] Furthermore, the importance of preserved myocardial oxidative metabolism as both a descriptor and a determinant of the capacity for functional recovery of myocardium subjected to ischemia and reperfusion has been demonstrated.[149]

Summary Points

- The successful growth of PET metabolic imaging will require advances in several areas. First, there will be a need for continued improvement in instrumentation design, both at the human level and at the level of imaging of small animals.
- Advances in PET detector design and postdetector electronics will result in improved counting statistics that should improve the ability to perform more complex compartmental modeling, permitting more complete characterization of the metabolism for a given substrate.
- Rapid advances are occurring in small animal imaging, with PET systems achieving a spatial resolution <1 mm. Moreover, smaller hybrid systems such as PET/MRI are being developed that will permit the near-simultaneous assessment of perfusion (with MRI) and metabolism (PET).
- A key need is the development of new radiopharmaceuticals that will provide a more comprehensive understanding of myocardial substrate metabolism. New radiopharmaceuticals are required to image "upstream" at key regulation sites such as for substrate transport (i.e., GLUT 1 and GLUT 4) or substrate switching (i.e., AMPK or PPARα). Others are needed for the interrogation of other key aspects of carbohydrate metabolism such as lactate or pyruvate metabolism.
- Similarly, radiopharmaceuticals are needed to delineate the differential contribution of plasma triglycerides and fatty acids to myocardial fatty acid metabolism.
- Novel radiopharmaceuticals also need to be developed that assess the downstream effects of altered myocardial substrate use, such as the activation of the nitric oxide system or the induction of apoptosis.
- Ultimately, radiopharmaceuticals labeled with longer-lived PET radionuclides ([18]F = ~110 minutes or [76]B = ~16 hours) that image the relevant metabolic pathways will need to be developed. In this way, large-scale trials can be performed that assess the diagnostic accuracy and prognostic value of a metabolic pathway or evaluate the efficacy of a new therapy designed to manipulate myocardial substrate use.

Acknowledgments

This work was supported by NIH grants PO1-HL13581, RO1-HL69100, RO1-HL73120, and RO1-AG15466.

References

1. Kelly DP. PPAR signaling in the control of cardiac energy metabolism. *Trends Cardiovasc Med.* 2000;10:238–245.
2. Goodwin GW, Taylor CS, Taegtmeyer H. Regulation of energy metabolism of the heart during acute increase in heart work. *J Biol Chem.* 1998;273:29530–29539.

3. Goodwin GW, Ahmad F, Doenst T, Taegtmeyer H. Energy provision from glycogen, glucose, and fatty acids on adrenergic stimulation of isolated working rat hearts. *Am J Physiol.* 1998;274(Pt 2):H1239–H1247.

4. Depre C, Vanoverschelde JJ, Taegtmeyer H. Glucose for the heart. *Circulation.* 1999;99: 578–588.

5. Stanley WC, Lopaschuck GD, Hall JL, McCormack JG. Regulation of myocardial carbohydrate metabolism under normal and ischaemic conditions. *Cardiovasc Res.* 1997; 33:243–257.

6. Taegtmeyer H, Roberts AFC, Raine AEG. Energy metabolism in reperfused heart muscle. *J Am Coll Cardiol.* 1985;6:864–870.

7. Heyndricks GR, Wijns W, Vogelaers D, Degrieck Y, Bol A, Vandeplassche G. Recovery of regional contractile function and oxidative metabolism in stunned myocardium induced by 1-hour circumflex coronary artery stenosis in chronically instrumented dogs. *Circ Res.* 1993;72:901–913.

8. Myears DW, Sobel BE, Bergmann SR. Substrate use in ischemic and reperfused canine myocardium: quantitative considerations. *Am J Physiol Heart Circ Physiol.* 1987;253: H107–H114.

9. Taegtmeyer H, Overturf ML. Effects of moderate hypertension on cardiac function and metabolism in the rabbit. *Hypertension.* 1988;11:416–426.

10. Sack MN, Rader TA, Park S, Bastin J, McCune SA, Kelly DP. Mitochondrial fatty acid oxidation enzyme gene expression is downregulated in the failing heart. *Circulation.* 1996;94:2837–2842.

11. Chaitman BR, Pepine CJ, Parker JO, et al. Effects of ranolazine with atenolol, amlodipine, or diltiazem on exercise tolerance and angina frequency in patients with severe chronic angina: a randomized controlled trial. *JAMA.* 2004;291:309–316.

12. Iida H, Rhodes CG, Araujo LI, et al. Noninvasive quantification of regional myocardial metabolic rate for oxygen by use of $^{15}O_2$ inhalation and positron emission tomography: theory, error analysis, and application in humans. *Circulation.* 1996;94:792–807.

13. Yamamoto Y, de Silva R, Rhodes CG, et al. Noninvasive quantification of regional myocardial metabolic rate of oxygen by $^{15}O_2$ inhalation and positron emission tomography: experimental validation. *Circulation.* 1996;94:808–816.

14. Laine H, Katoh C, Luotolahti M. Myocardial oxygen consumption is unchanged but efficiency is reduced in patients with essential hypertension an left ventricular hypertrophy. *Circulation.* 1999;l100:2425–2430.

15. Ukkonen H, Knuuti J, Katoh C, et al. Use of [^{11}C]acetate and [^{15}O]O_2 PET for the assessment of myocardial oxygen utilization in patients with chronic myocardial infarction. *Eur J Nucl Med.* 2001;28:334–339.

16. Armbrecht JJ, Buxton DB, Schelbert HR. Validation of [1–^{11}C]acetate as a tracer for noninvasive assessment of oxidative metabolism with positron emission tomography in normal, ischemic, postischemic, and hyperemic canine myocardium. *Circulation.* 1990;81: 1594–1605.

17. Brown M, Marshall DR, Sobel BE, Bergmann SR. Delineation of myocardial oxygen utilization with carbon-11-labeled acetate. *Circulation.* 1987;76:687–696.

18. Brown MA, Myears DW, Bergmann SR. Noninvasive assessment of canine myocardial oxidative metabolism with carbon-11 acetate and positron emission tomography. *J Am Coll Cardiol.* 1988;12:1054–1063.

19. Buck A, Wolpers G, Hutchins GD, et al. Effect of carbon-11-acetate recirculation on estimates of myocardial oxygen consumption by PET. *J Nucl Med.* 1991;32:1950–1957.

20. Sun KT, Yeatman A, Buxton DB, et al. Simultaneous measurement of myocardial oxygen consumption and blood flow using [1-carbon-11] acetate. *J Nucl Med.* 1998;39: 272–280.

21. Beanlands RSB, Bach DS, Raylman R, et al. Acute effects of dobutamine on myocardial oxygen consumption and car5diac efficiency measured using carbon-11 acetate kinetics in patients with dilated cardiomyopathy. *J Am Coll Cardiol.* 1993;22:1389–1398.

22. Davila-Roman VG, Vedala G, Herrero P, et al. Altered myocardial fatty acid and glucose metabolism in idiopathic dilated cardiomyopathy. *J Am Coll Cardiol.* 2002;40: 271–277.

23. Hutchins GD, Chen T, Carlson KA, et al. PET imaging of oxidative metabolism abnormalities in sympathetically denervated canine myocardium. *J Nucl Med.* 1999;40:846–853.

24. Martin GV, Caldwell JH, Graham MM, et al. Noninvasive detection of hypoxic myocardium using fluorine-18-fluoromisonidazole and positron emission tomography. *J Nucl Med*. 1992;33:2202–2208.

25. Martin GV, Caldwell JH, Rasey JS, Grunbaum Z, Cerqueira M, Krohn KA. Enhanced binding of the hypoxic cell marker [3H]fluoromisonidazole in ischemic myocardium. *J Nucl Med*. 1989;30:194–201.

26. Shelton ME, Dence CS, Hwang DR, Herrero P, Welch MJ, Bergmann SR. In vivo delineation of myocardial hypoxia during coronary occlusion using fluorine-18 fluoromisonidazole and positron emission tomography: a potential approach for identification of jeopardized myocardium. *J Am Coll Cardiol*. 1990;16:477–485.

27. Shelton ME, Dence CS, Hwang DR, Welch MJ, and Bergmann SR. Myocardial kinetics of fluorine-18 misonidazole: a marker of hypoxic myocardium. *J Nucl Med*. 1989;30:351–358.

28. Nunn A, Linder K, Strauss HW. Nitroimidazoles and imaging hypoxia. *Eur J Nucl Med*. 1995;22:265–280.

29. Dearling JLJ, Lewis JS, Mullen GED, Welch MJ, Blower MJ. Copper bis(thio-semicarbazone) complexes as hypoxia imaging agents: Structure-activity relationships. *J Biol Inorg Chem*. 2002;7:249–259.

30. Fujibayashi Y, Taniuchi H, Yonekura Y, Ohtani H, Konishi J, Yokoyama A. Copper-62-ATSM: a new hypoxia imaging agent with high membrane permeability and low redox potential. *J Nucl Med*. 1997;38:1155–1160.

31. Lewis JS, McCarthy DW, McCarthy TJ, Fujibayashi Y, Welch MJ. Evaluation of ^{64}Cu-ATSM in vivo and in vitro in a hypoxic tumor model. *J Nucl Med*. 1999;40:177–183.

32. Lewis JS, Herrero P, Sharp TL, et al. Delineation of hypoxia in canine myocardium using PET and copper(II)-diacetyl-bis(N[4]-methylthiosemicarbazone). *J Nucl Med*. 2002;43:1557–1569.

33. Lerch RA, Bergmann SR, Sobel BE. Delineation of myocardial fatty acid metabolism with positron emission tomography. In: Bergmann SR, Sobel BE, eds. *Positron Emission Tomography of the Heart*. New York: Futura Publishing; 1992:129–152.

34. Schon HR, Schelbert HR, Robinson G, et al. C-11 labeled palmitic acid for the noninvasive evaluation of regional myocardial fatty acid metabolism with positron-computed tomography I. kinetics of C-11 palmitic acid in normal myocardium. *Am Heart J*. 1982;103:532–547.

35. Lerch RA, Bergmann SR, Ambos HD, Welch MJ, Ter-Pogossian MM, Sobel BE. Effect of flow-independent reduction of metabolism on regional myocardial clearance of ^{11}C-palmitate. 1982;65:731–738.

36. Bergmann SR, Weinheimer CJ, Markham J, Herrero P. Quantitation of myocardial fatty acid metabolism using PET. *J Nucl Med*. 1995;37:1723–1730.

37. Fox KA, Abendschein DR, Ambos HD, Sobel BE, Bergmann SR. Efflux of metabolized and nonmetabolized fatty acid from canine myocardium. Implications for quantifying myocardial metabolism tomographically. *Circ Res*. 1985;57:232–243.

38. DeGrado TR. Synthesis of 14(R,S)-[^{18}F]fluoro-6-thia-heptadecanoic acid (FTHA). *J Labelled Comp Radiopharm*. 1991;29:989–995.

39. DeGrado TR, Stocklin G, Coenen HH. 14(R,S)-[^{18}F]fluoro-6-thia-heptadecanoic acid (FTHA): evaluation in mouse of a new in vivo probe of myocardial utilization of long-chain fatty acids. *J Nucl Med*. 1991;32:1888–1896.

40. Ebert A, Herzog H, Stocklin GL, et al. Kinetics of 14(R,S)-fluorine-18-fluoro-6-thia-heptadecanoic acid in normal human hearts at rest, during exercise and after dipyridamole injection. *J Nucl Med*. 1994;35:51–56.

41. Maki MT, Haaparanta M, Nuutila P, et al. Free fatty acid uptake in the myocardium and skeletal muscle using fluorine-18-fluoro-6-thia-heptadecanoic acid. *J Nucl Med*. 1998;39:1320–1327.

42. Schultz G, Vom Dahl J, Kaiser HJ, et al. Imaging of beta-oxidation by static PET with 14(R, S)-[^{18}F]-fluoro-6-thiaheptadecanoic acid (FTHA) in patients with advanced coronary heart disease; a comparison with [18]FDG-PET and ^{99m}Tc-MIBI SPECT. *Nucl Med Commun*. 1996;17:1057–1064.

43. Renstrom B, Rommelfanger S, Stone CK, et al. Comparison of fatty acid tracers FTHA and BMIPP during myocardial ischemia and hypoxia. *J Nucl Med*. 1998;39:1684–1689.

44. DeGrado TR, Wang S, Holden JE, Nickles RJ, Taylor M, Stone CK. Synthesis and preliminary evaluation of ^{18}F-labeled 4-thia palmitate as a PET tracer of myocardial fatty acid oxidation. *Nucl Med Biol.* 2000;27:221–231.

45. Phelps ME, Hoffman EJ, Selin C, et al. Investigation of [^{18}F]2-fluoro-2-deoxyglucose for the measure of myocardial glucose metabolism. *J Nucl Med.* 1978;19:1311–1319.

46. Ratib O, Phelps ME, Huang SC, Henze E, Selin CE, Schelbert HR. Positron tomography with deoxyglucose for estimating local myocardial glucose metabolism. *J Nucl Med.* 1982;23:577–586.

47. Herrero P, Dence CS, Sharp TL, Welch MJ, Gropler RJ. Impact of reversible trapping of tracer and the presence of blood metabolites on measurement of myocardial glucose utilization performed by PET and ^{18}F-fluorodeoxyglucose using the Patlak method. *Nucl Med Biol.* 2004;31:883–892.

48. Krivokapich J, Huang SC, Selin CE, Phelps ME. Fluorodeoxyglucose rate constants, lumped constant, and glucose metabolic rate in rabbit heart. *Am J Physiol Heart Circ Physiol.* 1987;252:H777–H787.

49. Choi Y, Brunken RC, Hawkins RA, et al. Factors affecting myocardial 2-[F-18]fluoro-2-deoxy-D-glucose uptake in positron emission tomography studies of normal humans. *Eur J Nucl Med.* 1993;20:308–318.

50. Knuuti MJ, Nuutila P, Ruotsalainen U, et al. Euglycemic hyperinsulinemic clamp and oral glucose load in stimulating myocardial glucose utilization during positron emission tomography. *J Nucl Med.* 1992;33:1255–1262.

51. Choi Y, Hawkins RA, Huang SC, et al. Parametric images of myocardial metabolic rate of glucose generated from dynamic cardiac PET and 2-[^{18}F]fluoro-2-deoxy-d-glucose studies. *J Nucl Med.* 1991;32:733–738.

52. Gambhir SS, Schwaiger M, Huang SC, et al. Simple noninvasive quantification method for measuring myocardial glucose utilization in humans employing positron emission tomography and fluorine-18 deoxyglucose. *J Nucl Med.* 1989;30:359–366.

53. Krivokapich J, Huang SC, Selin CE, Phelps ME. Fluorodeoxyglucose rate constants, lumped constant, and glucose metabolic rate in rabbit heart. *Am J Physiol Heart Circ Physiol.* 1987;252:H777–H787.

54. Gropler RJ, Siegel BA, Lee KJ, et al. Nonuniformity in myocardial accumulation of gluorine-18-fluorodeoxyglucose in normal fasted humans. *J Nucl Med.* 1990;31:1749–1756.

55. Iozzo P, Chareonthaitawee P, Di Terlizzi M, Betteridge DJ, Ferrannini E, Camici PG. Regional myocardial blood flow and glucose utilization during fasting and physiological hyperinsulinemia in humans. *Am J Physiol Endocrinol Metab.* 2002;282:E1163–E1171.

56. Botker HE, Bottcher M, Schmitz O, et al. Glucose uptake and lumped constant variability in normal human hearts determined with [^{18}F] fluorodeoxyglucose. *J Nucl Cardiol.* 1997;4:125–132.

57. Hariharan R, Bray M, Ganim R, Doenst T, Goodwin GW, and Taegtmeyer H. Fundamental limitations of [^{18}F]2-deoxy-2-fluoro-D-glucose for assessing myocardial glucose uptake. *Circulation.* 1995;91:2435–2444.

58. Hashimoto K, Nishimura T, Imahashi KI, Yamaguchi H, Hori M, Kusuoka H. Lumped constant for deoxyglucose is decreased when myocardial glucose uptake is enhanced. *Am J Physiol Heart Circ Physiol.* 1999;276:H129–H133.

59. Marshall RC, Powers-Risius P, Heusman RH, et al. Estimating glucose metabolism using glucose analogs and two tracer kinetic models in isolated rabbit hearts. *Am J Physiol Heart Circ Physiol.* 1998;275:H668–H679.

60. McFalls EO, Baldwin D, Marx D, Fashingbauer P, Ward HB. Effect of regional hyperemia on myocardial uptake of 2-deoxy-[^{18}F]fluoro-D-glucose. *Am J Physiol Endocrinol Metab.* 2000;278:96–102.

61. Botker HE, Goodwin GW, Holden JE, Doenst T, Gjedde A, Taegtmeyer H. Myocardial glucose uptake measured with fluorodeoxyglucose: a proposed method to account for variable lumped constants. *J Nucl Med.* 1999;40:1186–1196.

62. Herrero P, Weinheimer CJ, Dence C, Oellerich WF, Gropler RJ. Quantification of myocardial glucose utilization by PET and 1-carbon-11-glucose. *J Nucl Cardiol.* 2002;9:5–14.

63. Herrero P, Sharp TL, Dence C, Haraden BM, Gropler RJ. Comparison of 1–[11]C-glucose and ^{18}F-FDG for quantifying myocardial glucose use with PET. *J Nucl Med.* 2002;43:1530–1541.

64. Herrero P, Kisrieva-Ware Z, Dence CS, et al. Measurement of myocardial glucose metabolism and glycogen storage with 1-carbon-11-glucose by PET and kinetic modeling. Paper presented at: 2nd Annual Meeting of the Society for Heart and Vascular Metabolism; 2004; Quebec, Canada.

65. Bergmann SR, Fox KAA, Geltman EM, Sobel BE. Positron emission tomography of the heart. *Prog Cardiovasc Dis.* 1985;28:165–194.

66. Herrero P, Dence CS, Kisrieva-Ware Z, Eisenbeis P, Welch MJ, Gropler RJ. Measurement of myocardial kinetics of L-3[C-11]lactic acid. *J Nucl Med.* 2004;45:579.

67. Abu-Erreish GM, Neely JR, Whitmer JT, Whitman V, Sanadi DR. Fatty acid oxidation by isolated perfused working hearts of aged rats. *Am J Physiol.* 1977;232:E258–E262.

68. McMillin JB, Taffet GE, Taegtmeyer H, Hudson EK, Tate CA. Mitochondrial metabolism and substrate competition in the aging Fischer rat heart. *Cardiovasc Res.* 1993;27:2222–2228.

69. Odiet, JA, Boerrigter M, Wei JY. Carnitine palmitoyl transferase-I activity in the aging-mouse heart. *Mech Ageing Dev* 79:127–136,1995.

70. Iemitsu M, Miyauchi T, Maeda S, et al. Age-induced decrease in the PPAR-α level in hearts improved by exercise training. *Am J Physiol Heart Circ Physiol.* 2002;283: H1750–H1760.

71. Kates AM, Herrero P, Dence C, et al. Impact of aging on substrate metabolism by the human heart. *J Am Coll Cardiol.* 2003;41:293–299.

72. Soto P, Herrero P, Kowalski R, et al. Impact of aging on dobutamine-induced changes in myocardial substrate utilization. *Am J Physiol.* 2003;285:H2158–H2164.

73. Grist M, Wambolt RB, Bondy GP, English DR, Allard MF. Estrogen replacement stimulates fatty acid oxidation and impairs post-ischemic recovery of hearts from ovariectomized female rats. *Can J Physiol Pharmacol.* 2002;80:1001–1007.

74. Djouadi F, Weinheimer CJ, Saffitz JE, et al. A gender-related defect in lipid metabolism and glucose homeostasis in peroxisome proliferator-activated receptor alpha-deficient mice. *J Clin Invest.* 1998;102:1083–1091.

75. Herrero P, Soto PF, Dence CS, et al. Impact of hormone replacement on myocardial fatty acid metabolism: potential role of estrogen. *J Nucl Cardiol.* 2005;35:679–685.

76. Roe CR, Coates PM. Mitochondrial fatty acid oxidation disorders. In: Scriver CR, Beaudet AI, Sly WS, et al, eds. *The Metabolic and Molecular Bases of Inherited Disease.* New York: McGraw-Hill; 1995:1501–1533.

77. Blair E, Redwood C, Ashrafian H, et al. Mutations in the gamma(2) subunit of AMP-activated protein kinase cause familial hypertrophic cardiomyopathy: evidence for the central role of energy compromise in disease pathogenesis. *Hum Mol Genet.* 2001;10: 1215–1220.

78. Rupp H, Jacob R. Metabolically-modulated growth and phenotype of the rat heart. *Eur Heart J.* 1992;13:56–61.

79. Barger PM, Kelly DP. PPAR signaling in the control of cardiac energy metabolism. *Trends Cardiovasc Med.* 2000;10:238–245.

80. Barger PM, Kelly DP. Fatty acid utilization in the hypertrophied and failing heart: molecular regulatory mechanisms. *Am J Med Sci.* 1999;318:36–42.

81. Jamshidi Y, Montgomery HE, Hense HW, et al. Peroxisome proliferator-activated receptor alpha gene regulates left ventricular growth in response to exercise and hypertension. *Circulation.* 2002;105:950–955.

82. de las Fuentes L, Herrero P, Peterson LR, Kelly DP, Gropler RJ, Davila-Roman VG. Myocardial fatty acid metabolism: independent predictor of left ventricular mass in hypertensive heart disease. *Hypertension.* 2003;41:83–87.

83. Beanlands RS, Armstrong WF, Hicks RJ, et al. The effects of afterload reduction on myocardial carbon 11-labeled acetate kinetics and noninvasively estimated mechanical efficiency in patients with dilated cardiomyopathy. *J Nucl Cardiol.* 1994;1:3–16.

84. El Alaoui-Talibi Z, Landormy A, Loireau A, Morovec J. Fatty acid oxidation and mechanical performance of volume overloaded rat hearts. *Am J Physiol.* 1992;262: H1068–H1074.

85. Allard MF, Schonekess BO, Henning SL, et al. Contribution of oxidative metabolism and glycolysis to ATP production in hypertrophied hearts. *Am J Physiol.* 1994;267: H742–H750.

86. Wittels B, Spann JF Jr. Defective lipid metabolism in the failing heart. *J Clin Invest.* 1968;47:1787–1794.

87. Kantor PF, Robertson MA, Coe JY, Lopaschuk GD. Volume overload hypertrophy of the newborn heart slows the maturation of enzymes involved in the regulation of fatty acid metabolism. *J Am Coll Cardiol.* 1999;33:1724–1734.

88. Lompre AM, Schwartz K, Albis A, et al. Myosin isozymes redistribution in chronic heart overloading. *Nature.* 1979;282:105–107.

89. Buttrick PM, Kaplan M, Leinwand LA, et al. Alterations in gene expression in the rat heart after chronic pathological and physiological loads. *J Mol Cell Cardiol.* 1994;26: 61–67.

90. Massie BM, Schaefer S, Garcia J, et al. Myocardial high-energy phosphate and substrate metabolism in swine with moderate left ventricular hypertrophy. *Circulation.* 1995;91: 1814–1823.

91. Liao R, Nascimben L, Friedrich J, Gwathmey JK, Ingwall JS. Decreased energy reserve in an animal model of dilated cardiomyopathy. Relationship to contractile performance. *Circ Res.* 1996;78:893–902.

92. Neubauer S, Horn M, Cramer M, et al. Myocardial phosphocreatinine-to-ATP ratio is a predictor of mortality in patients with dilated cardiomyopathy. *Circulation.* 1997;96: 2190–2196.

93. Chiu HC, Kovacs A, Ford DA, et al. A novel mouse model of lipotoxic cardiomyopathy. *J Clin Invest.* 2001;107:318–822.

94. Nikolaidis LA, Elahi D, Hentosz T, et al. Recombinant glucagon-like peptide-1 increases myocardial glucose uptake and improves left ventricular performance in conscious dogs with pacing-induced dilated cardiomyopathy. *Circulation.* 2004;110:955–961.

95. Hasenfuss G, Maier LS, Hermann H-P, et al. Influence of pyruvate on contractile performance and Ca^{2+} cycling in isolated failing human myocardium. *Circulation.* 2002;105: 194–199.

96. Goldstein RA, Klein MS, Welch MJ, Sobel BE. External assessment of myocardial metabolism with C-11 palmitate in vivo. *J Nucl Med.* 1980;21:342–348.

97. Eisenberg JD, Sobel BE, Geltman EM. Differentiation of ischemic from nonischemic cardiomyopathy with positron emission tomography. *Am J Cardiol.* 1987;59:1410–1414.

98. Kelly DP, Mendelsohn NJ, Sobel BE, Bergmann SR. Detection and assessment by positron emission tomography of a genetically determined defect in myocardial fatty acid utilization (long-chain Acyl-CoA dehydrogenase deficiency). *Am J Cardiol.* 1993;71: 738–744.

99. Davila-Roman VG, Vedala G, Herrero P, et al. Altered fatty acid and glucose metabolism in idiopathic dilated cardiomyopathy. *J Am Coll Cardiol.* 2002;40:271–277.

100. Taylor M, Wallhaus TR, DeGrado TR, et al. An evaluation of myocardial fatty acid and glucose uptake using PET with [^{18}F]fluoro-6-thia-heptadecanoic acid and [^{18}F]FDG in patients with congestive heart failure. *J Nucl Med.* 2001;42:55–62.

101. Wallhaus TR, Taylor M, DeGrado TR, et al. Myocardial free fatty acid and glucose use after carvedilol treatment in patients with congestive heart failure. *Circulation.* 2001; 103:2441–2446.

102. Stolen KQ, Kemppainen J, Ukkonen H, et al. Exercise training improves biventricular oxidative metabolism and left ventricular efficiency in patients with dilated cardiomyopathy. *J Am Coll Cardiol.* 2003;41:460–467.

103. Sundell J, Engblom E, Koistinen J, et al. The effects of cardiac resynchronization therapy on left ventricular function, myocardial energetics, and metabolic reserve in patients with dilated cardiomyopathy and heart failure. *J Am Coll Cardiol.* 2004;43:1027–1033.

104. Nowak B, Sinha AM, Schaefer WM, et al. Cardiac resynchronization therapy homogenizes myocardial glucose metabolism and perfusion in dilated cardiomyopathy and left bundle branch block. *J Am Coll Cardiol.* 2003;41:1523–1528.

105. Beanlands RSB, Nahmias C, Gordon E, et al. The effects of β₁-blockade on oxidative metabolism and the metabolic cost of ventricular work in patients with left ventricular dysfunction: a double-blind, placebo-controlled, positron-emission tomography study. *Circulation.* 2000;102:2070–2075.

106. Hasegawa S, Kusuoka H, Maruyama K, Nishimura T, Hori M, Hatazawa J. Myocardial positron emission computed tomographic images obtained with fluorine-18 fluoro-2-deoxyglucose predict the response of idiopathic dilated cardiomyopathy patients to beta-blockers. *J Am Coll Cardiol.* 2004;43:224–233.

107. Kannel WB, Hjortland M, Castelli WP. Role of diabetes in congestive heart failure: the Framingham study. *Am J Cardiol.* 1974;34:29–34.

108. Rubler S, Dlugash J, Yuceoglu YZ, Kumral T, Branwood AW, Grishman A. New type of cardiomyopathy associated with diabetic glomerulosclerosis. *Am J Cardiol.* 1972;30: 595–602.
109. Rodrigues B, Cam MC, McNeill JH. Myocardial substrate metabolism: implications for diabetic cardiomyopathy. *J Mol Cell Cardiol.* 1995;27:169–179.
110. Stanley WC, Lopaschuck GD, McCormack JG. Regulation of energy substrate metabolism in the diabetic heart. *Cardiovasc Res.* 1997;34:25–33.
111. Avogaro A, Nosadini R, Doria A, et al. Myocardial metabolism in insulin-deficient diabetic humans without coronary artery disease. *Am J Physiol.* 1990;258:E606–E618.
112. Kerbey AL, Vary TC, Randle PJ. Molecular mechanisms regulating myocardial glucose oxidation. *Basic Res Cardiol.* 1985;80:93–96.
113. Randle PJ, Priestman DA, Mistry S, Halsall A. Mechanisms modifying glucose oxidation in diabetes mellitus. *Diabetologia.* 1994;37:S155–S161.
114. Huisamen B, van Zyl M, Keyser A, Lochner A. The effects of insulin and beta-adrenergic stimulation on glucose transport, glut 4 and PKB activation in the myocardium of lean and obese noninsulin dependent diabetes mellitus rats *Mol Cell Biochem.* 2001;223: 15–25.
115. Razeghi P, Young ME, Cockrill TC, Frazier OH, Taegtmeyer H. Downregulation of myocardial myocyte enhancer factor 2C and myocyte enhancer factor 2C-regulated gene expression in diabetic patients with nonischemic heart failure *Circulation.* 2002;106: 407–411.
116. Ungar I, Gilbert M, Siegel A, et al. Studies on myocardial metabolism IV myocardial metabolism in diabetes. *Am J Med.* 1955;18:385–396.
117. Randle P, Sugden P, Kerbey A, et al. Regulation of pyruvate oxidation and the conservation of glucose. *Biochem Soc Symp.* 1978;43:47–67.
118. Wu P, Inskeep K, Bowker-Kinley M, et al. Mechanism responsible for inactivation of skeletal muscle pyruvate dehydrogenase complex in starvation and diabetes. *Diabetes.* 1999;48:1593–1599.
119. Chen V, Ianuzzo C, Fong B, et al. The effects of acute and chronic diabetes on myocardial metabolism in rats. *Diabetes.* 1984;33:1078–1084.
120. Stroedter D, Schmidt T, Bretzel R, et al. Glucose metabolism and left ventricular dysfunction are normalized by insulin and islet transplantation in mild diabetes in the rat. *Acta Diabetol.* 1995;32:235–243.
121. Giffin M, Arthur G, Choy PC, Man RYK. Lysophosphatidyl choline metabolism and cardiac arrhythmias. *Can J Physiol.* 1988;66:185–189.
122. Sparagna GC, Hickson-Bick DL. Cardiac fatty acid metabolism and the induction of apoptosis. *Am J Med Sci.* 1999;318:15–23.
123. Vatner SF, Hittinger L. Coronary vascular mechanisms involved in decompensation from hypertrophy to heart failure. *J Am Coll Cardiol.* 1993;22:34A-40A.
124. Finck BN, Lehman JJ, Leone TC, et al. The cardiac phenotype induced by PPARα overexpression mimics that caused by diabetes mellitus. *J Clin Invest.* 2002;109:121–130.
125. Herrero P, Cassady D, Kisrieva-Ware Z, Srinivasan M, McGill J, Gropler RJ. Myocardial fatty acid oxidation is increased in patients with insulin dependent diabetes mellitus. *J Nucl Med.* 2002;43:510.
126. Herrero P, Srinivasan M, Cassady DS, Kisrieva-Ware Z, McGill J, Gropler RJ. Impact of increased lipid delivery on myocardial fatty acid oxidation in type 1 diabetics. *Circulation.* 2002;106:II-478.
127. Nuutila P, Knuuti J, Ruotsalainen U, et al. Insulin resistance is localized to skeletal but not heart muscle in type 1 diabetes. *Am J Physiol.* 1993;258:E756–E762.
128. vom Dahl J, Herman WH, Hicks RJ, et al. Myocardial glucose uptake in patients with insulin-dependent diabetes mellitus assessed quantitatively by dynamic positron emission tomography. *Circulation.* 1993;88:395–404.
129. Iozzo P, Chareonthaitawee P, Dutka D, Betteridge DJ, Ferrannini E, Camici PG. Independent association of type 2 diabetes and coronary artery disease with myocardial insulin resistance. *Diabetes.* 2002;51:3020–3024.
130. Monti LD, Landoni C, Setola E, et al. Myocardial insulin resistance associated with chronic hypertriglyceridemia and increased FFA levels in Type 2 diabetic patients. *Am J Physiol Heart Circ Physiol.* 2004;287:H1225–H1231.

131. Hallsten K, Virtanen KA, Lonnqvist F, et al. Enhancement of insulin-stimulated myocardial glucose uptake in patients with Type 2 diabetes treated with rosiglitazone. *Diabet Med.* 2004;21:1280–1287.
132. Zhou YT, Grayburn P, Karim A, et al. Lipotoxic heart disease in obese rats: implications for human obesity. *Proc Natl Acad Sci U S A.* 2000;97:1784.
133. Berk PD, Zhou SL, Kiang CL, et al. Uptake of long chain free fatty acids is selectively up-regulated in adipocytes of Zucker rats with genetic obesity and noninsulin-dependent diabetes mellitus. *J Biol Chem.* 1997;272;8830.
134. Luiken JJ, Arumugam Y, Dyck DJ, et al. Increased rates of fatty acid uptake and plasmalemmal fatty acid transporters in obese Zucker rats. *J Biol Chem.* 2001;276:40567.
135. Commerford SR, Pagliassotti MJ, Melby CL, et al. Fat oxidation, lipolysis, and free fatty acid cycling in obesity-prone and obesity-resistant rats. *Am J Physiol.* 2000;279:E875.
136. Peterson LR, Herrero P, Schechtman KB, et al. Effect of obesity and insulin resistance on myocardial substrate metabolism and efficiency in young women. *Circulation.* 2004;109:2191–2196.
137. Lee L, Horowitz J, Frenneaux M. Metabolic manipulation in ischemic heart disease, a novel approach to treatment. *Eur Heart J.* 2004;25:634–641.
138. Mody FV, Singh BN, Mohiuddin IH, et al. Trimetazidine-induced enhancement of myocardial glucose utilization in normal and ischemic myocardial tissue: an evaluation by positron emission tomography. *Am J Cardiol.* 1998;82:42K–49K.
139. Delbeke D, Lorenz CH, Votaw JR, et al. Estimation of left ventricular mass and infarct size from nitrogen-13-ammonia PET images based on pathological examination of explanted human hearts. *J Nucl Med.* 1993;34:826–833.
140. Geltman EM, Biello D, Welch MJ, Ter-Pogossian MM, Roberts R, Sobel BE. Characterization of nontransmural myocardial infarction by positron emission tomography. *Circulation.* 1982;65:747–755.
141. Bing RJ. The metabolism of the heart. *Harvey Lect.* 1955;50:27–70.
142. Neely JR, Morgan HE. Relationship between carbohydrate metabolism and energy balance of heart muscle. *Ann Rev Physiol.* 1974;36:413–459.
143. Desvergne B, Wahli W. Peroxisome proliferator-activated receptors: Nuclear control of metabolism. *Endocr Rev.* 1999;20:649–688.
144. Vanoverschelde JL, Melin JA, Bol A, et al. Regional oxidative metabolism in patients after recovery from reperfused anterior myocardial infarction. Relation to regional blood flow and glucose uptake. *Circulation.* 1992;85:9–21.
145. Weiss ES, Ahmed SA, Welch MJ, Williamson JR, Ter-Pogossian MM, Sobel BE. Quantification of infarction in cross sections of canine myocardium in vivo with positron emission transaxial tomography and ^{11}C-palmitate. *Circulation.* 1977;55:66–73.
146. Walsh MN, Geltman EM, Brown MA, et al. Noninvasive estimation of regional myocardial oxygen consumption by positron emission tomography with carbon-11 acetate in patients with myocardial infarction. *J Nucl Med.* 1989;30:1798–1808.
147. Henes CG, Bergmann SR, Perez JE, Sobel BE, Geltman EM. The time course of restoration of nutritive perfusion, myocardial oxygen consumption, and regional function after coronary thrombolysis. *Coron Artery Dis.* 1989;1:687–696.
148. Knabb RM, Bergmann SR, Fox KA, Sobel BE. The temporal pattern of recovery of myocardial perfusion and metabolism delineated by positron emission tomography after coronary thrombolysis. *J Nucl Med.* 1987;28:1563–1570.
149. Gropler RJ, Siegel BA, Sampathkumaran K, et al. Dependence of recovery of contractile function on maintenance of oxidative metabolism after myocardial infarction. *J Am Coll Cardiol.* 1992;19:989–997.

18 Myocardial Viability Assessment with PET and PET/CT

Marcelo F. Di Carli

Left ventricular (LV) function is a well-established and powerful predictor of outcome after myocardial infarction (MI).[1] Indeed, the occurrence of severe LV systolic dysfunction (i.e., LV ejection fraction <35%) post-MI, especially when combined with heart failure, is associated with very poor survival if treated with medical therapy alone.[2] In selected patients, high-risk surgical revascularization appears to afford long-term survival benefit.[3] However, selection of patients with severe LV dysfunction for high-risk revascularization remains controversial.

In some patients with coronary artery disease (CAD), LV dysfunction results from myocardial infarction with attendant necrosis and scar formation. However, it is now clear that in many patients, such myocardial dysfunction may be reversible with revascularization; this condition is otherwise referred to as hibernating[4] and/or stunned[5] myocardium. Consequently, the distinction of LV dysfunction caused by fibrosis from that arising from viable but dysfunctional myocardium is a diagnostic issue with important implications for patients with low ejection fraction. In these patients, severe heart failure may be attributed to severe, widespread hibernation or stunning (or both) rather than to necrosis of a critical mass of myocardium.[6] Failure to identify patients with these potentially reversible causes of heart failure may lead to progressive cellular damage, heart failure, and death.

Pathophysiology of Ischemic LV Dysfunction

For many years, the presence of chronic LV dysfunction occurring at rest in patients with CAD was thought to represent myocardial infarction and, thus, irreversible damage. However, it is now clear that myocardium that has been subjected to acute or chronic ischemia may remain viable and demonstrate prolonged alterations in regional and global LV function that can be improved with revascularization. Such reversible contractile dysfunction may be caused by myocardial stunning[5] or hibernation.[4]

Myocardial stunning is a reversible state of regional contractile dysfunction that can occur after restoration of coronary blood flow following a brief episode of ischemia despite the absence of necrosis.[5] Stunned myocardium has been described in animals[7] and subsequently documented in humans,[8] where it is considered to play a role in the prolonged contractile dysfunction seen in patients undergoing reperfusion therapy for acute myocardial infarction, following attacks of unstable angina, and in some patients with exercise-induced ischemia.[8] Although commonly regarded as an acute phenomenon, stunned myocardium may also occur in patients with chronic coronary stenoses who experience recurrent episodes of ischemia (symptomatic or asymptomatic) in the same territory.[8] The latter mechanism is probably the most common form of stunning in patients with chronic LV dysfunction due to CAD. Myocardial stunning is considered a form of reperfusion injury, whereby reintroduction of oxygen after a period of ischemia induces a transient calcium overload that damages the contractile apparatus.[9] The postischemic contractile abnormality is fully reversible provided that recurrent ischemia (followed by stunning) does not occur and sufficient time is allowed for the myocardium to recover.

Myocardial hibernation refers to a state of persistent LV dysfunction associated with chronically reduced blood flow but preserved viability.[4] This chronic downregulation in contractile function at rest is thought to represent a protective mechanism whereby the heart reduces its oxygen requirements to ensure myocyte survival. However, this protective mechanism can result in a considerable amount of myocardium that is rendered hypocontractile, and, thus, it may contribute to overall LV dysfunction.[10]

There is considerable controversy regarding the mechanisms that lead to these states of altered systolic function. In the new paradigm, stunning and hibernation represent a continuum (Figure 18.1).[11] Initially, the presence of a flow-limiting coronary artery stenosis leads to a reduction in coronary vasodilator reserve with preserved resting coronary blood flow. The reduced flow reserve in turn results in episodes of ischemia during periods of increased oxygen demand. Ultimately, these transient, recurrent episodes of ischemia lead to a state of persistent LV dysfunction (so-called repetitive stunning). As the severity of coronary stenosis increases, coronary vasodilator reserve becomes critically reduced and resting coronary blood flow eventually falls. The presence of resting hypoperfusion marks the transition from repetitive stunning to hibernation.[11] The varying degree of flow deficit underlying these two conditions likely explains the distinct morphological changes present in stunned[12] and hibernating[13,14] myocytes. This precarious balance between perfusion and viability in hibernating myocardium cannot be maintained indefinitely, and myocardial necrosis ultimately occurs if blood flow is not restored.

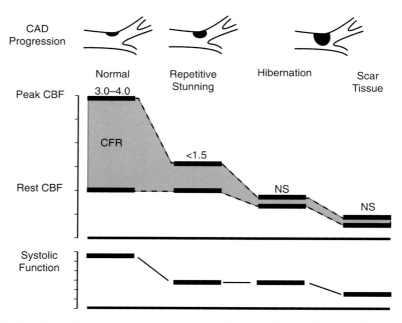

FIGURE 18.1. Schematic of the changes in myocardial perfusion leading to LV dysfunction in patients with CAD. (Courtesy of Dr. Heinrich R. Schelbert, UCLA School of Medicine.)

Methods for Assessing Myocardial Viability with PET

18F-Fluorodeoxyglucose

The physiologic basis and rationale for the use of fluorine-18 fluorodeoxyglucose (^{18}F-FDG) to assess myocardial glucose metabolism as an index of tissue viability were discussed in detail in Chapter 17.

Imaging Protocols

Because dysfunctional myocardium that improves functionally after revascularization must retain sufficient blood flow and metabolic activity to sustain myocyte viability, the combined assessment of regional myocardial perfusion and glucose metabolism appears most attractive for delineating myocardial viability (Figure 18.2). With this approach, regional myocardial perfusion is first evaluated. Since information regarding the magnitude of stress-induced ischemia and information regarding resting viability are both important for management decisions, the ideal approach should include both rest and stress perfusion imaging. However, the selection of the approach (i.e., rest vs stress/rest) should be tailored to the clinical question being addressed in an individual patient.

Regional glucose uptake is then assessed with FDG (a marker of exogenous glucose uptake), providing an index of myocardial metabolism and, thus, cell viability. After intravenous administration, FDG traces the initial transport of glucose across the myocyte membrane and its subsequent hexokinase-mediated phosphorylation to FDG-6-phosphate.[15] Since the latter is a poor substrate for further metabolism and is rather impermeable to the cell membrane, it becomes virtually trapped in the myocardium.

Patient Preparation for FDG Imaging

As mentioned above, utilization of energy-producing substrates by the heart muscle is largely a function of their concentration in plasma and hormone levels (especially

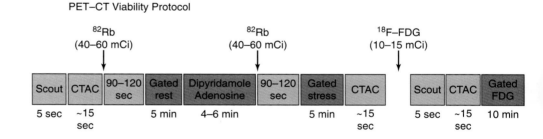

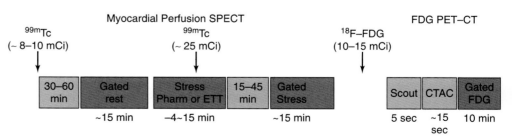

FIGURE 18.2. Myocardial viability protocols using PET/CT and the hybrid SPECT/PET/CT approach.

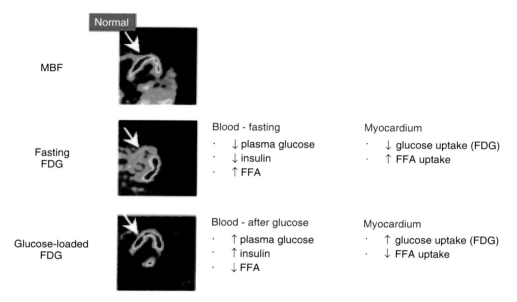

FIGURE 18.3. Changes in FDG uptake in normal myocardium in the fasting and glucose-loaded states. Under fasting conditions, FDG uptake in normal myocardium (arrow) is decreased due to the relatively low glucose and insulin levels and high free fatty acid levels. After glucose loading, the relative increase in plasma glucose stimulates the release of endogenous insulin, which in turn decreases the plasma levels of free fatty acids and facilitates the transport and utilization of FDG by the normal myocytes. The overestimation of the magnitude of viability in the lateral wall in the fasting state due to the lack of tracer uptake in normal (reference) myocardium compared to the glucose-loaded state is noteworthy.

plasma insulin, insulin/glucagon ratio, growth hormone, and catecholamines) and of oxygen availability for oxidative metabolism. For a detailed step-by-step description of the available methods for FDG imaging, the reader should review the guidelines for PET imaging published by the American Society of Nuclear Cardiology and the Society of Nuclear Medicine.[16]

These approaches for FDG imaging include:

- *Fasting:* Fasting is the simplest method because it does not require any substrate manipulation. With this approach, ischemic but viable tissue shows as a hot spot due to the preferential free fatty acid (FFA) utilization by normal (nonischemic) myocardium. While imaging interpretation would seem straightforward, the lack of tracer uptake in normal (reference) myocardium may occasionally lead to an overestimation of the amount of residual viability within a dysfunctional territory (Figure 18.3). Indeed, the predictive accuracy of this approach is lower[17] than that of the glucose-loaded approach.[18]

- *Oral or intravenous glucose loading:* Glucose loading is the most commonly used approach to FDG imaging (Figure 18.4). The goal of glucose loading is to stimulate the release of endogenous insulin to decrease the plasma levels of FFA and to facilitate the transport and utilization of FDG. Patients are usually fasted for at least 6 hours and then receive an oral or intravenous glucose load. Most patients require the administration of intravenous (IV) insulin to maximize myocardial FDG uptake. With this approach, image quality is generally of diagnostic quality and the reported diagnostic accuracy very good.[18]

- *Hyperinsulinemic-euglycemic clamp:* The hyperinsulinemic-euglycemic clamp approach is technically demanding and time-consuming (Figure 18.4). However, it provides the highest and most consistent image quality.[19] Based on the reported predictive accuracies, however, this does not necessarily translate into improved

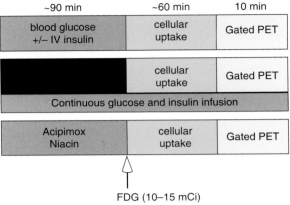

FIGURE 18.4. Timeline of protocols for patient preparation before FDG imaging.

predictions of functional outcome.[20] Because it is technically demanding, most laboratories reserve this approach for challenging conditions (e.g., diabetes and severe congestive heart failure).

- *Free fatty acid inhibition:* Acipimox and niacin are both nicotinic acid derivatives that inhibit peripheral lipolysis, thereby reducing plasma FFA levels and, indirectly, forcing a switch to preferential myocardial glucose utilization. These drugs are usually given 60 to 90 minutes prior to FDG administration (Figure 18.4). The approach is practical and provides consistent image quality.[19,21] However, Acipimox is not available for clinical use in the United States.

Myocardial Perfusion and Glucose-loaded FDG Patterns

Using the sequential perfusion-FDG approach, 4 distinct perfusion-metabolism patterns can be observed in dysfunctional myocardium:

1. Normal perfusion associated with normal FDG uptake
2. Reduced perfusion associated with preserved or enhanced FDG uptake (so-called perfusion-metabolism mismatch), which reflects myocardial viability (Figure 18.5)
3. Proportional reduction in perfusion and FDG uptake (so-called perfusion-metabolism match), which reflects nonviable myocardium (Figure 18.5)
4. Normal or near-normal perfusion with reduced FDG uptake (so-called reversed perfusion-metabolism mismatch) (Figures 18.5 and 18.6)[22,23]

The patterns of normal perfusion and metabolism or of a PET mismatch identify potentially reversible myocardial dysfunction; the PET match pattern identifies irreversible myocardial dysfunction. The reversed perfusion-FDG mismatch has been described in the context of repetitive myocardial stunning[22] and in patients with left bundle branch block.[23] Quantitation of regional myocardial perfusion and FDG tracer uptake and their difference can be helpful to objectively assess the magnitude of viability (Figure 18.7).

Special Considerations for the Hybrid Myocardial Perfusion SPECT and FDG PET Approach

In current clinical practice, FDG PET images are often performed and interpreted in combination with SPECT myocardial perfusion images (Figure 18.2). The interpretation of the specific viability patterns shown in Figures 18.5 and 18.6 should be performed carefully, especially when comparing nonattenuation-corrected SPECT

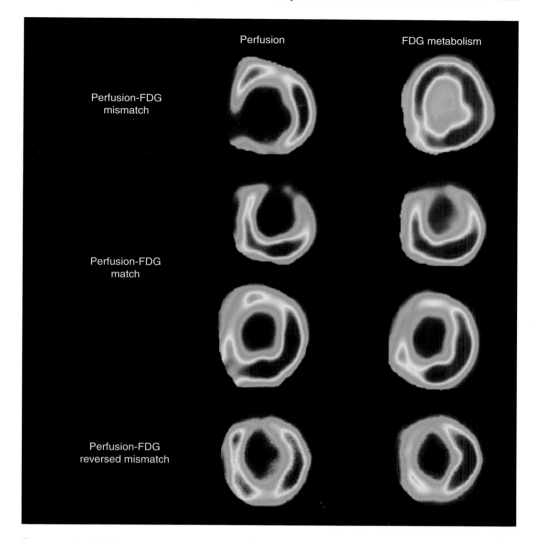

Perfusion   FDG metabolism

Perfusion-FDG
mismatch

Perfusion-FDG
match

Perfusion-FDG
reversed mismatch

FIGURE 18.5. Midventricular short axis slices of myocardial perfusion (obtained with ^{13}N-ammonia) and FDG uptake illustrating tissue viability patterns following glucose loading. (Reprinted from Di Carli M. Advances in positron emission tomography. J Nucl Cardiol, 11:719–32, Copyright 2004, with permission from The American Society of Nuclear Cardiology.)

myocardial perfusion images with attenuation-corrected FDG PET images. Myocardial regions showing an excessive reduction in tracer concentration due to attenuation artifacts on the perfusion images, such as the inferior wall or the anterior wall in females, may result in falsely positive perfusion-FDG mismatches. Two approaches have proved useful for overcoming this limitation. First, because assessment of viability is relevant only in myocardium with regional contractile dysfunction, gated SPECT or gated PET images offer a means for determining whether apparent perfusion defects are associated with abnormal regional wall motion. Second, quantitative analysis of regional myocardial perfusion using polar map displays that are compared to tracer- and (for SPECT images) gender-specific databases may be a useful aid to the visual interpretation.

Gated Imaging to Assess LV Volumes and Function

FDG PET provides excellent gated images (Figure 18.8), and the parameters of global and regional LV function derived from these images correlate closely with those obtained with magnetic resonance imaging (MRI).[24] As mentioned above,

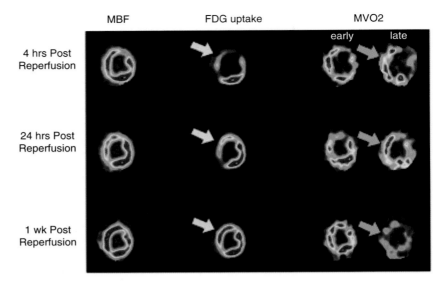

FIGURE 18.6. PET images of a dog heart in short-axis views obtained at corresponding mid-ventricular levels obtained postreperfusion after four 5-minute LAD coronary occlusions, each followed by 5 minutes of reperfusion. Images of blood flow (left column) were obtained with ^{13}N-ammonia and images of glucose metabolism (middle column) with FDG. Images of oxidative metabolism (reflecting regional myocardial oxygen consumption [MVO$_2$]; right column) were obtained with ^{11}C-acetate; the early phase denotes delivery of the tracer to the myocardium while the late phase represents regional washout of the tracer through the tricarboxylic acid cycle (myocardial oxidation). The top panel depicts corresponding midventricular short-axis sections of regional blood flow, glucose, and MVO$_2$ 4 hours postreperfusion. The flow images (left) demonstrate near-normal perfusion in the stunned regions (i.e., anterior and anteroseptum). However, stunned regions demonstrated reduced FDG utilization (arrow) and slow clearance of ^{11}C-acetate (impaired oxidation) relative to normal myocardium (lateral wall). The middle panel illustrates 1 day postreperfusion. Myocardial perfusion in stunned myocardium is near normal, glucose uptake (arrow) remains depressed, and the MVO$_2$ is still lower (arrow) than in normal myocardium. The bottom panel illustrates 1 week after reperfusion. Blood flow, glucose uptake, and MVO$_2$ are largely homogenous. Wall motion and metabolism demonstrated a parallel recovery with time. (Reprinted by permission of the Society of Nuclear Medicine from: MF Di Carli, P Prcevski, TP Singh, J Janisse, J Ager, O Muzik, and R Vander Heide. Myocardial blood flow, function, and metabolism in repetitive stunning. J Nucl Med. 2000;41:1227–1234. Figure 6.)

gated images are particularly useful when FDG PET patterns are interpreted in relation to nonattenuation-corrected SPECT perfusion images. In addition, measures of global LV function and remodeling (i.e., left ventricular ejection fraction [LVEF] and volumes) are also useful for predicting improvement in LV function after revascularization.[25] Indeed, increased LV volumes and cavity size are predictors of poor outcome in patients with ischemic cardiomyopathy who are undergoing coronary artery bypass graft (CABG). For example, a preoperative LV end-diastolic dimension ≥70 mm as assessed by echocardiography has been shown to be a marker of poor outcome after revascularization.[26] Similarly, others have shown that a preoperative LV end-systolic volume index (LVESVI) > 100 mL/m^2, as assessed by contrast left ventriculography, was a predictor of mortality and postoperative heart failure.[27] Patients with LVESVI > 100 mL/m^2 failed to improve regional and global LV function after CABG, resulting in lower survival and a higher probability of postoperative heart failure. Significantly, these poor results in patients with severe LV dilation were observed even in the patients with severe anginal symptoms, suggesting that progressive LV remodeling after myocardial infarction may limit the benefits of revascularization on ventricular function and survival even if there is evidence of viable (ischemic) myocardium.

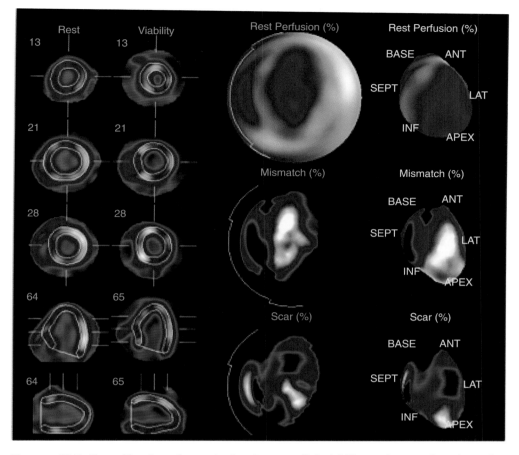

FIGURE 18.7. Quantification of magnitude of myocardial viability and scar using circumferential profile analysis.

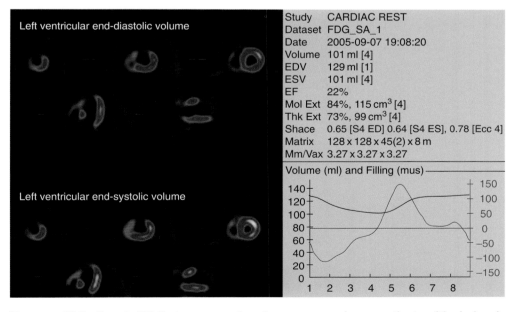

FIGURE 18.8. Gated FDG images and volume curves in a patient with ischemic cardiomyopathy.

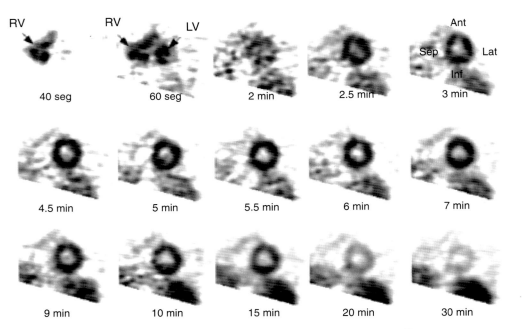

FIGURE 18.9. Serial mid-short-axis images following the administration of ^{11}C-acetate. Images were acquired for 30 minutes, starting at the time of ^{11}C-acetate injection. The first image demonstrates the first pass of the radioactive bolus through the right (RV) and left ventricular (LV) chambers. The subsequent images show the clearance of ^{11}C-acetate from the blood pool, followed by the uptake of the radiotracer in the myocardium and, finally, the washout of ^{11}C-acetate over time.

Carbon-11 Acetate

Physiologic Basis

The physiologic basis and rationale for the use of carbon-11 acetate (^{11}C-acetate) to assess myocardial oxidative metabolism as an index of tissue viability were discussed in detail in Chapter 17.

Imaging and Quantification of Myocardial Oxidative Metabolism

Serial imaging following the IV administration of ^{11}C-acetate demonstrates the passage of the radioactive bolus through the cardiac chambers, followed by the extraction and accumulation of the radiotracer in the myocardium and its clearance from the blood pool, and, finally, the clearance of the radiotracer from the myocardial tissue, reflecting the rate of oxidative metabolism (Figure 18.9). After an IV injection, ^{11}C-acetate is rapidly extracted from the circulation and enters the myocyte via facilitated transport. The first-pass extraction fraction is inversely related to coronary blood flow, with an average extraction of 63% under baseline conditions. The initial part (2 to 5 minutes) of the myocardial ^{11}C-acetate kinetics reflects tracer that has been delivered but not yet metabolized (oxidation), thereby representing regional myocardial perfusion.[28,29] Once in the myocyte, it is activated to ^{11}C-acetyl-CoA in the mitochondria, where it enters the tricarboxylic acid cycle (TCA) cycle and the oxidative phosphorylation and is converted into $^{11}CO_2$ and water.

The ^{11}C-acetate time-activity curve demonstrates a biexponential clearance from the myocardium, reflecting at least 2 metabolic compartments of different size and turnover rate. The rapid washout phase (expressed as k_{mono}) is linearly related to myocardial oxygen consumption; the slow phase appears to reflect the incorporation of ^{11}C-acetate into the lipid pool. The rapid tissue clearance rate (k_{mono}) is determined by monoexponential least-squares fitting of the initial portion of the time-activity curve. k_{mono} values are then compared to reference normal values and used to determine the amount of residual viability within a dysfunctional myocardial segment. The uptake and clearance of ^{11}C-acetate are affected by changes in regional blood flow and metabolism. For example, during ischemia there is a reduction in the initial uptake and the rapid clearance phase of ^{11}C-acetate that is proportional to the reduction in regional blood flow and oxidative metabolism.

Using PET for Predicting Functional Recovery

Myocardial Perfusion

Since timely restoration of nutritive perfusion to ischemic myocardium is crucial for cell survival, estimates of regional perfusion have been used for predicting functional recovery of dysfunctional myocardium. The experience using PET tracers of blood flow, including oxygen-15 water (^{15}O-water), ^{11}C-acetate, and nitrogen-13 ammonia (^{13}N-ammonia), for predicting recovery of function has been documented in 6 studies including 182 patients with LV dysfunction (Table 18.1).[30] Contractile dysfunction was predicted to be reversible after revascularization when regional blood flow was only mild or moderately reduced (>50% of normal) and irreversible when regional blood flow was severely reduced (<50% of normal). Using these criteria, the average positive predictive accuracy of blood flow estimates for predicting functional recovery after revascularization is 63% (range, 45% to 78%), whereas the average negative predictive accuracy is 63% (range, 45% to 100%). While normal or near-normal blood flow in a dysfunctional region served by a stenosed coronary artery indicates tissue viability and suggests that function can be improved with revascularization, a severe blood flow deficit generally (although not always) reflects mostly nonviable myocardium that is unlikely to show improved function with revascularization. However, blood flow deficits of intermediate severity are more difficult to interpret. They may represent the coexistence of extensive subendocardial necrosis with normal myocardium, a condition unlikely to show improved function with revascularization. Alternatively, they may reflect the coexistence of extensive areas of ischemic but viable with normal tissue, scar tissue, or both, a condition likely to show improved function with revascularization. In this situation, FDG imaging adds significant independent information for distinguishing reversible from irreversible myocardial dysfunction.[37] Patients with low ejection fraction and relatively normal perfusion at rest should undergo stress

TABLE 18.1. Predictive Values for Segmental Functional Recovery after Revascularization Using Estimates of Regional Myocardial Perfusion with PET

Author	N	LVEF %	Criteria for Viability	PPV % (Segs)	NPV % (Segs)	Diagnostic Accuracy
Gropler et al[31]	34	NR	ACE ± 2 SD	45 (34/75)	68 (28/41)	53 (62/116)
Maes et al[32]	20	48 ± 9	NH$_3$ > 50%	53 (10/19)	100 (1/1)	55 (11/20)
Grandin et al[33]	25	49 ± 11	NH$_3$ > 50%	78 (14/18)	57 (4/7)	72 (18/25)
Tamaki et al[34]	43	41	NH$_3$ > 50%	48 (47/98)	87 (28/32)	58 (75/130)
Wolpers et al[35]*	30	42 ± 11	MBF > 50%	78	85	—
Marinho et al[36]	30	35 ± 11	MBF ± 2 SD	55 (53/96)	45 (5/11)	54 (58/107)
Mean ± SD	182			63 ± 14	63 ± 28	58 ± 8

Abbreviations: N, number of patients; NR, not reported; LVEF, left ventricular ejection fraction; PPV, positive predictive value; NPV, negative predictive value; Segs, segments; ACE, ^{11}C-acetate; NH$_3$, ^{13}N-ammonia; MBF, myocardial blood flow (mL/min/g).
*Segmental data not reported.

imaging to determine whether reversible ischemia (followed by stunning) is the likely cause of LV dysfunction.

Measures of Myocardial Oxidative Metabolism

The experience with ^{11}C-acetate and PET for identifying viability and predicting functional recovery after revascularization has been documented in 5 studies, of which only 3 studies including 83 patients provided sufficient data to estimate predictive accuracies for regional functional recovery (Table 18.2). Of note, most of these studies come from the same institution,[38–40] indicating that assessment of myocardial viability using ^{11}C-acetate has had less widespread validation than the FDG PET approach. Relatively preserved quantitative measures of oxidative metabolism (based on k_{mono} values) in dysfunctional myocardial regions were predictive of improved function after revascularization, while severely decreased oxidative metabolism was predictive of irreversible damage. Using these criteria, the average positive predictive accuracy for predicting improved segmental function after revascularization is 72% (range, 62% to 88%), whereas the average negative predictive accuracy is 76% (range, 65% to 89%) (Table 18.2). Similar to regional perfusion measures, estimates of MVO_2 (which are closely coupled with myocardial perfusion) accurately predict functional outcome when they are either normal or severely decreased. In individual patients, intermediate reductions in estimates of MVO_2 are more difficult to interpret because they could represent nontransmural scar or hibernating myocardium. To overcome this limitation, it has been suggested that the magnitude of improvement (from baseline) in estimates for MVO_2 during low-dose dobutamine stimulation (a measure of myocardial "oxidative reserve") may be a more accurate predictor of functional recovery than PET measurements of MVO_2 performed at rest.[41] In 28 patients with chronic myocardial infarction and mild to moderate LV dysfunction, Hata et al demonstrated excellent discrimination (with virtually no overlap) between viable and nonviable myocardium using estimates of MVO_2 in response to low-dose dobutamine stimulation, assessed by ^{11}C-acetate and PET.[41]

Combined Myocardial Perfusion and FDG

The experience with the combined myocardial perfusion-FDG approach using PET or the PET/SPECT hybrid technique (SPECT perfusion with PET FDG imaging) has been documented in 17 studies including 462 patients (Table 18.3).[30] Contractile dysfunction was predicted to be reversible after revascularization in regions with increased FDG uptake or a perfusion-metabolism mismatch (Part VI, Case 9) and irreversible

TABLE 18.2. Predictive Values for Segmental Functional Recovery after Revascularization Using Estimates of Regional Myocardial MVO_2 with ^{11}C-Acetate and PET

Author	N	LVEF %	Criteria for Viability	PPV % (Segs)	NPV % (Segs)	Diagnostic Accuracy
Gropler et al[31]	34	NR	Mean $MVO_2 \pm 2$ SD	67 (40/60)	89 (50/56)	78 (90/116)
Rubin et al[40]	19	NR	Mean $MVO_2 \pm 2$ SD	88 (28/32)	73 (16/22)	81 (44/54)
Wolpers et al[35]*	30	42 ± 11	$MVO_2 > 0.09$/min	62	65	—
Mean ± SD	83			72 ± 14	76 ± 12	

Abbreviations: N, number of patients; NR, not reported; LVEF, left ventricular ejection fraction; PPV, positive predictive value; NPV, negative predictive value; Segs, segments.
*Segmental data not reported.

TABLE 18.3. Predictive Values for Segmental Functional Recovery after Revascularization Using Combined Estimates of Myocardial Perfusion and FDG Metabolism with PET

Author	N	LVEF %	Criteria for Viability	PPV % (Segs)	NPV % (Segs)	Diagnostic Accuracy
Tillisch et al[42]	17	32 ± 14	Mismatch	85 (35/41)	92 (24/26)	88 (59/67)
Tamaki et al[17]	22	NR	Mismatch	78 (18/23)	78 (18/23)	78 (36/46)
Tamaki et al[43]	11	NR	Mismatch	80 (40/50)	100 (0/6)	82 (46/56)
Carrel et al[44]	23	34	Mismatch	84 (16/19)	75 (3/4)	83 (19/23)
Lucignani et al[45]	14	38 ± 5	Mismatch	95 (37/39)	80 (12/15)	91 (49/54)
Gropler et al[38]	16	NR	Mismatch	79 (19/24)	83 (24/29)	81 (43/53)
Marwick et al[46]	16	NR	FDG > 2 SD	67 (25/37)	79 (38/48)	74 (63/85)
Gropler et al[31]	34	NR	FDG > 2 SD	52 (38/73)	81 (35/43)	63 (73/116)
Vanoverschelde et al[12]	12	55 ± 7	Mismatch	100 (12/12)	—	100 (12/12)
vom Dahl et al[47]	37	34 ± 10	Mismatch	53 (29/55)	86 (90/105)	74 (119/160)
Knuuti et al[48]	48	53 ± 11	FDG > 85%	70 (23/33)	93 (53/57)	84 (76/90)
Maes et al[32]	20	48 ± 9	Mismatch	75 (9/12)	75 (6/8)	75 (15/20)
Grandin et al[33]	25	49 ± 11	Mismatch	79 (15/19)	67 (4/6)	76 (19/25)
Tamaki et al[34]	43	41	FDG UI	76 (45/59)	91 (65/71)	85 (110/130)
Baer et al[49]	42	40 ± 13	FDG > 50%	72 (167/232)	91 (126/139)	79 (293/371)
vom Dahl et al[50]	52	47 ± 10	Mismatch	68 (19/28)	96 (25/26)	81 (44/54)
Wolpers et al[35]*	30	42 ± 11	FDG > 50%	78	85	—
Mean ± SD	462			76 ± 12	82 ± 14	79 ± 10

Abbreviations: N, number of patients; NR, not reported; LVEF, left ventricular ejection fraction; PPV, positive predictive value; NPV, negative predictive value; Segs, segments; UI, uptake index.
*Segmental data not reported.

in regions with reduced FDG uptake or a perfusion-metabolism match pattern (Part VI, Case 8). Using these criteria, the average positive predictive accuracy for predicting improved segmental function after revascularization is 76% (range, 52% to 100%), whereas the average negative predictive accuracy is 82% (range, 67% to 100%).

Using Viability Information in Patient Management

Predicting Improvement in LV Function

An important question in patients with severely depressed LV function is whether revascularization will provide a clinically meaningful improvement in global cardiac function that may translate into improved exercise capacity, symptoms, and survival. Several studies using different PET approaches have shown that the gain in global left ventricular systolic function after revascularization is related to the magnitude of viable myocardium assessed preoperatively (Table 18.4).[30]

These data demonstrate that clinically meaningful changes in global LV function can be expected after revascularization only in patients with relatively large areas of hibernating myocardium, stunned myocardium, or both (≥17% of the left ventricular mass). Similar results have been reported using estimates of myocardial scar with PET.[52] These results are in agreement with those obtained with SPECT,[53] dobutamine echocardiography,[54] and contrast-enhanced MRI.[55]

Applicability of Viability Data to Predictions of Functional Outcome

The goal of viability assessment in the setting of severe LV dysfunction post-MI is to identify patients in whom revascularization can potentially improve LV function, symptoms, and survival. Then viability assessment would be of critical clinical importance in patients with the highest clinical risk post-MI (i.e., LVEF < 30%), who would

TABLE 18.4. Relation Between the Extent of Viability and the Change in LV Ejection Fraction after Revascularization Using Combined Estimates of Myocardial Perfusion and FDG Metabolism with PET

Author	N	Criteria for Viability	Pre-LVEF %	Post-LVEF %
Tillisch et al[42]	17	Mismatch ≥ 25% LV	30 ± 11	45 ± 14
Carrel et al[44]	23	Mismatch ≥ 17% LV	34 ± 14	52 ± 11
Vanoverschelde et al[12]	12	Anterior wall mismatch	55 ± 7	65 ± 8
Maes et al[32]	20	Anterior wall mismatch	51 ± 11	60 ± 10
Grandin et al[33]	25	Mismatch ≥ 20% LV	51 ± 12	63 ± 18
Schwarz et al[13]	24	Anterior wall mismatch	44 ± 12	54 ± 9
Wolpers et al[35]	30	Anterior wall mismatch	39 ± 10	49 ± 17
vom Dahl et al[51]	82	Mismatch ≥1 CAT	46 ± 9	54 ± 11

Abbreviations: N, number of patients; LVEF, left ventricular ejection fraction; CAT, coronary artery territory.

derive the highest potential benefit from revascularization. However, more than 90% of the published data documenting the accuracy of noninvasive methods for diagnosing viability and predicting functional recovery have been obtained in patients with normal LV function or mild or moderate LV dysfunction (i.e., LVEF > 30%).[56] There have been only a limited number of studies with small numbers of patients (representing <10% of the published data) that document the diagnostic accuracy of methods for viability detection among patients with the highest risk.[56] This is important because the accuracy of noninvasive methods for predicting functional recovery after revascularization appears to decrease significantly with worsening LV function (Figure 18.10). Consequently, the direct extrapolation of the excellent results obtained in patients with regional or mild to moderate LV dysfunction to patients with very low ejection fraction is problematic, and it often results in suboptimal clinical results.

This may be related in part to the fact that predictions of functional recovery following revascularization using noninvasive methods have been largely based solely on the extent of viable myocardium before revascularization. The focus on viability information alone seems to ignore the multifactorial influences on improvement in LV function after revascularization.[58] From a clinical standpoint, it is likely that

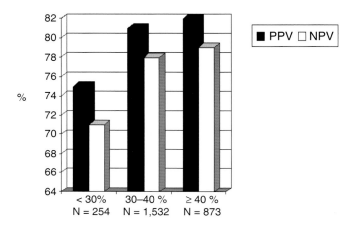

FIGURE 18.10. Accuracy of methods of viability assessment for predicting a change in LV function after revascularization by the level of LV ejection fraction before revascularization. PPV, positive predictive value; NPV, negative predictive value. (Reprinted from Di Carli MF, (57), with permission from The American Society of Nuclear Cardiology.)

relying even on the most accurate of these multiple indexes of tissue viability or its absence in isolation will lead to suboptimal prediction of outcomes.[58] It is now evident that multiple other factors—including the presence and magnitude of stress-induced ischemia, the stage of cellular degeneration within viable myocytes, the degree of LV remodeling, the timing and success of revascularization procedures, the adequacy of the target coronary vessels, and the timing of LV functional assessment after revascularization—can affect functional outcome after revascularization. Indeed, recent evidence suggests that integrating many of these factors that influence functional recovery after revascularization in multivariable models results in improved clinical predictions, as compared to approaches that are based on only a single index of tissue viability.[52] These issues are discussed in further detail in Chapter 21.

Predicting Improvement in Symptoms

An important challenge in the management of patients with poor cardiac function under consideration for bypass surgery is to identify those in whom revascularization can provide a significant alleviation of anginal and, especially, heart failure symptoms, which is often their primary functional limitation. In one study of 23 patients with LV dysfunction (LVEF: 35 ± 14%) and impaired functional capacity (70% in New York Heart Association class II-III), investigators have shown that the amount of viable myocardium before revascularization was predictive of a significant improvement in exercise parameters after revascularization.[60] In this study, peak rate-pressure product, maximal heart rate, and exercise capacity increased significantly after revascularization only in patients with multiple viable regions on preoperative PET imaging. Similarly, others have demonstrated a significant linear correlation between the global extent of a preoperative perfusion-metabolism PET mismatch (reflecting hibernating myocardium) and the percentage improvement in functional capacity after CABG in 36 patients with ischemic cardiomyopathy (LVEF: 28 ± 6%) (Figure 18.11).[6] In this study, a perfusion-metabolic PET mismatch involving ≥18% of the LV on quantitative analysis was associated with a sensitivity of 76% and a specificity of 78% for predicting a significant improvement in heart failure class following bypass surgery.

The notion that preoperative viability imaging may be able to identify patients with a high likelihood of improvement in LV function and heart failure symptoms is of great clinical importance, as it would also prevent costly rehospitalizations for decompensated heart failure. A recent study examined the interactions among the extent of

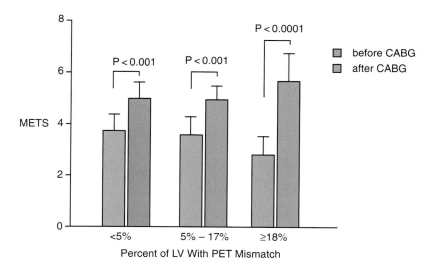

FIGURE 18.11. Relation between the anatomic extent of the perfusion-FDG PET mismatch (% of the LV) and the change in functional capacity (METS) after coronary artery bypass graft (CABG) in patients with severe LV dysfunction. (Based on data from Reference 6.)

preoperative viability, the mode of treatment (i.e., medical therapy vs CABG), and the frequency of hospital readmissions during a mean follow-up of 25 months after the PET scan in 99 patients with severe LV dysfunction (LVEF: 22 ± 6%).[60] This study reported that among patients with relatively large areas of viable myocardium preoperatively, high-risk revascularization provided a significant reduction in hospital readmissions for heart failure as compared to medical therapy alone (3% vs 31%, respectively). In contrast, hospital admissions for heart failure were similarly high regardless of the mode of treatment in patients without significant amounts of viability by PET (50% vs 48% for revascularization and medical therapy, respectively).

Stratifying Risk and Predicting Improvement in Survival

A major goal of viability imaging is to identify patients with low ejection fraction who are at the highest clinical risk, in whom revascularization may offer the greatest survival benefit. Table 18.5 summarizes the results of 5 published reports evaluating the risk of cardiovascular events in patients with viable myocardium treated medically compared to the risk in those without viable myocardium.[30] They included a total of 288 patients with CAD and moderate or severe LV dysfunction. Most of these patients had a history of myocardial infarction and multivessel CAD. In these studies, survival and recurrent clinical events (myocardial infarction, unstable angina, ventricular arrhythmia, and hospital readmissions) were evaluated for an average of 12 to 29 months.

The results of these studies showed that patients with viable myocardium had a consistently higher event rate than those without viable myocardium. The odds ratios were consistently >1 in all reports, suggesting an increased risk of a cardiac event for those subjects with viable myocardium treated medically. These data suggest that the presence of ischemic but viable myocardium as assessed by FDG PET seems to consistently identify patients with LV dysfunction who are at high risk for cardiac events when treated with medical therapy alone.

Figure 18.12 summarizes the results of 5 published reports evaluating the risk of cardiac events in 262 patients with hibernating myocardium treated medically compared with those undergoing revascularization. In all these studies, management decisions (i.e., revascularization or medical therapy) in patients with and without evidence of hibernating myocardium were made on clinical grounds. However, no significant differences in relevant clinical and angiographic variables known to affect

TABLE 18.5. Risk of Cardiac Events for Patients with Moderate-Severe LV Dysfunction and Hibernating Myocardium Compared with Those Without Hibernating Myocardium

Author	Year	Viability Assessment	Patients	LVEF %	FU (months)	OR	Lower 95% CI	Upper 95% CI
Eitzman et al[61]	1992	PET	42	34 ± 13	12	7.00	1.53	32.08
Di Carli et al[62]	1994	PET	50	24 ± 7	13	7.00	1.51	32.33
Lee et al[63]	1994	PET	61	38 ± 16	17	7.66	2.31	25.44
vom Dahl et al[51]	1997	Sestamibi/ FDG	77	≤50	29	1.21	0.22	6.51
Rohatgi et al[60]	2001	PET	58	22 ± 6	25	1.27	0.44	3.66

Abbreviations: LVEF, left ventricular ejection fraction; FU, follow-up (reflects reported average); OR, odds ratio; CI, confidence interval.

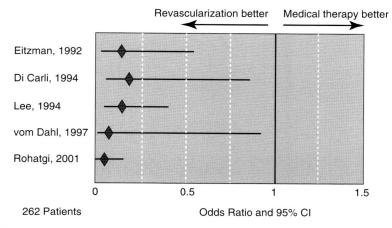

FIGURE 18.12. Relative risk of cardiovascular events (odds ratio) for patients with moderate-severe LV dysfunction and viable (hibernating) myocardium treated with revascularization compared with medical therapy. CI, confidence interval.

prognosis were found between these two groups. The results showed that the consistently poor event-free survival of patients with hibernating myocardium undergoing medical therapy was improved significantly and consistently by early referral to revascularization. The odds ratios were consistently <1 in all these reports. Interestingly, similar results have been reported by virtually every noninvasive imaging modality.

Summary Points

- PET imaging is an accurate and reproducible technique for the noninvasive evaluation of myocardial ischemia and viability.
- The FDG approach can be technically challenging, especially in patients with diabetes and congestive heart failure, and aggressive patient preparation is mandatory to optimize diagnostic accuracy. The available evidence suggests that this approach can provide accurate predictions of functional, symptomatic, and prognostic improvement after revascularization and thus improve management decisions in patients with poor cardiac function.
- Despite the robust and extensive body of evidence supporting the use of viability information for selecting patients for high-risk revascularization, several issues remain unresolved. There appears to be a rather significant reduction in the accuracy of viability testing, including PET, for predicting functional recovery in patients with severely depressed LV function (LVEF <30%). This is likely related to the fact that clinical predictions of functional recovery based on viability information alone are inadequate because they ignore the multifactorial influences affecting changes in LV function after revascularization.[58] Clinically important factors such as the degree of LV remodeling and the severity of morphological alterations within viable but dysfunctional myocytes (and likely others) may influence clinical outcomes even in the presence of relatively large areas of viable myocardium.[14,25,27,64]
- Future studies should focus on understanding the (likely) complex links between viability and ischemia and the molecular changes leading to altered myocyte function, progressive tissue damage, and LV remodeling. This type of information will be of great pathophysiological interest and will likely have important diagnostic implications.

References

1. Risk stratification and survival after myocardial infarction. *N Engl J Med*. 1983;309: 331–336.
2. Emond M, Mock MB, Davis KB, et al. Long-term survival of medically treated patients in the Coronary Artery Surgery Study (CASS) Registry. *Circulation*. 1994;90:2645–2657.
3. Baker D, Jones R, Hodges J, Massie BM, Konstam MA, Rose EA. Management of heart failure. III. The role of revascularization in the treatment of patients with moderate or severe left ventricular systolic dysfunction. *JAMA*. 1994;272:1528–1534.
4. Rahimtoola SH. The hibernating myocardium. *Am Heart J*. 1989;117:211–221.
5. Braunwald E, Kloner RA. The stunned myocardium: prolonged, postischemic ventricular dysfunction. *Circulation*. 1982;66:1146–1149.
6. Di Carli MF, Asgarzadie F, Schelbert HR, et al. Quantitative relation between myocardial viability and improvement in heart failure symptoms after revascularization in patients with ischemic cardiomyopathy. *Circulation*. 1995;92:3436–3444.
7. Heyndrickx GR, Millard RW, McRitchie RJ, Maroko PR, Vatner SF. Regional myocardial functional and electrophysiological alterations after brief coronary artery occlusion in conscious dogs. *J Clin Invest*. 1975;56:978–985.
8. Bolli R. Myocardial "stunning" in man. *Circulation*. 1992;86:1671–1691.
9. Kloner RA. Does reperfusion injury exist in humans? *J Am Coll Cardiol*. 1993;21: 537–545.
10. Rahimtoola SH. From coronary artery disease to heart failure: role of the hibernating myocardium. *Am J Cardiol*. 1995;75:16E–22E.
11. Canty JMJ, Fallavollita JA. Chronic hibernation and chronic stunning: a continuum. *J Nucl Cardiol*. 2000;7:509–527.
12. Vanoverschelde JL, Wijns W, Depre C, et al. Mechanisms of chronic regional postischemic dysfunction in humans. New insights from the study of noninfarcted collateral-dependent myocardium [see comments]. *Circulation*. 1993;87:1513–1523.
13. Schwarz ER, Schaper J, vom Dahl J, et al. Myocyte degeneration and cell death in hibernating human myocardium. *J Am Coll Cardiol*. 1996;27:1577–1585.
14. Elsasser A, Schlepper M, Klovekorn WP, et al. Hibernating myocardium: an incomplete adaptation to ischemia. *Circulation*. 1997;96:2920–2931.
15. Phelps ME, Hoffman EJ, Selin C, et al. Investigation of [18F]2-fluoro-2-deoxyglucose for the measure of myocardial glucose metabolism. *J Nucl Med*. 1978;19:1311–1319.
16. Bacharach SL, Bax JJ, Case J, et al. PET myocardial glucose metabolism and perfusion imaging with 18FDG, 13NH3 and 82Rb. Part 1—Guidelines for data acquisition and patient preparation. *J Nucl Cardiol*. 2003;10:543–556.
17. Tamaki N, Yonekura Y, Yamashita K, et al. Positron emission tomography using fluorine-18 deoxyglucose in evaluation of coronary artery bypass grafting. *Am J Cardiol*. 1989; 64:860–865.
18. Schoder H, Campisi R, Ohtake T, et al. Blood flow-metabolism imaging with positron emission tomography in patients with diabetes mellitus for the assessment of reversible left ventricular contractile dysfunction. *J Am Coll Cardiol*. 1999;33: 1328–1337.
19. Bax JJ, Veening MA, Visser FC, et al. Optimal metabolic conditions during fluorine-18 fluorodeoxyglucose imaging; a comparative study using different protocols. *Eur J Nucl Med*. 1997;24:35–41.
20. Pagano D, Bonser RS, Townend JN, Ordoubadi F, Lorenzoni R, Camici PG. Predictive value of dobutamine echocardiography and positron emission tomography in identifying hibernating myocardium in patients with postischaemic heart failure. *Heart*. 1998;79: 281–288.
21. Vitale GD, deKemp RA, Ruddy TD, Williams K, Beanlands RS. Myocardial glucose utilization and optimization of (18)F-FDG PET imaging in patients with non-insulin-dependent diabetes mellitus, coronary artery disease, and left ventricular dysfunction. *J Nucl Med*. 2001;42:1730–1736.
22. Di Carli MF, Prcevski P, Singh TP, et al. Myocardial blood flow, function, and metabolism in repetitive stunning. *J Nucl Med*. 2000;41:1227–1234.

23. Nowak B, Sinha AM, Schaefer WM, et al. Cardiac resynchronization therapy homogenizes myocardial glucose metabolism and perfusion in dilated cardiomyopathy and left bundle branch block. *J Am Coll Cardiol.* 2003;41:1523–1528.

24. Schaefer WM, Lipke CS, Nowak B, et al. Validation of an evaluation routine for left ventricular volumes, ejection fraction and wall motion from gated cardiac FDG PET: a comparison with cardiac magnetic resonance imaging. *Eur J Nucl Med Mol Imaging.* 2003;30:545–553.

25. Yamaguchi A, Ino T, Adachi H, Mizuhara A, Murata S, Kamio H. Left ventricular end-systolic volume index in patients with ischemic cardiomyopathy predicts postoperative ventricular function. *Ann Thorac Surg.* 1995;60:1059–1062.

26. Louie HW, Laks H, Milgalter E, et al. Ischemic cardiomyopathy. Criteria for coronary revascularization and cardiac transplantation. *Circulation.* 1991;84:III290–III295.

27. Yamaguchi A, Ino T, Adachi H, et al. Left ventricular volume predicts postoperative course in patients with ischemic cardiomyopathy. *Ann Thorac Surg.* 1998;65:434–438.

28. Chan SY, Brunken RC, Phelps ME, Schelbert HR. Use of the metabolic tracer carbon-11-acetate for evaluation of regional myocardial perfusion. *J Nucl Med.* 1991;32:665–672.

29. Gropler RJ, Siegel BA, Geltman EM. Myocardial uptake of carbon-11-acetate as an indirect estimate of regional myocardial blood flow. *J Nucl Med.* 1991;32:245–251.

30. Di Carli MF. Predicting improved function after myocardial revascularization. *Curr Opin Cardiol.* 1998;13:415–424.

31. Gropler RJ, Geltman EM, Sampathkumaran K, et al. Comparison of carbon-11-acetate with fluorine-18-fluorodeoxyglucose for delineating viable myocardium by positron emission tomography. *J Am Coll Cardiol.* 1993;22:1587–1597.

32. Maes A, Borgers M, Flameng W, et al. Assessment of myocardial viability in chronic coronary artery disease using technetium-99m sestamibi SPECT. *J Am Coll Cardiol.* 1997;29:62–68.

33. Grandin C, Wijns W, Melin JA, et al. Delineation of myocardial viability with PET. *J Nucl Med.* 1995;36:1543–1552.

34. Tamaki N, Kawamoto M, Tadamura E, et al. Prediction of reversible ischemia after revascularization. Perfusion and metabolic studies with positron emission tomography. *Circulation.* 1995;91:1697–1705.

35. Wolpers HG, Burchert W, van den Hoff J, Weinhardt R, Meyer GJ, Lichtlen PR. Assessment of myocardial viability by use of 11C-acetate and positron emission tomography. Threshold criteria of reversible dysfunction. *Circulation.* 1997;95:1417–1424.

36. Marinho NV, Keogh BE, Costa DC, Lammerstma AA, Ell PJ, Camici PG. Pathophysiology of chronic left ventricular dysfunction. New insights from the measurement of absolute myocardial blood flow and glucose utilization. *Circulation.* 1996;93:737–744.

37. Di Carli MF, Asgarzadie F, Schelbert HR, Brunken RC, Rokhsar S, Maddahi J. Relation of myocardial perfusion at rest and during pharmacologic stress to the PET patterns of tissue viability in patients with severe left ventricular dysfunction. *J Nucl Cardiol.* 1998;5:558–566.

38. Gropler RJ, Geltman EM, Sampathkumaran K, et al. Functional recovery after coronary revascularization for chronic coronary artery disease is dependent on maintenance of oxidative metabolism. *J Am Coll Cardiol.* 1992;20:569–577.

39. Gropler RJ, Bergmann SR. Flow and metabolic determinants of myocardial viability assessed by positron-emission tomography. *Coron Artery Dis.* 1993;4:495–504.

40. Rubin PJ, Lee DS, Davila-Roman VG, et al. Superiority of C-11 acetate compared with F-18 fluorodeoxyglucose in predicting myocardial functional recovery by positron emission tomography in patients with acute myocardial infarction. *Am J Cardiol.* 1996;78:1230–1235.

41. Hata T, Nohara R, Fujita M, et al. Noninvasive assessment of myocardial viability by positron emission tomography with 11C acetate in patients with old myocardial infarction. *Circulation.* 1996;94:1834–1841.

42. Tillisch J, Brunken R, Marshall R, et al. Reversibility of cardiac wall-motion abnormalities predicted by positron tomography. *N Engl J Med.* 1986;314:884–888.

43. Tamaki N, Ohtani H, Yamashita K, et al. Metabolic activity in the areas of new fill-in after thallium-201 reinjection: comparison with positron emission tomography using fluorine-18-deoxyglucose. *J Nucl Med.* 1991;32:673–678.

44. Carrel T, Jenni R, Haubold-Reuter S, Von Schulthess G, Pasic M, Turina M. Improvement in severely reduced left ventricular function after surgical revascularization in patients with preoperative myocardial infarction. *Eur J Cardiothorac Surg.* 1992;6: 479–484.

45. Lucignani G, Schwaiger M, Melin J, Fazio F. Assessing hibernating myocardium: an emerging cost-effectiveness issue [editorial]. *Eur J Nucl Med.* 1997;24:1337–1341.

46. Marwick TH, MacIntyre WJ, Lafont A, Nemec JJ, Salcedo EE. Metabolic responses of hibernating and infarcted myocardium to revascularization. A follow-up study of regional perfusion, function, and metabolism. *Circulation.* 1992;85:1347–1353.

47. vom Dahl J, Eitzman DT, al-Aouar ZR, et al. Relation of regional function, perfusion, and metabolism in patients with advanced coronary artery disease undergoing surgical revascularization. *Circulation.* 1994;90:2356–2366.

48. Knuuti MJ, Saraste M, Nuutila P, et al. Myocardial viability: fluorine-18-deoxyglucose positron emission tomography in prediction of wall motion recovery after revascularization. *Am Heart J.* 1994;127:785–796.

49. Baer FM, Voth E, Deutsch HJ, et al. Predictive value of low dose dobutamine transesophageal echocardiography and fluorine-18 fluorodeoxyglucose positron emission tomography for recovery of regional left ventricular function after successful revascularization. *J Am Coll Cardiol.* 1996;28:60–69.

50. vom Dahl J, Altehoefer C, Sheehan FH, et al. Recovery of regional left ventricular dysfunction after coronary revascularization. Impact of myocardial viability assessed by nuclear imaging and vessel patency at follow-up angiography. *J Am Coll Cardiol.* 1996;28: 948–958.

51. vom Dahl J, Altehoefer C, Sheehan FH, et al. Effect of myocardial viability assessed by technetium-99 m-sestamibi SPECT and fluorine-18-FDG PET on clinical outcome in coronary artery disease. *J Nucl Med.* 1997;38:742–748.

52. Beanlands RS, Ruddy TD, deKemp RA, et al. Positron emission tomography and recovery following revascularization (PARR-1): the importance of scar and the development of a prediction rule for the degree of recovery of left ventricular function. *J Am Coll Cardiol.* 2002;40:1735–1743.

53. Ragosta M, Beller GA, Watson DD, Kaul S, Gimple LW. Quantitative planar rest-redistribution 201Tl imaging in detection of myocardial viability and prediction of improvement in left ventricular function after coronary bypass surgery in patients with severely depressed left ventricular function. *Circulation.* 1993;87:1630–1641.

54. Perrone-Filardi P, Pace L, Prastaro M, et al. Dobutamine echocardiography predicts improvement of hypoperfused dysfunctional myocardium after revascularization in patients with coronary artery disease. *Circulation.* 1995;91:2556–2565.

55. Kim RJ, Wu E, Rafael A, et al. The use of contrast-enhanced magnetic resonance imaging to identify reversible myocardial dysfunction. *N Engl J Med.* 2000;343:1445–1453.

56. Bax JJ, Poldermans D, Elhendy A, Boersma E, Rahimtoola SH. Sensitivity, specificity, and predictive accuracies of various noninvasive techniques for detecting hibernating myocardium. *Curr Probl Cardiol.* 2001;26:141–186.

57. Di Carli MF. The quest for myocardial viability: Is there a role for nitrate-enhanced imaging? *J Nucl Cardiol.* 2003;10:696–699.

58. Di Carli MF, Hachamovitch R, Berman D. The art and science of predicting post-revascularization improvement in LV function in patients with severely depressed LV function [editorial]. *J Am Coll Cardiol.* 2002;40:1744–1747.

59. Marwick TH, Nemec JJ, Lafont A, Salcedo EE, MacIntyre WJ. Prediction by postexercise fluoro-18 deoxyglucose positron emission tomography of improvement in exercise capacity after revascularization. *Am J Cardiol.* 1992;69:854–859.

60. Rohatgi R, Epstein S, Henriquez J, et al. Utility of positron emission tomography in predicting cardiac events and survival in patients with coronary artery disease and severe left ventricular dysfunction. *Am J Cardiol.* 2001;87:1096–1099, A6.

61. Eitzman D, al-Aouar Z, Kanter HL, et al. Clinical outcome of patients with advanced coronary artery disease after viability studies with positron emission tomography [see comments]. *J Am Coll Cardiol.* 1992;20:559–565.

62. Di Carli MF, Davidson M, Little R, et al. Value of metabolic imaging with positron emission tomography for evaluating prognosis in patients with coronary artery disease and left ventricular dysfunction. *Am J Cardiol.* 1994;73:527–533.

63. Lee KS, Marwick TH, Cook SA, et al. Prognosis of patients with left ventricular dysfunction, with and without viable myocardium after myocardial infarction. Relative efficacy of medical therapy and revascularization. *Circulation.* 1994;90:2687–2694.
64. Beanlands RS, Hendry PJ, Masters RG, deKemp RA, Woodend K, Ruddy TD. Delay in revascularization is associated with increased mortality rate in patients with severe left ventricular dysfunction and viable myocardium on fluorine 18-fluorodeoxyglucose positron emission tomography imaging. *Circulation.* 1998;98:II51–II56.

19 Myocardial Perfusion, Viability, and Functional Assessment with Contrast CT

Martin J. Lipton

Rationale for CT

Computed tomography (CT) can acquire high-resolution cross-sectional images of geometrically precise tomographic sections of the whole heart and thorax during one breath hold. It has the potential not only for measuring cardiac chamber size, shape, and dynamics but also for displaying the myocardial wall itself and providing estimates of myocardial wall dimensions including wall thickness, thickening, mass, and integrity on a regional and global basis. Consequently, contrast cardiac CT can provide useful information regarding myocardial viability and LV remodeling that could be of clinical value in the management of patients with heart failure.

Multidetector electrocardiogram (ECG)-gated CT (MDCT) has become widely available only in the last few years, but these multipurpose whole-body scanners are currently being used in the heart for routine clinical CT angiography (CTA) of coronary artery morphology. However, early feasibility studies have demonstrated a much greater potential for functional cardiac CT; during the past 2 years, gated MDCT is increasingly being applied to examine left ventricular morphology and function. The following paragraphs discuss feasibility and describe how cardiac CT applications could develop in the future for evaluating cardiac remodeling and viability.

Assessing Myocardial Blood Flow

The requirements for cellular viability include intact cell membrane function to maintain electrochemical gradients, preserved metabolic activity to generate high-energy phosphates, and residual myocardial blood flow to deliver substrates and remove the metabolites resulting from the metabolic processes. Thus, CT-based assessment of myocardial blood flow may provide useful information regarding myocyte viability.

Measurements of regional CT attenuation changes over time allow quantitation of tissue perfusion and of blood flow through blood vessels and cardiac chambers (Figure 19.1).[1,2] Ringertz et al showed that carotid blood flow could be assessed by CT.[3] Garrett et al validated CT measurement of cardiac output and also showed that this technique was comparable to oximetry.[4] Rumberger at al demonstrated the utility and potential of CT for quantitative regional myocardial perfusion.[5] Regional myocardial perfusion measured by CT at rest and during pharmacologically induced stress compared favorably with radioactive microspheres (Figure 19.2).[6]

FIGURE 19.1. (A) Myocardial perfusion curve generated over lateral wall from a patient with a previous anterior myocardial infarction. Curve analysis provides peak height. Blood flow (F/V) in any myocardial region can be calculated as the ratio of the peak of the time-density curve in that area (P) to the area under the aorta or left ventricle time-density curve (A), which is representative of cardiac output. HU, Hounsfield units.

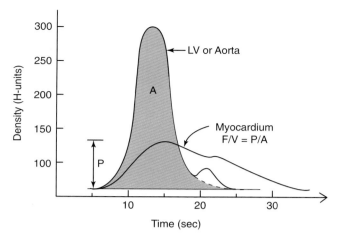

The principle of measuring blood flow using tomographic imaging with indicator dilution theory has been applied to radiotracer methods and typically requires repetitive samplings of a region of interest to generate a gamma-variant fit to the data. Using CT, this can be accomplished for any organ, as described by Jaschke et al.[2] In the case of the myocardium, diastolic images are obtained at the same anatomic levels of the heart on either every beat or every other cardiac cycle, depending on heart rate. The curve is fitted on data collected during the first 15 seconds before there is recirculation (Figure 19.1). The accuracy of CT measurements of myocardial blood flow using intravenous agents is influenced by the well-recognized effects of contrast medium and mixing as well as many other factors.[7,8] Validation studies of myocardial perfusion with conventional MDCT-ECG-gated scanners, which have sufficient temporal resolution, are also now possible.[9]

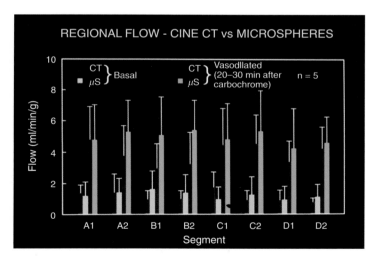

FIGURE 19.2. Comparison of electron beam computed tomography (EBCT) measurements of regional myocardial perfusion with microspheres in a series of dogs. Four areas of interest were identified at 2 LV levels on CT images during sequential scans triggered at end diastole to minimize motion. Chromonar was administered to provide data for each of 8 regions at rest and during maximal vasodilatation. The microspheres were injected simultaneously and the results graphed as illustrated in pairs for resting and stress states by region. The error bars illustrate the excellent correlation achieved. (Reproduced from Reference 6 with permission.)

Assessing Myocardial Ischemia and Infarction

Since myocardial perfusion is pivotal to the prognosis of patients sustaining an acute myocardial infarct (AMI), the assessment of microvascular flow following reperfusion therapy is of great importance. Indeed, Gibson et al established that patients with both normal epicardial coronary blood flow and normal tissue perfusion are at extremely low risk of death.[10]

Myocardial perfusion is currently evaluated primarily by nuclear imaging techniques.[11–13] However, magnetic resonance imaging (MRI), contrast echocardiography,[14–16] and, more recently, gated MDCT can also provide this information.[17,18]

Early attempts at recognizing and quantifying myocardial ischemia and infarction with CT were confined to in vitro studies of either excised or in situ arrested canine hearts.[19–27] Doherty et al explored the detection and quantitation of myocardial ischemia and infarction in vivo using transmission CT in a series of 28 dogs.[28] Upon intravenous (IV) contrast administration, myocardial regions distal to an occluded coronary artery showed as areas of reduced contrast opacification (so-called cold-spot imaging) compared to normal remote myocardium (Figure 19.3). The interpretation of these "cold spots" must be temporally related to the time of coronary occlusion. They are not specific markers for myocardial infarction per se. Early after a coronary occlusion they reflect primarily reduced tissue perfusion, whereas their appearance late after a prolonged occlusion reflects primarily scar tissue formation and attendant necrosis.

These early studies also demonstrated the value of delayed imaging after 5 to 20 minutes following contrast administration for differentiating acutely infarcted from

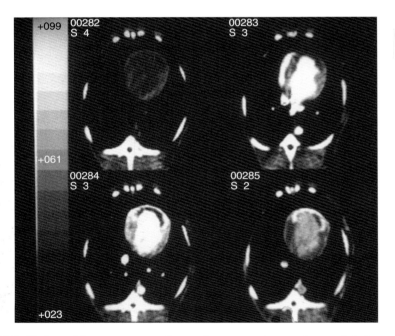

FIGURE 19.3. Early and late contrast medium enhancement in a canine model of acute myocardial infarction. This figure shows four 4.8-second, 1-cm-thick scans following an intravenous bolus of 20 mL of contrast medium at the level of the ventricular cavities in a dog with a heart rate of 114 beats per minute. This animal has a 2-day-old anteroseptal myocardial infarction produced by permanent ligation of the left anterior descending coronary artery. The left upper panel shows the precontrast scan, which is followed by contrast enhancement of both ventricles in the right upper panel. The area that appears to be less well opacified (black), in the right upper and left lower panels, represents the area of myocardial blood flow deficit. The scan in the right lower panel was obtained 10 minutes later through the same level without further contrast medium injection. The hypoperfused region is now dramatically profiled by contrast medium entrapment relative to surrounding healthy myocardium, which is less enhanced due to normal washout.

FIGURE 19.4. Comparison of CT and autopsy measurements of infarct area in individual tomographic slices. The excellent correlation is due partly to the presumption of transmural infarcts, which simplifies the boundary placement task for both the CT and autopsy area calculations. (Reprinted from Doherty PW, et al. Detection and quantitation of myocardial infarction in vivo using transmission computed tomography. Circulation. 1981;63(3):597–606, with permission.)

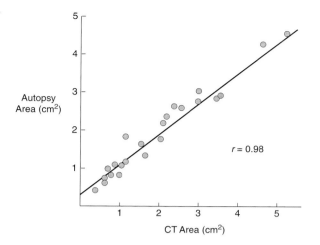

dysfunctional but viable myocardium. Indeed, the studies by Doherty demonstrated that washout of contrast medium was slower in infarcted than in normal myocardium (Figure 19.3). However, delayed contrast enhancement (so-called hot-spot imaging) could not be demonstrated consistently and reliably until 24 hours after ligation. As with MRI, delayed contrast enhancement appears to be a good marker for the presence of myocardial scar. This finding is not seen when the coronary artery is transiently occluded for as long as 10 minutes.[29] These early studies demonstrated that the quantitative extent of myocardial scar assessed by contrast CT correlates well with the corresponding infarct area determined by pathology (Figure 19.4). These observations have been confirmed in both experimental and clinical models of acute and chronic myocardial infarction (Figure 19.5).[30,31]

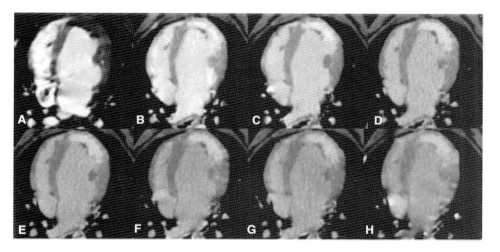

FIGURE 19.5. Axial temporal image series demonstrating postreperfusion contrast agent kinetics after 150-mL injection of contrast. The first image (A) represents the first-pass image during contrast agent injection. Note that the signal density of the infarct in the first pass is substantially lower than that of the remote myocardium and indicates a subendocardial microvascular obstruction. Five minutes after injection (B), the signal density of the damaged myocardial region is significantly greater than that of the remote myocardium and washes out over time. As can be appreciated from (B), the infarct becomes well delineated and reaches peak enhancement at 5 minutes after injection and then washes out in proportion to the chamber (blood pool) and remote myocardial signal. (Reproduced from Reference 31 with permission.)

Mechanism of Delayed Contrast Enhancement

Delayed contrast enhancement with CT was observed in the late 1970s and was also reported with MRI when this technique became available in the early 1980s. Gadolinium was approved for patient use in Europe before FDA approval in America. Hence, early contrast-enhanced MRI studies in myocardial infarction were initially performed in Germany. However, it was not until recently that Kim et al popularized hyperenhancement with MRI using newer scanners and described the implications of this finding on management decisions after myocardial infarction.[32]

The mechanism causing the initial hypodense central zone of an infarct on first pass of the contrast agent (iodine or gadolinium) followed by delayed contrast hyperenhancement of the infarct border zone seen with CT and MRI is thought to be associated with the same pathophysiology, although this theory has been the source of considerable debate.

Intravenously delivered contrast agents entering the vascular space normally enter and are confined to the extracellular compartment. However, ischemic injury of the myocytes changes the distribution. Rehwald et al noted that the sarcolemmal membrane of the myocytes appears ruptured in this setting when studied by electron microscopy.[33] Skioldebrand et al demonstrated the development of increased interstitial spaces between collagen bundles in dense scar tissue of chronic healing infarcts.[34] Accumulation of contrast agent may occur within these "vascular lakes," while healthy myocardium demonstrates normal washout. A similar phenomenon has been postulated for MRI.[32]

Kramer et al used a single-slice non-gated CT scanner to study 19 patients with ST elevation myocardial infarction (MI) 3 to 29 days postinfarction.[18] Areas of infarction were characterized by low contrast attenuation compared with normal myocardium on the first passage of contrast agent. The infarct area was measured using planimetry at each anatomical scan level. Delayed contrast enhancement occurred in some, but not all, patients and was seen as a halo of increased density in the border zone between normal and infarcted myocardium. There was time-dependent variation in the density of the infarcted region and surrounding myocardium following contrast administration. In some patients, this edge became indistinct in terms of density due to changes in both the infarct region and surrounding myocardium. This was explained on the basis of heterogeneity due to patchy islands of ischemic and necrotic tissue.

More recently, Koyama et al confirmed these early observations in 58 patients with ST-elevation MI undergoing successful percutaneous coronary reperfusion.[17] Gated contrast CT was performed within 48 hours of coronary reperfusion. Patients underwent a 2-phase contrast-enhanced CT with images being acquired following intravenous contrast at 45 seconds and again at 7 minutes. In this study, the authors described 3 enhancement patterns: In pattern 1, there was no perfusion defect in the first phase, and there was late enhancement without residual perfusion defect (reflecting complete restoration of tissue perfusion with a very small area of subendocardial scar). In pattern 2, there was a perfusion defect in the early phase with a concomitant area of late enhancement without residual perfusion deficit in the late phase. In pattern 3, there was a perfusion defect in the early phase with a concomitant area of late enhancement with residual perfusion defect in the late phase (denoting an area of infarction with severe microvascular obstruction after epicardial reperfusion).

The variability in enhancement pattern was attributed to variability in the extent of microvascular damage. As expected, LV functional recovery was observed in patients with pattern 1 and to some extent in those with pattern 2. However, no functional recovery was observed among patients with pattern 3. That is, they might not have complete reperfusion at the microvascular level, while those patients who did not have an early or a residual perfusion defect (pattern 1) might experience a complete recovery of left ventricular function, which might be indicative of successful

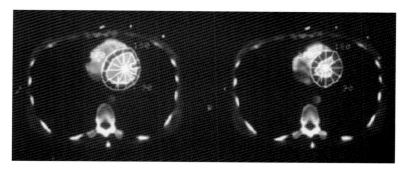

FIGURE 19.6. Geometric radial analysis of regional wall thickness and cavity volume change during the cardiac cycle on the short axis obtained by EBCT. (Reprinted from Boxt LM, et al. Computed tomography for assessment of cardiac chambers, valves, myocardium and pericardium. Cardiology Clinics; 21(4):561–585, Copyright 2003, with permission from Elsevier.)

reperfusion at both the epicardial and the microvascular level. These observations are consistent with those reported by MRI.[35,36]

Assessing LV Geometry, Volumes, and Mass as Measures of LV Remodeling

Prognosis following AMI is closely related to the extent of myocardial necrosis and the degree of contractile dysfunction of the left ventricle. Since endocardial and epicardial borders can be well depicted by ECG-gated MDCT (Figure 19.6), the same CT data set acquired for coronary CTA can also be used to measure both systolic and diastolic LV function (Figure 19.7).[37] Therefore, myocardial wall thickness, thickening, and LV volumetric indices can be estimated by CT.

Myocardial infarction, especially when extensive and transmural, can produce alterations in both the infarcted and noninfarcted regions that result in changes in LV architecture known as LV remodeling.[38–40] In addition to the early thinning and elongation that occurs in the infarcted myocardium (infarct expansion), secondary changes occur in the noninfarcted zone characterized by a time-dependent associated increase in the end-diastolic length of viable myocytes that contribute to the overall process of LV enlargement.[39] Although this acute increase in cavity size tends to maintain pump function, this process usually leads to progressive ventricular dilation, heart failure, and decreased survival. Thus, measures of LV function and remodeling are important in the evaluation of the patient with heart failure.

Ventricular remodeling may be associated with compensatory hypertrophy of normal myocardium on a regional basis. Complications of acute MI include

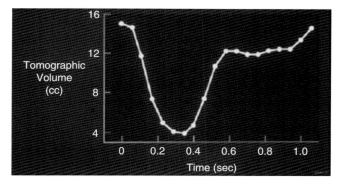

FIGURE 19.7. An example of how volume curves can be plotted from CT images to provide tomographic volumes of cardiac chambers at sequential levels. (Reproduced from Reference 37 with permission from The American College of Cardiology Foundation.)

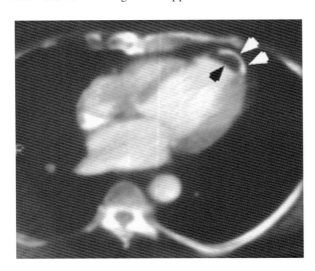

FIGURE 19.8. A non-ECG gated CT scan 8 mm thick in a patient 10 months following an acute anterior myocardial infarction. Note the anterior calcified aneurysm (white arrowheads) with black nonenhanced thrombus adjacent to it (black arrowhead) and a sharp linear distinction of the left ventricular apex. In addition, note typical compensatory hypertrophy along the lateral wall and relative thinning of the anteroseptal region. (Reprinted from Boxt LM, et al. Computed tomography for assessment of cardiac chambers, valves, myocardium and pericardium. Cardiology Clinics; 21(4):561–585, Copyright 2003, with permission from Elsevier.)

pericarditis with effusion, LV aneurysm formation, intracavity thrombus, and mitral insufficiency with enlargement of the left atrium either from dysfunction of the mitral valve apparatus itself or from ventricular cavity dilatation resulting in abnormal vector pull of an otherwise normal valve structure. As shown in Figure 19.8, CT can identify and monitor LV remodeling and the sequelae of myocardial infarction.

Regional and Global LV Function

Regional wall motion using ECG-gated single-slice CT was validated against echocardiography by Bouchard et al in a series of patients with documented anterior or posterior myocardial infarction.[41] The site of prior myocardial infarction was correctly identified in 21 of 22 patients. CT evaluation of right ventricular function has also been examined; it has outperformed echo in a series of patients with emphysema, as might be expected, indicating the potential complementary role that CT can play in this patient population.[42]

Global LV function has been examined by CT and the results correlated with MRI.[43] Interobserver variation for all volume measurements was acceptable, being in the 5% to 8% range. Left ventricular ejection fraction (LVEF) showed substantial agreement with values obtained from MRI. However, mean values for end-diastolic and end-systolic volumes appeared to be underestimated by MDCT. Other investigators have since shown the feasibility of MDCT for evaluating LV function, and the results showed good agreement with other imaging modalities.[44]

During the past 18 months, several studies have been reported in which global and regional LV function was estimated by gated 16-MDCT and the results were validated against MRI. Mahnken et al concluded that CT allows reliable LV volume measurements.[45] Boll et al examined the effects of heart rate and software on the validity and reproducibility of both CT and MRI using a set of volumetric phantoms for 10 patients referred for concurrent 16-MDCT and MRI cardiac evaluation performed on the same day.[46] This study showed that for all methods of data-set analysis, intraobserver variability was below 2% and unrelated to the magnitude of measurement. High accuracy was reported in the phantom. In patients, CT showed maximum variability at heart rates below 60 beats per minute, while for MRI data sets this occurred above 90 beats per minute. These authors concluded that CT and MRI data sets allowed an interchangeable utilization of volumetric analysis tools. Other studies, for example, that of Schlosser et al, measured LV function and mass derived from retrospectively ECG-gated 16-MDCT coronary data sets and compared the results in 18 patients referred for CTA with MRI.[47] As in other investigations, there was no significant difference found for ejection fraction between CT and MRI.[48–52]

LV and RV Volumes

Reiter et al performed a study in dogs assessing the determination of left ventricular stroke volume by EBCT compared with that derived simultaneously, using either a chronically implanted and calibrated aortic electromagnetic flow probe or careful assessment with established thermodilution techniques.[53] Electrocardiographically triggered scans were acquired in the movie mode nearly simultaneously from the cardiac apex through the base in the short axis during intravenous slow injection of iodinated contrast. Stroke volume was then calculated as the difference between end-diastolic (peak of R wave) and end-systolic (smallest cavity) volumes, again using a modification of Simpson's rule. Similar results have been reported in patients.[54]

Figure 19.9 shows 25 separate determinations of left ventricular stroke volume. These data confirm the precision of stroke volume determinations by EBCT even in the presence of acute myocardial infarction. If left ventricular stroke volume can be quantitated by CT, then by inference, determinations of end-diastolic and end-systolic volume should be, likewise, quantitative. Studies done using casts of canine left ventricles have previously shown the accuracy of static estimates of left ventricular volume by conventional CT.[23]

Simultaneous determination of right ventricular volumes is possible with the estimation of left ventricular mass and volumes.[53] As an addition to the studies of left ventricular volume noted above, Reiter et al also determined right ventricular stroke volumes by planimetry of the tomographic end-diastolic and end-systolic CT scans and the modified Simpson's rule (Figure 19.10). Application of this method then makes no assumptions as to right (or left) ventricular geometry as is commonly used for contrast angiography. Calculated right ventricular stroke volume compared absolutely with the left ventricular stroke volumes. As with the left ventricular volume calculations, inter- and intraobserver variability was minimal. The direct measurement of right ventricular volume by CT was expected based on studies of right ventricular casts.[55]

In conclusion, dynamic CT can be used to provide highly quantitative data regarding left and right ventricular volumes provided careful attention is paid to proper border definition. It can also measure segmental variability of left ventricular function.[53,56,57] These studies with EBCT have important implications for MDCT. Once the temporal resolution of MDCT improves, similar measurements in terms of accuracy and precision should be possible with this technique, irrespective of low or high heart rates. Furthermore, pharmacological interventions could then become

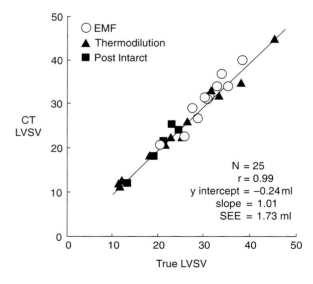

FIGURE 19.9. Comparison of true left ventricular stroke volume determined by either electromagnetic flow meter or thermodilution technique in the canine, with calculations of left ventricular stroke volume as determined by EBCT. (Reproduced from Reference 53 with permission.)

possible. Lanzer et al demonstrated the feasibility of performing CT in these circumstances.[58]

Assessment of LV remodeling requires precise measurements of cardiac morphology and function. Earlier EBCT longitudinal studies provided insight into the potential applications of MDCT for patient management. Notably, EBCT studies of patients with AMI showed findings similar to those in animals. These CT appearances correspond in general to those described by Koyama with MDCT.[17] Similarly, early validation CT studies have also been successfully performed in patients for regional and global myocardial analysis, as well as CT quantitation of regional wall motion abnormalities with exercise.[59–61] In the future, MDCT can be expected to provide accurate measurements of ventricular function in a routine clinical setting.

LV Mass

Precise cardiac border (edge) definition and contour placement is essential for accurate quantitation of left ventricular anatomy and function. A quantitative method of cardiac edge detection for CT was developed initially for the determination of left ventricular wall thickness and mass by Skioldebrand et al[62] and was applied to EBT by Feiring et al.[63] This technique defines the absolute placement of the cardiac edge at a CT density (Hounsfield scale) halfway between the density of the myocardium and adjacent structures. This requires evaluation of the CT numbers of the left and right ventricular cavities, anterior chest wall, lung, and adjacent myocardium.

Placement of the endocardial and epicardial surfaces, as a direct and straightforward application of this full-width/half-maximum method noted above, is aided by an operator-defined, computer-assisted, semiautomated edge-definition program, much of which was developed in the standard EBCT data analysis software. The operator determines the placement of the cardiac edge by defining the center level of the CT number range (window) that constitutes the density of the endocardial or epicardial surfaces. The software then outlines the contour and determines the absolute value of the area within. Minor vagaries in computer-aided placement of the cardiac edge can be corrected by the operator using a trackball device. Global measurements of left ventricular mass and volumes are performed at the data analysis console or workstation following definition of left ventricular endocardial and epicardial contours at each level from apex to aortic root.

Calculation of left ventricular mass was made using the modified Simpson's rule and knowledge of the scanning target geometry by subtracting the endocardial volume from the epicardial volume and multiplying by the myocardial mass. Comparison between left ventricular mass in situ and that calculated by EBCT in vivo showed

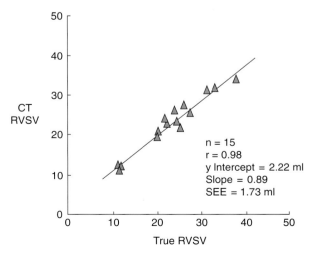

n = 15
r = 0.98
y Intercept = 2.22 ml
Slope = 0.89
SEE = 1.73 ml

FIGURE 19.10. True right ventricular stroke volume compared with CT calculation of right ventricular stroke volume in the dog. (Reproduced from Reference 53 with permission.)

FIGURE 19.11. Comparison of absolute postmortem myocardial mass of the canine left ventricle with in vivo determination using EBCT. (Reproduced from Reference 63 with permission.)

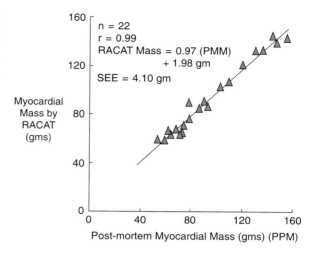

excellent correlation (Figure 19.11). Additionally, inter- and intraobserver variability has been assessed and the technique has been found to be highly reproducible.[63] Left ventricular mass measured by EBT has also shown very good correlation with two-dimensional echocardiography.[64]

Summary Points

- The focus to date of MDCT has been primarily on CT applications in the heart for evaluating cardiac anatomy, notably for displaying the coronary artery morphology and measuring coronary artery calcification, plaque characterization, and atherosclerotic luminal stenosis.
- The temporal resolution of MDCT has limited functional CT studies of the heart. However, if the temporal resolution of MDCT continues to be improved, there will be a compelling argument for undertaking further functional CT validation studies.
- Feasibility of CT has already been established by EBCT for general cardiac diagnosis. Modifications for MDCT include improved software methods for postprocessing ECG-gated scan data and higher-speed CT hardware for faster image acquisition, both of which are being developed now.
- Modern EBT is also evolving and continuously being refined so that new generations of these scanners have exposure times of 50 milliseconds or less. Radiation is a recognized concern, and the exposure dose is well characterized for coronary CTA. Contrast medium is also a significant issue.
- In comparing the value of competing cardiac imaging modalities, their availability, published diagnostic validation studies, convenience, procedure time, safety, comfort level (of patients and physicians), and cost are all critical. The degree of acceptance and the accuracy with which specific patient management questions can be definitively answered are crucial issues in determining which diagnostic procedure to perform. However, the jury is still out regarding the ultimate role of CT in the diagnosis of heart disease; certainly the great potential of cardiac CT has not yet been fully realized.[65]

References

1. Jaschke W, Cogan MG, Sievers R, Gould R, Lipton MJ. Measurement of renal blood flow by cine computed tomography. *Kidney Int.* 1987;31:1038–1042.
2. Jaschke W, Gould RG, Assimakopoulos PA, Lipton MJ. Flow measurements with a high-speed computed tomography scanner. *Med Phys.* 1987;14:238–243.

3. Ringertz HG, Jaschke W, Sievers R, Lipton MJ. Relative carotid blood flow measurements in dogs by high-speed CT. A preliminary study. *Invest Radiol.* 1987;22:960–964.

4. Garrett JS, Lanzer P, Jaschke W, et al. Measurement of cardiac output by cine computed tomography. *Am J Cardiol.* 1985;56:657–661.

5. Rumberger JA, Feiring AJ, Lipton MJ, Higgins CB, Ell SR, Marcus ML. Use of ultrafast computed tomography to quantitate regional myocardial perfusion: a preliminary report. *J Am Coll Cardiol.* 1987;9:59–69.

6. Gould RG, Lipton MJ, McNamara MT, Sievers RE, Koshold S, Higgins CB. Measurement of regional myocardial blood flow in dogs by ultrafast CT. *Invest Radiol.* 1988;23: 348–353.

7. Lanzer P, Dean PB, Lipton MJ, Sievers R, Botvinick E, Higgins CB. Effects of intravenous administration of a new nonionic dimeric contrast medium on the coronary circulation. Comparison with monomeric ionic and nonionic media. *Invest Radiol.* 1985;20: 746–750.

8. Lipton MJ, Higgins CB, Wiley AA, Angell WW, Barry WH. The effect of contrast media on the isolated perfused canine heart. *Invest Radiol.* 1978;13:519–522.

9. Koyama Y, Mochizuki T, Higaki J. Computed tomography assessment of myocardial perfusion, viability, and function. *J Magn Reson Imaging.* 2004;19:800–815.

10. Gibson CM, Cannon CP, Murphy SA, et al. Relationship of TIMI myocardial perfusion grade to mortality after administration of thrombolytic drugs. *Circulation.* 2000;101: 125–130.

11. Abe M, Kazatani Y, Fukuda H, Tatsuno H, Habara H, Shinbata H. Left ventricular volumes, ejection fraction, and regional wall motion calculated with gated technetium-99m tetrofosmin SPECT in reperfused acute myocardial infarction at super-acute phase: comparison with left ventriculography. *J Nucl Cardiol.* 2000;7:569–574.

12. Di Carli MF. Predicting improved function after myocardial revascularization. *Curr Opin Cardiol.* 1998;13:415–424.

13. Di Carli MF, Asgarzadie F, Schelbert HR, et al. Quantitative relation between myocardial viability and improvement in heart failure symptoms after revascularization in patients with ischemic cardiomyopathy. *Circulation.* 1995;92:3436–3444.

14. Bogaert J, Maes A, Van de Werf F, et al. Functional recovery of subepicardial myocardial tissue in transmural myocardial infarction after successful reperfusion: an important contribution to the improvement of regional and global left ventricular function. *Circulation.* 1999;99:36–43.

15. Lepper W, Hoffmann R, Kamp O, et al. Assessment of myocardial reperfusion by intravenous myocardial contrast echocardiography and coronary flow reserve after primary percutaneous transluminal coronary angioplasty [correction of angiography] in patients with acute myocardial infarction. *Circulation.* 2000;101:2368–2374.

16. Watzinger N, Lund GK, Higgins CB, Wendland MF, Weinmann HJ, Saeed M. The potential of contrast-enhanced magnetic resonance imaging for predicting left ventricular remodeling. *J Magn Reson Imaging.* 2002;16:633–640.

17. Koyama Y, Matsuoka H, Mochizuki T, et al. Assessment of reperfused acute myocardial infarction with two-phase contrast-enhanced helical CT: prediction of left ventricular function and wall thickness. *Radiology.* 2005;235:804–811.

18. Kramer PH, Goldstein JA, Herkens RJ, Lipton MJ, Brundage BH. Imaging of acute myocardial infarction in man with contrast-enhanced computed transmission tomography. *Am Heart J.* 1984;108:1514–1523.

19. Abrams HL, McNeil BJ. Medical implications of computed tomography ("CAT scanning") (second of two parts). *N Engl J Med.* 1978;298:310–318.

20. Adams DF, Hessel SJ, Judy PF, Stein JA, Abrams HL. Computed tomography of the normal and infarcted myocardium. *AJR Am J Roentgenol.* 1976;126:786–791.

21. Alfidi RJ, Haaga J, Meaney TF, et al. Computed tomography of the thorax and abdomen: a preliminary report. *Radiology.* 1975;117:257–264.

22. Gray WR Jr, Parkey RW, Buja LM, et al. Computed tomography: in vitro evaluation of myocardial infarction. *Radiology.* 1977;122:511–513.

23. Lipton MJ, Hayashi TT, Boyd D, Carlsson E. Measurement of left ventricular cast volume by computed tomography. *Radiology.* 1978;127:419–423.

24. Lipton MJ, Herfkens RJ, Boyd DP, Fuchs WA. Contrast enhancement and dynamic scanning of the heart. In: Fuchs WA, ed. *Contrast Enhancement in Body Computerized Tomography.* New York: Georg Thieme Verlag Stuttgart; 1981:57–70.

25. Siemers PT, Higgins CB, Schmidt W, Ashburn W, Hagan P. Detection, quantitation and contrast enhancement of myocardial infarction utilizing computerized axial tomography: comparison with histochemical staining and 99mTc-pyrophosphate imaging. *Invest Radiol.* 1978;13:103–109.

26. Ter-Pogossian MM, Weiss ES, Coleman RE, Sobel BE. Computed tomography of the heart. *AJR Am J Roentgenol.* 1976;127:79–90.

27. Wittenberg J, Powell WM Jr, Dinsmore RE, Miller SW, Maturi RA. Computerized tomography of ischemic myocardium: quantitation of extent and severity of edema in an in vitro canine model. *Invest Radiol.* 1977;12:215–223.

28. Doherty PW, Lipton MJ, Berninger WH, Skioldebrand CG, Carlsson E, Redington RW. Detection and quantitation of myocardial infarction in vivo using transmission computed tomography. *Circulation.* 1981;63:597–606.

29. Ringertz HG, Palmer RG, Lipton MJ, Carlsson E. CT attenuation ratio of myocardium and blood pool in the normal and infarcted canine heart. *Acta Radiol Diagn (Stockh).* 1983;24:11–16.

30. Gerber BL, Belge B, Legros GJ, et al. Characterization of acute and chronic myocardial infarcts by multidetector computed tomography. Comparison with contrast-enhanced magnetic resonance. *Circulation.* 2006;113:823–833.

31. Lardo AC, Cordeiro MA, Silva C, et al. Contrast-enhanced multidetector computed tomography viability imaging after myocardial infarction: characterization of myocyte death, microvascular obstruction, and chronic scar. *Circulation.* 2006;113:394–404.

32. Kim RJ, Wu E, Rafael A, et al. The use of contrast-enhanced magnetic resonance imaging to identify reversible myocardial dysfunction. *N Engl J Med.* 2000;343:1445–1453.

33. Rehwald WG, Fieno DS, Chen EL, Kim RJ, Judd RM. Myocardial magnetic resonance imaging contrast agent concentrations after reversible and irreversible ischemic injury. *Circulation.* 2002;105:224–229.

34. Skioldebrand CG, Lipton MJ, Redington RW, Berninger WH, Wallace A, Carlsson E. Myocardial infarction in dogs, demonstrated by non-enhanced computed tomography. *Acta Radiol Diagn (Stockh).* 1981;22:1–8.

35. Wu KC, Kim RJ, Bluemke DA, et al. Quantification and time course of microvascular obstruction by contrast-enhanced echocardiography and magnetic resonance imaging following acute myocardial infarction and reperfusion. *J Am Coll Cardiol.* 1998;32:1756–1764.

36. Wu KC, Zerhouni EA, Judd RM, et al. Prognostic significance of microvascular obstruction by magnetic resonance imaging in patients with acute myocardial infarction. *Circulation.* 1998;97:765–772.

37. Rumberger JA, Weiss RM, Feiring AJ, et al. Patterns of regional diastolic function in the normal human left ventricle: an ultrafast computed tomographic study. *J Am Coll Cardiol.* 1989;14:119–126.

38. McKay RG, Pfeffer MA, Pasternak RC, et al. Left ventricular remodeling after myocardial infarction: a corollary to infarct expansion. *Circulation.* 1986;74:693–702.

39. Pfeffer MA, Braunwald E. Ventricular remodeling after myocardial infarction. Experimental observations and clinical implications. *Circulation.* 1990;81:1161–1172.

40. Sutton MG, Sharpe N. Left ventricular remodeling after myocardial infarction: pathophysiology and therapy. *Circulation.* 2000;101:2981–2988.

41. Bouchard A, Lipton MJ, Farmer DW, et al. Evaluation of regional ventricular wall motion by ECG-gated CT. *J Comput Assist Tomogr.* 1987;11:969–974.

42. Himelman RB, Abbott JA, Lipton MJ, et al. Cine computed tomography compared with echocardiography in the evaluation of cardiac function in emphysema. *Am J Card Imaging.* 1988;2:283–291.

43. Halliburton SS, Petersilka M, Schvartzman PR, Obuchowski N, White RD. Evaluation of left ventricular dysfunction using multiphasic reconstructions of coronary multislice computed tomography data in patients with chronic ischemic heart disease: validation against cine magnetic resonance imaging. *Int J Cardiovasc Imaging.* 2003;19:73–83.

44. Juergens KU, Fischbach R. Left ventricular function studied with MDCT. *Eur Radiol.* 2006;16:342–357.

45. Mahnken AH, Koos R, Katoh M, et al. Sixteen-slice spiral CT versus MR imaging for the assessment of left ventricular function in acute myocardial infarction. *Eur Radiol.* 2005;15:714–720.

46. Boll DT, Gilkeson RC, Merkle EM, Fleiter TR, Duerk JL, Lewin JS. Functional cardiac CT and MR: effects of heart rate and software applications on measurement validity. *J Thorac Imaging.* 2005;20:10–16.

47. Schlosser T, Pagonidis K, Herborn CU, et al. Assessment of left ventricular parameters using 16-MDCT and new software for endocardial and epicardial border delineation. *AJR Am J Roentgenol.* 2005;184:765–773.

48. Heuschmid M, Rothfuss JK, Schroeder S, et al. Assessment of left ventricular myocardial function using 16-slice multidetector-row computed tomography: comparison with magnetic resonance imaging and echocardiography. *Eur Radiol.* 2006;16:551–559.

49. Hundt W, Siebert K, Wintersperger BJ, et al. Assessment of global left ventricular function: comparison of cardiac multidetector-row computed tomography with angiocardiography. *J Comput Assist Tomogr.* 2005;29:373–381.

50. Kim TH, Hur J, Kim SJ, et al. Two-phase reconstruction for the assessment of left ventricular volume and function using retrospective ECG-gated MDCT: comparison with echocardiography. *AJR Am J Roentgenol.* 2005;185:319–325.

51. Salm LP, Schuijf JD, de Roos A, et al. Global and regional left ventricular function assessment with 16-detector row CT: comparison with echocardiography and cardiovascular magnetic resonance. *Eur J Echocardiogr.* 2006;7:308–314.

52. Woodard PK. Science to practice: can multi-detector row spiral CT be used to assess left ventricular function? *Radiology.* 2005;236:1–2.

53. Reiter SJ, Rumberger JA, Feiring AJ, Stanford W, Marcus ML. Precision of measurements of right and left ventricular volume by cine computed tomography. *Circulation.* 1986;74:890–900.

54. Macmillan RM, Rees MR. Measurement of right and left ventricular volumes in human by cine computed tomography: comparison to biplane cineangiography. *Am J Card Imag.* 1988;2:214–219.

55. Ringertz HG, Rodgers B, Lipton MJ, Cann C, Carlsson E. Assessment of human right ventricular cast volume by CT and angiocardiography. *Invest Radiol.* 1985;20:29–32.

56. Feiring AJ, Rumberger JA, Reiter SJ, et al. Sectional and segmental variability of left ventricular function: experimental and clinical studies using ultrafast computed tomography. *J Am Coll Cardiol.* 1988;12:415–425.

57. Lipton MJ, Farmer DW, Killebrew EJ, et al. Regional myocardial dysfunction: evaluation of patients with prior myocardial infarction with fast CT. *Radiology.* 1985;157:735–740.

58. Lanzer P, Garrett J, Lipton MJ, et al. Quantitation of regional myocardial function by cine computed tomography: pharmacologic changes in wall thickness. *J Am Coll Cardiol.* 1986;8:682–692.

59. Caputo G, Gould R, Dery R, et al. Ultrafast CT evaluation of exercise induced ischemia: a feasibility study. *Dynamic Cardiovasc Imaging.* 1989;2:110–119.

60. Lipton MJ, Rumberger JA. Exercise ultrafast computed tomography: preliminary findings on its role in diagnosis and prognosis of coronary artery disease. *J Am Coll Cardiol.* 1989;13:1082–1084.

61. Roig E, Chomka EV, Castaner A, et al. Exercise ultrafast computed tomography for the detection of coronary artery disease. *J Am Coll Cardiol.* 1989;13:1073–1081.

62. Skioldebrand CG, Lipton MJ, Mavroudis C, Hayashi TT. Determination of left ventricular mass by computed tomography. *Am J Cardiol.* 1982;49:63–70.

63. Feiring AJ, Rumberger JA, Reiter SJ, et al. Determination of left ventricular mass in dogs with rapid-acquisition cardiac computed tomographic scanning. *Circulation.* 1985;72:1355–1364.

64. Diethelm L, Simonson JS, Dery R, Gould RG, Schiller NB, Lipton MJ. Determination of left ventricular mass with ultrafast CT and two-dimensional echocardiography. *Radiology.* 1989;171:213–217.

65. Boxt LM, Lipton MJ, Kwong RY, Rybicki F, Clouse ME. Computed tomography for assessment of cardiac chambers, valves, myocardium and pericardium. *Cardiol Clin.* 2003;21:561–585.

20 Assessment of Myocardial Viability by Cardiac MRI

Raymond Y. Kwong

Fundamental Physical Properties of MRI

Current clinical magnetic resonance imaging (MRI) techniques are based on detection of protons (^{1}H) that are bound to mostly water and macromolecules (such as in fat or protein) of the body. ^{1}H is very abundant in the body, and this property provides adequate signal-to-noise ratio for image generation at the magnetic field strengths (B_0) of current clinical MRI scanners (1.5 Tesla). The single positively charged proton itself functions much like a tiny tissue magnet inside a magnetic field. When a patient is placed in an MRI scanner, each proton aligns with the magnetic field and spins around its axis (a process known as precession) at a frequency defined by the magnitude of the magnetic field in Tesla. When a given direction and magnitude of the B_0 magnetic field are manipulated by applying a secondary magnetic field (radiofrequency pulse), the protons within a part of the body of imaging interest can then be "excited." These excited protons release a specific magnetic resonance signal (known as free induction decay) that contains structural and physical information on the tissues being imaged. To create an MR image, a set of gradient coils in the MRI provides the relevant three-dimensional spatial coordinates (x, y, and z) and detects the intensity of the magnetic resonance signal in each of the coordinates. Utilizing the fast speed of modern computers for data acquisition and digital processing, static or dynamic magnetic resonance images that provide crucial information of tissue functions can be rapidly acquired.

Cardiac MRI Approaches to the Assessment of Myocardial Viability

Ventricular Function, Chamber Size, and Myocardial Mass

A number of clinical studies have documented the strong associations of global ventricular function, volume, and myocardial mass to clinical outcomes in patients with coronary artery disease (CAD).[1,2] An accurate assessment of biventricular global and regional function can provide information about the extent of myocardial viability or ischemia and thus help planning of coronary intervention. To assess ventricular function and chamber sizes with the heart in constant motion, relatively high (<50 milliseconds) temporal and spatial (<2 mm) resolutions are required for accurate definition of cardiac anatomy and ventricular function. Cardiac magnetic resonance imaging

(CMR) is well validated by both in vitro and in vivo methods in quantifying global and regional ventricular functions, chamber sizes, and myocardial masses.[3–5] CMR is the current reference-standard imaging technique for assessment of myocardial function and morphology. The accuracy of CMR for measurement of global left and right ventricular volumes has been demonstrated by comparing CMR of ex vivo ventricles with the water displacement volume of casts of the ventricles.[4] Assessment of biventricular function and stroke volume have been validated in vivo by comparing them with the great vessel flows.[6] Assessment of myocardial mass has been validated against human autopsied hearts and in animals.[3,5]

Several technical advantages of CMR over other imaging modalities have made it the current gold-standard technique for assessing ventricular function and myocardial mass. Compared to two-dimensional (2D) or even three-dimensional (3D) echocardiography, the tomographic 3D imaging capability of CMR is not restricted by an acoustic imaging window, does not require the use of geometric assumptions, and provides superior delineation of the endocardial and epicardial borders.[7] Compared to nuclear imaging techniques such as single photon emission computed tomography (SPECT) and positron emission tomography (PET), CMR can more accurately assess biventricular function and myocardial morphology with superior spatial resolution, temporal resolutions, and tissue contrast. Widespread use of the steady-state free precession techniques for cine imaging[8] provides signal-to-noise ratio and myocardium-blood contrast that is superior to conventional gradient-echo techniques (Figures 20.1 and 20.2). One distinct feature of CMR is its excellent interstudy reproducibility in measuring ventricular function and myocardial mass compared to other imaging techniques. CMR is therefore well suited for noninvasive longitudinal follow-up of patients with heart failure and for myocardial remodeling research with small sample sizes.[9,10]

Delayed Myocardial Contrast Enhancement

Recent advances in hardware and pulse sequences have allowed accurate characterization of infarcted myocardium with high spatial resolution using a

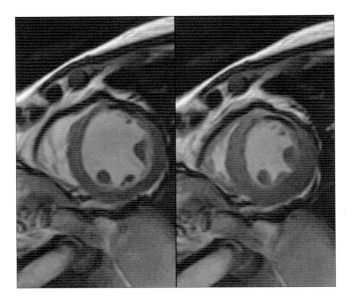

FIGURE 20.1. Steady-state free precession short-axis cine imaging of the heart. Structural details of the left ventricular myocardium during diastole (left) and systole (right) are provided from this CMR technique. Note the anterior akinesia in this patient who suffered from a previous myocardial infarction. This technique can assess myocardial structure and function at an in-plane spatial resolution of 1.5 mm, temporal resolution of 40 to 50 milliseconds, and high signal-to-noise ratio.

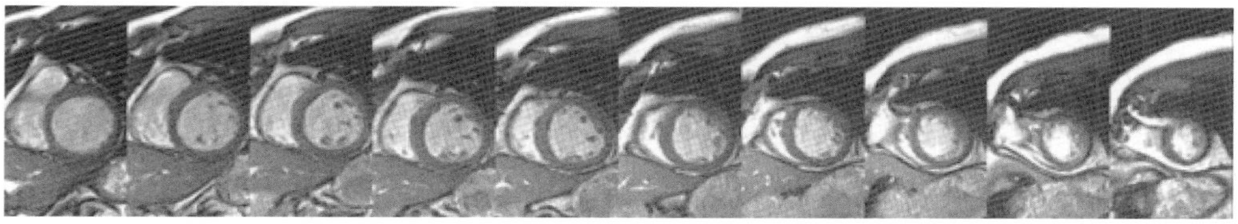

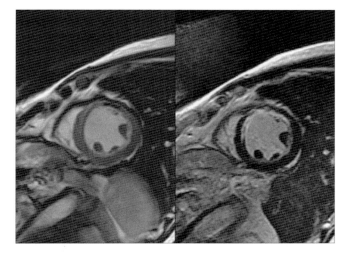

FIGURE 20.2. Volumetric quantitation of ventricular function, size, and myocardial mass by cine CMR. Using a tomographic technique, volumetric cine imaging of the heart without geometric assumption could be obtained over 3 to 4 minutes without the need for contrast injection. This CMR technique can be performed with or without patient breath holding.

contrast-enhanced technique known as late myocardial enhancement.[11] Using an inversion recovery pulse sequence to enhance tissue contrast, imaging of the infarcted myocardium at an in-plane spatial resolution of 1 to 2 mm is performed after injection of an intravenous dose of gadolinium-based contrast agent. The interstitial space in normal myocardial tissue allows little or no entry of the extracellular gadolinium contrast agent due to uniform tightly packed muscle. When this extracellular compartment is enlarged due to cellular rupture from myocardial infarction, entry of the extracellular gadolinium occurs and creates a strong enhancing effect in the region of myonecrosis on T1-weighted imaging. The maximal contrast created by the infiltration of gadolinium contrast in this technique is achieved after a delay of 10 to 20 minutes following contrast injection. With administration of a gadolinium-based contrast agent, this CMR technique images the myocardium with high tissue contrast at much higher spatial resolution (1.5 to 2 mm) than other conventional techniques (Figure 20.3).

Magnetic Resonance Spectroscopy

Beyond imaging of cardiac structure, function, and myocardial morphology, magnetic resonance spectroscopy (MRS) is a technique that can provide information regarding cellular metabolism and, thus, myocardial viability. Free energy for myocardial function in the form of adenosine triphosphate (ATP) is produced and stored primarily in mitochondria. Under the catalytic action of creatine kinase, phosphocreatine (PCr)

FIGURE 20.3. Contrast-enhanced late enhancement CMR imaging. Ten to 20 minutes after an intravenous administration of gadolinium-diethylenetriaminepentacetic acid (DTPA) contrast, infarcted myocardium matching the anterior akinetic segments demonstrate enhancement of signal intensity on average of 5 to 6 times that of the normal myocardium.

acts as a free-energy carrier between sites of free-energy production (e.g., mitochondria) with sites of free-energy consumption (e.g., myofibrils or ion transport channels at the cell membrane) through diffusion. Therefore, by quantifying the concentrations and ratios of PCr and ATP in a small volume of myocardium, phosphorus-31 (^{31}P) spectroscopy can assess myocardial energy metabolism and thus determine the integrity of myocyte function. Yabe et al were able to demonstrate that MRS could differentiate myocardial viability in patients who suffered an acute myocardial infarction by comparing them with evidence of viability by thallium redistribution.[12] Weiss et al demonstrated that the transient decrease in the phosphocreatine-to-ATP ratio was related to myocardial ischemia induced by hand-grip exercise.[13] However, the relative low concentration of high-energy phosphate molecules has resulted in a low signal-to-noise ratio and a limited sensitivity compared to other techniques. In addition, due to signal dropout as distance away from the surface coil increases, the ^{31}P MRS technique can assess only the anterior wall of the left ventricle. These limitations have currently hampered the clinical application of this technique. Creatine kinase reaction in the myocardium serves as the heart's main energy reserve. Proton (^{1}H) MRS has up to 20 times the sensitivity of ^{31}P MRS and can quantify both phosphorylated and unphosphorylated creatine in myocardium from any part of the left ventricle. Bottomley and Weiss et al developed and validated the technique using ^{1}H MRS with animal models of myocardial infarction and found that assessing regional depletion of myocardial creatine provides a metabolic method to distinguish healthy from infarcted nonviable myocardium (Figure 20.4).[14] Future work is needed to compare the relative merits of MRS and CMR imaging techniques.

Disadvantages of CMR include study contraindications such as the presence of hazardous metallic implants (pacemakers and defibrillators being most common) and patient claustrophobia. In addition, cardiac gating problems limit patients' ability for breath holding, and the presence of thoracic metals such as sternal wires or intracoro-

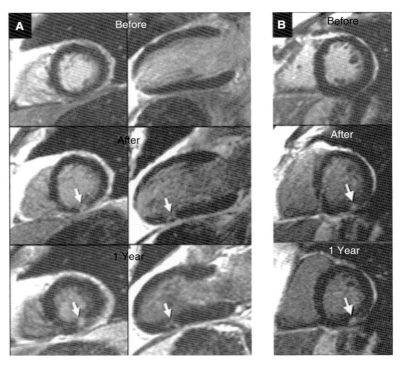

FIGURE 20.4. Sensitive detection of discrete myonecrosis secondary to percutaneous coronary intervention, without development of regional wall motion abnormality or Q waves on electroncardiogram (ECG). (Reprinted from Reference 19, with permission from Lippincott Williams and Wilkins.)

nary stents occasionally causes image-quality deterioration. In this author's experience, with proper premedication using a low-dose benzodiazepine, CMR can be performed safely and successfully in the majority of patients who report to be claustrophobic. Careful placement of thoracic gating leads can minimize the incidence of gating failure. By manipulating specific imaging parameters, metal artifacts can be minimized and technically adequate imaging data can be obtained during entirely free breathing in many patients who cannot breath hold due to their medical conditions.

CMR Assessment of Myocardial Changes After Acute Myocardial Infarction: Postinfarct Remodeling

Compared to all other noninvasive imaging modalities, CMR is the best suited to follow changes in postinfarct left ventricular geometry, ventricular global and regional function, myocardial perfusion, and infarct morphology. While many animal studies have used this imaging advantage for assessing the effects of pharmacological therapy of LV remodeling after acute infarction,[15–17] human studies using CMR are being performed with increasing frequency, capitalizing on the high precision of CMR imaging. While the efficacy of these pharmacological, interventional, or stem cell treatments need further study, CMR's capability is now recognized for quantifying cardiac function and infarct morphology for detecting treatment effects in a small patient sample size.

CMR Viability Imaging in Chronic CAD

CMR has proven to be highly sensitive in detecting the presence of small areas of myocardial scar from coronary artery disease. Because resting segmental function is inversely proportional to the transmural extent of myocardial infarction, segmental normokinesia or contractile reserve does not necessarily exclude the presence of regional endomyocardial necrosis.[18] Ricciardi et al studied a small group of patients without prior myocardial infarction who developed an average twofold elevation of serum creatine kinase-MB isoenzyme after percutaneous coronary intervention.[19] Contrast-enhanced delay enhancement techniques detected discrete myonecrosis in all the patients who were missed by cine wall motion imaging. In addition, the high resolution of CMR allows detection of subendocardial infarcts that are often missed by SPECT.[20] The clinical and prognostic implications of these findings are under active investigation.

Predicting Recovery of LV Function Following Coronary Revascularization

Wall Thickness and Contractile Reserve

Cine function CMR imaging at a resolution of 1.5 to 2 mm can characterize myocardial wall thickness and segmental and global left ventricular function with high accuracy and reproducibility.[21–23] Baer studied 43 patients with chronic infarction and mild LV dysfunction (mean left ventricular ejection fraction $42 \pm 10\%$) with dobutamine cine CMR before and 4 to 6 months after successful revascularization. An end-diastolic wall thickness cutoff of ≥ 5.5 mm (based on -2.5 SD from normal individuals) had a 92% sensitivity but only a 56% specificity for predicting recovery of segmental function after revascularization.[24–26] The limited predictive accuracy of segmental contractile recovery by end-diastolic wall thickness is not surprising since myocardial wall thickness often includes subendocardial irreversibly damaged myocardial tissue and a thinned epicardial rim of viable myocardium, which may not be sufficient to result in improved function after successful coronary revascularization.[25,26] Myocardial thickness has limited independent utility in predicting future segmental recovery also during the acute or subacute phase of myocardial infarction when local infarct remodeling is incomplete (up to 6 months post–acute infarction). In this setting, local edema and cellular infiltrates may increase regional wall thickness. Augmentation of regional contractility (i.e., improvement of wall thickening upon an inotropic challenge) in response to inotropic stimulus such as low-dose (5 to 10 µg/kg/min) dobutamine challenge has been well validated in identifying segmental viability from both the vast body of evidence from echocardiography and cine CMR.[24,27,28] Demonstration of segmental contractile reserve by cine CMR is a safe and reliable method for predicting recovery from coronary artery disease by either qualitative or quantitative methods. Baer et al also assessed the utility of a combined criterion of wall thickness and contractile reserve using cine CMR at rest and at low-dose dobutamine challenge to predict contractile recovery of any infarcted segments. Myocardial viability in an infarcted region was defined by a diastolic wall thickness of ≥5.5 mm and the presence of systolic wall thickening of ≥2 mm in at least 50% of the dysfunctional segments of the infarcted region. Although a resting wall thickness of ≥5.5 mm showed a high sensitivity for identifying viable myocardial segments (92%), their study showed a low specificity—56%. However, a physiological contractile reserve, as demonstrated by a systolic wall thickening of ≥2 mm, demonstrated an improved specificity and a preserved sensitivity in the prediction of segmental contractile recovery after revascularization (sensitivity 89%; specificity 94%).

Other similar studies consistently reported high specificity using contractile reserve by dobutamine CMR in identifying viable myocardial segments.[27,28] Geskin et al assessed the utility of low-dose dobutamine cine CMR in predicting myocardial viability in the early period after acute myocardial infarction.[29] In this study, quantitative analysis of segmental myocardial function was made possible with the use of magnetic resonance high-resolution tagging techniques, which allowed quantitation of the intramyocardial circumferential shortening and minimized the effect of through-plane motion on segmental contraction during low-dose dobutamine challenge (Figure 20.5). This study concluded that early after acute myocardial infarction, dysfunctional but viable myocardial segments can be identified by an exaggerated circumferential shortening in the subepicardial and midmyocardial layers compared to those of normal segments (Figure 20.6). One potential limitation exists in using only dobutamine cine contractile reserve in detecting segmental viability. Although excellent specificity for predicting segmental contractile recovery has been consistently reported, the sensitivity of low-dose dobutamine contractile reserve imaging has been in only the moderate range (50% to 76%) in segments with resting akinesia or dyskinesia.[28,30] This is attributed to the fact that in the presence of severe coronary stenosis and hypoperfusion, viable myocardial segments may fail to demonstrate contractile reserve with low-dose dobutamine due to rapid development of ischemia.[30]

Beyond detection of segmental myocardial viability, by further escalating the dobutamine infusion to achieve an adequate heart-rate response, cine CMR imaging can accurately detect myocardial ischemia. Nagel et al reported a sensitivity of 86% and a specificity of 86% using dobutamine stress cine CMR in detecting angiographically significant coronary artery disease.[7] Hundley et al reported similar utility in detecting coronary artery disease and also demonstrated strong prediction of adverse cardiac events by dobutamine cine CMR.[31,32]

Late Contrast Enhancement

While the concept of late enhancement observed in infarcted myocardium has long been recognized,[33] limitation in image quality has restricted the clinical application of contrast-enhanced CMR techniques until recent years. Over the past few years,

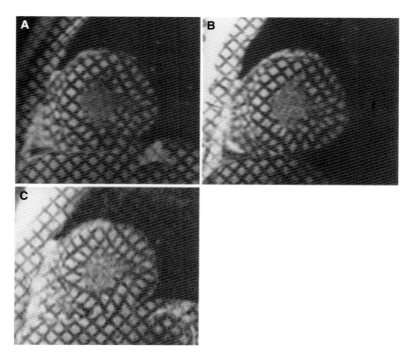

FIGURE 20.5. (A) End-systolic apical MR tagged short-axis image in a patient on day 5 after anterior MI. Right ventricular apex and interventricular septum lie from 6 o'clock to 9 o'clock positions on image, anterior wall from 9 o'clock to 12 o'clock, lateral wall from 12 o'clock to 3 o'clock, and inferior wall from 3 o'clock to 6 o'clock. The percent intramyocardial circumferential segment shortening (%S) was −3% in anterior wall, denoting stretching rather than shortening; 3% in septum (reduced compared with normal database); and 15% in lateral wall (also reduced). (B) End-systolic apical MR tagged short-axis image in same patient at end of $10\text{-}\mu g/kg^{-1}/min^{-1}$ dobutamine stage. Qualitatively, there is no more stretching in the anterior wall, but otherwise it is difficult to discern significant changes within other regions. Quantitatively, %S increased to 8% in anterior wall, 9% in septum, and 24% in lateral wall, all normal responses (≥5% increase). C, End-systolic apical MR tagged short-axis image in same patient at 8 weeks after MI. Function has improved all around short axis, and end-systolic cavity area is reduced. Quantitatively, %S has increased to 24% in anterior wall, 18% in septum, and 27% in lateral wall, all of which fall within range of normal. (Reprinted from Reference 29, with permission from Lippincott Williams and Wilkins.)

FIGURE 20.6. Quantification of percent intramyocardial circumferential segment shortening (%S) in 2 groups of regions, those with normal response (≥5% increase) to peak dobutamine and those with abnormal response (<5% increase) shown at baseline before dobutamine infusion (hatched bars) and at 8 weeks after infarction. Increase in %S from baseline to 8 weeks after MI in normal response group is significantly greater than that in abnormal response group ($p<0.04$). (Reprinted from Reference 29, with permission from Lippincott, Williams and Wilkins.)

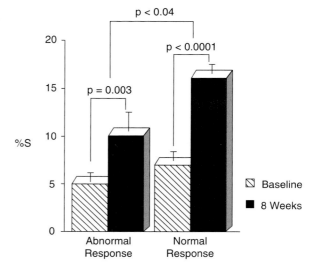

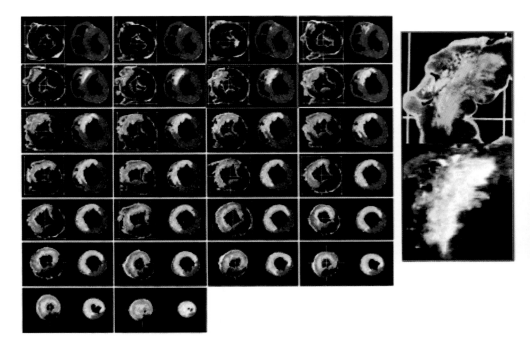

FIGURE 20.7. Comparison of ex vivo CMR images with triphenyl tetrazolium chloride (TTC)-stained slices in an animal at 3 days after myocardial infarction. Slices are arranged from base to apex starting at the upper left and advancing left to right, then top to bottom. At the right is a magnified view. (Reprinted from Reference 34, with permission from Lippincott Williams and Wilkins.)

advances in pulse sequence techniques, surface coils, and electrocardiogram (ECG) gating have resulted in substantial improvements in image quality of myocardial infarction by CMR delayed enhancement technique. Many animal and human studies have since demonstrated the utility of CMR contrast-enhanced delayed enhancement imaging technique in imaging myocardial infarction and in determining segmental viability. Quantitative assessments of the size and the transmural extent of myocardial infarction have been extensively validated in experimental animals. Kim et al utilized this technique in a study of 18 dogs and demonstrated that CMR accurately depicts histologically defined necrosis in both reperfused and nonreperfused myocardial infarction (Figure 20.7). On average, the tissue signal intensity of the infarcted myocardium is 5 to 6 times higher than that of normal tissue, which allows sensitive detection of myonecrosis and accurate delineation of the transmural extent of infarction.[20,34–38]

Kim et al also first reported the clinical utility of this technique in 804 dysfunctional myocardial segments from 50 patients with chronic coronary artery disease who underwent successful coronary revascularization.[35] A progressive, stepwise decrease in the likelihood of function recovery for a given segment was observed as the transmural extent of myocardial scar detected by contrast-enhanced CMR increased. It was further reported that the prediction of segmental functional recovery was even stronger in segments with resting akinesia or dyskinesia. For example, 88% of segments with <25% transmural extent of delayed enhancement improved contractile function, whereas only 4% of segments with >50% transmural extent of delayed contrast enhancement improved function after revascularization. Regions of myocardial scar on average demonstrated signal intensity of more than 500% of that of regions without delayed enhancement. In addition, the measured percentage of the left ventricle that demonstrated dysfunctional myocardium but without delayed enhancement was strongly related to improvement of both global and regional ventricular function after coronary revascularization.

Klein et al directly compared contrast-enhanced late enhancement CMR to PET imaging in 23 patients with severe global left ventricular dysfunction (left ventricular ejection fraction 28 ± 9%).[39] While late enhancement CMR closely correlated to areas of decreased flow and FDG metabolism (perfusion-metabolic matched defect) by PET, contrast-enhanced CMR identified subendocardial scar tissue more frequently than PET imaging did, reflecting CMR's higher spatial resolution. Similar results were reported when contrast-enhanced CMR was compared to SPECT.[20]

Two single-center studies systematically assessed the relative merits of dobutamine cine CMR and late enhancement techniques.[40,41] Motoyasu et al performed low-dose dobutamine cine CMR and late enhancement in 23 patients within 1 month after acute myocardial infarction and predicted superior receiver operating characteristic (ROC) by the dobutamine cine CMR technique over the late enhancement technique (ROC area under the curve of 0.87 by cine CMR vs 0.78 by late enhancement technique).[40] Wellnhofer et al assessed 29 patients prior to and 3 months after coronary revascularization with both low-dose dobutamine cine imaging and late enhancement imaging and reported similar findings.[41] While controversy remains whether dobutamine cine CMR or the late enhancement technique provides more comprehensive assessment of myocardial viability in the planning of mechanical coronary revascularization, this author's interpretation of the current evidence suggests that both techniques provide physiological significance and can be complementary in specific patient cases. Low-dose dobutamine cine imaging enjoys vastly greater prognostic experience over both dobutamine echocardiography and CMR.[42,43] The high specificity from low-dose dobutamine cine imaging provides a physiologic assessment of the midmyocardial and subepicardial contractile reserve, particularly in segments with subendocardial infarction involving less than 75% of the transmural extent.[29,41] In this author's opinion, patients with multiple comorbidities at very high procedural risks can benefit from the physiologic information obtained from low-dose dobutamine cine contractile reserve assessment. In this clinical setting, an imaging technique with an excellent specificity is needed to justify the risk of the coronary revascularization procedure. On the other hand, late enhancement technique provides high sensitivity (in contrast to dobutamine cine contractile reserve) in the prediction of contractile recovery in segments with resting akinesia or dyskinesia. It is simple to perform without the need for dobutamine challenge in patients with significant coronary stenosis. While late enhancement imaging provides a stepwise prediction of the likelihood of contractile recovery as well as improvement in global left ventricular function, a transmural extent of ≥75% rules out segmental contractile recovery with high certainty. For these reasons, this author's CMR center routinely performs both late enhancement technique and low-dose dobutamine challenge whenever feasible.

Even if functional improvement after revascularization is considered to be a relevant clinical endpoint of myocardial viability, it cannot be overemphasized that patients' benefits to coronary revascularization probably extend much beyond recovery of segmental contractile function. Samady et al demonstrated significant improvement of postrevascularization patient survival despite a lack of left ventricular functional improvement.[44] Although it remains unproven, it is conceivable that restoration of normal coronary perfusion by mechanical revascularization may offer prognostic advantages by mechanisms such as protection against infarction/ischemia in other stenotic coronary arterial territory and improved electrical stability in the peri-infarct zone. After an acute myocardial infarction, late patency of the infarct-related artery is also important since it may lessen the burden of adverse ventricular remodeling in the postinfarction period.[45] Therefore, other factors such as coexisting comorbidities, likelihood of successful myocardial reperfusion from revascularization, and procedural risk must be included in conjunction with the diagnostic information from viability imaging in evaluating the risk-benefit ratio of mechanical coronary revascularization.

Summary Points

- CMR is an accurate clinical method that provides useful physiological and prognostic information for the planning of invasive coronary intervention in patients with coronary artery disease.
- Combining structural and functional information of the left ventricle at rest and during inotropic dobutamine stress, the physiologic contractile reserve and the likelihood of benefit from revascularization can be determined.
- During the same imaging session, the transmural extent of the infarcted myocardium can also be determined, which provides a sensitive and stepwise estimate of segmental contractile recovery.
- In this author's experience, these techniques provide complementary assessment of myocardial physiology and morphology that is highly accurate for the prediction of benefits in patient outcome and in cardiac function.
- With more efficient image acquisition due to advances in hardware and pulse sequence techniques with or without contrast administration, a CMR examination that takes less than 1 hour is generally well tolerated by most patients; it has now become a routine clinical tool in many tertiary-care centers.
- In addition to the absence of ionizing radiation, the use of hypoallergenic nonnephrotoxic contrast agents in CMR also provide an additional level of safety in patients with allergic potentials or renal dysfunction.
- Magnetic resonance spectroscopy demands a high degree of technical expertise and specialized equipment; however, it provides a unique assessment of myocardial energy metabolism that can determine the status of myocardial viability.

References

1. Borow KM, Green LH, Mann T, et al. End-systolic volume as a predictor of postoperative left ventricular performance in volume overload from valvular regurgitation. *Am J Med.* 1980;68:655–663.
2. White HD, Norris RM, Brown MA, Brandt PW, Whitlock RM, Wild CJ. Left ventricular end-systolic volume as the major determinant of survival after recovery from myocardial infarction. *Circulation.* 1987;76:44–51.
3. Bloomgarden DC, Fayad ZA, Ferrari VA, Chin B, Sutton MG, Axel L. Global cardiac function using fast breath-hold MRI: validation of new acquisition and analysis techniques. *Magn Reson Med.* 1997;37:683–692.
4. Longmore DB, Klipstein RH, Underwood SR, et al. Dimensional accuracy of magnetic resonance in studies of the heart. *Lancet.* 1985;1:1360–1362.
5. Myerson SG, Bellenger NG, Pennell DJ. Assessment of left ventricular mass by cardiovascular magnetic resonance. *Hypertension.* 2002;39:750–755.
6. Firmin DN, Nayler GL, Klipstein RH, Underwood SR, Rees RS, Longmore DB. In vivo validation of MR velocity imaging. *Comput Assist Tomogr.* 1987;11:751–756.
7. Nagel E, Lehmkuhl HB, Bocksch W, et al. Noninvasive diagnosis of ischemia-induced wall motion abnormalities with the use of high-dose dobutamine stress MRI: comparison with dobutamine stress echocardiography. *Circulation.* 1999;99:763–770.
8. Barkhausen J, Ruehm SG, Goyen M, Buck T, Laub G, Debatin JF. MR evaluation of ventricular function: true fast imaging with steady-state precession versus fast low-angle shot cine MR imaging: feasibility study. *Radiology.* 2001;219:264–269.
9. Grothues F, Moon JC, Bellenger NG, Smith GS, Klein HU, Pennell DJ. Interstudy reproducibility of right ventricular volumes, function, and mass with cardiovascular magnetic resonance. *Am J Cardiol.* 2004;147:218–223.
10. Grothues F, Smith GC, Moon JC, et al. Comparison of interstudy reproducibility of cardiovascular magnetic resonance with two-dimensional echocardiography in normal subjects and in patients with heart failure or left ventricular hypertrophy. *Am Heart J.* 2002;90:29–34.
11. Simonetti OP, Kim RJ, Fieno DS, et al. An improved MR imaging technique for the visualization of myocardial infarction. *Radiology.* 2001;218:215–223.

12. Yabe T, Mitsunami K, Inubushi T, Kinoshita M. Quantitative measurements of cardiac phosphorus metabolites in coronary artery disease by 31P magnetic resonance spectroscopy. *Circulation*. 1995;92:15–23.

13. Weiss RG, Bottomley PA, Hardy CJ, Gerstenblith G. Regional myocardial metabolism of high-energy phosphates during isometric exercise in patients with coronary artery disease. *N Engl J Med*. 1990;323:1593–1600.

14. Bottomley PA, Weiss RG. Non-invasive magnetic-resonance detection of creatine depletion in non-viable infarcted myocardium. *Lancet*. 1998;351:714–718.

15. Kramer CM, Ferrari VA, Rogers WJ, et al. Angiotensin-converting enzyme inhibition limits dysfunction in adjacent noninfarcted regions during left ventricular remodeling. *J Am Coll Cardiol*. 1996;27:211–217.

16. McDonald KM, Rector T, Carlyle PF, Francis GS, Cohn JN. Angiotensin-converting enzyme inhibition and beta-adrenoceptor blockade regress established ventricular remodeling in a canine model of discrete myocardial damage. *J Am Coll Cardiol*. 1994;24: 1762–1768.

17. Saeed M, Wendland MF, Seelos K, Masui T, Derugin N, Higgins CB. Effect of cilazapril on regional left ventricular wall thickness and chamber dimension following acute myocardial infarction: in vivo assessment using MRI. *Am Heart J*. 1992;123:1472–1480.

18. Meza MF, Kates MA, Barbee RW, et al. Combination of dobutamine and myocardial contrast echocardiography to differentiate postischemic from infarcted myocardium. *J Am Coll Cardiol*. 1997;29:974–984.

19. Ricciardi MJ, Wu E, Davidson CJ, et al. Visualization of discrete microinfarction after percutaneous coronary intervention associated with mild creatine kinase-MB elevation. *Circulation*. 2001;103:2780–2783.

20. Wagner A, Mahrholdt H, Holly TA, et al. Contrast-enhanced MRI and routine single photon emission computed tomography (SPECT) perfusion imaging for detection of sub-endocardial myocardial infarcts: an imaging study. *Lancet*. 2003;361:374–379.

21. Alfakih K, Plein S, Thiele H, Jones T, Ridgway JP, Sivananthan MU. Normal human left and right ventricular dimensions for MRI as assessed by turbo gradient echo and steady-state free precession imaging sequences. *J Magn Reson Imaging*. 2003;17:323–329.

22. Grebe O, Kestler HA, Merkle N, et al. Assessment of left ventricular function with steady-state-free-precession magnetic resonance imaging. Reference values and a comparison to left ventriculography. *Z Cardiol*. 2004;93:686–695.

23. Kacere RD, Pereyra M, Nemeth MA, Muthupillai R, Flamm SD. Quantitative assessment of left ventricular function: steady-state free precession MR imaging with or without sensitivity encoding. *Radiology*. 2005;235:1031–1035.

24. Baer FM, Theissen P, Schneider CA, et al. Dobutamine magnetic resonance imaging predicts contractile recovery of chronically dysfunctional myocardium after successful revascularization. *J Am Coll Cardiol*. 1998;31:1040–1048.

25. Reimer KA, Jennings RB. The "wavefront phenomenon" of myocardial ischemic cell death. II. Transmural progression of necrosis within the framework of ischemic bed size (myocardium at risk) and collateral flow. *Lab Invest*. 1979;40:633–644.

26. Reimer KA, Lowe JE, Rasmussen MM, Jennings RB. The wavefront phenomenon of ischemic cell death. 1. Myocardial infarct size vs duration of coronary occlusion in dogs. *Circulation*. 1977;56:786–794.

27. Dendale PA, Franken PR, Waldman GJ, et al. Low-dosage dobutamine magnetic resonance imaging as an alternative to echocardiography in the detection of viable myocardium after acute infarction. *Am Heart J*. 1995;130:134–140.

28. Sandstede JJ, Bertsch G, Beer M, et al. Detection of myocardial viability by low-dose dobutamine cine MR imaging. *Magn Reson Imaging*. 1999;17:1437–1443.

29. Geskin G, Kramer CM, Rogers WJ, et al. Quantitative assessment of myocardial viability after infarction by dobutamine magnetic resonance tagging. *Circulation*. 1998;98:217–223.

30. Gunning MG, Anagnostopoulos C, Knight CJ, et al. Comparison of 201Tl, 99mTc-tetrofosmin, and dobutamine magnetic resonance imaging for identifying hibernating myocardium. *Circulation*. 1998;98:1869–1874.

31. Hundley WG, Hamilton CA, Thomas MS, et al. Utility of fast cine magnetic resonance imaging and display for the detection of myocardial ischemia in patients not well suited for second harmonic stress echocardiography. *Circulation*. 1999;100:1697–1702.

32. Hundley WG, Morgan TM, Neagle CM, Hamilton CA, Rerkpattanapipat P, Link KM. Magnetic resonance imaging determination of cardiac prognosis. *Circulation.* 2002;106: 2328–2333.

33. Wesbey GE, Higgins CB, McNamara MT, et al. Effect of gadolinium-DTPA on the magnetic relaxation times of normal and infarcted myocardium. *Radiology.* 1984;153:165–169.

34. Kim RJ, Fieno DS, Parrish TB, et al. Relationship of MRI delayed contrast enhancement to irreversible injury, infarct age, and contractile function. *Circulation.* 1999;100: 1992–2002.

35. Kim RJ, Wu E, Rafael A, et al. The use of contrast-enhanced magnetic resonance imaging to identify reversible myocardial dysfunction. *N Engl J Med.* 2000;343:1445–1453.

36. Fieno DS, Kim RJ, Chen EL, Lomasney JW, Klocke FJ, Judd RM. Contrast-enhanced magnetic resonance imaging of myocardium at risk: distinction between reversible and irreversible injury throughout infarct healing. *J Am Coll Cardiol.* 2000;36:1985–1991.

37. Oshinski JN, Yang Z, Jones JR, Mata JF, French BA. Imaging time after Gd-DTPA injection is critical in using delayed enhancement to determine infarct size accurately with magnetic resonance imaging. *Circulation.* 2001;104:2838–2842.

38. Rehwald WG, Fieno DS, Chen EL, Kim RJ, Judd RM. Myocardial magnetic resonance imaging contrast agent concentrations after reversible and irreversible ischemic injury. *Circulation.* 2002;105:224–229.

39. Klein C, Nekolla SG, Bengel FM, et al. Assessment of myocardial viability with contrast-enhanced magnetic resonance imaging: comparison with positron emission tomography. *Circulation.* 2002;105:162–167.

40. Motoyasu M, Sakuma H, Ichikawa Y, et al. Prediction of regional functional recovery after acute myocardial infarction with low dose dobutamine stress cine MR imaging and contrast enhanced MR imaging. *J Cardiovasc Magn Reson.* 2003;5:563–574.

41. Wellnhofer E, Olariu A, Klein C, et al. Magnetic resonance low-dose dobutamine test is superior to SCAR quantification for the prediction of functional recovery. *Circulation.* 2004;109:2172–2174.

42. Marwick TH, Case C, Sawada S, et al. Prediction of mortality using dobutamine echocardiography. *J Am Coll Cardiol.* 2001;37:754–760.

43. Poldermans D, Fioretti PM, Boersma E, et al. Long-term prognostic value of dobutamine-atropine stress echocardiography in 1737 patients with known or suspected coronary artery disease: a single-center experience. *Circulation.* 1999;99:757–762.

44. Samady H, Elefteriades JA, Abbott BG, Mattera JA, McPherson CA, Wackers FJ. Failure to improve left ventricular function after coronary revascularization for ischemic cardiomyopathy is not associated with worse outcome. *Circulation.* 1999;100:1298–1304.

45. Kondo H, Suzuki T, Fukutomi T, et al. Effects of percutaneous coronary arterial thrombectomy during acute myocardial infarction on left ventricular remodeling. *Am J Cardiol.* 2004;93:527–531.

21 Comparison of Imaging Modalities in the Assessment of Myocardial Viability

James E. Udelson, John Finley IV, and Vasken Dilsizian

Since initial reports that regional myocardial dysfunction is not always irreversible, the assessment of whether dysfunctional myocardial tissue or regions contain predominantly viable myocytes has become an important research and clinical issue for noninvasive imaging. Imaging of myocardial perfusion, myocyte cell membrane integrity, regional myocardial metabolism, and contractile reserve has provided important insights into the pathophysiology of hibernating and stunned myocardium. From a clinical perspective, the wealth of data built by many clinical investigators over the years has made noninvasive imaging of myocardial viability an important factor in treatment decisions for patients with heart failure, chronic coronary artery disease (CAD), and left ventricular (LV) dysfunction. Some of the historical milestones in this field are listed in Table 21.1.

Several sources are available that analyze the literature on the predictive value of noninvasive imaging modalities for regional functional recovery or other outcomes in patients with chronic CAD and LV dysfunction.[1–3] In this review, we will evaluate the strengths and weaknesses of the various imaging modalities that have been studied to assess viability, in the context of the clinical endpoints being addressed.

Historical Perspective: The Retrospective Recognition of Viable Dysfunctional Myocardium

Prior to the 1980s, impaired LV function at rest was predominantly thought to represent an irreversible process. The introduction and subsequent growth of the concepts of stunned and hibernating myocardium in the mid-1970s to early 1980s dramatically changed the application of noninvasive techniques in guiding therapeutic decisions for revascularization.

In 1975, Heyndrickx and coworkers showed that impaired regional mechanical function following coronary occlusions could persist for hours without myocardial infarction.[4] Following a plethora of experimental and clinical studies, delayed recovery of contractile function following a period of ischemia was termed *stunned myocardium*.[5] Interestingly, the concept of hibernating myocardium arose initially

TABLE 21.1. Historical Points in the Evolution of Assessment of Myocardial Viability

- Late 1970s to early 1980s: Retrospective studies recognizing that dysfunctional myocardium may improve function after revascularization by CABG
- Early to mid-1980s: Description of hibernating myocardium; potential prospective identification by invasive observations of improved regional function by left ventriculogram after nitroglycerin or with postextrasystolic potentiation
- Mid-1980s: Initial recognition that all "fixed defects" are not all representative of infarct and that quantitative analysis of the degree of ^{201}Tl uptake within fixed defects correlated with the probability of improved perfusion after CABG; opened the possibility that radionuclide imaging could prospectively identify potential improvement in perfusion or function, noninvasively
- Mid-1980s: Initial description of reversible resting ^{201}Tl defects and potential implications
- Late 1980s: Prospective noninvasive evaluation of the probability of postrevascularization functional recovery by PET imaging of perfusion and metabolism
- Late 1980s: Beginning of the evolution of ^{201}Tl imaging protocols to optimize assessment of viability, including late redistribution imaging
- Late 1980s to early 1990s: Initial reports of ^{201}Tl reinjection to optimize assessment of viability
- Early 1990s: Reports of contractile reserve by dobutamine echocardiography to assess viability
- Early to mid-1990s: Further evolution and understanding of ^{201}Tl protocols, including quantitative assessment of defect severity after reinjection
- Early to mid-1990s: Evaluation of other PET tracers and techniques, including imaging of fatty acids and tissue perfusible index
- Mid-1990s: Initial reports of the use of technetium-99m agents for assessing viability in animal models and in humans
- Mid-1990s: Biopsy and tissue studies correlating SPECT and PET imaging parameters and dobutamine echocardiography with direct measures of tissue or myocyte viability
- Mid- to late 1990s: Numerous reports on predicting functional recovery; initial reports on predicting other endpoints after revascularization, including improved symptoms and survival, as well as the prognostic importance of the presence of viability
- Mid- to late 1990s: Nitrate-enhanced imaging for ^{201}Tl and technetium-99m agents
- Late 1990s: Importance of incorporating evaluation of inducible ischemia into viability evaluation
- Late 1990s: Reports of contrast echocardiography to assess microvascular integrity
- Late 1990s to early 2000s: Other techniques, such as NOGA mapping and hyperenhancement cardiac MR imaging, emerge
- Mid-2000s: Concepts from hyperenhancement MR imaging applied to cardiac CT

from clinical rather than experimental observations.[6,7] In patients with chronic ischemic heart disease undergoing coronary artery bypass graft (CABG) surgery, improvements in both regional and global left ventricular function were often observed at rest.[8,9] Approximately one third of patients with preoperative LV dysfunction manifest significant increases in ventricular function after CABG, with normalization of ejection fraction in approximately one fourth of patients.[10]

Current understanding supports the concept that the myocardium has several mechanisms of acute and chronic adaptation to a temporary or sustained reduction in coronary blood flow, known as stunning, hibernation, and ischemic preconditioning.[11] These responses to ischemia preserve sufficient energy to protect the structural and functional integrity of the cardiac myocyte. In contrast to programmed cell death, or apoptosis, the term *programmed cell survival* has been used to describe the commonality among myocardial stunning, hibernation, and ischemic preconditioning, despite their distinct pathophysiology.[12]

From the mid-1970s to the early 1980s, a number of methods were introduced to assess regional LV contractile reserve in asynergic regions during invasive contrast or noninvasive radionuclide ventriculography. These included enhanced regional contractile reserve during nitroglycerin administration,[13] during postextrasystolic potentiation,[14] during low-dose catecholamine infusion,[15] or immediately postexercise.[16] However, none of these methods gained widespread clinical enthusiasm. In the meantime, thallium-201 (^{201}Tl) myocardial perfusion imaging, which was introduced in 1975 for detecting CAD, gained momentum as a viability probe for differentiating viable from scarred myocardium. Experimental studies showed that extraction of ^{201}Tl across the cell membrane was unaffected by hypoxia, chronic hypoperfusion (hibernation), or postischemic dysfunction (stunning), unless irreversible injury (scarred myocardium) is present. When it became possible to evaluate contractile reserve noninvasively, using dobutamine echocardiography, the technique gained more widespread attention.

Evolution of Understanding Appropriate Endpoints for Viability Studies

In parallel with the numerous studies in the 1980s reporting the retrospective observation of improved regional and/or global LV function in some patients following revascularization, seminal investigations reported the prospective identification and prediction of viability by noninvasive radionuclide imaging. Gibson and colleagues[17] used planar ^{201}Tl imaging to demonstrate that preoperative ^{201}Tl uptake patterns could be used to predict the probability of regionally improved perfusion after bypass surgery. In this study, postoperative improvement in perfusion in an initially abnormally perfused region was used as the marker or endpoint of regional tissue viability to be predicted.

Subsequently, Tillisch and coworkers, using positron emission tomography (PET) imaging of myocardial blood flow and glucose metabolism,[18] published the seminal data predicting improved regional function postrevascularization, in regions that were dysfunctional preoperatively. Following that publication, analysis of performance characteristics (usually positive and negative predictive values) for predicting improved regional function became the standard performance metric for viability studies. Fewer studies evaluated a change in global LV function (ejection fraction [EF]), though it could be argued that changes in LVEF would be more relevant to patient-related outcomes.

Regional or global functional recovery after revascularization represents a convenient endpoint for study and, particularly with the case of changes in regional function, provides many analytic data points even with relatively few patients (as the LV is divided into 9, 17, 20, or even 40 segments per patient). Although such an analysis can provide very relevant physiologic information regarding comparative aspects of different techniques for assessing viability, recovery of regional or global function may be an incomplete descriptor with regard to patient-related outcomes.[19] A significant improvement in LVEF is likely to be associated with favorable clinical and prognostic outcomes, but revascularization may conceivably be associated with many favorable clinical effects even in the absence of ventricular functional improvement. Such favorable effects may include relief of ischemic or heart failure symptoms, improved exercise tolerance related to diminished inducible ischemia or improved diastolic function, stabilization (or reversal) of remodeling and stabilization of the electrophysiologic milieu, and prevention of myocardial infarction.[19,20] A very important observation in this regard was published by Samady et al,[21] who reported that in a group of patients with LV dysfunction undergoing bypass surgery, long-term survival was similar regardless of whether LVEF increased after revascularization. These data suggested that improvement in regional or global LV function, or both, is a sufficient but not necessary condition for improved patient outcome after revascularization and broadens the potential for outcome assessment in viability studies.

In parallel with that observation, studies through the mid- to late 1990s and beyond have focused more on the performance characteristics of the noninvasive viability signals to predict outcomes more directly related to the patient, that is, improvement in symptoms and various components of short- or longer-term natural history outcomes. This approach is indeed appropriate, as the usual clinical purpose of assessing the presence and extent of myocardial viability in a patient with CAD and LV dysfunction is to select those patients who will benefit from revascularization.

Viability and Functional Recovery

The gold standard for imaging viability of dysfunctional myocardium in many early studies was recovery of regional or segmental function after revascularization. In the seminal report of Tillisch and colleagues,[18] PET imaging in dysfunctional myocardium had positive and negative predictive values of 85% and 92%, respectively. Subsequent reports examined the utility of ^{201}Tl reinjection,[22] rest-redistribution ^{201}Tl imaging,[23] and the use of the technetium-99 (^{99m}Tc) agents sestamibi[24] and tetrofosmin.[25] A pooled analysis of studies reporting the performance of ^{18}F-FDG PET, ^{201}Tl stress-redistribution-reinjection imaging, ^{201}Tl rest-redistribution imaging, ^{99m}Tc sestamibi single photon emission computed tomography (SPECT) imaging, and dobutamine echocardiography[2] suggested high sensitivity (83% to 90%) and modest specificity (54% to 81%) for the prediction of recovery of regional function. Radionuclide imaging had in general higher sensitivity, while imaging of contractile reserve by dobutamine echocardiography had higher specificity, and PET was slightly more accurate overall.

There have been relatively fewer studies addressing improvement in global LV function after revascularization. These studies uniformly indicate that the presence of a critical or threshold mass of viable myocardium is necessary for improvement in global LV function after revascularization. Using PET, in a study by Tillisch et al,[18] LV ejection fraction improved from $30 \pm 11\%$ to $45 \pm 14\%$ in patients with 2 or more viable segments in a 15-segment LV model. Ragosta and colleagues[23] reported that in patients with severely depressed LV function, the presence of viability in at least 7 of 15 segments by quantitative rest-redistribution planar ^{201}Tl imaging was predictive of a substantial improvement in global function (LVEF from $29 \pm 7\%$ to $41 \pm 11\%$) following CABG. Both studies demonstrated lack of improvement in global LV function when a lesser extent of viability was present prior to revascularization.

The influence of the extent of viability in heart failure patients on the recovery of global function following medical therapy has also been assessed. In the CHRISTMAS trial,[26] the extent of hibernating myocardium defined noninvasively by SPECT sestamibi imaging correlated with the magnitude of LVEF increase seen after treatment with carvedilol.

An issue that complicates the use of regional functional recovery as a gold standard is that the timing of functional recovery is not uniform after revascularization. It has been suggested that LV function may continue to improve for many months following revascularization; therefore, a single assessment, if not timed optimally, may underestimate the full extent of functional recovery.[27]

Viability and Remodeling

Although recovery of regional or global function or both is a relevant physiologic gold standard, revascularization may confer benefits beyond and besides functional recovery, including attenuation of progressive ventricular remodeling. Resting regional function is primarily determined by endocardial thickening, which is unlikely to improve despite partially preserved myocardial viability in patients who have suffered nontransmural myocardial infarction.[28–30] In such patients, preserved viability in the outer layers of the myocardium could prevent progressive LV dilatation, despite the lack of any improvement in resting function following revascularization. From the post-MI and heart failure literature, the prevention or reversal of adverse ventricular remodeling appears to be an important determinant of long-term natural history outcomes, and strategies that prevent or reverse remodeling generally have very favorable effects on that natural history.[31]

The relationship between infarct-zone viability and remodeling has been studied in animal models. Alhaddad and colleagues[32] created left coronary artery occlusions in rats randomized to permanent occlusion or 2, 8, or 16 hours of occlusion followed by reperfusion. On morphometric and histologic analyses performed 2 weeks later, the benefits of reperfusion on infarct expansion were related primarily to preservation and hypertrophy of small islets of viable myocytes located in the subepicardium of the scar, and progressively diminished with increasing periods of coronary ligation. Using a rodent model of MI, Hochman and Bulkley showed that even a small rim of viable epicardial myocardium may prevent or mitigate infarct expansion.[33]

The relative amounts of viable and necrotic myocardium within an infarct zone following MI vary widely but have been shown to be important determinants of subsequent LV remodeling.[34] Even in the presence of a high-grade stenosis or occlusion in the IRA, myocardial perfusion via collaterals can maintain infarct zone viability for prolonged periods.[35]

Relatively few studies have examined the assessment of regional viability to predict the outcome of revascularization or medical therapy on LV remodeling. An important achievement in this regard was the study of 56 patients with severe ischemic LV dysfunction by Senior and colleagues.[36] These investigators assessed viability (by nitrate-enhanced ^{201}Tl as well as nitrate-enhanced ^{99m}Tc-sestamibi imaging) at baseline, as well as LV function, size, and geometry before and again 21 months after physician-directed treatment with revascularization or medical therapy. In patients who had at least 5 viable segments in a 12-segment model (by either tracer), revascularization was associated with a prevention of remodeling, improvement in LVEF, and prevention of increasing sphericity compared to follow-up on medical therapy. On longer-term follow-up (out to 40 months), these changes with revascularization were associated with improved New York Heart Association symptom class and better survival. Thus, noninvasive evaluation of viability identified patients with ischemic cardiomyopathy in whom a strategy of revascularization was associated with both very favorable structural LV changes (prevention of remodeling) and favorable natural history outcomes.

More recently, gadolinium-enhanced cardiac magnetic resonance (CMR) imaging has been used to predict the response of the LV to an intervention in terms of both ejection fraction and volumes, that is, remodeling. Bello and colleagues reported that the response of the LV in patients with either ischemic or nonischemic cardiomyopathy to treatment with carvedilol was predicted by the degree of hyperenhancement (representing fibrosis or scarring) on CMR imaging (Figure 21.1). On multivariable analysis, the degree of scarring by CMR was an independent predictor of the carvedilol-induced change in ejection fraction, LV end-diastolic volume index, and LV end-systolic volume index.[37]

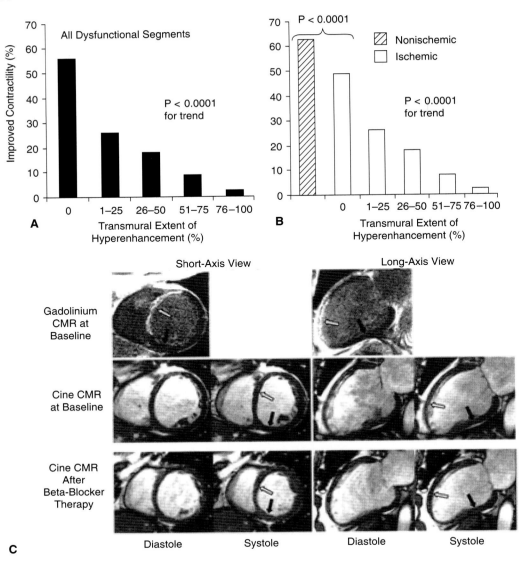

FIGURE 21.1. Evidence that the degree of scarring by hyperenhancement CMR imaging is related to improvement in regional function (as well as remodeling) even with medical therapy in patients with ischemic or nonischemic cardiomyopathy. In panels A and B, the transmural extent of hyperenhancement (by gadolinium CMR, x-axis) is related to the probability of improved regional function after β-blocker therapy (on the y-axis). Panel A represents all patients in the study, while in panel B, the patients are separated into those with ischemic (open bars) and nonischemic (closed bar) cardiomyopathy. The more hyperenhancement, the lower the likelihood of improved regional contractility. In panel C, gadolinium CMR images are shown in the top row, with evidence of gadolinium uptake consistent with fibrosis and nonviability in the anterior wall and septum (white arrows), but no gadolinium uptake in the inferior wall. In the cine CMR images before β-blocker therapy (second row) and after such therapy (third row), there is no improvement in function in the anterior wall and septum (white arrows), but improved regional function in the inferior wall, best seen as greater wall thickness at end-systole. (From Reference 37, modified and reprinted with permission.)

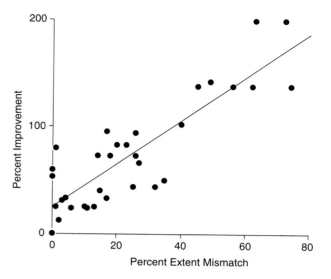

FIGURE 21.2. Relation between the extent (% LV myocardium, x-axis) showing viability on PET imaging (flow-metabolism mismatch) and change in functional status after CABG (percent improvement from baseline, y-axis), reflecting improvement in symptomatic status after revascularization. There is a strong, significant correlation, suggesting that the PET viability data provided a signal of the potential *magnitude* of the symptomatic benefit from revascularization. (Adapted from Reference 38 with permission.)

Viability and Improvement in Heart Failure Symptoms

In a seminal study of 36 patients with ischemic cardiomyopathy (mean LVEF 28 ± 6%), Di Carli and colleagues[38] found that the magnitude of improvement in heart failure symptoms after CABG was correlated with the preoperative extent of viable myocardium as determined by PET perfusion-metabolism mismatch. Patients with evidence of viability involving ≥18% of the LV myocardium had the greatest improvement in their functional status. While previous studies demonstrated significant improvements in functional status following surgical revascularization in ischemic cardiomyopathy,[39,40] this was the first study to establish a direct correlation between the magnitude of preserved myocardial viability and the magnitude of improvement in functional status (Figure 21.2).

Since the publication of those data, many reports have confirmed the concept that noninvasive imaging of viability can predict the degree of symptomatic improvement in such patients in studies involving PET,[41] SPECT imaging of ^{201}Tl or ^{99m}Tc-sestamibi,[36] as well as in identification of contractile reserve by dobutamine echocardiography.[42] Taken together, these data suggest that the extent of dysfunctional, ischemic viable myocardium in heart failure patients can be used as a potential marker of the symptomatic benefit that will accrue secondary to revascularization. As revascularization in patients with significant LV dysfunction is high-risk revascularization, the data suggest that viability imaging information can provide a signal of the potential benefit to inform the risk-benefit equation.

Viability and Survival

An issue of even greater clinical relevance is the role of the presence of viable myocardium in the survival advantage offered by revascularization for patients with ischemic LV dysfunction. Management decisions are vexing in these patients, balancing the high perioperative mortality imposed by severe LV dysfunction[43] with the potential for significant improvement in symptoms, functional status, and survival. In the important first studies to examine outcomes of medical therapy versus revascularization and the influence of retained viability, Eitzman and colleagues,[44] as well as Di Carli and coworkers,[45] concordantly reported on patients with ischemic cardiomyopathy studied with PET imaging. Among patients exhibiting a PET

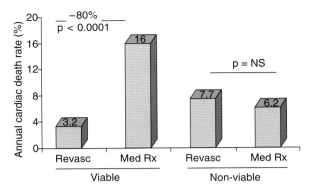

FIGURE 21.3. Annual cardiac death rates (y-axis) for patients with and without myocardial viability and the influence of the subsequent treatment strategy of revascularization or medical therapy (x-axis). Among patients with viability by noninvasive imaging treated medically, there is a 16%/year death rate, a very-high-risk group. There is an almost 80% reduction in mortality for similar patients with viability treated by revascularization ($p < 0.0001$, left two bars). Among patients without substantial myocardial viability, there is no significant difference in mortality with revascularization versus medical therapy (right two bars). (Adapted from Allman KC, et al. (1), with permission from The American College of Cardiology Foundation.)

perfusion-metabolism mismatch pattern and classified as predominantly viable, survival was significantly higher following surgical revascularization than during medical therapy. In contrast, among patients with predominantly nonviable myocardium by PET, there was no survival benefit of revascularization compared to medical therapy.

The strength of conclusions that may be drawn from those important initial papers is limited by the small numbers of patients, raising the possibility of erroneous statistical significance or lack of significance. Since those initial publications however, more than 20 similarly designed observational studies have been published and a meta-analysis of these studies has been reported[1]. This pooled analysis consisted of 3088 patients in 24 studies reporting viability using radionuclide imaging, PET, or dobutamine echocardiography, and long-term survival after revascularization or medical therapy. In patients with predominant viability, follow-up on medical therapy was associated with very high risk, a 16% annual mortality. In similar patients, revascularization was associated with an 80% reduction in annual mortality (16% vs 3.2%, $p < 0.0001$), compared with medical therapy (Figure 21.3). Patients with the most severe LV dysfunction derived the greatest benefit from revascularization; that is, with worsening LVEF, the survival benefit associated with revascularization of patients with viable myocardium increased proportionately. The data suggested that the presence of viable myocardium, as defined by noninvasive imaging in patients with heart failure, is a marker for very high natural history risk, and that risk appears to be significantly reduced by revascularization. These conclusions must be viewed in the context of the limitations of pooling observational cohort studies, which may bring into play unevaluable selection biases when meta-analyzing published literature. More definitive conclusions may result from the ongoing Surgical Treatment of Ischemic Heart Disease (STICH) trial, which is randomizing heart-failure patients without angina to revascularization or no revascularization; subsets of patients will have noninvasive imaging of viability prior to randomization.

Since the report by Allman et al,[1] other studies using ^{99m}Tc-sestamibi imaging or dobutamine echocardiography have shown concordant results[36,46–48] that, in patients with ischemic cardiomyopathy, the presence of myocardial viability consistently predicts improved survival following revascularization.

Viability and Short-Term Management Implications

The original description of hibernating myocardium suggested that it was an adaptive, steady state, potentially reversible with revascularization. Since that time, however, several reports have suggested that progressive structural as well as clinical deterioration may be occurring in that pathophysiologic setting, with more advanced structural changes being associated with less favorable improvement after revascularization. In a comprehensive, seminal study, Elsasser et al[49] described 38 patients with hibernating myocardium. On myocardial biopsies they found evidence of disorganization of the contractile and cytoskeletal proteins, dedifferentiation (expression of more fetal proteins), and changes in the extracellular matrix with evidence of reparative fibrosis. Patients with more advanced abnormalities had less improvement in regional and global function after revascularization. These investigators suggested that hibernation was an "incomplete adaptation to ischemia," and that, once it was identified, prompt revascularization should occur.

Consistent with this concept are data from Beanlands et al,[50] who reported that after identification of patients with ischemic cardiomyopathy who had significant viable myocardium by PET imaging, substantial delay in revascularization was associated with mortality during that delay and with absence of postrevascularization LV functional improvement, compared to similar patients undergoing more prompt revascularization.

These important studies have significant practical implications, suggesting that identification of patients with substantial ischemia and viability are not only at long-term risk, but also at risk in the short term as well, and that optimal reversibility of LV dysfunction and improvement in symptoms and outcome are dependent on prompt referral for revascularization.

Incorporating viability information into the database available for decision making regarding revascularization can also provide insight into the early and intermediate-term postoperative course. Haas et al[51] reported on two groups of patients with ischemic cardiomyopathy referred for bypass surgery: one group was selected on clinical and angiographic criteria, while the second group had PET imaging performed as part of the evaluation and selection process. The group in which PET informed the clinical decision had a less complicated postoperative course, less need for perioperative inotropic support, as well as lower in-hospital and 12-month mortality. These important data support the concept that viability information can assist in the selection of patients with the most optimal potential outcome of revascularization.

Evolution of Understanding Appropriate Analytic Techniques for Viability Studies

In contrast to the literature on imaging for detection of CAD or risk stratification, in which visual and semiquantitative segmental scoring have been the predominant analytic methodologies, the viability literature almost from the beginning has often incorporated quantitative techniques to more precisely report imaging patterns. The seminal study in this regard was reported by Gibson et al,[17] using quantitative analysis of the degree of ^{201}Tl uptake in planar images. This study provided the initial recognition that "fixed defects" are not all representative of infarct, in that regions with preoperative fixed defects could often demonstrate improved or even normal stress/redistribution ^{201}Tl uptake postoperatively. Moreover, quantitative analysis of the degree of ^{201}Tl uptake within fixed defects correlated with the probability of improved perfusion after CABG. These important data opened the possibility that radionuclide imaging could prospectively identify potential improvement in perfusion or function, noninvasively.

Subsequently, many other reports explored and validated the importance of quantitative analysis. Dilsizian and colleagues[22] used both visual and quantitative analysis to demonstrate the importance of ^{201}Tl reinjection in identifying myocardial viability. These investigators also reported that the quantitative magnitude of increase in ^{201}Tl uptake after reinjection was by itself an important determinant of the probability of viability and potential recovery of function.[52] Quantitative analysis of the degree of tracer uptake, as opposed to simply presence or absence, was also shown to be important for the use of ^{99m}Tc sestamibi for assessing viability.[24,53]

A key concept that has emerged from the use of quantitative analysis of tracer uptake in viability studies is that tracer uptake represents a continuous signal rather than a dichotomous signal. That is, tracer uptake is a biologic signal that reflects the full spectrum of how much tissue viability is present in a dysfunctional region, from completely retained viability ("transmural hibernation") to transmural infarct/scar, and all admixtures in between. This concept has been confirmed by a series of studies, correlating tracer uptake with direct examination of tissue viability from myocardial biopsy samples.[54–56]

Zimmermann and coworkers[56] performed myocardial biopsies of dysfunctional anterior wall zones during bypass surgery in patients who had undergone planar thallium scintigraphy with thallium reinjection prior to operation. There was a very good correlation between the quantitated thallium regional activity within the anterior wall from the planar images following reinjection and the percent fibrosis within the biopsy specimens of those same walls (Figure 21.4). Similarly, in patients with chronic ischemic cardiomyopathy undergoing pretransplantation stress-redistribution-reinjection SPECT ^{201}Tl scintigraphy, patterns of ^{201}Tl defects correlated with the posttransplantation extent and distribution of collagen replacement.[57] The higher collagen content in irreversible thallium regions was associated with lower wall thickness and more severe cross-sectional coronary artery narrowing when compared with reversible and normal thallium regions.[57] These data suggest that quantitative analysis of ^{201}Tl uptake indeed reflects the degree of regional tissue viability.

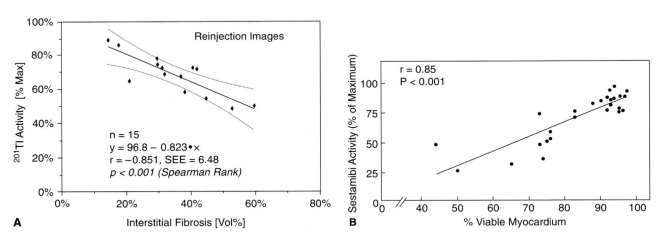

FIGURE 21.4. Relation between quantitated tracer uptake and histologic measures of viability. In panel A, the relation of preoperative quantitated ^{201}Tl activity after reinjection (y-axis, as a percentage of peak counts) from planar imaging, is compared to the percentage of interstitial fibrosis (an inverse measure of viability), taken from biopsy samples of dysfunctional anterior walls during CABG surgery. There is a strong correlation. In panel B, the relation of preoperative quantitated SPECT ^{99m}Tc-sestamibi activity (after a rest high-dose injection) is compared to the percentage of viability similarly taken from biopsy samples of dysfunctional anterior walls during CABG surgery. There is a strong direct correlation, with the same correlation coefficient as the ^{201}Tl study. Both these studies documented that tracer uptake is a continuum, which correlates with the direct extent of tissue viability. (From References 54 [panel B] and 56 [panel A], with permission.)

Two key studies examined this issue using ^{99m}Tc-sestamibi. Medrano and colleagues[55] injected sestamibi at rest in patients with severe ischemic cardiomyopathy just prior to heart transplantation. Following explantation of the recipient's severely dysfunctional heart, these investigators found that the magnitude of sestamibi defect severity (on imaging of the sliced pathologic specimens of the explanted heart) was closely correlated to the percentage of scarring within those same segments on pathologic examination (Figure 21.4). In addition, well counting of myocardial specimens for sestamibi activity also correlated well with the presence of viable myocardium by microscopy. These data suggest that even in the setting of severe ischemic cardiomyopathy (average LVEF 24 ± 6%) and dysfunctional territories supplied by severely stenosed coronary arteries, quantitative sestamibi activity correlated well with the magnitude of preserved regional tissue viability within dysfunctional territories. The data on sestamibi defect severity were, however, gathered from imaging specimens of the already explanted heart, leaving open the question of whether these elegant data could indeed be generalized to in vivo clinical planar or SPECT imaging.

However, two subsequent studies, by Dakik and colleagues,[54] as well as by Maes and coworkers,[57] demonstrated that similar data could indeed be derived from SPECT imaging in vivo. In both studies, 30 patients with severe LAD stenosis and significant anterior wall dysfunction underwent resting sestamibi SPECT imaging and the data were analyzed using quantitative polar maps. There was a very good correlation between the quantitated sestamibi activity within the anterior wall from the preoperative SPECT images and the percent fibrosis seen in the biopsy specimens. These investigators concluded that the magnitude of sestamibi uptake is inversely related to the amount of interstitial fibrosis (and thus directly related to the magnitude of preserved tissue viability) and that ^{99m}Tc-sestamibi activity reflects not only flow but also regional tissue viability. These data are concordant with animal studies suggesting that in low-flow territories, sestamibi activity is higher than one would expect based on behavior of a pure flow tracer.[23]

These concepts of quantitative analysis have been applied to hyperenhancement CMR imaging. In a seminal study, Kim and coworkers demonstrated that the quantitated evaluation of the extent of transmural or nontransmural scarring in a dysfunction region, analyzed by gadolinium-enhanced CMR images, was directly related to the probability of functional recovery after revascularization,[58] analogous to previously published radionuclide studies.

The data from all these studies emphasize the concept that noninvasive assessment of regional viability in dysfunctional myocardium by any methodology, whether interrogating perfusion, metabolism, contractile reserve, or degree of scarring, should be viewed as a continuum of values related to the degree of tissue viability and intact myocytes. Analytically, in published studies, quantitative cut points, such as 50% or 60% of peak uptake or extent of transmural scar, are used to distinguish "viable" (above that cut point) from "nonviable" (below that cut point) regions. It is important to note that such cut points are necessary for determining performance characteristics such as positive and negative predictive values. In light of the biopsy studies, however, whether functional recovery occurs following revascularization is related to the mass of preserved myocardial tissue, and threshold or cut points of regional isotope activity or degree of hyperenhancement will merely reflect that sufficient mass of tissue.

The concept that "viability" is a continuous function, which relates not only to the mass of preserved myocytes but also extends to endpoints such as the probability of functional recovery; that is, the greater the amount of viability in a dysfunctional region, the greater the probability of functional recovery after revascularization. This principle has been demonstrated for ^{201}Tl imaging,[59] ^{99m}Tc sestamibi imaging,[24,60] for PET evaluation of metabolic activity,[60,61] as well as for hyperenhancement CMR imaging.[58]

Assessment of Viability Versus Assessment of Inducible Ischemia

A relatively unexplored issue in the analysis of viability studies is the relative importance of assessing "pure" viability (as evaluated by resting tracer uptake, resting metabolic activity, extent of hyperenhancement, or contractile reserve to low-dose inotropic stimulation) compared to assessment of inducible ischemia using a stress-rest approach. Most studies evaluating the radionuclide techniques for assessing viability, for instance, have focused on analysis of resting tracer uptake (as with ^{201}Tl, sestamibi) or tetrofosmin or evidence of preserved metabolic activity at rest (by FDG or C-11 acetate). In some patients, however, nontransmural infarction may have occurred with preservation of some degree of viability in the setting of a noncritically stenosed vessel. In this setting, evidence of uptake of the single photon tracers or metabolic activity by FDG may result in "intermediate" values, such that the role of revascularization is not clear. When this occurs, assessment of stress-induced ischemia appears to provide additional important information. In an important study, Kitsiou and coworkers demonstrated that the finding of stress-induced ischemia (a reversible perfusion defect) was a more powerful predictor of recovery of function than a "fixed" defect with a similar degree of resting tracer activity[62] (Figure 21.5A). Subsequently, Pasquet and colleagues[63] showed that among patients with CAD and LV dysfunction, evidence of stress-induced ischemia by SPECT was an important prognostic factor in a multivariate analysis even when rest viability information was known. Moreover, stress-induced ischemia by radionuclide imaging correlated with a favorable effect of revascularization on outcomes more powerfully than viability data alone.

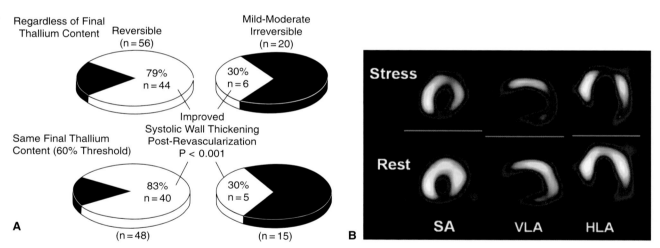

FIGURE 21.5. A, Pie chart demonstrating postrevascularization functional outcome of asynergic regions in relation to prerevascularization ^{201}Tl patterns of reversible defects and mild-to-moderate irreversible defects using a stress-redistribution-reinjection protocol. In the top panel, the probability of functional recovery after revascularization was much higher if ischemia was demonstrated in contrast to a mild-to-moderate irreversible defect. In the bottom panel, among segments with a final ^{201}Tl content of at least 60% of peak (that is, even at a similar mass of viable myocardial tissue as reflected by the final thallium content), the presence of inducible ischemia was associated with an increased likelihood of functional recovery. (Adapted from Reference 62 with permission.) B, Selected short-axis (SA), vertical long-axis (VLA) and horizontal long-axis (HLA) images at stress and rest from a patient with severe ischemic cardiomyopathy, advanced heart-failure symptoms, and minimal anginal symptoms, being considered for CABG. LVEF was 23% from the ECG-gated SPECT analysis in this 81-year-old diabetic. Coronary angiography demonstrated severe 3-vessel CAD, with technically bypassable vessels. On rest imaging (bottom row), there is substantial tracer uptake in all areas except the inferobasal wall, suggesting retained viability. Given the magnitude of risk associated with CABG, however (based on age, LV function, presence of diabetes), and the severity of the LV dysfunction and the LV size, the clinicians requested more information. The stress images (top row) confirm that there is extensive inducible ischemia in the anterior, apical, lateral, and inferoapical walls. The extent of ischemia suggests substantial potential benefit from revascularization.

Conceptually, similar data have been shown using echocardiography as well as CMR imaging. In a series of patients with ischemic cardiomyopathy studied before and after revascularization, Afridi and colleagues, using low- as well as high-dose dobutamine echocardiography, demonstrated that a "biphasic" response (contractile reserve at low dose, with worsening function at higher doses, presumably reflecting viability and inducible ischemia, respectively) had the optimal predictive value for predicting functional recovery, compared to other patterns of response.[64] Wellnhofer et al have shown that the discriminatory ability of CMR imaging for assessment of functional recovery is enhanced by incorporating evidence of regional responsiveness to dobutamine, over and above the assessment of scar extent alone by hyperenhancement imaging.[65]

Thus, the data from use of multiple imaging modalities suggest the following concept: in settings where evidence of resting tracer uptake, metabolic activity, extent of hyperenhancement, or degree of contractile reserve falls into an intermediate range (where the probability of recovery of function or improved outcome is itself intermediate), addition of stress imaging to assess for the presence of stress-induced ischemia may be helpful for informing the clinical decision making regarding revascularization (Figure 21.5B).

Important Differences Among Noninvasive Testing Modalities

The different noninvasive modalities available to assess myocardial viability interrogate distinct pathophysiologic myocyte and myocardial processes. The SPECT radionuclide tracers examine myocyte cell membrane integrity, and dobutamine echocardiography assesses regional ventricular contractile reserve. PET images identify myocardial blood flow and metabolism, while MR hyperenhancement imaging identifies scarred myocardium. Despite these distinctions, there have not been major differences identified among the modalities that would suggest consistently major differences in driving patient management. A comparison of the imaging properties of the various modalities relevant to assessment of viability is shown in Table 21.2.

How the modalities compare with one another for clinical assessment of viability has been evaluated in a number of ways. Many published studies have compared two or more of the modalities directly (or head-to-head) in the same population of patients. A summary of such studies is shown in Table 21.3. The following concepts can be gleaned from these published data:

- Most of the studies involve small numbers of patients.
- Most of the patients included in these studies have only mild to moderate degrees of LV dysfunction.
- The endpoint, or gold standard, used for "viability" varies widely. In some cases, the gold standard may be simply another imaging modality, itself subject to variability that is often unaccounted for.
- In almost all the studies, the LV is divided into many segments for comparative analysis (data not shown in Table 21.3). This enhances the number of data points but creates an artificial situation in which "significant" differences between modalities may be based on very small areas of the LV that may not be clinically relevant for differential patient outcomes.
- The evaluated performance characteristics vary widely within the individual studies and among patients. The performance characteristics of an individual modality also vary widely among studies, influenced in part by choice of endpoint.
- When such comparative analysis is based on multiple segments within the same patient, statistical correction for repeated measures within the same patient that are likely to be highly correlated should be performed. This is rarely done in these studies.

TABLE 21.2. Comparison of Viability Imaging Modalities

Viability Techniques	Advantages	Disadvantages
SPECT	—Availability	—Low energy tracers —Low spatial resolution —Lack of built-in attenuation correction
PET	—Built-in attenuation correction —High energy tracers	—Limited availbility —High costs —Complexity
MRI	—Temporal and spatial resolution —Provide simultaneous information on anatomy, function, and perfusion —Superior spatial resolution —better reproducibility —not dependent on anatomy or examiner	—difficulty obtaining quality images in diabetics —Lower temporal resolution —Need for breath-holding sequences during acquisition —Poor images with irregular rhythms and implantable metallic devices
Echocardiography	—Availability —Less technical —Low relative cost	—Limited by qualitative assessment —High interobserver and intercenter variation —Difficulty obtaining adequate acoustic windows

Abbreviations: SPECT-single positron emission computed tomography; PET-fluorine 18 deoxyglucose-positron emission tomography; MRI-cardiac magnetic resonance imaging

- Soon after initial validation studies of CMR, it began to be used as a gold standard.

More comprehensive analyses of comparative performance of the imaging modalities have included pooled or meta-analysis of the published literature, as well as randomized trials. In a pooled analysis of studies reporting on rates of regional functional recovery, Bax et al[2] reported that the radionuclide agents are more sensitive and dobutamine echocardiography is more specific, with PET having slightly higher overall accuracy for predicting functional recovery. Cardiac MRI hyperenhancement data published so far appear similar[65] in general.

In the meta-analysis by Allman et al,[1] there was no difference in the reduction of death in patients with viable myocardium treated by revascularization, whether viability was identified by single-photon radionuclide agents, PET, or dobutamine echocardiography.

The most rigorous method for identifying any difference in modalities is a randomized trial. In an elegant study, Siebelink et al[93] reported on patients with CAD and LV dysfunction in whom information on the presence and extent of viability was needed to make a decision regarding revascularization. Patients were randomized to have that information provided by stress/rest SPECT sestamibi imaging or by PET imaging, with the decision-making clinical blinded to the modality providing the viability information. There was no difference in the proportion of patients sent to revascularization, and, more important, there was no difference in the long-term outcomes between the 2 randomization groups.

These data together suggest that all the noninvasive testing modalities can provide important information on viability to inform management decisions, and major differences, sufficient to result in differential long-term outcomes, among the modalities in that regard are not apparent.

The following concepts summarize of the strengths and weaknesses of the various imaging modalities:

TABLE 21.3. Comparative Viability Studies

Reference	Subjects	Modality	Reference Modality	Endpoint-Viability Criteria	Sensitivity	Specificity	NPV	PPV
Gerber et al[66]	39 patients with ischemic LV dysfunction (mean EF 33% ± 10%)	FDG PET	Echo	Mismatch	0.75	0.67	0.63	0.78
		Low-dose dobutamine echo	Echo	Increased wall motion and thickening	0.71	0.89	0.65	0.89
Baer et al[67]	42 patients with ischemic LV dysfunction (mean EF 40% ± 13%)	FDG PET	Echo	Normal FDG uptake (>50% of maximum)	0.92	0.88	0.88	0.92
		Low-dose dobutamine echo	Echo	Increased wall motion and thickening	0.96	0.69	0.92	0.83
Pagano et al[68]	30 patients with ischemic LV dysfunction (mean EF 25% ± 7%)	FDG PET	Echo	rMGU	0.99	0.33	0.96	0.66
		Low-dose dobutamine echo	Echo	Increased wall motion and thickening	0.61	0.63	0.55	0.68
Marzullo et al[69]	14 patients with ischemic LV dysfunction (mean EF 36% ± 7%)	201Tl rest-redistribution (planar)	Echo	Activity late (>55%)	0.86	0.92	0.77	0.95
		Low-dose dobutamine echo	Echo	Increased wall motion	0.82	0.94	0.73	0.95
		99mTc-sestamibi scintigraphy (without addition of nitrates) (planar)	Echo	Activity (>54%)	0.75	0.84	0.64	0.90

(Continued)

TABLE 21.3. *Continued*

Reference	Subjects	Modality	Reference Modality	Endpoint-Viability Criteria	Sensitivity	Specificity	NPV	PPV
Alfieri et al[70]	13 patients with ischemic LV dysfunction (mean EF 35% ± 8%)	^{201}Tl rest-redistribution (SPECT)	Echo	Defect reversibility	0.94	0.64	0.70	0.92
		Low-dose dobutamine echo	Echo	Increased wall motion and thickening	0.91	0.78	0.76	0.92
Charney et al[71]	14 patients with CAD	^{201}Tl rest-redistribution (SPECT)	Echo	Activity late	0.95	0.85	0.92	0.90
		Low-dose dobutamine echo	Echo	Increased wall motion and thickening	0.71	0.93	0.74	0.92
Arnese et al[72]	38 patients with ischemic LV dysfunction (mean EF 31%)	^{201}Tl rest-redistribution (SPECT)	Echo	Increased wall motion and thickening			0.94	0.30
		Low-dose dobutamine echo	Echo	Increased wall motion and thickening	0.74	0.96	0.93	0.85
Haque et al[73]	26 patients with ischemic LV dysfunction (mean EF 43% ± 14%)	^{201}Tl rest-redistribution (SPECT)	Echo	Increased wall motion and thickening			1.00	0.85
		Low-dose dobutamine echo	Echo	Increased wall motion and thickening	0.86	0.94	0.89	0.93
Senior et al[74]	22 patients with ischemic LV dysfunction (mean EF 26% ± 8%)	^{201}Tl rest-redistribution (planar/ SPECT)	Echo	Activity late	0.92	0.78	0.80	0.91
		Low-dose dobutamine echo	Echo	Increased wall motion	0.87	0.82	0.73	0.92

Study	Patients	Technique		Criteria				
Vanoverschelde et al[75]	73 patients with ischemic LV dysfunction (mean EF 36% ±12%)	Low-dose dobutamine echo	Echo	Increased wall motion and thickening at low dose	0.94	0.80	0.80	0.94
		201Tl rest-redistribution (SPECT)	Echo	Increased wall motion and thickening	0.48	0.79		
Kostopoulos et al[76]	31 patients with ischemic LV dysfunction (mean EF 41% ±6%)	Low-dose dobutamine echo	Echo	Increased wall motion and thickening at low dose	0.71	0.86	0.80	0.79
		201Tl rest-redistribution (SPECT)	Echo	Increased wall motion and thickening	0.71	0.90		
Bax et al[77]	17 patients with ischemic LV dysfunction (mean EF 36% ±11%)	Low-dose dobutamine echo	Echo	Increased wall motion and thickening	0.93	0.89	0.94	0.86
		201Tl rest-redistribution (SPECT)	Echo	Increased wall motion and thickening	0.40	0.93		
		Low-dose dobutamine echo	Echo	Increased wall motion	0.49	0.91	0.63	0.85
Perrone-Filardi et al[59]	18 patients with ischemic LV dysfunction (mean EF 43% ±12%)	201Tl rest-redistribution (SPECT)	Echo	Activity late (>55%) and defect reversibility (>12%)	0.72	1.00	0.22	1.00
		Low-dose dobutamine echo	Echo	Increased wall motion and thickening at low dose	0.91	0.67	0.83	0.79
Qureshi et al[78]	34 patients with CAD	201Tl redistribution on (SPECT)	Echo	Activity late (>60%)	0.45	0.94	0.56	0.90
		Low-dose dobutamine echo	Echo	Biphasic response/ worsening	0.63	0.90	0.82	0.76

(Continued)

TABLE 21.3. *Continued*

Reference	Subjects	Modality	Reference Modality	Endpoint-Viability Criteria	Sensitivity	Specificity	NPV	PPV
Nagueh et al[79]	19 patients with ischemic LV dysfunction (mean EF 38% ± 13%)	201Tl redistribution (SPECT)	Echo	Activity (>60%)	0.91	0.43	0.87	0.54
		High-dose dobutamine echo	Echo	Biphasic response	0.68	0.83	0.82	0.70
Pace et al[80]	46 patients with ischemic LV dysfunction (mean EF 40% ± 11%)	201Tl redistribution (SPECT)	Echo	Activity (>65%); reversibility (>12%)	0.76	0.74	0.76	0.74
		Low-dose dobutamine echo	Echo	Increased wall motion and thickening	0.52	0.87	0.80	0.65
Gunning et al[25]	30 patients with ischemic LV dysfunction (mean EF 24% ± 8%)	201Tl redistribution (SPECT)	MRI	Activity late (>60%)	0.72	0.58	0.76	0.53
		Low-dose dobutamine echo	MRI	Increased systolic thickening	0.50	0.81	0.71	0.63
		99mTc-tetrofosmin scintigraphy (without addition of nitrates) SPECT	MRI	Activity (>64%)	0.63	0.62	0.72	0.53
Sicari[81]	57 patients with ischemic LV dysfunction (mean EF 31% ± 11%)	201Tl redistribution	Echo	Activity late (>55%)	0.87	0.61	0.79	0.74
		Low-dose dobutamine echo	Echo	Increased wall motion	0.82	0.93	0.80	0.94

Study	Patients	Test	Modality	Criterion				
Gunning et al[82]	15 patients with ischemic LV dysfunction (mean EF 23% ±8%)	99mTc-tetrofosmin scintigraphy (without addition of nitrates) SPECT	MRI	Activity (>55%)	0.62	0.61	0.69	0.53
		201Tl redistribution (SPECT)	MRI	Activity late (>55%)	0.71	0.64	0.75	0.58
Cornel et al[83]	91 patients with ischemic LV dysfunction (mean EF 32% ±11%)	Low-dose dobutamine echo	Echo	Increased wall motion and thickening	0.92	0.62	0.08	0.05
	61 patients with ischemic LV dysfunction (mean EF 33%)	High-dose dobutamine echo	Echo	Biphasic response	0.83	0.89	0.92	0.75
Udelson et al[24]	18 patients with ischemic LV dysfunction (mean EF 34% ±10%)	201Tl redistribution (SPECT)	Echo	Activity late (>60%)	0.88	0.83	0.92	0.75
		99mTc-sestamibi scintigraphy (without addition of nitrates) (SPECT)	Echo	Activity (>60%)	0.94	0.86	0.96	0.80
Sciagra et al[84]	29 patients with ischemic LV dysfunction (mean EF 35% ±7%)	201Tl redistribution (SPECT)	Echo	Activity (>60%); reversibility (>10%)	0.78	0.58	0.70	0.68
	35 patients with ischemic LV dysfunction (mean EF 36% ±8%)	99mTc-tetrofosmin scintigraphy (postnitrates) SPECT	Rest postnitrate MIBI	Activity (>65%); reversibility (after nitrate)	0.77	0.77	0.74	0.79

(Continued)

TABLE 21.3. *Continued*

Reference	Subjects	Modality	Reference Modality	Endpoint-Viability Criteria	Sensitivity	Specificity	NPV	PPV
Matsunari et al[85]	25 patients with ischemic LV dysfunction (mean EF 42% ± 8%)	[201]Tl redistribution (SPECT)	RNV	Activity (>55%); reversibility (>10%)	0.92	0.33	0.71	0.69
		^{99m}Tc-tetrofosmin scintigraphy (without addition of nitrates) SPECT	RNV	Activity (>50%)	0.96	0.30	0.82	0.69
Maes et al[57]	23 patients with ischemic LV dysfunction (mean EF 40% ± 13%)	^{99m}Tc-sestamibi scintigraphy (without addition of nitrates) (SPECT) FDG PET	RNV	Activity (>50%) Mismatch, NP	0.92 0.83	0.60 0.91	0.86 0.83	0.75 0.91
Giorgetti et al[86]	21 patients with CAD and severe LVEF dysfunction (EF 29% ± 6%)	^{99m}Tc-tetrofosmin scintigraphy (without addition of nitrates) SPECT	MRI	Activity (>40%)	0.86	0.56		
		^{99m}Tc-tetrofosmin scintigraphy (postnitrates) SPECT	MRI	Activity (>51%)	0.89	0.78		

Study	Patient population	Test	Reference	Criterion				
Baer et al[87]	35 patients with LV dysfunction (mean EF 42%)	Rest MRI with preserved EDWT	FDG PET	FDG uptake >50% in a region with normal wall motion as assessed by left ventriculography	0.72	0.89	0.66	0.91
		MRI with dobutamine stress	FDG PET	FDG uptake >50% in a region with normal wall motion as assessed by left ventriculography	0.81	0.95	0.75	0.96
		Rest MRI with preserved EDWT AND/OR MRI with dobutamine stress	FDG PET	FDG uptake >50% in a region with normal wall motion as assessed by left ventriculography	0.88	0.87	0.82	0.92
Baer et al[88]	43 patients with ischemic LV dysfunction (mean EF 41%)	MRI with dobutamine stress	MRI	Regional wall motion abnormality and LV thickness	0.89	0.94	0.83	0.96
		Rest MRI with preserved EDWT	MRI	Regional wall motion abnormality and LV thickness (EDWT<5.5mm = scar)	0.92	0.56	0.82	0.78
Kim et al[58]	41 patients with ischemic LV dysfunction (mean EF 43%)	MRI with DHE	MRI (pre/postrevascularization)	Segmental wall thickness	0.97	0.44		
Lauerma et al[89]	11 patients with ischemic heart failure–multivessel CAD s/p CABG	MRI with dobutamine stress	MRI	Regional wall motion abnormality and LV thickness	0.79	0.93		
		Rest MRI with preserved EDWT	MRI	Regional wall motion abnormality and LV thickness	0.97	0.96		
		MRI with DHE	MRI	Regional wall motion abnormality and LV thickness	0.62	0.98		
		FDG PET	MRI	Regional wall motion abnormality and LV thickness	0.81	0.86		

(Continued)

TABLE 21.3. *Continued*

Reference	Subjects	Modality	Reference Modality	Endpoint-Viability Criteria	Sensitivity	Specificity	NPV	PPV
Selvanayagam et al[90]	52 patients with CAD undergoing multivessel CABG (mean EF 62% ± 12%)	MRI with DHE	MRI (pre/post-CABG)	Regional wall motion abnormality	0.95	0.26	0.69–0.72	0.73–0.81
Wellnhofer et al[65]	29 patients with ischemic LV dysfunction (mean EF 32% ± 8%)	MRI with DHE	MRI	Regional wall motion abnormality/transmurality of scar	0.90	0.52		
		MRI with dobutamine stress	MRI	Regional wall motion abnormality/transmurality of scar	0.75	0.93		
Gutberlet et al[91]	27 patients with ischemic LV dysfunction (mean EF 29% ± 9%)	Rest MRI with preserved EDWT	^{201}Tl rest-redistribution (SPECT)	Nonreversibility/delayed enhancement in an area >50% of entire segment/ED WT <6mm = scar	0.94	0.36	0.65	0.83
		MRI with DHE	^{201}Tl rest-redistribution (SPECT)	Nonreversibility/delayed enhancement in an area >50% of entire segment/ED WT <6mm = scar	0.93	0.39	0.65	0.83
		MRI with dobutamine stress	^{201}Tl rest-redistribution (SPECT)	Nonreversibility/delayed enhancement in an area >50% of entire segment/ED WT <6mm = scar	0.84	0.50	0.49	0.85

	Modality	Study	Criteria				
	Rest MRI with preserved EDWT	Recovery of contractile function 6 months after CABG	Nonreversibility delayed enhancement in an area >50% of entire segment/ED WT <6mm = scar	0.96	0.35	0.57	0.90
	MRI with DHE	Recovery of contractile function 6 months after CABG	Nonreversibility/ delayed enhancement in an area >50% of entire segment/ED WT <6mm = scar	0.99	0.94	0.94	0.99
	MRI with dobutamine stress	Recovery of contractile function 6 months after CABG	Nonreversibility/ delayed enhancement in an area >50% of entire segment/ED WT <6mm = scar	0.88	0.90	0.56	0.98
	201Tl rest-redistribution (SPECT)	Recovery of contractile function 6 months after CABG	Nonreversibility/ delayed enhancement in an area >50% of entire segment/ED WT <6mm = scar	0.86	0.68	0.44	0.94
Bodi et al[92]	Rest MRI with preserved EDWT (>5.5mm)	40 patients with ischemic LV dysfunction (mean EF 49% ± 13%)	MRI	Regional wall motion abnormality and LV thickness	0.95	0.21	0.87	0.43
	MRI with dobutamine stress		MRI	Regional wall motion abnormality and LV thickness	0.42	0.93	0.72	0.78

Abbreviations: NPV, negative predictive value; PPV, positive predictive value; LV, left ventricle; EF, ejection fraction; FDG PET, fluorine-18 deoxyglucose positron emission tomography; echo, echocardiogram; rMGU, regional myocardial glucose utilization; CAD, coronary artery disease; SPECT, single positron emission computed tomography; MRI, cardiac magnetic resonance imaging; MIBI, sestimibi; RNV, radionucleotide ventriculography; CV, contrast ventriculography; NP, normal perfusion; DHE, delayed hyperenhancement with gadolinium; CABG, coronary artery bypass grafting; EDWT, end-diastolic wall thickness.

Single-Photon Radionuclide Imaging

Strengths

- Modality provides strong validation for the central concept that quantitated tracer uptake on planar or SPECT imaging represents the magnitude of regional tissue viability.
- Modality provides strong validation of performance characteristics for predicting all viability-related outcomes.
- Quantitative analysis tools are widely available and easily applied.
- Assessment of stress-induced ischemia is straightforward to incorporate.

Weaknesses

- Most literature involves patients with only moderate LV dysfunction.
- Partial volume or recovery coefficient effects would likely limit usefulness and negative predictive value in patients with severe LV dysfunction and thinner walls, patients in whom clinical decisions regarding revascularization are most challenging.
- As the LV is larger and more dilated, attenuation issues become more important. Data on attenuation correction effects are very limited.

Dobutamine Echocardiography

Strengths

- Modality provides strong validation for the central concept that contractile reserve represents a threshold magnitude of regional tissue viability.
- Modality provides strong validation of performance characteristics for predicting all viability-related outcomes.
- Modality is easily applied, even at the bedside.

Weaknesses

- Quantitation is not routine. Visual analysis is challenging to the nonexpert.
- Various patterns (biphasic response, further improvement with high-dose dobutamine, for instance) may coexist in the same patient, complicating interpretation.
- Most literature involves patients with only moderate LV dysfunction.
- Little exploration has been done regarding influence of remodeled but viable myocardium on predictive values.
- Images are limited by windows. Use of contrast for cavity enhancement has not been extensively explored as yet.
- Use of contrast for microvascular integrity has not been well explored as yet and is challenging to interpret.

Metabolic Imaging by PET

Strengths

- Modality provides strong validation for the central concept that tracer uptake represents the magnitude of preserved tissue metabolic activity.
- Modality provides strong(est) validation of performance characteristics for predicting all viability-related outcomes.
- Quantitative analysis tools are available.
- Higher-energy emissions make application to patients with more dilated LV and thinner walls more tenable, though this is still relatively unexplored in the literature.
- "Mismatch" concept of perfusion and metabolism is likely able to differentiate viable hibernating myocardium from viable remodeled myocardium, but as yet this is not well explored.

Weaknesses

- Though equipment is now more widely available, expertise to perform high-quality viability studies is less available.
- Modality is technically more complex to perform with high quality.
- Metabolic imaging is technically challenging in diabetics.
- Incremental need for and value of using perfusion imaging as well as metabolic imaging have not been clearly established for various clinical scenarios.

Gadolinium Hyperenhancement CMR Imaging

Strengths

- Modality provides strong validation for the central concept that enhanced areas of the myocardium represent the magnitude of regional scarring.
- Modality affords the ability to supply high-quality imaging of function and viability using different sequences.
- Modality is conceptually the most applicable of the techniques to patients with more dilated LVs and more severe degrees of LV dysfunction, with thinner walls.
- To date, validation is limited to predicting regional and global function improvement.

Weaknesses

- Though equipment is now widely available at medical centers, technical expertise to perform and interpret hyperenhancement imaging is not yet widespread.
- Modality is sensitive to acquisition timing.
- The need for stress-induced ischemia information over and above information on resting viability information is not well established.
- It is technically challenging to obtain ischemia information.
- Perfusion imaging is as yet not fully validated.

Representative images of the various modalities are shown in Figure 21.6.

Caveats Regarding Application of the Viability Literature to Clinical Decision Making for Revascularization

The published literature documenting the performance characteristics of viability imaging techniques for predicting functional recovery or improvement in symptoms by its nature reflects patients who have been selected for revascularization, often on clinical grounds, who then undergo viability imaging. In other cases, patient selection for revascularization is predicated on the results from viability imaging. Thus, in either scenario, potential is created for pre- or posttest referral bias to influence the performance characteristics being measured.

Perhaps the most important caveat regarding application of the viability literature to actual clinical practice involves the potential extrapolation of the literature to patient subsets that have more advanced degrees of LV dysfunction or more concomitant complicating conditions. Most of the studies in the literature involve patients with LVEF values in the 25% to 35% range (or higher in many studies). Particularly in centers where patients are being referred for evaluation for heart transplant, where high-risk revascularization might be considered an option based on viability information, it would be expected that the range of LVEF among such patients would be distinctly lower. Whether the imaging tests perform in a similar manner among patients with more dilated, dysfunctional ventricles has not been carefully studied. Moreover,

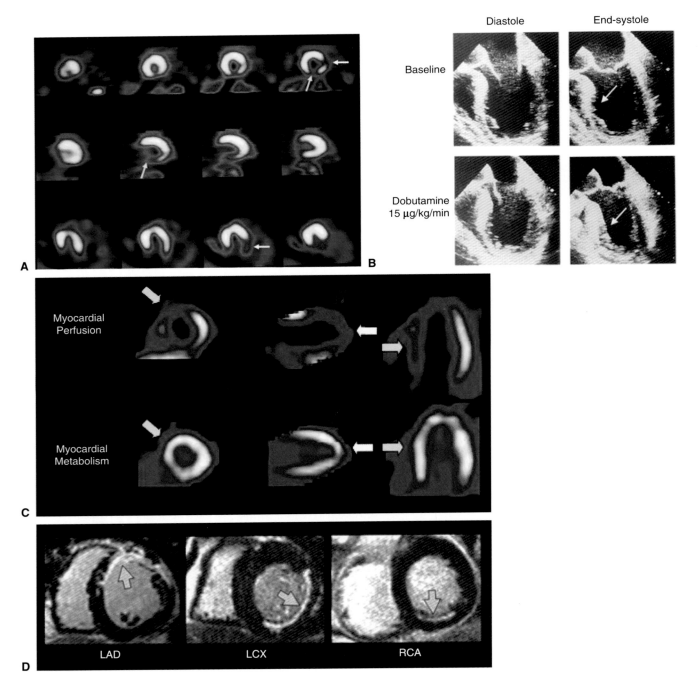

FIGURE 21.6. A-D. Images representing viability information provided by (A) SPECT imaging of tracer uptake, (B) dobutamine echocardiography. (B, Reprinted with permission from Panza JA, Dilsizian V, Laurienzo JM, et al. Relation between thalium uptake and contractile response to dobutamine: Implications regarding myocardial viability in patients with chronic coronary artery disease and left ventricular dysfunction. Circ Feb, 1995;91:996–998.) (C) PET imaging of preserved glucose metabolism and impaired perfusion, and (D) gadolinium hyperenhancment CMR imaging. In panel A, there is substantial uptake of sestamibi in most regions of the LV, save for reduced uptake in the inferior wall (yellow arrow) and part of the lateral wall (white arrow), suggesting reduced viability in those areas. In panel B, reduced wall thickening is seen in the septum in these still frames, from diastole to systole at baseline (top row). During infusion of dobutamine, contractile reserve is demonstrated, with improved wall thickening during systole (bottom row). (Reproduced from Reference 94 with permission.) In panel C, PET images of perfusion (top row) and glucose metabolism are shown in the short axis (SA), vertical long axis (VLA) and horizontal long axis (HLA). There are perfusion defects in the septum (yellow arrows), anterior wall (red arrows), and apex (white arrow). All these areas show preserved glucose metabolism and thus PET "mismatch," consistent with ischemic, viable myocardium. (Courtesy of Marcelo Di Carli MD). In panel D, gadolinium-enhanced CMR images are shown from patients with infarct in the LAD territory (left panel), in the LCX territory (middle panel), and in the RCA territory (right panel). Gadolinium uptake (arrows) denotes areas of infarct/fibrosis. (D, Copyright © 2000 Massachusetts Medical Society. All rights reserved. Reprinted from Kim RJ, Wu E, Rafael A, et al. The use of contrast-enhanced magnetic resonance imaging to identify reversible myocardial dysfunction. N Eng J Med. 2000;343:1445–1453.)

although one might expect that PET or CMR imaging would be superior to SPECT or dobutamine echocardiography in patients with very dilated ventricles and generally thinner walls,[95] this has been evaluated only in small cohorts of patients (Figure 21.7).

Predicting recovery of regional and particularly global LV function in the setting of significant valvular heart disease may also be problematic. Studies of changes in regional or global LV function after revascularization usually exclude such patients from analysis, based on the complicating effect of mitral valve replacement or repair on the studied outcome, for instance. Thus, information on viability and its incorporation into benefit-risk decision-making equations should be assessed in the context of both the published literature and the individual situation at hand. Finally, as the published literature emanates from expert centers, it is important to factor in local expertise and experience in selecting the test modality for assessing viability.

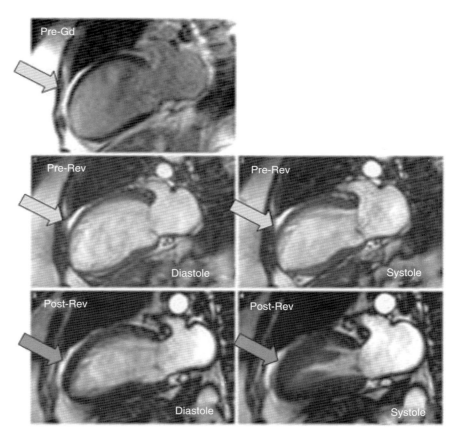

FIGURE 21.7. Example of viability information provided by hyperenhancement CMR imaging in a patient with severe LV dysfunction, a very dilated LV, and a thin anterior wall and apex (blue arrows). Conventionally, such a thin wall would be considered likely scarred. However, there is absence of hyperenhancement (top row, Pre-Gd) image with no areas of brightness throughout the anterior wall and apex. In the images following revascularization (bottom row), there is dramatic recovery of function (red arrows), consistent with complete viability. The thinness of the anterior wall and apex makes it somewhat unlikely that the single photon tracers and SPECT imaging would have been able to accurately report the status of regional viability in this case. (Reprinted from Reference 96, with permission.)

Areas for Future Research

As seen in the admittedly incomplete historical chronology in Table 21.1, there has been an enormous volume of literature exploring the use of imaging techniques for assessment of myocardial viability over the last 20 to 25 years. There are, however, issues that remain underexplored. Such issues include:

- What is the true prevalence of viability or ischemia in a large, unselected heart-failure population?
- How well do all the techniques extrapolate to patients with more severe LV dysfunction, given more contemporary PET techniques (such as new crystals), SPECT attenuation correction, and advancing CMR technology?
- How often does the analysis of stress-induced ischemia add incremental information to analysis of resting tracer uptake or resting metabolic activity, particularly when the latter are in the "intermediate" range?
- Can more comprehensive outcome modeling be done for patients with ischemic cardiomyopathy, analogous to contemporary data for patients with CAD incorporating clinical, demographic, and stress test factors with imaging variables to more precisely model natural history outcomes?
- How is the viability information to be used in the setting of more complex decision making for revascularization, with concomitant valvular disease, for instance?
- Can we improve identification of remodeled myocardium that is viable by SPECT and PET but not capable of improving function, by incorporating new imaging probes, such as angiotensin-converting enzyme imaging,[97] that may identify physiologic signals of irreversible remodeling?
- Can the late gadolinium hyperenhancement CMR imaging concepts and data be reproduced using more widely available and technically less complex cardiac CT imaging, allowing comprehensive assessment of coronary anatomy incorporated in analysis of regional and global function as well as tissue viability?

Summary Points

- Major achievements in the study of noninvasive imaging techniques for assessing viability have shed light on the interesting and complex pathophysiologic processes of hibernation and stunning and advanced the use of imaging to inform patient management decisions and improve outcomes.
- The clinical literature on the use of noninvasive imaging to assess myocardial viability has evolved from predicting improvement in regional LV function to predicting patient-related outcomes, including heart-failure symptom improvement, survival, and differential outcomes with revascularization.
- Patients with heart failure, LV dysfunction, and a significant extent of ischemic viable myocardium are a very-high-risk subset. A substantial body of data demonstrates that risk to be reduced by revascularization. Among patients with predominantly nonviable myocardium, there appears no clear advantage to revascularization. Ongoing randomized trials may add to and refine our understanding of these issues.
- Substantial evidence suggests that noninvasive imaging of myocardial ischemia and viability can provide important prognostic information in patients with heart failure and LV dysfunction and can predict the potential benefit of revascularization.

References

1. Allman KC, Shaw LJ, Hachamovitch R, Udelson JE. Myocardial viability testing and impact of revascularization on prognosis in patients with coronary artery disease and left ventricular dysfunction: a meta-analysis. *J Am Coll Cardiol.* 2002;39:1151–1158.

2. Bax JJ, Wijns W, Cornel JH, Visser FC, Boersma E, Fioretti PM. Accuracy of currently available techniques for prediction of functional recovery after revascularization in patients with left ventricular dysfunction due to chronic coronary artery disease: comparison of pooled data. *J Am Coll Cardiol.* 1997;30:1451–1460.

3. Di Carli MF. Assessment of myocardial viability after myocardial infarction. *J Nucl Cardiol.* 2002;9:229–235.

4. Heyndrickx GR, Millard RW, McRitchie RJ, Maroko PR, Vatner SF. Regional myocardial functional and electrophysiological alterations after brief coronary artery occlusion in conscious dogs. *J Clin Invest.* 1975;56:978–985.

5. Braunwald E, Kloner RA. The stunned myocardium: prolonged, postischemic ventricular dysfunction. *Circulation.* 1982;66:1146–1149.

6. Diamond GA, Forrester JS, deLuz PL, Wyatt HL, Swan HJ. Post-extrasystolic potentiation of ischemic myocardium by atrial stimulation. *Am Heart J.* 1978;95:204–209.

7. Rahimtoola SH. A perspective on the three large multicenter randomized clinical trials of coronary bypass surgery for chronic stable angina. *Circulation.* 1985;72:V123–V135.

8. Dilsizian V, Bonow RO, Cannon RO 3rd, et al. The effect of coronary artery bypass grafting on left ventricular systolic function at rest: evidence for preoperative subclinical myocardial ischemia. *Am J Cardiol.* 1988;61:1248–1254.

9. Rees G, Bristow JD, Kremkau EL, et al. Influence of aortocoronary bypass surgery on left ventricular performance. *N Engl J Med.* 1971;284:1116–1120.

10. Bonow RO, Dilsizian V. Thallium 201 for assessment of myocardial viability. *Semin Nucl Med.* 1991;21:230–241.

11. Wijns W, Vatner SF, Camici PG. Hibernating myocardium. *N Engl J Med.* 1998;339:173–181.

12. Taegtmeyer H. *Myocardial Viability: A Clinical and Scientific Treatise.* Armonk, NY: Futura Publishing Company Inc; 2000.

13. Helfant RH, Pine R, Meister SG, Feldman MS, Trout RG, Banka VS. Nitroglycerin to unmask reversible asynergy. Correlation with post coronary bypass ventriculography. *Circulation.* 1974;50:108–113.

14. Popio KA, Gorlin R, Bechtel D, Levine JA. Postextrasystolic potentiation as a predictor of potential myocardial viability: preoperative analyses compared with studies after coronary bypass surgery. *Am J Cardiol.* 1977;39:944–953.

15. Horn HR, Teichholz LE, Cohn PF, Herman MV, Gorlin R. Augmentation of left ventricular contraction pattern in coronary artery disease by an inotropic catecholamine. The epinephrine ventriculogram. *Circulation.* 1974;49:1063–1071.

16. Rozanski A, Berman D, Gray R, et al. Preoperative prediction of reversible myocardial asynergy by postexercise radionuclide ventriculography. *N Engl J Med.* 1982;307:212–216.

17. Gibson RS, Watson DD, Taylor GJ, et al. Prospective assessment of regional myocardial perfusion before and after coronary revascularization surgery by quantitative thallium-201 scintigraphy. *J Am Coll Cardiol.* 1983;1:804–815.

18. Tillisch J, Brunken R, Marshall R, et al. Reversibility of cardiac wall-motion abnormalities predicted by positron tomography. *N Engl J Med.* 1986;314:884–888.

19. Bonow RO. Identification of viable myocardium. *Circulation.* 1996;94:2674–2680.

20. Udelson JE. Steps forward in the assessment of myocardial viability in left ventricular dysfunction. *Circulation.* 1998;97:833–838.

21. Samady H, Elefteriades JA, Abbott BG, Mattera JA, McPherson CA, Wackers FJ. Failure to improve left ventricular function after coronary revascularization for ischemic cardiomyopathy is not associated with worse outcome. *Circulation.* 1999;100:1298–1304.

22. Dilsizian V, Rocco TP, Freedman NM, Leon MB, Bonow RO. Enhanced detection of ischemic but viable myocardium by the reinjection of thallium after stress-redistribution imaging. *N Engl J Med.* 1990;323:141–146.

23. Ragosta M, Beller GA, Watson DD, Kaul S, Gimple LW. Quantitative planar rest-redistribution 201Tl imaging in detection of myocardial viability and prediction of

improvement in left ventricular function after coronary bypass surgery in patients with severely depressed left ventricular function. *Circulation*. 1993;87:1630–1641.

24. Udelson JE, Coleman PS, Metherall J, et al. Predicting recovery of severe regional ventricular dysfunction. Comparison of resting scintigraphy with 201Tl and 99mTc-sestamibi. *Circulation*. 1994;89:2552–2561.

25. Gunning MG, Anagnostopoulos C, Knight CJ, et al. Comparison of 201Tl, 99mTc-tetrofosmin, and dobutamine magnetic resonance imaging for identifying hibernating myocardium. *Circulation*. 1998;98:1869–1874.

26. Cleland JG, Pennell DJ, Ray SG, et al. Myocardial viability as a determinant of the ejection fraction response to carvedilol in patients with heart failure (CHRISTMAS trial): randomised controlled trial. *Lancet*. 2003;362:14–21.

27. Rahimtoola SH. The hibernating myocardium. *Am Heart J*. 1989;117:211–221.

28. Kaul S. There may be more to myocardial viability than meets the eye. *Circulation*. 1995; 92:2790–2793.

29. Lieberman AN, Weiss JL, Jugdutt BI, et al. Two-dimensional echocardiography and infarct size: relationship of regional wall motion and thickening to the extent of myocardial infarction in the dog. *Circulation*. 1981;63:739–746.

30. Myers JH, Stirling MC, Choy M, Buda AJ, Gallagher KP. Direct measurement of inner and outer wall thickening dynamics with epicardial echocardiography. *Circulation*. 1986; 74:164–172.

31. Udelson JE, Konstam MA. Relation between left ventricular remodeling and clinical outcomes in heart failure patients with left ventricular systolic dysfunction. *J Cardiac Failure*. 2003;8:S465–S471.

32. Alhaddad IA, Kloner RA, Hakim I, Garno JL, Brown EJ. Benefits of late coronary artery reperfusion on infarct expansion progressively diminish over time: relation to viable islets of myocytes within the scar. *Am Heart J*. 1996;131:451–457.

33. Hochman JS, Bulkley BH. Pathogenesis of left ventricular aneurysms: an experimental study in the rat model. *Am J Cardiol*. 1982;50:83–88.

34. Senior R, Lahiri A, Kaul S. Effect of revascularization on left ventricular remodeling in patients with heart failure from severe chronic ischemic left ventricular dysfunction. *Am J Cardiol*. 2001;88:624–629.

35. Sabia PJ, Powers ER, Ragosta M, Sarembock IJ, Burwell LR, Kaul S. An association between collateral blood flow and myocardial viability in patients with recent myocardial infarction. *N Engl J Med*. 1992;327:1825–1831.

36. Senior R, Kaul S, Raval U, Lahiri A. Impact of revascularization and myocardial viability determined by nitrate-enhanced Tc-99m sestamibi and Tl-201 imaging on mortality and functional outcome in ischemic cardiomyopathy. *J Nucl Cardiol*. 2002;9:454–462.

37. Bello D, Shah DJ, Farah GM, et al. Gadolinium cardiovascular magnetic resonance predicts reversible myocardial dysfunction and remodeling in patients with heart failure undergoing beta-blocker therapy. *Circulation*. 2003;108:1945–1953.

38. Di Carli MF, Asgarzadie F, Schelbert HR, et al. Quantitative relation between myocardial viability and improvement in heart failure symptoms after revascularization in patients with ischemic cardiomyopathy. *Circulation*. 1995;92:3436–3444.

39. Coles JG, Del Campo C, Ahmed SN, et al. Improved long-term survival following myocardial revascularization in patients with severe left ventricular dysfunction. *J Thorac Cardiovasc Surg*. 1981;81:846–850.

40. Kron IL, Flanagan TL, Blackbourne LH, Schroeder RA, Nolan SP. Coronary revascularization rather than cardiac transplantation for chronic ischemic cardiomyopathy. *Ann Surg*. 1989;210:348–352; discussion 352–354.

41. Marwick TH, Zuchowski C, Lauer MS, Secknus MA, Williams J, Lytle BW. Functional status and quality of life in patients with heart failure undergoing coronary bypass surgery after assessment of myocardial viability. *J Am Coll Cardiol*. 1999;33:750–758.

42. Bax JJ, Poldermans D, Elhendy A, et al. Improvement of left ventricular ejection fraction, heart failure symptoms and prognosis after revascularization in patients with chronic coronary artery disease and viable myocardium detected by dobutamine stress echocardiography. *J Am Coll Cardiol*. 1999;34:163–169.

43. Mickleborough LL, Maruyama H, Takagi Y, Mohamed S, Sun Z, Ebisuzaki L. Results of revascularization in patients with severe left ventricular dysfunction. *Circulation*. 1995;92: II73–II79.

44. Eitzman D, al-Aouar Z, Kanter HL, et al. Clinical outcome of patients with advanced coronary artery disease after viability studies with positron emission tomography. *J Am Coll Cardiol.* 1992;20:559–565.
45. Di Carli MF, Davidson M, Little R, et al. Value of metabolic imaging with positron emission tomography for evaluating prognosis in patients with coronary artery disease and left ventricular dysfunction. *Am J Cardiol.* 1994;73:527–533.
46. Chaudhry FA, Tauke JT, Alessandrini RS, Vardi G, Parker MA, Bonow RO. Prognostic implications of myocardial contractile reserve in patients with coronary artery disease and left ventricular dysfunction. *J Am Coll Cardiol.* 1999;34:730–738.
47. Sawada S, Bapat A, Vaz D, et al. Incremental value of myocardial viability for prediction of long-term prognosis in surgically revascularized patients with left ventricular dysfunction. *J Am Coll Cardiol.* 2003;42:2099–2105.
48. Sciagra R, Pellegri M, Pupi A, et al. Prognostic implications of Tc-99m sestamibi viability imaging and subsequent therapeutic strategy in patients with chronic coronary artery disease and left ventricular dysfunction. *J Am Coll Cardiol.* 2000;36:739–745.
49. Elsasser A, Schlepper M, Klovekorn WP, et al. Hibernating myocardium: an incomplete adaptation to ischemia. *Circulation.* 1997;96:2920–2931.
50. Beanlands RS, Hendry PJ, Masters RG, deKemp RA, Woodend K, Ruddy TD. Delay in revascularization is associated with increased mortality rate in patients with severe left ventricular dysfunction and viable myocardium on fluorine 18-fluorodeoxyglucose positron emission tomography imaging. *Circulation.* 1998;98:II51–II56.
51. Haas F, Haehnel CJ, Picker W, et al. Preoperative positron emission tomographic viability assessment and perioperative and postoperative risk in patients with advanced ischemic heart disease. *J Am Coll Cardiol.* 1997;30:1693–1700.
52. Dilsizian V, Freedman NM, Bacharach SL, Perrone-Filardi P, Bonow RO. Regional thallium uptake in irreversible defects. Magnitude of change in thallium activity after reinjection distinguishes viable from nonviable myocardium. *Circulation.* 1992;85:627–634.
53. Dilsizian V, Arrighi JA, Diodati JG, et al. Myocardial viability in patients with chronic coronary artery disease. Comparison of 99mTc-sestamibi with thallium reinjection and [18F]fluorodeoxyglucose. *Circulation.* 1994;89:578–587.
54. Dakik HA, Howell JF, Lawrie GM, et al. Assessment of myocardial viability with 99mTc-sestamibi tomography before coronary bypass graft surgery: correlation with histopathology and postoperative improvement in cardiac function. *Circulation.* 1997;96:2892–2898.
55. Medrano R, Lowry RW, Young JB, et al. Assessment of myocardial viability with 99mTc sestamibi in patients undergoing cardiac transplantation. A scintigraphic/pathological study. *Circulation.* 1996;94:1010–1017.
56. Zimmermann R, Mall G, Rauch B, et al. Residual 201Tl activity in irreversible defects as a marker of myocardial viability. Clinicopathological study. *Circulation.* 1995;91:1016–1021.
57. Maes AF, Borgers M, Flameng W, et al. Assessment of myocardial viability in chronic coronary artery disease using technetium-99m sestamibi SPECT. Correlation with histologic and positron emission tomographic studies and functional follow-up. *J Am Coll Cardiol.* 1997;29:62–68.
58. Kim RJ, Wu E, Rafael A, et al. The use of contrast-enhanced magnetic resonance imaging to identify reversible myocardial dysfunction. *N Engl J Med.* 2000;343:1445–1453.
59. Perrone-Filardi P, Pace L, Prastaro M, et al. Assessment of myocardial viability in patients with chronic coronary artery disease. Rest-4-hour-24-hour 201Tl tomography versus dobutamine echocardiography. *Circulation.* 1996;94:2712–2719.
60. Altehoefer C, vom Dahl J, Biedermann M, et al. Significance of defect severity in technetium-99m-MIBI SPECT at rest to assess myocardial viability: comparison with fluorine-18-FDG PET. *J Nucl Med.* 1994;35:569–574.
61. Tamaki N, Kawamoto M, Tadamura E, et al. Prediction of reversible ischemia after revascularization. Perfusion and metabolic studies with positron emission tomography. *Circulation.* 1995;91:1697–1705.
62. Kitsiou AN, Srinivasan G, Quyyumi AA, Summers RM, Bacharach SL, Dilsizian V. Stress-induced reversible and mild-to-moderate irreversible thallium defects: are they equally accurate for predicting recovery of regional left ventricular function after revascularization? *Circulation.* 1998;98:501–508.

63. Pasquet A, Robert A, D'Hondt AM, Dion R, Melin JA, Vanoverschelde JL. Prognostic value of myocardial ischemia and viability in patients with chronic left ventricular ischemic dysfunction. *Circulation.* 1999;100:141–148.

64. Afridi I, Kleiman NS, Raizner AE, Zoghbi WA. Dobutamine echocardiography in myocardial hibernation. Optimal dose and accuracy in predicting recovery of ventricular function after coronary angioplasty. *Circulation.* 1995;91:663–670.

65. Wellnhofer E, Olariu A, Klein C, et al. Magnetic resonance low-dose dobutamine test is superior to SCAR quantification for the prediction of functional recovery. *Circulation.* 2004;109:2172–2174.

66. Gerber BL, Vanoverschelde JL, Bol A, et al. Myocardial blood flow, glucose uptake, and recruitment of inotropic reserve in chronic left ventricular ischemic dysfunction. Implications for the pathophysiology of chronic myocardial hibernation. *Circulation.* 1996;94:651–659.

67. Baer FM, Voth E, Deutsch HJ, et al. Predictive value of low dose dobutamine transesophageal echocardiography and fluorine-18 fluorodeoxyglucose positron emission tomography for recovery of regional left ventricular function after successful revascularization. *J Am Coll Cardiol.* 1996;28:60–69.

68. Pagano D, Bonser RS, Townend JN, Ordoubadi F, Lorenzoni R, Camici PG. Predictive value of dobutamine echocardiography and positron emission tomography in identifying hibernating myocardium in patients with postischaemic heart failure. *Heart.* 1998;79:281–288.

69. Marzullo P, Parodi O, Reisenhofer B, et al. Value of rest thallium-201/technetium-99m sestamibi scans and dobutamine echocardiography for detecting myocardial viability. *Am J Cardiol.* 1993;71:166–172.

70. Alfieri O, La Canna G, Giubbini R, Pardini A, Zogno M, Fucci C. Recovery of myocardial function. The ultimate target of coronary revascularization. *Eur J Cardiothorac Surg.* 1993;7:325–330; discussion 330.

71. Charney R, Schwinger ME, Chun J, et al. Dobutamine echocardiography and resting-redistribution thallium-201 scintigraphy predicts recovery of hibernating myocardium after coronary revascularization. *Am Heart J.* 1994;128:864–869.

72. Arnese M, Cornel JH, Salustri A, et al. Prediction of improvement of regional left ventricular function after surgical revascularization. A comparison of low-dose dobutamine echocardiography with 201Tl single-photon emission computed tomography. *Circulation.* 1995;91:2748–2752.

73. Haque T, Furukawa T, Takahashi M, Kinoshita M. Identification of hibernating myocardium by dobutamine stress echocardiography: comparison with thallium-201 reinjection imaging. *Am Heart J.* 1995;130:553–563.

74. Senior R, Glenville B, Basu S, et al. Dobutamine echocardiography and thallium-201 imaging predict functional improvement after revascularisation in severe ischaemic left ventricular dysfunction. *Br Heart J.* 1995;74:358–364.

75. Vanoverschelde JL, D'Hondt AM, Marwick T, et al. Head-to-head comparison of exercise-redistribution-reinjection thallium single-photon emission computed tomography and low dose dobutamine echocardiography for prediction of reversibility of chronic left ventricular ischemic dysfunction. *J Am Coll Cardiol.* 1996;28:432–442.

76. Kostopoulos KG, Kranidis AI, Bouki KP, et al. Detection of myocardial viability in the prediction of improvement in left ventricular function after successful coronary revascularization by using the dobutamine stress echocardiography and quantitative SPECT rest-redistribution-reinjection 201Tl imaging after dipyridamole infusion. *Angiology.* 1996;47:1039–1046.

77. Bax JJ, Cornel JH, Visser FC, et al. Prediction of recovery of myocardial dysfunction after revascularization. Comparison of fluorine-18 fluorodeoxyglucose/thallium-201 SPECT, thallium-201 stress-reinjection SPECT and dobutamine echocardiography. *J Am Coll Cardiol.* 1996;28:558–564.

78. Qureshi U, Nagueh SF, Afridi I, et al. Dobutamine echocardiography and quantitative rest-redistribution 201Tl tomography in myocardial hibernation. Relation of contractile reserve to 201Tl uptake and comparative prediction of recovery of function. *Circulation.* 1997;95:626–635.

79. Nagueh SF, Vaduganathan P, Ali N, et al. Identification of hibernating myocardium: comparative accuracy of myocardial contrast echocardiography, rest-redistribution thallium-

201 tomography and dobutamine echocardiography. *J Am Coll Cardiol.* 1997;29:985–993.

80. Pace L, Perrone-Filardi P, Mainenti P, et al. Combined evaluation of rest-redistribution thallium-201 tomography and low-dose dobutamine echocardiography enhances the identification of viable myocardium in patients with chronic coronary artery disease. *Eur J Nucl Med.* 1998;25:744–750.

81. Sicari R, Varga A, Picano E, Borges AC, Gimelli A, Marzullo P. Comparison of combination of dipyridamole and dobutamine during echocardiography with thallium scintigraphy with thallium scintigraphy to improve viability detection. *Am J Cardiol.* 1999;83:6–10.

82. Gunning MG, Anagnostopoulos C, Davies G, et al. Simultaneous assessment of myocardial viability and function for the detection of hibernating myocardium using ECG-gated 99Tcm-tetrofosmin emission tomography: a comparison with 201Tl emission tomography combined with cine magnetic resonance imaging. *Nucl Med Commun.* 1999;20:209–214.

83. Cornel JH, Bax JJ, Elhendy A, Poldermans D, Vanoverschelde JL, Fioretti PM. Predictive accuracy of echocardiographic response of mildly dyssynergic myocardial segments to low-dose dobutamine. *Am J Cardiol.* 1997;80:1481–1484.

84. Sciagra R, Santoro GM, Bisi G, Pedenovi P, Fazzini PF, Pupi A. Rest-redistribution thallium-201 SPECT to detect myocardial viability. *J Nucl Med.* 1998;39:384–390.

85. Matsunari I, Fujino S, Taki J, et al. Quantitative rest technetium-99m tetrofosmin imaging in predicting functional recovery after revascularization: comparison with rest-redistribution thallium-201. *J Am Coll Cardiol.* 1997;29:1226–1233.

86. Giorgetti A, Pingitore A, Favilli B, Kusch A, Lombardi M, Marzullo P. Baseline/postnitrate tetrofosmin SPECT for myocardial viability assessment in patients with postischemic severe left ventricular dysfunction: new evidence from MRI. *J Nucl Med.* 2005;46:1285–1293.

87. Baer FM, Voth E, Schneider CA, Theissen P, Schicha H, Sechtem U. Comparison of low-dose dobutamine-gradient-echo magnetic resonance imaging and positron emission tomography with [18F]fluorodeoxyglucose in patients with chronic coronary artery disease. A functional and morphological approach to the detection of residual myocardial viability. *Circulation.* 1995;91:1006–1015.

88. Baer FM, Theissen P, Schneider CA, et al. Dobutamine magnetic resonance imaging predicts contractile recovery of chronically dysfunctional myocardium after successful revascularization. *J Am Coll Cardiol.* 1998;31:1040–1048.

89. Lauerma K, Niemi P, Hanninen H, et al. Multimodality MR imaging assessment of myocardial viability: combination of first-pass and late contrast enhancement to wall motion dynamics and comparison with FDG PET-initial experience. *Radiology.* 2000;217:729–736.

90. Selvanayagam JB, Kardos A, Francis JM, et al. Value of delayed-enhancement cardiovascular magnetic resonance imaging in predicting myocardial viability after surgical revascularization. *Circulation.* 2004;110:1535–1541.

91. Gutberlet M, Frohlich M, Mehl S, et al. Myocardial viability assessment in patients with highly impaired left ventricular function: comparison of delayed enhancement, dobutamine stress MRI, end-diastolic wall thickness, and Tl201-SPECT with functional recovery after revascularization. *Eur Radiol.* 2005;15:872–880.

92. Bodi V, Sanchis J, Lopez-Lereu MP, et al. Usefulness of a comprehensive cardiovascular magnetic resonance imaging assessment for predicting recovery of left ventricular wall motion in the setting of myocardial stunning. *J Am Coll Cardiol.* 2005;46:1747–1752.

93. Siebelink HM, Blanksma PK, Crijns HJ, et al. No difference in cardiac event-free survival between positron emission tomography-guided and single-photon emission computed tomography-guided patient management: a prospective, randomized comparison of patients with suspicion of jeopardized myocardium. *J Am Coll Cardiol.* 2001;37:81–88.

94. Panza JA, Dilsizian V, Laurienzo JM, Curiel RV, Katsiyiannis PT. Relation between thallium uptake and contractile response to dobutamine. Implications regarding myocardial viability in patients with chronic coronary artery disease and left ventricular dysfunction. *Circulation.* 1995;91:990–998.

95. Srinivasan G, Kitsiou AN, Bacharach SL, Bartlett ML, Miller-Davis C, Dilsizian V. [18F]fluorodeoxyglucose single photon emission computed tomography: can it replace PET

and thallium SPECT for the assessment of myocardial viability? *Circulation.* 1998; 97:843–850.

96. John AS, Dreyfus GD, Pennell DJ. Images in cardiovascular medicine. Reversible wall thinning in hibernation predicted by cardiovascular magnetic resonance. *Circulation.* 2005;111:e24–e25.

97. Dilsizian V, Shirani J, Lee YHC, et al. Specific binding of [18F] fluorobenzoyl-lisinopril to angiotensin converting enzyme in human heart tissue of ischemic cardiomyopathy. *Circulation.* 2001;104:II–694.

22 Role of Imaging Cardiac Innervation and Receptors in Heart Failure

Takahiro Higuchi, Markus Schwaiger, and Frank M. Bengel

Involvement of the sympathetic nervous system in congestive heart failure is characterized by a vicious circle, where reduced cardiac output results in neurohumoral activation. The hyperadrenergic state in turn causes desensitization and downregulation of cardiac β-adrenergic receptors and alterations of postsynaptic signal transduction, which further impair myocardial performance. Alterations of presynaptic cardiac sympathetic innervation are also involved in this pathophysiologic process. Reduction of presynaptic catecholamine reuptake increases overexposure to catecholamines further and thereby contributes to disease progression.

Positron emission tomography (PET) provides noninvasive information about global and regional myocardial autonomic innervation. This technique has substantially facilitated and refined the study of the heart's nervous system in health and disease, and has significantly contributed to a continuous improvement of the understanding of heart failure pathophysiology. Owing to high spatial and temporal resolution and routine attenuation correction, tracer kinetics can be defined in detail and absolute quantification is feasible. Radiolabeled catecholamines and catecholamine analogues are available that are well understood with regard to their tracer physiologic properties. Additionally, receptor ligands have been introduced that can be combined with presynaptic tracers to gain unique insights into mechanisms of myocardial biology and pathology.

This chapter summarizes currently available information on the use of cardiac PET imaging of autonomic innervation in the failing heart. First, a brief overview on biology of the sympathetic nervous system, along with available PET tracers, is given. Then, specific results in heart failure are summarized and put into the perspective of available additional experimental and clinical evidence.

The Cardiac Autonomic Nervous System

Regulation of cardiac function is essentially achieved by the cardiac muscle fiber length and its tension as an expression of ventricular volume and pressure, through the operation of Starling's law of the heart.[1,2] In addition, it is well known that the autonomic nervous system plays an important role in cardiac adaptation to the varying demands of daily life.[3-5] The central nervous system collects information about blood pressure, flow, and chemical milieu via receptors located in the left ventricle, carotid sinus, and aortic arch, connected with afferent neurons.[6] Based on the collected information, the autonomic nervous system then controls the rate, speed, and pattern of heart contraction via efferent neurons. Additionally, autonomic nervous regulation is also influenced by circulating hormonal factors[7] such as catecholamines[8] and angiotensin II (Figure 22.1).[9,10]

The central component of the cardiac autonomic nerve system is located in the medulla[11,12] and forms network loops with sensory afferent and efferent neurons. It consists of the sympathetic and parasympathetic systems, with their major neurotransmitters norepinephrine and acetylcholine, respectively.[13] These two systems mainly have opposing actions in their influence on cardiovascular physiology.[14,15]

Sympathetic nerve fibers are well distributed throughout the entire myocardium. They travel along epicardial vascular structures and penetrate the myocardium as coronary vessels do. In the presynaptic ending of sympathetic nerves, the sympathetic neurotransmitter norepinephrine is generated from tyrosine via dihydroxyphenylalanine and dopamine,[16–19] is imported to vesicles by energy-requiring vesicular monoamine transporter (VMAT), and is stored in the vesicles.[19] When a firing impulse arrives at the synaptic ending, voltage-dependent calcium channels open and norepinephrine is released to the synaptic cleft via exocytosis.[20] Only a small part of the norepinephrine in the cleft binds to adrenoreceptors on cardiac myocytes.[19] Most of the norepinephrine is reabsorbed into nerve endings via the presynaptic uptake-1 transporter.[21] A part of the absorbed norepinephrine is used again, and the other part is metabolized by monoamine oxidase (MAO) to 3,4-hydroxyphenylglycol (DHPG).[19,22] Because nerve endings do not contain catechol-o-methyltransferase (COMT),[23] most DHPG in the systemic circulation is believed to have a neural source. There is another reuptake mechanism into nonneuronal tissue mediated by the so-called uptake-2 transporter.[24] Norepinephrine that is taken up into nonneuronal tissue is metabolized to 3-methoxy-4-hydroxyphenylglycol (MHPG) via normetanephrine (NMN) by COMT and MAO.[25] Only a small fraction of norepinephrine released into the neural cleft spills over into vascular space. This fraction can be measured as norepinephrine level in coronary sinus vein blood.[26] In addition to neuronal stimulation, there are a number of regulatory mechanisms by presynaptic receptors, including α_2-adrenergic receptor, which provide negative feedback for exocytosis (Figure 22.2).[27]

Adrenergic receptors are guanine-nucleotide-binding protein (G-protein)-coupled receptors[28] and are classified into subtypes according to pharmacologic tissue effects or molecular biology. β-adrenergic receptors are abundant and uniformly distributed throughout the heart. β-adrenergic receptors are further classified into the subtypes β_1 and β_2. The ratio between β_1 and β_2 is approximately $5:1$ in healthy human heart.[29–31] α-adrenergic receptors are predominantly found in the vasculature but are also present in myocardium and constitute 15% of the total myocardial adrenergic receptors. α_1-adrenergic receptors are present postsynaptically, and α_2-adrenergic receptors are present both postsynaptically and presynaptically.[32]

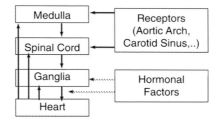

FIGURE 22.1. Schematic presentation of cardiac autonomic nerve pathway. The major central cardiac autonomic nerve system is located in the medulla and forms network loops with afferent and efferent neurons. This system controls cardiac function via efferent neurons based on the collected information via afferent neurons from receptors including aortic arch, carotid sinus, and heart. It is also influenced by many circulating hormonal factors.

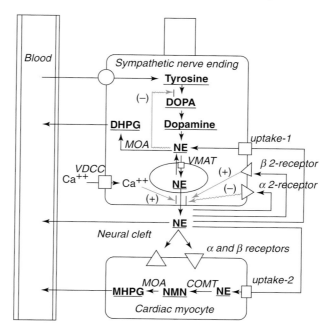

FIGURE 22.2. Cardiac sympathetic nerve ending. Sympathetic neurotransmitter norepinephrine is generated in synaptic nerve endings and stored in vesicles. At neuronal stimulation, norepinephrine is released into the synaptic cleft and partly binds to adrenoreceptors on the cardiac myocyte. Remaining norepinephrine is reabsorbed into nerve endings via uptake-1 transporter or into myocyte via uptake-2 transporter. Apart from neuronal stimulation, adrenergic receptors on the nerve ending provide negative and positive feedback for exocytosis. DOPA, dihydroxyphenylalanine; NE, norepinephrine, NMN, normetanephrine; MHPG, 3-methoxy-4-hydroxyphenylglycol; VMAT, vesicular amine transporter; DHPG, 3,4-hydroxyphenylglycol; MOA, monoamine oxidase; COMT, catechol-o-methyltransferase; VDDC, voltage-dependent calcium channel.

The parasympathetic nervous system acts predominantly against the effects of sympathetic function and is essential for maintaining homeostasis of heart function.[15,33] Parasympathetic neurons are distributed mainly in the atria and conduction nodules.[34] The density of parasympathetic neurons within myocardium is low compared to that of sympathetic nerves, rendering them a difficult target for nuclear imaging. Acetylcholine is the main neurotransmitter in parasympathetic neurons and is synthesized from choline in nerve endings. It is transported via the vesicular acetylcholine transporter (VAChT) into storage vesicles. Upon nerve stimulation, acetylcholine is then released from nerve terminals to the neural cleft[35] and binds to muscarinic receptors (M2-subtype) on the myocardium to activate changes in cardiac ion channel function.[36]

PET Tracers for Imaging Innervation and Receptors

Presynaptic Sympathetic Innervation

PET techniques provide noninvasive information about global and regional myocardial autonomic innervation.[37–43] Common PET tracers for presynaptic sympathetic innervation are either true catecholamines or catecholamine analogues (Table 22.1). Radiolabeled true neurotransmitters follow the entire metabolic pathways; analogues resist specific steps of metabolism. The specificity for the presynaptic uptake-1 transporter and vesicular storage inside the nerve terminal varies among currently available tracers.

TABLE 22.1. PET Radiopharmaceuticals for Clinical Neuronal Imaging

Tracer	Biologic Target
[11]C-hydroxyephedrine	Presynaptic catecholamine uptake
[11]C-epinephrine	Presynaptic catecholamine uptake and storage
[11]C-phenylephrine	Presynaptic catecholamine uptake and metabolism
F-18 fluorodopamine	Presynaptic sympathetic function

Carbon-11 (^{11}C)-meta-hydroxyephedrine (HED) is a norepinephrine analogue and is the most frequently used PET tracer for sympathetic neuronal imaging in human studies (Figure 22.3).[44-49] It is synthesized by N-methylation of metaraminol with ^{11}C-methyl iodide, which reliably yields HED at approximately 95% radiochemical and 98% chemical purity.[50] Plasma HED is transported into cardiac sympathetic nerve terminals via the uptake-1 mechanism in a fashion similar to norepinephrine, but it is metabolically resistant to MAO and COMT enzymes.[51] A validation study in pigs by Rosenspire et al showed that less than 5% of metabolites of HED remain in the heart 30 minutes after intravenous injection.[50] Although HED is not metabolized by neuronal degradation, it is slowly metabolized by liver tissue, and some radioactive metabolites appear in blood. In another rat experiment, selective neuronal uptake-1 blockage with desipramine resulted in a 92% reduction in HED myocardial tracer accumulation.[50] Norepinephrine treatment increased clearance rate without changing initial uptake, suggesting competitive inhibition of neuronal uptake or accelerated neuronal release or both.[52] Although vesicular storage seems to occur, binding inside vesicles is low due to a higher lipophilicity of HED compared to norepinephrine. These results from animal validation studies suggest that the retention of HED is highly dependent on reuptake by the norepinephrine transporter.

[11]C-epinephrine (EPI) is a more physiologic tracer than HED for evaluation of reuptake, vesicular storage, and metabolism in sympathetic presynaptic nerve terminals. EPI has been used in a few clinical studies.[48,53] It is synthesized from norepinephrine by direct methylation with ^{11}C-methyl iodide or ^{11}C-methyl triflate.

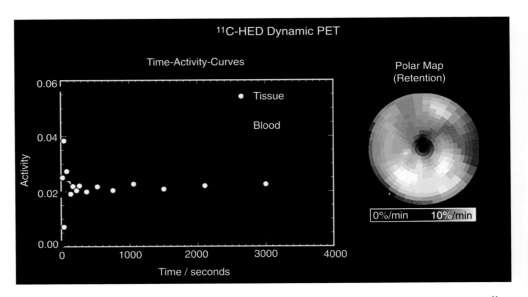

FIGURE 22.3. Dynamic PET study using the presynaptic sympathetic tracer ^{11}C-hydroxyephedrine (HED). Shown are representative time-activity curves for blood and myocardial tissue after tracer injection on the left, along with a polar map of quantitatively determined HED retention on the right, obtained in a normal individual.

Radiochemical and chemical purities are approximately 98% and 97%, respectively.[54] Plasma EPI is rapidly transported into cardiac sympathetic nerve terminals via uptake-1 and stored in terminal vesicles in a fashion similar to that of norepinephrine. It is vulnerable to cytosolic MAO degradation. In isolated perfused rat hearts, inhibition of uptake-1 by desipramine and reserpine demonstrated a decrease in myocardial uptake and retention of EPI by 91% and 95%, respectively, compared to controls.[55] However, the tracer washout acceleration by uptake-1 blockage is less in EPI compared to HED.[55] These results indicate that EPI is a tracer of neuronal uptake and vesicular storage while HED largely reflects uptake-1 only. In a clinical study, healthy volunteers and patients after heart transplantation were investigated using both EPI and HED.[53] Radiolabeled metabolites in blood at 20 minutes after injection were 82% and 47% for EPI and HED, respectively. However, the metabolite-corrected myocardial retention fraction of EPI was higher than that of HED. Difference between patients and a normal control group was larger for EPI than for HED. These results from clinical validation studies indicate that EPI may be more suitable for the study of neuronal integrity.

[11]C-phenylephrine (PHEN) is a norepinephrine analogue that is structurally similar to HED but is metabolized by MAO. PHEN is a sympathomimetic amine that is synthesized from direct methylation of m-octopamine with either ^{11}C-CH$_3$I or ^{11}C-CFSO$_3$CH$_3$, achieving high specific activity.[56] Biodistribution studies indicate that the initial uptake of PHEN in rat heart is approximately half that of HED.[56] Washout occurring from 5 to 60 minutes is higher for PHEN (50%) compared to HED (20%).[56] The heart neuronal selectivity determined by desipramine blockade of neuronal uptake is less for PHEN (76%) compared to HED.[56] Pretreatment with the MAO A inhibitor clorgyline resulted in higher PHEN retention in the rat heart.[56] Validation PET studies in healthy volunteers showed reduced retention and a half-life of approximately 60 minutes, while HED remained constant in myocardium.[51,57] These comparative animal and human PET experiments indicate that PHEN washout mainly reflects MAO activity.

In summary, the available ^{11}C-labeled tracers, including HED, EPI, and PHEN, thus reflect different mechanisms of norepinephrine metabolism in sympathetic nerve endings. These tracers can be combined to identify differential effects of disease on processes of norepinephrine uptake, vesicular storage, and metabolism in presynaptic adrenergic nerve terminals.

F-18 fluorodopamine (FDA) is another norepinephrine analogue that has been used for PET imaging of sympathetic innervation and function in humans.[58-62] It is labeled with F-18 (half-life, 110 minutes) so that tracer clearance from the heart can be surveyed over a longer period of time than with ^{11}C-labeled tracers (half-life, 20 minutes). Chirakal et al introduced a direct radiofluorination method of FDA to obtain high specific activity suitable for cardiac neuronal studies.[63] Plasma FDA is imported via the uptake-1 mechanism into sympathetic nerve endings and transported into storage vesicles, where it is β-hydroxylated to F-18 fluoronorepinephrine. Animal experimental data showed that pretreatment with despramine or tomoxetine markedly reduced cardiac uptake.[64] Comparative studies of the kinetics of FDA and fluoronorepinephrine revealed a faster myocardial washout for fluorodopamine.[62] These data suggest that myocardial radioactivity clearance after fluorodopamine injection is largely attributed to inefficient β-hydroxylation and subsequent degradation by neuronal MAO.

Presynaptic Parasympathetic Innervation

F-18 fluoroethoxybenzovesamicol (FEOBV) is a specific tracer that binds to the acetylcholine transporter on parasympathetic neurons. Kinetic experiments in isolated perfused rat hearts demonstrated high extraction and rapid washout of unbound tracer within 5 minutes.[65] However, specific binding in isolated perfused rat hearts was low, and nonspecific binding was high.[65] Additionally, there was considerable flow dependency of uptake[65] so that the usefulness of the tracer for clinical cardiac PET imaging was considered low. These results emphasize that, in contrast to sympathetic neurons, PET imaging of cardiac parasympathetic neurons is complicated, not only because density of cholinergic neurons within the ventricular myocardium is low. Design of a cholinergic tracer is difficult because the parasympathetic neurotransmitter mechanism is highly specific for acetylcholine, and cholinergic substances are very rapidly metabolized in blood. These factors have contributed to a persistent lack of established tracers for presynaptic parasympathetic innervation in heart.

Postsynaptic Autonomic Receptors

Several postsynaptic receptor ligands have been labeled and proposed as positron-emitting radioisotopes for cardiac imaging (Table 22.2). However, the clinical use of receptor-targeted tracers has been limited to a few studies and still faces significant challenges.[66] High specific binding, high affinity and hydrophilicity to avoid binding to internalized inactive receptors, lack of pharmacologic effects, and finally a simple and reliable tracer synthesis are requirements that must be met for a widespread application of receptor ligands for cardiac PET.

The hydrophilic nonselective β-adrenoreceptor antagonist ^{11}C-CGP12177 is still the most widely used tracer for adrenergic receptor imaging.[67–71] Synthesis of this tracer is not simple and requires ^{11}C-phosgen as a precursor, which has prevented a broader clinical application until now.[72] CGP12177 has high specific affinity and fast plasma clearance, suggesting feasibility for clinical imaging.[73] A graphical method that circumvents issues related to metabolites has been established for quantification in humans.[74] This approach requires a dual-injection protocol with doses of high and low specific activity.[74] β-adrenergic receptor density (B_{max}) measured by ^{11}C-CGP12177 PET correlated well with in vitro measurement from myocardial samples in healthy volunteers and patients with congestive cardiomyopathy.[71]

[11]C-CGP12388 is a recently introduced, nonselective β-adrenergic receptor antagonist (Figure 22.4). ^{11}C-CGP12388 can be labeled more easily than CGP12177 via a 1-pot procedure using $2-$[11]C-acetone.[72] It is also hydrophilic, even more so than ^{11}C-CGP12177, and the biodistribution and retention of CGP12388 are reported to be similar to those of CGP12177.[75] Studies in isolated perfused rat heart have shown that there is no significant difference between the B_{max} and total distribution volume (DVtot) under high-flow and low-flow conditions. DVtot was strongly reduced by β-adrenergic blockade using propranolol, and the B_{max} correlated significantly with in vitro values.[75] B_{max} estimated in 6 healthy human volunteers with ^{11}C-CGP12388 demonstrated values similar to those of ^{11}C-CGP12177.[76]

[11]C-GB67 is an analogue of the α_1-adrenergic receptor antagonist prazosin and is a tracer for myocardial α-adrenoceptor imaging.[77] It has been labeled by ^{11}C-methylation of N-desmethylamido-GB67.[78] Studies in rats demonstrated rapid plasma clearance of radioactivity.[78] Uptake was blocked with nonselective α-adrenergic receptor antagonists and only partially blocked with high-dose α_2-antagonists and β-antagonists, suggesting high selectivity for myocardial α_1-adrenoceptors.[78] In a clinical

TABLE 22.2. PET Radiopharmaceuticals for Clinical Receptor Imaging

Tracer	Biologic Target
[11]C-CGP12177	β-adrenergic receptor (nonselective)
[11]C-CGP12388	β-adrenergic receptor (nonselective)
[11]C-GB67	α-adrenergic receptor
[11]C-MQNB	Muscarinic receptor

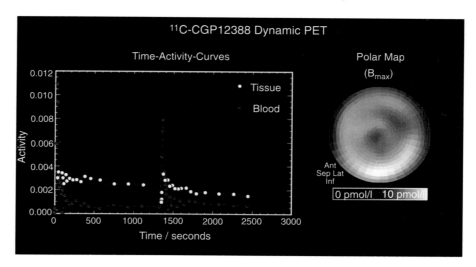

FIGURE 22.4. Dynamic PET study using the postsynaptic sympathetic tracer ^{11}C-CGP12388. Shown are representative time-activity curves for blood and myocardial tissue after dual tracer injection on the left, along with a polar map of quantitatively determined β-adrenoceptor density (B_{max}) on the right, obtained after graphical analysis in a normal individual.

validation study in two male human volunteers, ^{11}C-GB67 PET imaging demonstrated high myocardial uptake.[78] These results suggest that the tracer is promising for further evaluation. A variety of other subtype-specific or nonspecific tracers for adrenergic receptors have been tested experimentally but were found to be not suitable for clinical imaging, mainly due to high nonspecific binding or lipophilicity.

[11]C-methylquinuclidinyl benzilate (MQNB) is a tracer for parasympathetic muscarinic receptors. It is a nonmetabolized lipophilic and specific antagonist for muscarinic receptors. MQNB is synthesized with ^{11}C-methyl iodide from [11]$C-CO_2$ and quinuclidinyl benzilate and purified with HPLC.[79] Studies in dogs showed similar decreases of MQNB uptake in vivo and in vitro at baseline and after treatment with an irreversible acetylcholinesterase inhibitor.[80] PET studies in healthy volunteers demonstrated rapid plasma clearance and heart uptake mainly in the ventricular septum and in the left ventricular wall, while the atria were not visualized.[81] Additionally, MQNB concentrations in the ventricular septum were found to be highest when the heart rate at the time of injection was low, indicating the relation between a low-affinity conformational state of the receptor and predominant vagal stimulation.[81]

Other Cardiac Receptor Systems

In addition to the autonomic nervous system, there are other attractive targets for myocardial receptor imaging. They include the endothelin, opioid, adenosine, and angiotensin receptor systems, which are all thought to play a role in cardiovascular pathophysiology.

Endothelin (ET) is a potent vasoconstrictive peptide; its elevation has been reported in patients with chronic heart failure.[82–84] ET-1, one of the three isoforms of ET, is thought to play an important role in regulation of vascular function.[84] ET-1 pathophysiologic actions are mediated via binding with two receptor subtypes, ET_A and ET_B.[85] The ET_A receptor is located on vascular smooth muscle cells and mediates vasoconstriction. The ET_B receptor is located on both vascular smooth muscle and endothelial cells. In contrast to ET_A receptor bioactivity, the ET_B receptor on endothelial cells mediates vasodilation and growth inhibition indirectly through stimulation of nitric oxide and prostacyclin production. These ET receptors are frequently found in the heart and are thought to be markedly involved in the pathophysiologic mechanisms underlying heart failure.[85] ^{11}C-L-735037, a ^{11}C-labeled antagonist for ET_A and ET_B receptors, was evaluated in a dog study.[86] PET imaging showed high uptake in the left ventricular wall and reduced uptake after ET_A inhibitor infusion.[86] F-18 SB209670 is another, fluorine-labeled tracer for ET receptor imaging. In vivo studies in rats using an animal PET scanner demonstrated visualization of uptake in the rat heart.[87]

The opioid peptide receptor (OPR) is a well-established member of the G-protein-coupled receptor (GPCR) superfamily that is involved in regulating cardiac contractility, energy metabolism, and myocyte survival or death.[88–90] Animal models of heart failure showed activation of the opioid system, and opioid receptor-blocking agents may exert beneficial cardiovascular effects in heart failure.[88,89,91] ^{11}C-carfentanil and ^{11}C-N-methyl-naltindole are selective radioligands for mu and delta opioid receptor subtypes, respectively.[92] Initial PET studies with both tracers in humans showed homogeneous visualization of the heart and a decrease in the myocardial distribution volume in blocking studies with naloxone.[92]

These examples, although preliminary and limited to few studies, show that targeting of other, nonautonomic receptors may be feasible and may indicate some potential for further studies. But challenges similar to those in imaging of autonomic receptors, which are related to specific binding, affinity, hydrophilicity, and lack of pharmacologic effects and reliable synthesis, do exist and need to be addressed before a clinical establishment.

Imaging of Autonomic Nerve Function in Heart Failure

Dysfunction of the autonomic nervous system is an inherent feature of the failing heart.[93] The pathophysiologic importance of alterations of the autonomic system has been increasingly emphasized, and pharmacologic intervention using β-adrenergic blockers has become a standard feature of heart-failure therapy.[94] Autonomic nerve dysfunction is thought to be related to progression of heart failure through direct effects on the myocardium and through activation of other hormonal systems such as the renin-angiotensin system. PET imaging has contributed significantly to improving understanding of the role of autonomic innervation in the failing heart.

Presynaptic Sympathetic Innervation in Heart Failure

A huge body of experimental and clinical data has proven that sympathetic tone is increased in heart failure.[26,93,95,96] High levels of circulating norepinephrine are observed, and increased sympathetic nerve activity has been directly identified by clinical microneurography.[97,98] Eisenhofer et al investigated cardiac norepinephrine turnover in patients with chronic heart failure using tritiated norepinephrine. Baseline plasma norepinephrine levels, DHPG levels, and DHPG production rate were higher, but synthesis of norepinephrine itself did not change. Both norepinephrine release and reuptake were increased, but the efficacy of reuptake was reduced.[99] These data suggested that norepinephrine spillover is increased approximately 4 times, and cardiac norepinephrine store is reduced approximately 50% compared to that of normal subjects.[99] Reduction of functioning local presynaptic catecholamine uptake sites thus is likely to increase the myocardial overexposure to catecholamines.

The involvement of presynaptic sympathetic innervation in the pathophysiologic alterations occurring in the failing heart was further confirmed by PET and ^{11}C-HED in clinical studies. Vesalainen et al evaluated HED uptake in 30 patients with stable New York Heart Association (NYHA) class II and III heart failure due to coronary artery disease ($n = 24$) or dilated cardiomyopathy ($n = 6$), and in 10 healthy controls.

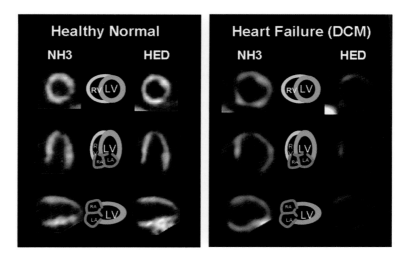

FIGURE 22.5. PET images of myocardial perfusion (by use of N-13 ammonia [NH₃]) and presynaptic sympathetic innervation (by use of ¹¹C-hydroxyephedrine [HED]) in a healthy normal individual (left) and in a patient with heart failure due to idiopathic dilated cardiomyopathy (right). Note the significant reduction of HED uptake in the failing heart when compared to perfusion tracer uptake in the same heart and when compared to the normal individual.

Global myocardial HED retention in all heart-failure patients was significantly reduced compared to normals (Figure 22.5). In addition, reduced HED retention was proportional to the response of systolic pressure to head-tilt and baroreflex control of heart rate.[100] These results suggest interaction between abnormal myocardial innervation and blood pressure maintenance. In another study, reduced global myocardial HED retention was reported to correlate with clinical markers of heart failure such as impaired ejection fraction and NYHA class as well as with elevation of plasma catecholamine levels.[101,102] Overall oxidative metabolism, determined by ¹¹C-acetate PET, was not directly correlated with impaired presynaptic innervation, but a significant correlation with impaired myocardial efficiency was identified.[101,103]

Regional patterns of myocardial sympathetic dysinnervation were described in 29 patients with NYHA class II-III heart failure due to dilated cardiomyopathy.[102] Significant reduction was found especially in the distal myocardium and reached a maximum in the apical and distal inferior segments. Another interesting study by Ungerer et al[104] in patients with terminal heart failure demonstrated significant correlation of in vivo measured regional HED retention with ex vivo determined downregulation of uptake-1 carriers in tissue samples from explanted hearts after transplantation.

Probably due to the mechanisms described above, the severity of alterations of sympathetic innervation seems to be closely related to progression of heart failure and patient outcome. Using nuclear imaging, this was first suggested by studies using single photon emission computed tomography (SPECT) with the catecholamine analogue I-123 MIBG.[105-107] Consistently, Pietila et al found that reduced global HED retention as determined by PET was also a predictor of adverse outcome (death or cardiac transplantation) in 46 patients with NYHA class II-III heart failure due to dilated cardiomyopathy and coronary artery disease.[49] Another study reported by Pietila demonstrated beneficial improvements with exercise training.[108] Although obtained in a limited number of patients, these data suggest potential clinical usefulness of neuronal imaging for determining prognosis and monitoring therapy.

Postsynaptic Receptors and Heart Failure

The hyperadrenergic state in congestive heart failure causes desensitization and downregulation of cardiac β-adrenergic receptors, along with alterations of postsynaptic signal transduction, which impair myocardial performance.[109–111] In vitro experimental data have confirmed a reduction of postsynaptic β-adrenergic receptor density (downregulation) and an impairment of receptor function (uncoupling), while the inactivating postsynaptic β-adrenergic receptor kinase-1 was elevated.[112] Additionally, the proportion of β-adrenergic receptor subtypes seems to change in heart failure, resulting in decreased density of β_1-receptors, but unchanged β_2-receptor status.[30,113]

Some PET studies with postsynaptic adrenergic receptor ligands were performed in heart failure. Merlet et al studied 8 normal subjects and 10 patients with idiopathic cardiomyopathy[114] and confirmed in vivo that left ventricular β-adrenergic receptor density was decreased (3.1 vs 6.6 pmol/mL, respectively). Using the alternative adrenergic receptor ligand ^{11}C-CGP12388, de Jong et al more recently also observed lower β-receptor density in patients with NYHA class II-III heart failure than in controls (5.4 vs 8.4 pmol/mL, respectively).[115]

The Parasympathetic Nervous System and Heart Failure

Based on the knowledge about impaired sympathetic innervation and the well-known, close interaction between sympathetic and parasympathetic innervation, it can already be assumed that parasympathetic innervation is also involved in heart failure pathophysiology. Indeed, changes of parasympathetic nerve activity have been described.[116] In some experimental and clinical studies, parasympathetic stimulation was shown to prevent pumping failure, cardiac remodeling, and life-threatening arrhythmias.[117] In advanced chronic heart failure, however, parasympathetic drive seems to be attenuated, and the resulting autonomic imbalance is thought to further promote disease progression.[117–119]

Changes in the density of ventricular muscarinic receptors have also been demonstrated. In an experimental study in dogs, Dunlap et al showed that muscarinic receptors are upregulated in heart failure induced by rapid pacing.[120] Le Guludec et al performed ^{11}C-MQNB PET studies in 20 patients with NYHA class II-IV heart failure due to idiopathic dilated cardiomyopathy and 12 controls.[121] Consistent with experimental data, they were able to show that in vivo muscarinic receptor density was significantly higher in patients than in controls (35 vs 26 pmol/mL), with no changes in affinity constants.

Summary Points

- The pivotal role of the autonomic nerve system in the control of cardiac function of heart failure has been known for decades and is still increasingly important.
- Advances in molecular pharmacology and recombinant DNA technology have allowed further insights into signal transduction and pre- and postsynaptic interaction. Progress in the field has often been achieved by in vitro studies and animal models. Although features in animal hearts and experimental disease models often reflect those in humans, the failing human heart still has some unique characteristics.[122]
- Advanced PET imaging techniques provide noninvasive, repeatable in vivo information on global and regional presynaptic neurotransmission and postsynaptic receptor function of the human heart. In addition, the spectrum of target molecules is continuously broadening and will allow for increasingly specific characterization.
- Autonomic innervation and receptor imaging with PET is thus a unique method with a strong future potential for providing profound insights into molecular pathophysiology, monitoring of treatment, and determination of individual outcomes.

References

1. Fukuda N, Granzier H. Role of the giant elastic protein titin in the Frank-Starling mechanism of the heart. *Curr Vasc Pharmacol.* 2004;2:135–139.
2. Katz AM. Molecular biology in cardiology, a paradigmatic shift. *J Mol Cell Cardiol.* 1988;20:355–366.
3. Luetscher JA, Boyers DG, Cuthbertson JG, McMahon DF. A model of the human circulation. Regulation by autonomic nervous system and renin-angiotensin system, and influence of blood volume on cardiac output and blood pressure. *Circ Res.* 1973;32(suppl 1):84–98.
4. Hellenbrand WK, Klassen GA, Armour JA, Sezerman O, Paton B. Autonomic nervous system regulation of epicardial coronary vein systolic and diastolic blood velocity as measured by a laser Doppler velocimeter. *Can J Physiol Pharmacol.* 1986;64:1463–1472.
5. Levy MN, Yang T, Wallick DW. Assessment of beat-by-beat control of heart rate by the autonomic nervous system: molecular biology techniques are necessary, but not sufficient. *J Cardiovasc Electrophysiol.* 1993;4:183–193.
6. Levy MN. Autonomic interactions in cardiac control. *Ann N Y Acad Sci.* 1990;601:209–221.
7. Randall DC, Evans JM, Billman GE, Ordway GA, Knapp CF. Neural, hormonal and intrinsic mechanisms of cardiac control during acute coronary occlusion in the intact dog. *J Auton Nerv Syst.* 1981;3:87–99.
8. Miura Y, Haneda T, Sato T, et al. Plasma catecholamine levels in the coronary sinus, aorta and femoral vein of subjects undergoing cardiac catheterization at rest and during exercise. *Jpn Circ J.* 1976;40:929–934.
9. Klug D, Robert V, Swynghedauw B. Role of mechanical and hormonal factors in cardiac remodeling and the biologic limits of myocardial adaptation. *Am J Cardiol.* 1993;71:46A–54A.
10. Liu JL, Zucker IH. Regulation of sympathetic nerve activity in heart failure: a role for nitric oxide and angiotensin II. *Circ Res.* 1999;84:417–423.
11. Pilowsky P, West M, Chalmers J. Renal sympathetic nerve responses to stimulation, inhibition and destruction of the ventrolateral medulla in the rabbit. *Neurosci Lett.* 1985;60:51–55.
12. Yen CT, Hwang JC, Su CK, Lin YF, Yang JM, Chai CY. Differential actions of the medial region of caudal medulla on autonomic nerve activities. *Clin Exp Pharmacol Physiol.* 1991;18:743–751.
13. Levy MN. Cardiac sympathetic-parasympathetic interactions. *Fed Proc.* 1984;43:2598–2602.
14. Zemaityte DJ, Varoneckas GA, Sokolov EN. Interaction between the parasympathetic and sympathetic divisions of the autonomic nervous system in cardiac rhythm regulation. *Hum Physiol.* 1985;11:208–215.
15. Sunagawa K, Kawada T, Nakahara T. Dynamic nonlinear vago-sympathetic interaction in regulating heart rate. *Heart Vessels.* 1998;13:157–174.
16. Jonsson G, Sachs C. Synthesis of noradrenaline from 3,4-dihydroxyphenylalanine (DOPA) and dopamine in adrenergic nerves of mouse atrium—effect of reserpine, monoamine oxidase and tyrosine hydroxylase inhibition. *Acta Physiol Scand.* 1970;80:307–322.
17. Tong JH, Smyth RG, Benoiton NL, D'Iorio A. In vivo studies on the conversion of m-tyrosine to 3,4-dihydroxyphenylalanine in the rat. *Can J Biochem.* 1977;55:1103–1107.
18. Udenfriend S, Dairman W. Regulation of norepinephrine synthesis. *Adv Enzyme Regul.* 1970;9:145–165.
19. Eisenhofer G, Kopin IJ, Goldstein DS. Catecholamine metabolism: a contemporary view with implications for physiology and medicine. *Pharmacol Rev.* 2004;56:331–349.
20. Wakade AR, Przywara DA, Bhave SV, Chowdhury PS, Bhave A, Wakade TD. Massive exocytosis triggered by sodium-calcium exchange in sympathetic neurons is attenuated by co-culture with cardiac cells. *Neuroscience.* 1993;55:813–821.
21. Goldstein DS, Brush JE, Jr., Eisenhofer G, Stull R, Esler M. In vivo measurement of neuronal uptake of norepinephrine in the human heart. *Circulation.* 1988;78:41–48.
22. Smith CB. The role of monoamine oxidase in the intraneuronal metabolism of norepinephrine released by indirectly-acting sympathomimetic amines or by adrenergic nerve stimulation. *J Pharmacol Exp Ther.* 1966;151:207–220.

23. Scheinin M, Karhuvaara S, Ojala-Karlsson P, Kallio A, Koulu M. Plasma 3,4-dihydroxyphenylglycol (DHPG) and 3-methoxy-4-hydroxyphenylglycol (MHPG) are insensitive indicators of alpha 2-adrenoceptor mediated regulation of norepinephrine release in healthy human volunteers. *Life Sci.* 1991;49:75–84.

24. Clarke DE, Jones CJ, Linley PA. Histochemical fluorescence studies on noradrenaline accumulation by Uptake 2 in the isolated rat heart. *Br J Pharmacol.* 1969;37:1–9.

25. Oeltmann T, Carson R, Shannon JR, Ketch T, Robertson D. Assessment of O-methylated catecholamine levels in plasma and urine for diagnosis of autonomic disorders. *Auton Neurosci.* 2004;116:1–10.

26. Hasking GJ, Esler MD, Jennings GL, Burton D, Johns JA, Korner PI. Norepinephrine spillover to plasma in patients with congestive heart failure: evidence of increased overall and cardiorenal sympathetic nervous activity. *Circulation.* 1986;73:615–621.

27. Hein L, Altman JD, Kobilka BK. Two functionally distinct alpha2-adrenergic receptors regulate sympathetic neurotransmission. *Nature.* 1999;402:181–184.

28. Insel PA. Adrenergic receptors. Evolving concepts on structure and function. *Am J Hypertens.* 1989;2:112S–118S.

29. von der Leyen H, Steinfath M, Hecht A, et al. Changes in cardiac beta 1- and beta 2-adrenoceptor densities after human cardiac transplantation: relation to transplant coronary vasculopathy and pretransplantation disease. *Am Heart J.* 1992;124:686–693.

30. Steinfath M, Lavicky J, Schmitz W, Scholz H, Doring V, Kalmar P. Regional distribution of beta 1- and beta 2-adrenoceptors in the failing and nonfailing human heart. *Eur J Clin Pharmacol.* 1992;42:607–611.

31. Heitz A, Schwartz J, Velly J. Beta-adrenoceptors of the human myocardium: determination of beta 1 and beta 2 subtypes by radioligand binding. *Br J Pharmacol.* 1983;80:711–717.

32. Williams RS, Dukes DF, Lefkowitz RJ. Subtype specificity of alpha-adrenergic receptors in rat heart. *J Cardiovasc Pharmacol.* 1981;3:522–531.

33. Kawada T, Ikeda Y, Sugimachi M, et al. Bidirectional augmentation of heart rate regulation by autonomic nervous system in rabbits. *Am J Physiol.* 1996;271:H288–H295.

34. Johnson TA, Gray AL, Lauenstein JM, Newton SS, Massari VJ. Parasympathetic control of the heart. I. An interventriculo-septal ganglion is the major source of the vagal intracardiac innervation of the ventricles. *J Appl Physiol.* 2004;96:2265–2272.

35. Paton WD, Vizi ES, Zar MA. The mechanism of acetylcholine release from parasympathetic nerves. *J Physiol.* 1971;215:819–848.

36. Harvey RD, Belevych AE. Muscarinic regulation of cardiac ion channels. *Br J Pharmacol.* 2003;139:1074–1084.

37. Melon P, Schwaiger M. Imaging of metabolism and autonomic innervation of the heart by positron emission tomography. *Eur J Nucl Med.* 1992;19:453–464.

38. Schwaiger M, Beanlands R, vom Dahl J. Metabolic tissue characterization in the failing heart by positron emission tomography. *Eur Heart J.* 1994;15(suppl D):14–19.

39. Raffel DM, Wieland DM. Assessment of cardiac sympathetic nerve integrity with positron emission tomography. *Nucl Med Biol.* 2001;28:541–559.

40. Carrio I. Cardiac neurotransmission imaging. *J Nucl Med.* 2001;42:1062–1076.

41. Bengel FM, Schwaiger M. Assessment of cardiac sympathetic neuronal function using PET imaging. *J Nucl Cardiol.* 2004;11:603–616.

42. Langer O, Halldin C. PET and SPET tracers for mapping the cardiac nervous system. *Eur J Nucl Med Mol Imaging.* 2002;29:416–434.

43. Machac J. Cardiac positron emission tomography imaging. *Semin Nucl Med.* 2005;35:17–36.

44. Schwaiger M, Hutchins GD, Kalff V, et al. Evidence for regional catecholamine uptake and storage sites in the transplanted human heart by positron emission tomography. *J Clin Invest.* 1991;87:1681–1690.

45. Bengel FM, Ueberfuhr P, Hesse T, et al. Clinical determinants of ventricular sympathetic reinnervation after orthotopic heart transplantation. *Circulation.* 2002;106:831–835.

46. Bengel FM, Ueberfuhr P, Schiepel N, Nekolla SG, Reichart B, Schwaiger M. Effect of sympathetic reinnervation on cardiac performance after heart transplantation. *N Engl J Med.* 2001;345:731–738.

47. Mazzadi AN, Andre-Fouet X, Duisit J, et al. Cardiac retention of [11C]HED in genotyped long QT patients: a potential amplifier role for severity of the disease. *Am J Physiol Heart Circ Physiol.* 2003;285:H1286–H1293.

48. Bengel FM, Ueberfuhr P, Ziegler SI, Nekolla S, Reichart B, Schwaiger M. Serial assessment of sympathetic reinnervation after orthotopic heart transplantation. A longitudinal study using PET and C-11 hydroxyephedrine. *Circulation.* 1999;99: 1866–1871.

49. Pietila M, Malminiemi K, Ukkonen H, et al. Reduced myocardial carbon-11 hydroxyephedrine retention is associated with poor prognosis in chronic heart failure. *Eur J Nucl Med.* 2001;28:373–376.

50. Rosenspire KC, Haka MS, Van Dort ME, et al. Synthesis and preliminary evaluation of carbon-11-meta-hydroxyephedrine: a false transmitter agent for heart neuronal imaging. *J Nucl Med.* 1990;31:1328–1334.

51. Raffel DM, Corbett JR, del Rosario RB, et al. Clinical evaluation of carbon-11-phenylephrine: MAO-sensitive marker of cardiac sympathetic neurons. *J Nucl Med.* 1996;37:1923–1931.

52. DeGrado TR, Hutchins GD, Toorongian SA, Wieland DM, Schwaiger M. Myocardial kinetics of carbon-11-meta-hydroxyephedrine: retention mechanisms and effects of norepinephrine. *J Nucl Med.* 1993;34:1287–1293.

53. Munch G, Nguyen NT, Nekolla S, et al. Evaluation of sympathetic nerve terminals with [(11)C]epinephrine and [(11)C]hydroxyephedrine and positron emission tomography. *Circulation.* 2000;101:516–523.

54. Chakraborty PK, Gildersleeve DL, Jewett DM, et al. High yield synthesis of high specific activity R-(-)-[11C]epinephrine for routine PET studies in humans. *Nucl Med Biol.* 1993;20:939–944.

55. Nguyen NT, DeGrado TR, Chakraborty P, Wieland DM, Schwaiger M. Myocardial kinetics of carbon-11-epinephrine in the isolated working rat heart. *J Nucl Med.* 1997;38:780–785.

56. Del Rosario RB, Jung YW, Caraher J, Chakraborty PK, Wieland DM. Synthesis and preliminary evaluation of [11C]-(-)-phenylephrine as a functional heart neuronal PET agent. *Nucl Med Biol.* 1996;23:611–616.

57. Raffel DM, Corbett JR, del Rosario RB, et al. Sensitivity of [11C]phenylephrine kinetics to monoamine oxidase activity in normal human heart. *J Nucl Med.* 1999;40: 232–238.

58. Singleton A, Gwinn-Hardy K, Sharabi Y, et al. Association between cardiac denervation and parkinsonism caused by alpha-synuclein gene triplication. *Brain.* 2004;127:768–772.

59. Li ST, Holmes C, Kopin IJ, Goldstein DS. Aging-related changes in cardiac sympathetic function in humans, assessed by 6-18F-fluorodopamine PET scanning. *J Nucl Med.* 2003;44:1599–1603.

60. Li ST, Tack CJ, Fananapazir L, Goldstein DS. Myocardial perfusion and sympathetic innervation in patients with hypertrophic cardiomyopathy. *J Am Coll Cardiol.* 2000;35: 1867–1873.

61. Goldstein DS, Holmes C, Stuhlmuller JE, Lenders JW, Kopin IJ. 6-[18F]fluorodopamine positron emission tomographic scanning in the assessment of cardiac sympathoneural function—studies in normal humans. *Clin Auton Res.* 1997;7:17–29.

62. Goldstein DS, Eisenhofer G, Dunn BB, et al. Positron emission tomographic imaging of cardiac sympathetic innervation using 6-[18F]fluorodopamine: initial findings in humans. *J Am Coll Cardiol.* 1993;22:1961–1971.

63. Chirakal R, Coates G, Firnau G, Schrobilgen GJ, Nahmias C. Direct radiofluorination of dopamine: 18F-labeled 6-fluorodopamine for imaging cardiac sympathetic innervation in humans using positron emission tomography. *Nucl Med Biol.* 1996;23:41–45.

64. Ding YS, Fowler JS, Gatley SJ, Logan J, Volkow ND, Shea C. Mechanistic positron emission tomography studies of 6-[18F]fluorodopamine in living baboon heart: selective imaging and control of radiotracer metabolism using the deuterium isotope effect. *J Neurochem.* 1995;65:682–690.

65. DeGrado TR, Mulholland GK, Wieland DM, Schwaiger M. Evaluation of (-)[18F]fluoro ethoxybenzovesamicol as a new PET tracer of cholinergic neurons of the heart. *Nucl Med Biol.* 1994;21:189–195.

66. Elsinga PH, van Waarde A, Visser TJ, Vaalburg W. Visualization of beta-Adrenoceptors Using PET. *Clin Positron Imaging.* 1998;1:81–94.

67. Link JM, Stratton JR, Levy W, et al. PET measures of pre- and post-synaptic cardiac beta adrenergic function. *Nucl Med Biol.* 2003;30:795–803.

68. Schafers M, Lerch H, Wichter T, et al. Cardiac sympathetic innervation in patients with idiopathic right ventricular outflow tract tachycardia. *J Am Coll Cardiol*. 1998;32: 181–186.

69. Lefroy DC, de Silva R, Choudhury L, et al. Diffuse reduction of myocardial beta-adrenoceptors in hypertrophic cardiomyopathy: a study with positron emission tomography. *J Am Coll Cardiol*. 1993;22:1653–1660.

70. Wichter T, Schafers M, Rhodes CG, et al. Abnormalities of cardiac sympathetic innervation in arrhythmogenic right ventricular cardiomyopathy: quantitative assessment of presynaptic norepinephrine reuptake and postsynaptic beta-adrenergic receptor density with positron emission tomography. *Circulation*. 2000;101:1552–1558.

71. Ungerer M, Weig HJ, Kubert S, et al. Regional pre- and postsynaptic sympathetic system in the failing human heart–regulation of beta ARK-1. *Eur J Heart Fail*. 2000;2:23–31.

72. Elsinga PH, van Waarde A, Jaeggi KA, Schreiber G, Heldoorn M, Vaalburg W. Synthesis and evaluation of (S)-4-(3-(2′-[11C]isopropylamino)-2-hydroxypropoxy) -2H-benzimidazol -2-one ((S)-[11C]CGP 12388) and (S)-4-(3-((1′-[18F]-fluoroisopropyl)amino)-2-hydroxypropoxy) -2H- benzimidazol-2-one ((S)-[18F]fluoro-CGP 12388) for visualization of beta-adrenoceptors with positron emission tomography. *J Med Chem*. 1997;40:3829–3835.

73. Law MP. Demonstration of the suitability of CGP 12177 for in vivo studies of beta-adrenoceptors. *Br J Pharmacol*. 1993;109:1101–1109.

74. Delforge J, Mesangeau D, Dolle F, et al. In vivo quantification and parametric images of the cardiac beta-adrenergic receptor density. *J Nucl Med*. 2002;43:215–226.

75. Momose M, Reder S, Raffel DM, et al. Evaluation of cardiac beta-adrenoreceptors in the isolated perfused rat heart using (S)-11C-CGP12388. *J Nucl Med*. 2004;45:471–477.

76. Doze P, Elsinga PH, van Waarde A, et al. Quantification of beta-adrenoceptor density in the human heart with (S)-[11C]CGP 12388 and a tracer kinetic model. *Eur J Nucl Med Mol Imaging*. 2002;29:295–304.

77. Pike VW, Law MP, Osman S, et al. Selection, design and evaluation of new radioligands for PET studies of cardiac adrenoceptors. *Pharm Acta Helv*. 2000;74:191–200.

78. Law MP, Osman S, Pike VW, et al. Evaluation of [11C]GB67, a novel radioligand for imaging myocardial alpha 1-adrenoceptors with positron emission tomography. *Eur J Nucl Med*. 2000;27:7–17.

79. Kassiou M, Mardon K, Katsifis AG, et al. Radiosynthesis of [123I]N-methyl-4-iododexetimide and [123I]N-methyl-4-iodolevetimide: in vitro and in vivo characterisation of binding to muscarinic receptors in the rat heart. *Nucl Med Biol*. 1996;23:147–153.

80. Valette H, Syrota A, Fuseau C. Down-regulation of cardiac muscarinic receptors induced by di-isopropylfluorophosphate. *J Nucl Med*. 1997;38:1430–1433.

81. Syrota A, Comar D, Paillotin G, et al. Muscarinic cholinergic receptor in the human heart evidenced under physiological conditions by positron emission tomography. *Proc Natl Acad Sci U S A*. 1985;82:584–588.

82. Bennett RT, Jones RD, Morice AH, Smith CF, Cowen ME. Vasoconstrictive effects of endothelin-1, endothelin-3, and urotensin II in isolated perfused human lungs and isolated human pulmonary arteries. *Thorax*. 2004;59:401–407.

83. Zolk O, Bohm M. The role of the cardiac endothelin system in heart failure. *Nephrol Dial Transplant*. 2000;15:758–760.

84. Pousset F, Isnard R, Lechat P, et al. Prognostic value of plasma endothelin-1 in patients with chronic heart failure. *Eur Heart J*. 1997;18:254–258.

85. Kobayshi T, Miyauchi T, Sakai S, et al. Down-regulation of ET(B) receptor, but not ET(A) receptor, in congestive lung secondary to heart failure. Are marked increases in circulating endothelin-1 partly attributable to decreases in lung ET(B) receptor-mediated clearance of endothelin-1? *Life Sci*. 1998;62:185–193.

86. Aleksic S, Szabo Z, Scheffel U, et al. In vivo labeling of endothelin receptors with [(11)C]L-753,037: studies in mice and a dog. *J Nucl Med*. 2001;42:1274–1280.

87. Johnstrom P, Harris NG, Fryer TD, et al. (18)F-Endothelin-1, a positron emission tomography (PET) radioligand for the endothelin receptor system: radiosynthesis and in vivo imaging using microPET. *Clin Sci (Lond)*. 2002;103(suppl 48):4S-8S.

88. Oldroyd KG, Gray CE, Carter R, et al. Activation and inhibition of the endogenous opioid system in human heart failure. *Br Heart J*. 1995;73:41–48.

89. Imai N, Kashiki M, Woolf PD, Liang CS. Comparison of cardiovascular effects of mu- and delta-opioid receptor antagonists in dogs with congestive heart failure. *Am J Physiol.* 1994;267:H912–H917.
90. Sakamoto S, Liang CS. Opiate receptor inhibition improves the blunted baroreflex function in conscious dogs with right-sided congestive heart failure. *Circulation.* 1989;80:1010–1015.
91. Liang CS, Imai N, Stone CK, Woolf PD, Kawashima S, Tuttle RR. The role of endogenous opioids in congestive heart failure: effects of nalmefene on systemic and regional hemodynamics in dogs. *Circulation.* 1987;75:443–451.
92. Villemagne PS, Dannals RF, Ravert HT, Frost JJ. PET imaging of human cardiac opioid receptors. *Eur J Nucl Med Mol Imaging.* 2002;29:1385–1388.
93. Kaye D, Esler M. Sympathetic neuronal regulation of the heart in aging and heart failure. *Cardiovasc Res.* 2005;66:256–264.
94. Sauls JL, Rone T. Emerging trends in the management of heart failure: Beta blocker therapy. *Nurs Clin North Am.* 2005;40:135–148.
95. Esler M, Lambert G, Brunner-La Rocca HP, Vaddadi G, Kaye D. Sympathetic nerve activity and neurotransmitter release in humans: translation from pathophysiology into clinical practice. *Acta Physiol Scand.* 2003;177:275–284.
96. Daly PA, Sole MJ. Myocardial catecholamines and the pathophysiology of heart failure. *Circulation.* 1990;82:I35–I43.
97. Andersson KE. Adrenergic mechanisms in congestive heart failure. *Acta Med Scand Suppl.* 1986;707:37–44.
98. Ferrari R, Ceconi C, Curello S, Visioli O. The neuroendocrine and sympathetic nervous system in congestive heart failure. *Eur Heart J.* 1998;19(suppl F):F45–F51.
99. Eisenhofer G, Friberg P, Rundqvist B, et al. Cardiac sympathetic nerve function in congestive heart failure. *Circulation.* 1996;93:1667–1676.
100. Vesalainen RK, Pietila M, Tahvanainen KU, et al. Cardiac positron emission tomography imaging with [11C]hydroxyephedrine, a specific tracer for sympathetic nerve endings, and its functional correlates in congestive heart failure. *Am J Cardiol.* 1999;84:568–574.
101. Bengel FM, Permanetter B, Ungerer M, Nekolla SG, Schwaiger M. Relationship between altered sympathetic innervation, oxidative metabolism and contractile function in the cardiomyopathic human heart; a non-invasive study using positron emission tomography. *Eur Heart J.* 2001;22:1594–1600.
102. Hartmann F, Ziegler S, Nekolla S, et al. Regional patterns of myocardial sympathetic denervation in dilated cardiomyopathy: an analysis using carbon-11 hydroxyephedrine and positron emission tomography. *Heart.* 1999;81:262–270.
103. Bengel FM, Ueberfuhr P, Ziegler SI, et al. Non-invasive assessment of the effect of cardiac sympathetic innervation on metabolism of the human heart. *Eur J Nucl Med.* 2000;27:1650–1657.
104. Ungerer M, Weig HJ, Kubert S, et al. Regional pre- and postsynaptic sympathetic system in the failing human heart-regulation of beta ARK-1. *Eur J Heart Fail.* 2000;2:23–31.
105. Momose M, Kobayashi H, Iguchi N, et al. Comparison of parameters of 123I-MIBG scintigraphy for predicting prognosis in patients with dilated cardiomyopathy. *Nucl Med Commun.* 1999;20:529–535.
106. Hattori N, Schwaiger M. Metaiodobenzylguanidine scintigraphy of the heart: what have we learnt clinically? *Eur J Nucl Med.* 2000;27:1–6.
107. Yamashina S, Yamazaki J. Role of MIBG myocardial scintigraphy in the assessment of heart failure: the need to establish evidence. *Eur J Nucl Med Mol Imaging.* 2004;31:1353–1355.
108. Pietila M, Malminiemi K, Vesalainen R, et al. Exercise training in chronic heart failure: beneficial effects on cardiac (11)C-hydroxyephedrine PET, autonomic nervous control, and ventricular repolarization. *J Nucl Med.* 2002;43:773–779.
109. Insel PA, Hammond HK. Beta-adrenergic receptors in heart failure. *J Clin Invest.* 1993;92:2564.
110. Lefkowitz RJ, Rockman HA, Koch WJ. Catecholamines, cardiac beta-adrenergic receptors, and heart failure. *Circulation.* 2000;101:1634–1637.
111. Liggett SB. Polymorphisms of beta-adrenergic receptors in heart failure. *Am J Med.* 2004;117:525–527.

112. Choi DJ, Koch WJ, Hunter JJ, Rockman HA. Mechanism of beta-adrenergic receptor desensitization in cardiac hypertrophy is increased beta-adrenergic receptor kinase. *J Biol Chem.* 1997;272:17223–17229.

113. Pitschner HF, Droege A, Mitze M, Schlepper M, Brodde OE. Down-regulated beta-adrenoceptors in severely failing human ventricles: uniform regional distribution, but no increased internalization. *Basic Res Cardiol.* 1993;88:179–191.

114. Merlet P, Delforge J, Syrota A, et al. Positron emission tomography with 11C CGP-12177 to assess beta-adrenergic receptor concentration in idiopathic dilated cardiomyopathy. *Circulation.* 1993;87:1169–1178.

115. de Jong RM, Blanksma PK, van Waarde A, van Veldhuisen DJ. Measurement of myocardial beta-adrenoceptor density in clinical studies: a role for positron emission tomography? *Eur J Nucl Med Mol Imaging.* 2002;29:88–97.

116. Shi H, Wang H, Li D, Nattel S, Wang Z. Differential alterations of receptor densities of three muscarinic acetylcholine receptor subtypes and current densities of the corresponding K+ channels in canine atria with atrial fibrillation induced by experimental congestive heart failure. *Cell Physiol Biochem.* 2004;14:31–40.

117. Azevedo ER, Parker JD. Parasympathetic control of cardiac sympathetic activity: normal ventricular function versus congestive heart failure. *Circulation.* 1999;100:274–279.

118. Floras JS. Clinical aspects of sympathetic activation and parasympathetic withdrawal in heart failure. *J Am Coll Cardiol.* 1993;22:72A–84A.

119. Binkley PF, Nunziata E, Haas GJ, Nelson SD, Cody RJ. Parasympathetic withdrawal is an integral component of autonomic imbalance in congestive heart failure: demonstration in human subjects and verification in a paced canine model of ventricular failure. *J Am Coll Cardiol.* 1991;18:464–472.

120. Dunlap ME, Bibevski S, Rosenberry TL, Ernsberger P. Mechanisms of altered vagal control in heart failure: influence of muscarinic receptors and acetylcholinesterase activity. *Am J Physiol Heart Circ Physiol.* 2003;285:H1632–H1640.

121. Le Guludec D, Cohen-Solal A, Delforge J, Delahaye N, Syrota A, Merlet P. Increased myocardial muscarinic receptor density in idiopathic dilated cardiomyopathy: an in vivo PET study. *Circulation.* 1997;96:3416–3422.

122. Brodde OE, Michel MC. Adrenergic and muscarinic receptors in the human heart. *Pharmacol Rev.* 1999;51:651–690.

Part V
Emerging Role of Molecular Imaging

23 Evaluating High-Risk, Vulnerable Plaques with Integrated PET/CT

Udo Hoffmann, Javed Butler, and Ahmed A. Tawakol

Is it estimated that approximately 19 million people around the world suffer from either acute coronary syndrome (ACS) or sudden cardiac death (SCD).[1,2] In the United States, approximately 540,000 individuals experience a myocardial infarction, and more than 515,000 deaths are caused by coronary artery disease (CAD) each year. A large proportion of these patients are asymptomatic and without clinically overt cardiovascular disease.[1,2] These data underscore the significance of early identification and treatment of these high-risk patients.

It is well documented that the majority of ACSs and SCDs result from the rupture of high-risk, vulnerable plaques that in most cases are not flow limiting prior to the acute event.[3] Plaque rupture and subsequent thrombotic occlusion of coronary vessels account for up to 70% of sudden coronary deaths.[2] Several plaque characteristics, including the size of the plaque, thickness of the fibrous cap and lipid core, as well as degree of plaque inflammation, are related to the risk of rupture and thrombosis that lead to subsequent adverse events.[4] While coronary angiography remains the cornerstone for the detection and treatment of occlusive coronary artery stenosis, more than 60% of myocardial infarctions are caused by atherosclerotic plaques that are associated with a luminal narrowing of less than 50%.[4] Thus, early detection of high-risk plaques may offer a novel target for detection and treatment of patients at high risk for coronary events.

Pathophysiology of Atherosclerotic Lesions

Early Atherosclerotic Lesions

One of the first measurable changes in the evolution of CAD is the development of endothelial cell dysfunction.[5] Many traditional risk factors for CAD are associated with endothelial dysfunction, including elevated low-density lipoprotein (LDL) cholesterol, smoking, hypertension, diabetes, advanced age, male gender, and a family history of premature coronary disease.[5] Several emerging risk factors have also been associated with abnormal endothelial function, including inflammation, hyperhomocysteinemia, and others.[6,7] The biochemical hallmark of endothelial dysfunction is a reduction in the bioavailability of nitric oxide (NO). This can be the result of increased metabolism or decreased production of NO or both.[8] Nitric oxide plays several important roles that are relevant to the pathophysiology of atherosclerosis. It is a potent antithrombotic agent on the endothelial surface (inhibits adhesion, activation, and aggregation of platelets); it reduces the adhesion and migration of leukocytes into the vessel wall; and it limits vascular smooth muscle cell proliferation and mediates local vasodilation.[7,9,10]

The normal coronary vessel intima is covered by endothelial cells and also contains muscle cells, macrophages, mast cells, and an extracellular matrix.[11] Nonobstructive intimal thickening is often seen in response to mechanical forces including pressure, stretch or tension, and shear stress. Such adaptations are common at bifurcations, as the shear and tensile stresses are not uniformly distributed.[12] However, diffuse thickening may develop in relatively straight arterial segments also with evenly distributed stresses. In the presence of other atherosclerotic stimuli, adaptive intimal thickening becomes prone to development of atherosclerosis.[13]

Fatty streaks represent an inflammatory reaction within the intima and consist of lipid-filled macrophages (foam cells) and T lymphocytes.[14] These tend to develop in regions with intact but dysfunctional endothelium, particularly in atherosclerosis-prone areas with preexisting intimal thickening. Hypercholesterolemia is associated with increased endothelial permeability and intimal retention of lipoproteins, among other inflammatory reactions.[15] The macrophages then engulf oxidized LDLs to become lipid-filled foam cells, a hallmark of fatty streaks.

Advanced Atherosclerotic Lesions

The development of atherosclerotic plaques is the hallmark of more advanced atherosclerosis. Plaques contain extracellular lipids, which are drawn both from blood and from the senescence of lipid-laden macrophages.[16] Plaque progression is also associated with proliferation of connective tissue produced by smooth muscle cells. Thus, the lipid content of plaques may vary considerably.

Leukocyte recruitment becomes important for the growth of the atherosclerotic plaque. Chemoattractant cytochines (such as monocyte chemoattractant protein-1 [MCP1]) are produced by the endothelium in response to oxidized LDL and other stimuli, which attracts leukocytes to the growing plaque. The ingress of macrophages and other inflammatory cells leads to the development of more foam cells and the release of additional inflammatory mediators. The resulting reaction produces additional chemoattractants that cause migration of smooth muscle cells from the media to the intima and also lead to the production of degradative enzymes such as metalloproteases. The arrival of fibroblasts in the intima may enhance collagen deposition into the plaque, making it more structurally stable. Conversely, the release of degradative enzymes results in breakdown of the collagen matrix and thinning of the fibrous cap, resulting in a structurally vulnerable plaque. The balance of plaque degradation and collagen deposition may therefore determine the structural integrity of the plaque.[17]

Calcium deposition within the atherosclerotic plaques is common and increases with age. Both lipid- and collagen-rich plaques may calcify.[18] As discussed in Chapter 13, the available evidence suggests that coronary calcification is a marker of overall atherosclerotic plaque burden but does not correlate with the degree of stenosis or its vulnerability for acute complications.[19–21] In fact, the heavily calcified plaques may represent a more stable form of atherosclerotic plaque than the noncalcified plaques.[22]

An important aspect of plaque progression is the manner by which it causes vessel remodeling. Growth of the atherosclerotic plaque could result in positive (outward) remodeling, whereby the lumen of the plaque is preserved, or negative (inward) remodeling, whereby the vessel lumen is compromised. Plaques responsible for stable angina often cause severe luminal narrowing due to negative remodeling.[23–29] On the other hand, atherosclerotic plaques that cause fatal thrombosis are more frequently positively remodeled.[30]

High-Risk Plaque

An advanced plaque that is at high risk of rupturing may be referred to as a "vulnerable plaque" or a "high-risk plaque."[31–37] It is well documented that the majority of acute myocardial infarctions result from complication of plaques (erosion, rupture, and thrombosis) that in most cases did not cause flow limitation prior to the acute event.[31,38–40] From autopsy studies, it has been shown that the histological characteristics of these plaques include a thin fibrous cap, an underlying lipid core, and abundance of inflammatory cells.[31,40–46] Moreover, recent evidence demonstrates that the inflammatory cells within the atheroma, especially macrophages, release matrix degradation proteins that weaken the plaque, thereby rendering it susceptible to rupture.[47] Epidemiological data lend further support to the concept that inflammation plays an especially important role in the events that result in plaque rupture.[48]

Several additional plaque characteristics have been associated with plaque rupture. Positive arterial remodeling, paucity of collagen synthesis, lack of smooth muscle cells, and excess of degradative enzymes are all commonly cited.[14,40,49] Additionally, macrophage apoptosis not only may accelerate enlargement of the lipid pool but also may be a source of the procoagulant tissue factor.[50] Neovascularization, which is often present at the base of advanced plaques, may play an active role in the recruitment of proinflammatory cells and, thus, contribute to the progression of the plaque. Even in the presence of plaque surface integrity, small hemorrhages are common in these neovascularized areas.[42,51]

Detection of Nonocclusive Atherosclerotic Disease

The current strategies for prediction of cardiovascular risk do not include morphological information on the presence and severity of coronary artery disease. Clinical approaches emphasize traditional risk factors such as the patient's age and sex and the presence and extent of established, modifiable coronary risk factors such as hypertension, hyperlipidemia, diabetes mellitus, and cigarette smoking in the prediction and reduction of coronary risk.[52] Risk-prediction algorithms, such as the Framingham Heart Study coronary risk score, have been shown to be a valid, generalizable tool for risk prediction, and current treatment guidelines have incorporated traditional risk factors, risk-factor algorithms, or both into recommendations for initiation of drug therapy for hypertension and hyperlipidemia.[52–54] Despite optimal use of traditional risk-stratification tools, mortality and morbidity due to coronary artery disease remain massive.

Invasive Approaches

There are multiple invasive modalities that have been used to assess coronary plaques. Although they are precise and elegant, common disadvantages of invasive approaches include their high cost, their small but measurable associated morbidity and mortality, and the fact that these procedures are justified only in intermediate- to high-risk symptomatic patients.

Coronary Angiography

Coronary angiography currently is the gold standard for diagnosing occlusive coronary artery disease. Although irregular coronary lumen suggests plaque burden, this technology has significant limitations for nonstenotic plaque detection, including lack of data regarding the vessel wall and composition of the plaque. In diffuse coronary disease, coronary angiography underestimates the severity of plaque burden. Moreover, one cannot detect positive remodeling seen in the early stages of plaque development.[55] Thus, absence of significant coronary artery disease by cardiac catheterization does not rule out the presence of nonobstructive coronary atherosclerotic plaque.

Coronary Angiography with Intravascular Ultrasound

These deficiencies can be overcome by introducing an intravascular ultrasound (IVUS) probe in the coronary arteries.[56] These catheter-based ultrasound devices provide cross-sectional images of the coronary artery lumen and wall with an in-plane resolution of 80 to 150 µm. This method has been shown to be highly accurate to detect coronary atherosclerotic plaque ex vivo, compared to histology,[57–60] as well as in patients.[61] IVUS can accurately quantify plaque burden[61] and remodeling of the coronary artery wall, measure distensibility of plaques,[62,63] and monitor effects of lipid-lowering therapy.[64,65] Some researchers suggest that IVUS can distinguish fibrous, lipid, and calcified regions.[66,67] Based on plaque echogenecity, coronary plaques can then be divided into three groups: highly echo reflective (calcified), hyperechoic (with fibrosis or microcalcification), and hypoechoic (thrombotic or lipid laden). Because IVUS is an invasive technique, however, it can be used clinically only in patients undergoing coronary angiography.

Optical Coherence Tomography

Optical coherence tomography (OCT) is an invasive investigational method similar to IVUS that uses light interferometry to visualize subsurface structure in biological tissue.[68] Objective OCT criteria are highly sensitive and specific for characterizing different types of atherosclerotic plaques.[69] In particular, high contrast and spatial resolution (10 to 20 µm) enable OCT to differentiate plaque into fibrous, lipid, and calcified components.

Other Invasive Approaches

Other invasive methods to assess coronary plaques include angioscopy (allows direct visualization of the plaque surface), thermography (assesses plaque temperature), Raman spectroscopy, and near-infrared spectroscopy (both techniques assess plaque composition).[69–75]

A noninvasive method for visualization and quantification of atherosclerotic plaque burden within the entire coronary artery tree could provide the ability to observe the natural history of coronary artery disease and to assess the response of coronary atherosclerotic plaque to medical therapy such as lipid-lowering therapy. If successful, such a method would provide new insight into coronary artery disease and would have the potential to improve risk stratification for coronary events.

Noninvasive Approaches

Endothelial Function Testing

Several techniques have been used to assess endothelial function. Most serve as bioassays of nitric oxide bioavailability by measuring vasodilation that results from endothelial release of NO. A commonly employed method is brachial artery ultrasonography.[7,9] With this technique and others, endothelial dysfunction can be identified as impairment in the endothelium-dependent vasodilation that is related to the presence of atherosclerotic risk factors such as dyslipidemia, diabetes, hypertension, and smoking. In addition, endothelial dysfunction has been shown to predict coronary events in patient groups independent of risk factors and has been suggested to account for acute coronary syndrome in patients without occlusive coronary disease.[72,76] However, this measurement is highly variable and may not be used to predict individual patient risk.

Detecting Carotid Intima-Media Thickness

Vascular ultrasonography and magnetic resonance imaging (MRI), also discussed in Chapter 24, are capable of detecting intimal thickening. A large body of literature demonstrates that increased carotid intima-media thickness (IMT) correlates with cardiovascular risk factors[77,78] and is an independent predictor of myocardial infarction and stroke.[79,80]

Positron Emission Tomography

The high-risk, vulnerable atherosclerotic plaque differs metabolically from stable atherosclerotic plaques. Accordingly, metabolic imaging is an attractive candidate technology for differentiating vulnerable plaques from stable plaques. Several targets within the vulnerable plaque have the potential to be imaged, such as the inflammatory components, enzymatic activity, integrins, and apoptosis. Plaque inflammation is a particularly attractive target for detection and characterization of vulnerable plaque because inflammation plays such a prominent role in the development, progression, rupture, and thrombosis of plaques.

Positron emission tomography (PET) imaging with fluorine-18 fluorodeoxyglucose (^{18}F-FDG) is a well-tolerated, noninvasive technique that has been used extensively in humans to detect neoplasms, autoimmune disease, and infections.[81–86] The enhanced FDG activity associated with such foci is often due to the increased FDG uptake of the associated inflammatory cells such as macrophages.[82,87,88]

Relatively high uptake of FDG by macrophages, an index of plaque inflammation, may be the result of two important factors: (1) macrophages have relatively high metabolic rates,[89] and (2) macrophages do not store glycogen and therefore rely on external glucose as a source of fuel for the hexose monophosphate shunt pathway.[90–92] When macrophages are activated, their glucose consumption increases further. The mechanistic basis for enhanced glucose uptake following macrophage activation is not well established. Increases in glycolytic rate[85,89] and increased expression and translocation of glucose transporters are other possible mechanisms.[90,93–96]

FDG PET Imaging of Atherosclerotic Plaques

Preclinical Models

Several groups have shown that FDG accumulates in experimental atherosclerotic lesions[97–99] and that the accumulation can be measured noninvasively by PET.[97,98] A commonly employed animal model, the balloon-injured, cholesterol-fed New Zealand white rabbit, results in an aorta full of atherosclerotic plaques with varying degrees of inflammation. Using such models, researchers have shown that FDG accumulation in inflamed atherosclerotic plaques approaches 20 times that which is seen in noninflamed arteries, which enables noninvasive detection of the inflamed plaques.[98] Moreover, since FDG uptake in those plaques correlates with inflammation, the measured FDG uptake can be used as an index of plaque inflammation. From these studies, it also becomes evident that computed tomography (CT) (or another structural imaging method such as MR) needs to be performed in conjunction with PET to map the metabolic signals derived from PET onto the vasculature.

Clinical Observations

Vascular FDG uptake has been reported in humans with diseases associated with vessel wall inflammation such as Takayasu arteritis, giant cell arteritis, polymyalgia rheumatica, and nonspecific aortitis.[100-103] More recently, Rudd and colleagues demonstrated increased FDG uptake in symptomatic, unstable plaques compared to asymptomatic lesions.[104] In a related ex vivo experiment, that same group reported accumulation of FDG within macrophage-rich areas of excised human carotid arteries.[104]

Similar data have also been reported by our group.[105] Patients with carotid stenosis who were scheduled for carotid endarterectomy surgery underwent PET imaging (3 hours after 25 mCi FDG administration). Patients additionally underwent either CT or MRI imaging for structural delineation of their carotid plaques. PET images were then coregistered with the MR or CT images, and carotid plaque uptake of FDG was determined. Less than 1 month later, subjects underwent carotid endarterectomy, at which time carotid specimens were collected and examined for macrophage staining. Carotid FDG uptake was subsequently compared to macrophage density (determined histologically).

Approximately 30% of carotid specimens had histological evidence of significant inflammation. FDG uptake determined by PET correlated with macrophage staining of plaques (Figures 23.1–23.3). Furthermore, FDG uptake correlated *negatively* with fibrous plaques ($r = -0.76$; $p < 0.01$). This demonstrates that carotid plaque inflammation may be assessed noninvasively with FDG PET, as validated by histology.

Future Directions in PET Imaging of Vulnerable Plaques

In addition to the imaging of extracardiac vessels, ^{18}F-FDG may potentially be used to characterize coronary arterial plaques. There are several potential obstacles to coronary imaging: the relatively small plaque size relative to the spatial resolution of PET, the increased mobility of coronary vessels compared to the carotids, and the relatively high myocardial uptake of ^{18}F-FDG.[106-108] However, several possible solutions exist, including the emergence of better PET/CT instrumentation and the use of simple techniques to suppress myocardial FDG uptake. Indeed, several groups are currently investigating the role of FDG PET in coronary plaque characterization.

Perhaps more important are the ongoing efforts to develop novel tracers directed at the vulnerable plaque. Much of that work to date has involved the development of tracers for use in single photon emission computed tomography (SPECT), with the expectation that PET analogues will be developed for those tracers that prove successful in SPECT imaging. To that end, tracers targeting apoptosis,[109] the purine

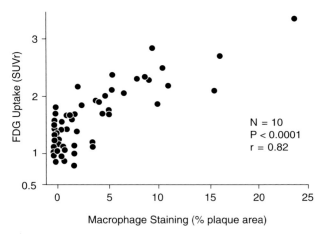

FIGURE 23.1. Correlation between PET measurement of FDG uptake (SUVr) in carotid plaques, reflecting inflammation, and histological evidence of macrophage infiltration ($r = 0.82$; $p < 0.0001$).

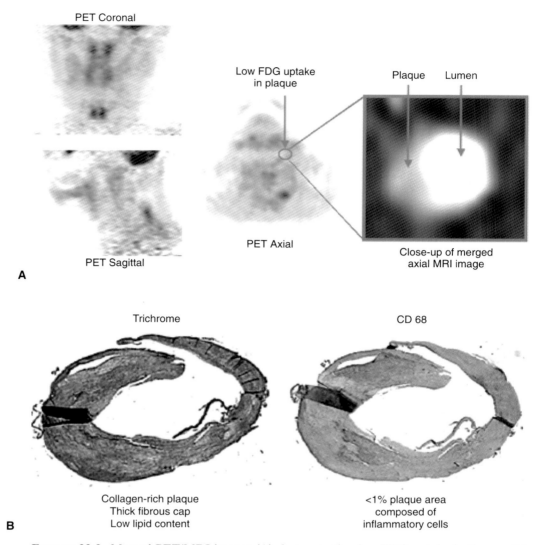

FIGURE 23.2. Merged PET/MRI images (A) demonstrating low FDG uptake in the carotid plaque that was subsequently removed during surgery. The corresponding histology (B) demonstrates a collagen-rich plaque with a thick fibrous cap and low lipid content (trichrome stain). The corresponding CD 68 stain demonstrates rare macrophage infiltration. These histological features are consistent with a metabolically stable and potentially clinically stable plaque.

receptor,[110] the integrin receptor,[111] and abnormal smooth muscle cell proliferation,[112] among others, are being studied.

Summary Points

- PET and CT provide complementary information about atherosclerotic plaques.
- Integrated PET/CT imaging of plaques is a powerful tool for plaque characterization that may prove clinically useful for the detection of vulnerable atherosclerotic plaques.
- Rapid advances in instrumentation and tracer development are expected to further improve plaque characterization. This imaging technology may result in the ability to detect plaques that are at the highest risk of rupturing and thus enable a change in therapy that could prevent a clinical event.

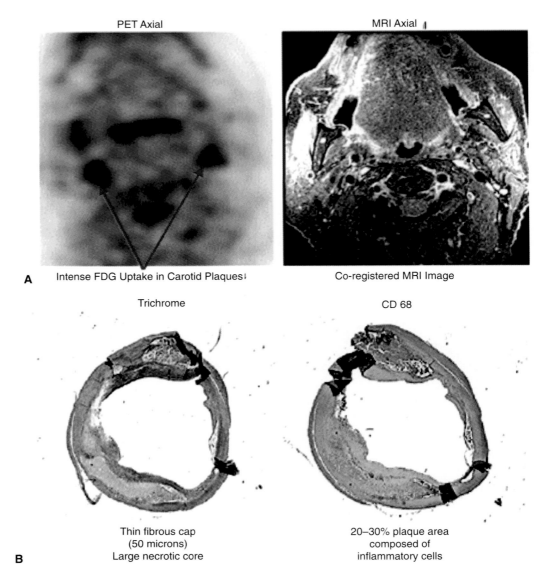

FIGURE 23.3. Merged PET/MRI images (A) demonstrating intense FDG uptake in the plaques of both carotid arteries, subsequently removed during surgery. The corresponding histology (B) demonstrates a plaque with a thin fibrous cap (50 μm) and large necrotic core (trichrome stain). The corresponding CD 68 stain demonstrates intense macrophage infiltration. These histological features are consistent with a metabolically active plaque, presumably vulnerable to rupture. Notably, the SUVr measured in this plaque was the highest of the 10 patients studied, and the histological evidence of inflammation was likewise highest of all plaques that were analyzed.

References

1. Myerburg RJ, Interian A Jr, Mitrani RM, Kessler KM, Castellanos A. Frequency of sudden cardiac death and profiles of risk. *Am J Cardiol.* 1997;80:10F–19F.
2. Naghavi M, Libby P, Falk E, et al. From vulnerable plaque to vulnerable patient: a call for new definitions and risk assessment strategies: Part I. *Circulation.* 2003;108: 1664–1672.
3. Falk E, Shah PK, Fuster V. Coronary plaque disruption. *Circulation.* 1995;92:657–671.
4. Virmani R, Kolodgie FD, Burke AP, Farb A, Schwartz SM. Lessons from sudden coronary death: a comprehensive morphological classification scheme for atherosclerotic lesions. *Arterioscler Thromb Vasc Biol.* 2000;20:1262–1275.

5. Verma S, Anderson TJ. Fundamentals of endothelial function for the clinical cardiologist. *Circulation*. 2002;105:546–549.

6. Biegelsen ES, Loscalzo J. Endothelial function and atherosclerosis. *Coron Artery Dis*. 1999;10:241–256.

7. Tawakol A, Omland T, Gerhard M, Wu JT, Creager MA. Hyperhomocyst(e)inemia is associated with impaired endothelium-dependent vasodilation in humans. *Circulation*. 1997;95:1119–1121.

8. Tawakol A, Forgione MA, Stuehlinger M, et al. Homocysteine impairs coronary microvascular dilator function in humans. *J Am Coll Cardiol*. 2002;40:1051–1058.

9. Gerhard M, Walsh BW, Tawakol A, et al. Estradiol therapy combined with progesterone and endothelium-dependent vasodilation in postmenopausal women. *Circulation*. 1998;98:1158–1163.

10. Loscalzo J. Nitric oxide and vascular disease. *N Engl J Med*. 1995;333:251–253.

11. Stary HC, Chandler AB, Glagov S, et al. A definition of initial, fatty streak, and intermediate lesions of atherosclerosis. A report from the Committee on Vascular Lesions of the Council on Arteriosclerosis, American Heart Association. *Circulation*. 1994;89: 2462–2478.

12. Stary HC, Blankenhorn DH, Chandler AB, et al. A definition of the intima of human arteries and of its atherosclerosis-prone regions. A report from the Committee on Vascular Lesions of the Council on Arteriosclerosis, American Heart Association. *Circulation*. 1992;85:391–405.

13. Schwartz SM, deBlois D, O'Brien ER. The intima. Soil for atherosclerosis and restenosis. *Circ Res*. 1995;77:445–465.

14. Libby P. Inflammation in atherosclerosis. *Nature*. 2002;420:868–874.

15. McGill HC Jr, McMahan CA, Malcom GT, Oalmann MC, Strong JP. Effects of serum lipoproteins and smoking on atherosclerosis in young men and women. The PDAY Research Group. Pathobiological Determinants of Atherosclerosis in Youth. *Arterioscler Thromb Vasc Biol*. 1997;17:95–106.

16. Stary HC, Chandler AB, Glagov S, et al. A definition of initial, fatty streak, and intermediate lesions of atherosclerosis. A report from the Committee on Vascular Lesions of the Council on Arteriosclerosis, American Heart Association. *Arterioscler Thromb*. 1994;14:840–856.

17. Libby P. Molecular bases of the acute coronary syndromes. *Circulation*. 1995;91: 2844–2850.

18. Abedin M, Tintut Y, Demer LL. Vascular calcification: mechanisms and clinical ramifications. *Arterioscler Thromb Vasc Biol*. 2004;24:1161–1170.

19. Moselewski F, Ropers D, Pohle K, et al. Comparison of measurement of cross-sectional coronary atherosclerotic plaque and vessel areas by 16-slice multidetector computed tomography versus intravascular ultrasound. *Am J Cardiol*. 2004;94:1294–1297.

20. Sangiorgi G, Rumberger JA, Severson A, et al. Arterial calcification and not lumen stenosis is highly correlated with atherosclerotic plaque burden in humans: a histologic study of 723 coronary artery segments using nondecalcifying methodology. *J Am Coll Cardiol*. 1998;31:126–133.

21. Virmani R, Burke AP, Farb A, Kolodgie FD. Pathology of the unstable plaque. *Prog Cardiovasc Dis*. 2002;44:349–356.

22. Beckman JA, Ganz J, Creager MA, Ganz P, Kinlay S. Relationship of clinical presentation and calcification of culprit coronary artery stenoses. *Arterioscler Thromb Vasc Biol*. 2001;21:1618–1622.

23. Achenbach S, Daniel WG. Imaging of coronary atherosclerosis using computed tomography: current status and future directions. *Curr Atheroscler Rep*. 2004;6:213–218.

24. Burke AP, Kolodgie FD, Farb A, Weber D, Virmani R. Morphological predictors of arterial remodeling in coronary atherosclerosis. *Circulation*. 2002;105:297–303.

25. Hong MK, Park SW, Lee CW, et al. Intravascular ultrasound findings of negative arterial remodeling at sites of focal coronary spasm in patients with vasospastic angina. *Am Heart J*. 2000;140:395–401.

26. Kotani J, Mintz GS, Castagna MT, et al. Intravascular ultrasound analysis of infarct-related and non-infarct-related arteries in patients who presented with an acute myocardial infarction. *Circulation*. 2003;107:2889–2893.

27. Nakamura M, Nishikawa H, Mukai S, et al. Impact of coronary artery remodeling on clinical presentation of coronary artery disease: an intravascular ultrasound study. *J Am Coll Cardiol.* 2001;37:63–69.

28. Schoenhagen P, Ziada KM, Kapadia SR, Crowe TD, Nissen SE, Tuzcu EM. Extent and direction of arterial remodeling in stable versus unstable coronary syndromes: an intravascular ultrasound study. *Circulation.* 2000;101:598–603.

29. Worthley SG, Helft G, Zaman AG, Fuster V, Badimon JJ. Atherosclerosis and the vulnerable plaque—imaging: part II. *Aust N Z J Med.* 2000;30:704–710.

30. Bezerra HG, Higuchi ML, Gutierrez PS, et al. Atheromas that cause fatal thrombosis are usually large and frequently accompanied by vessel enlargement. *Cardiovasc Pathol.* 2001;10:189–196.

31. Davies MJ. Acute coronary thrombosis—the role of plaque disruption and its initiation and prevention. *Eur Heart J.* 1995;16(suppl L):3–7.

32. Fuster V. Human lesion studies. *Ann N Y Acad Sci.* 1997;811:207–224; discussion 224–225.

33. Libby P, Schoenbeck U, Mach F, Selwyn AP, Ganz P. Current concepts in cardiovascular pathology: the role of LDL cholesterol in plaque rupture and stabilization. *Am J Med.* 1998;104:14S–18S.

34. Lusby RJ, Ferrell LD, Ehrenfeld WK, Stoney RJ, Wylie EJ. Carotid plaque hemorrhage. Its role in production of cerebral ischemia. *Arch Surg.* 1982;117:1479–1488.

35. Muller JE, Stone PH, Turi ZG, et al. Circadian variation in the frequency of onset of acute myocardial infarction. *N Engl J Med.* 1985;313:1315–1322.

36. Muller JE, Tofler GH, Stone PH. Circadian variation and triggers of onset of acute cardiovascular disease. *Circulation.* 1989;79:733–743.

37. Shah PK. Pathophysiology of plaque rupture and the concept of plaque stabilization. *Cardiol Clin.* 1996;14:17–29.

38. Abela GS, Picon PD, Friedl SE, et al. Triggering of plaque disruption and arterial thrombosis in an atherosclerotic rabbit model. *Circulation.* 1995;91:776–784.

39. Davies MJ. Detecting vulnerable coronary plaques. *Lancet.* 1996;347:1422–1423.

40. Davies MJ, Woolf N, Rowles P, Richardson PD. Lipid and cellular constituents of unstable human aortic plaques. *Basic Res Cardiol.* 1994;89(suppl 1):33–39.

41. Burke AP, Farb A, Malcom GT, Liang YH, Smialek J, Virmani R. Coronary risk factors and plaque morphology in men with coronary disease who died suddenly. *N Engl J Med.* 1997;336:1276–1282.

42. Davies MJ, Thomas A. Thrombosis and acute coronary-artery lesions in sudden cardiac ischemic death. *N Engl J Med.* 1984;310:1137–1140.

43. Farb A, Burke AP, Tang AL, et al. Coronary plaque erosion without rupture into a lipid core. A frequent cause of coronary thrombosis in sudden coronary death. *Circulation.* 1996;93:1354–1363.

44. Golledge J, Cuming R, Ellis M, Davies AH, Greenhalgh RM. Carotid plaque characteristics and presenting symptom. *Br J Surg.* 1997;84:1697–1701.

45. Kolodgie FD, Burke AP, Farb A, et al. The thin-cap fibroatheroma: a type of vulnerable plaque: the major precursor lesion to acute coronary syndromes. *Curr Opin Cardiol.* 2001;16:285–292.

46. Virmani R, Farb A, Burke AP. Risk factors in the pathogenesis of coronary artery disease. *Compr Ther.* 1998;24:519–529.

47. Libby P. What have we learned about the biology of atherosclerosis? The role of inflammation. *Am J Cardiol.* 2001;88:3J–6J.

48. Ridker PM, Glynn RJ, Hennekens CH. C-reactive protein adds to the predictive value of total and HDL cholesterol in determining risk of first myocardial infarction. *Circulation.* 1998;97:2007–2011.

49. Virmani R, Burke AP, Kolodgie FD, Farb A. Vulnerable plaque: the pathology of unstable coronary lesions. *J Interv Cardiol.* 2002;15:439–446.

50. Shah PK. Plaque disruption and thrombosis: potential role of inflammation and infection. *Cardiol Rev.* 2000;8:31–39.

51. O'Brien KD, McDonald TO, Chait A, Allen MD, Alpers CE. Neovascular expression of E-selectin, intercellular adhesion molecule-1, and vascular cell adhesion molecule-1 in human atherosclerosis and their relation to intimal leukocyte content. *Circulation.* 1996; 93:672–682.

52. Wilson PW, D'Agostino RB, Levy D, Belanger AM, Silbershatz H, Kannel WB. Prediction of coronary heart disease using risk factor categories. *Circulation*. 1998;97: 1837–1847.

53. Boden WE. Therapeutic implications of recent ATP III guidelines and the important role of combination therapy in total dyslipidemia management. *Curr Opin Cardiol*. 2003;18: 278–285.

54. Gotto AM. NCEP ATP III guidelines incorporate global risk assessment. *Am J Manag Care*. 2003;Suppl. 1:3.

55. Glagov S, Weisenberg E, Zarins CK, Stankunavicius R, Kolettis GJ. Compensatory enlargement of human atherosclerotic coronary arteries. *N Engl J Med*. 1987;316: 1371–1375.

56. Tuzcu EM, Kapadia SR, Tutar E, et al. High prevalence of coronary atherosclerosis in asymptomatic teenagers and young adults: evidence from intravascular ultrasound. *Circulation*. 2001;103:2705–2710.

57. Gussenhoven EJ, Essed CE, Frietman P, et al. Intravascular ultrasonic imaging: histologic and echographic correlation. *Eur J Vasc Surg*. 1989;3:571–576.

58. Gussenhoven EJ, Essed CE, Lancee CT, et al. Arterial wall characteristics determined by intravascular ultrasound imaging: an in vitro study. *J Am Coll Cardiol*. 1989;14: 947–952.

59. Nishimura RA, Edwards WD, Warnes CA, et al. Intravascular ultrasound imaging: in vitro validation and pathologic correlation. *J Am Coll Cardiol*. 1990;16:145–154.

60. Potkin BN, Bartorelli AL, Gessert JM, et al. Coronary artery imaging with intravascular high-frequency ultrasound. *Circulation*. 1990;81:1575–1585.

61. Nissen SE, Yock P. Intravascular ultrasound: novel pathophysiological insights and current clinical applications. *Circulation*. 2001;103:604–616.

62. Carlier SG, de Korte CL, Brusseau E, Schaar JA, Serruys PW, van der Steen AF. Imaging of atherosclerosis. Elastography. *J Cardiovasc Risk*. 2002;9:237–245.

63. de Korte CL, van der Steen AF, Cepedes EI, et al. Characterization of plaque components and vulnerability with intravascular ultrasound elastography. *Phys Med Biol*. 2000;45: 1465–1475.

64. Matsuzaki M, Hiramori K, Imaizumi T, et al. Intravascular ultrasound evaluation of coronary plaque regression by low density lipoprotein-apheresis in familial hypercholesterolemia: the Low Density Lipoprotein-Apheresis Coronary Morphology and Reserve Trial (LACMART). *J Am Coll Cardiol*. 2002;40:220–227.

65. Schartl M, Bocksch W, Koschyk DH, et al. Use of intravascular ultrasound to compare effects of different strategies of lipid-lowering therapy on plaque volume and composition in patients with coronary artery disease. *Circulation*. 2001;104:387–392.

66. Mintz GS, Nissen SE, Anderson WD, et al. American College of Cardiology Clinical Expert Consensus Document on Standards for Acquisition, Measurement and Reporting of Intravascular Ultrasound Studies (IVUS). A report of the American College of Cardiology Task Force on Clinical Expert Consensus Documents. *J Am Coll Cardiol*. 2001;37: 1478–1492.

67. Nair A, Kuban BD, Tuzcu EM, Schoenhagen P, Nissen SE, Vince DG. Coronary plaque classification with intravascular ultrasound radiofrequency data analysis. *Circulation*. 2002;106:2200–2206.

68. Tearney GJ, Yabushita H, Houser SL, et al. Quantification of macrophage content in atherosclerotic plaques by optical coherence tomography. *Circulation*. 2003;107:113–119.

69. Yabushita H, Bouma BE, Houser SL, et al. Characterization of human atherosclerosis by optical coherence tomography. *Circulation*. 2002;106:1640–1645.

70. Botnar RM, Stuber M, Kissinger KV, Kim WY, Spuentrup E, Manning WJ. Noninvasive coronary vessel wall and plaque imaging with magnetic resonance imaging. *Circulation*. 2000;102:2582–2587.

71. Charash WE LR, Moreno PR, Purushothaman RK, Swain JA, O'Connor WN, Muller JE. Detection of simulated vulnerable plaque using a novel infrared spectroscopy catheter. *J Am Coll Cardiol*. 2000;35:38A.

72. Reddy KG, Nair RN, Sheehan HM, Hodgson JM. Evidence that selective endothelial dysfunction may occur in the absence of angiographic or ultrasound atherosclerosis in patients with risk factors for atherosclerosis. *J Am Coll Cardiol*. 1994;23:833–843.

73. Romer TJ, Brennan JF 3rd, Puppels GJ, et al. Intravascular ultrasound combined with Raman spectroscopy to localize and quantify cholesterol and calcium salts in atherosclerotic coronary arteries. *Arterioscler Thromb Vasc Biol.* 2000;20:478–483.

74. Stefanadis C, Diamantopoulos L, Vlachopoulos C, et al. Thermal heterogeneity within human atherosclerotic coronary arteries detected in vivo: a new method of detection by application of a special thermography catheter. *Circulation.* 1999;99:1965–1971.

75. Thieme T, Wernecke KD, Meyer R, et al. Angioscopic evaluation of atherosclerotic plaques: validation by histomorphologic analysis and association with stable and unstable coronary syndromes. *J Am Coll Cardiol.* 1996;28:1–6.

76. Neunteufl T, Heher S, Katzenschlager R, et al. Late prognostic value of flow-mediated dilation in the brachial artery of patients with chest pain. *Am J Cardiol.* 2000;86: 207–210.

77. Chambless LE, Heiss G, Folsom AR, et al. Association of coronary heart disease incidence with carotid arterial wall thickness and major risk factors: the Atherosclerosis Risk in Communities (ARIC) Study, 1987–1993. *Am J Epidemiol.* 1997;146:483– 494.

78. Davis PH, Dawson JD, Riley WA, Lauer RM. Carotid intimal-medial thickness is related to cardiovascular risk factors measured from childhood through middle age: the Muscatine Study. *Circulation.* 2001;104:2815–2819.

79. Bots ML, Hoes AW, Koudstaal PJ, Hofman A, Grobbee DE. Common carotid intima-media thickness and risk of stroke and myocardial infarction: the Rotterdam Study. *Circulation.* 1997;96:1432–1437.

80. O'Leary DH, Polak JF, Kronmal RA, Manolio TA, Burke GL, Wolfson SK Jr. Carotid-artery intima and media thickness as a risk factor for myocardial infarction and stroke in older adults. Cardiovascular Health Study Collaborative Research Group. *N Engl J Med.* 1999;340:14–22.

81. Deshmukh A, Scott JA, Palmer EL, Hochberg FH, Gruber M, Fischman AJ. Impact of fluorodeoxyglucose positron emission tomography on the clinical management of patients with glioma. *Clin Nucl Med.* 1996;21:720–725.

82. Fischman AJ, Thornton AF, Frosch MP, Swearinger B, Gonzalez RG, Alpert NM. FDG hypermetabolism associated with inflammatory necrotic changes following radiation of meningioma. *J Nucl Med.* 1997;38:1027–1029.

83. Hunter GJ, Choi NC, McLoud TC, Fischman AJ. Lung tumor metastasis to breast detected by fluorine-18-fluorodeoxyglucose PET. *J Nucl Med.* 1993;34:1571–1573.

84. Jones HA, Cadwallader KA, White JF, Uddin M, Peters AM, Chilvers ER. Dissociation between respiratory burst activity and deoxyglucose uptake in human neutrophil granulocytes: implications for interpretation of (18)F-FDG PET images. *J Nucl Med.* 2002;43:652–657.

85. Lorenzen J, Buchert R, Bohuslavizki KH. Value of FDG PET in patients with fever of unknown origin. *Nucl Med Commun.* 2001;22:779–783.

86. Sugawara Y, Gutowski TD, Fisher SJ, Brown RS, Wahl RL. Uptake of positron emission tomography tracers in experimental bacterial infections: a comparative biodistribution study of radiolabeled FDG, thymidine, L-methionine, 67Ga-citrate, and 125I-HSA. *Eur J Nucl Med.* 1999;26:333–341.

87. Kaim AH, Weber B, Kurrer MO, Gottschalk J, Von Schulthess GK, Buck A. Autoradiographic quantification of 18F-FDG uptake in experimental soft-tissue abscesses in rats. *Radiology.* 2002;223:446–451.

88. Kubota R, Kubota K, Yamada S, Tada M, Ido T, Tamahashi N. Microautoradiographic study for the differentiation of intratumoral macrophages, granulation tissues and cancer cells by the dynamics of fluorine-18-fluorodeoxyglucose uptake. *J Nucl Med.* 1994;35: 104–112.

89. Newsholme P, Newsholme EA. Rates of utilization of glucose, glutamine and oleate and formation of end-products by mouse peritoneal macrophages in culture. *Biochem J.* 1989;261:211–218.

90. Ahmed N, Kansara M, Berridge MV. Acute regulation of glucose transport in a monocyte-macrophage cell line: glut-3 affinity for glucose is enhanced during the respiratory burst. *Biochem J.* 1997;327(pt 2):369–375.

91. Kiyotaki C, Peisach J, Bloom BR. Oxygen metabolism in cloned macrophage cell lines: glucose dependence of superoxide production, metabolic and spectral analysis. *J Immunol.* 1984;132:857–866.

92. Rist RJ, Jones GE, Naftalin RJ. Effects of macrophage colony-stimulating factor and phorbol myristate acetate on 2-D-deoxyglucose transport and superoxide production in rat peritoneal macrophages. *Biochem J.* 1991;278(pt 1):119–128.

93. Bashan N, Burdett E, Hundal HS, Klip A. Regulation of glucose transport and GLUT1 glucose transporter expression by O2 in muscle cells in culture. *Am J Physiol.* 1992;262: C682–C690.

94. Berridge MV, Tan AS. Interleukin-3 facilitates glucose transport in a myeloid cell line by regulating the affinity of the glucose transporter for glucose: involvement of protein phosphorylation in transporter activation. *Biochem J.* 1995;305(pt 3):843–851.

95. Nefesh I, Bauskin AR, Alkalay I, Golembo M, Ben-Neriah Y. IL-3 facilitates lymphocyte hexose transport by enhancing the intrinsic activity of the transport system. *Int Immunol.* 1991;3:827–831.

96. Pasternak CA, Aiyathurai JE, Makinde V, et al. Regulation of glucose uptake by stressed cells. *J Cell Physiol.* 1991;149:324–331.

97. Ogawa M, Ishino S, Mukai T, et al. (18)F-FDG accumulation in atherosclerotic plaques: immunohistochemical and PET imaging study. *J Nucl Med.* 2004;45:1245–1250.

98. Tawakol A, Migrino RQ, Hoffmann U, et al. Noninvasive in vivo measurement of vascular inflammation with F-18 fluorodeoxyglucose positron emission tomography. *J Nucl Cardiol.* 2005;12:294–301.

99. Vallabhajosula S. Imaging atherosclerotic macrophage density by positron emission tomography using F-18-flurodeoxyglucose. *J Nucl Med.* 1996;37:38p.

100. Blockmans D, Maes A, Stroobants S, et al. New arguments for a vasculitic nature of polymyalgia rheumatica using positron emission tomography. *Rheumatology (Oxford).* 1999;38:444–447.

101. Derdelinckx I, Maes A, Bogaert J, Mortelmans L, Blockmans D. Positron emission tomography scan in the diagnosis and follow-up of aortitis of the thoracic aorta. *Acta Cardiol.* 2000;55:193–195.

102. Hara M, Goodman PC, Leder RA. FDG-PET finding in early-phase Takayasu arteritis. *J Comput Assist Tomogr.* 1999;23:16–18.

103. Meller J, Altenvoerde G, Munzel U, et al. Fever of unknown origin: prospective comparison of [18F]FDG imaging with a double-head coincidence camera and gallium-67 citrate SPET. *Eur J Nucl Med.* 2000;27:1617–1625.

104. Rudd JH, Warburton EA, Fryer TD, et al. Imaging atherosclerotic plaque inflammation with [18F]-fluorodeoxyglucose positron emission tomography. *Circulation.* 2002;105: 2708–2711.

105. Tawakol A, Migrino RQ, Bashian G, et al. FDG-PET provides a non-invasive index of carotid plaque inflammation in humans [abstract]. *J Nucl Med.* 2004;45:118P.

106. Gerber BL, Vanoverschelde JL, Bol A, et al. Myocardial blood flow, glucose uptake, and recruitment of inotropic reserve in chronic left ventricular ischemic dysfunction. Implications for the pathophysiology of chronic myocardial hibernation. *Circulation.* 1996;94: 651–659.

107. Melon PG, de Landsheere CM, Degueldre C, Peters JL, Kulbertus HE, Pierard LA. Relation between contractile reserve and positron emission tomographic patterns of perfusion and glucose utilization in chronic ischemic left ventricular dysfunction: implications for identification of myocardial viability. *J Am Coll Cardiol.* 1997;30:1651–1659.

108. Tawakol A, Skopicki HA, Abraham SA, et al. Evidence of reduced resting blood flow in viable myocardial regions with chronic asynergy. *J Am Coll Cardiol.* 2000;36: 2146–2153.

109. Johnson LL, Schofield L, Donahay T, Narula N, Narula J. 99mTc-annexin V imaging for in vivo detection of atherosclerotic lesions in porcine coronary arteries. *J Nucl Med.* 2005;46:1186–1193.

110. Elmaleh DR, Narula J, Babich JW, et al. Rapid noninvasive detection of experimental atherosclerotic lesions with novel 99mTc-labeled diadenosine tetraphosphates. *Proc Natl Acad Sci U S A.* 1998;95:691–695.

111. Blankenberg FG, Mari C, Strauss HW. Development of radiocontrast agents for vascular imaging: progress to date. *Am J Cardiovasc Drugs.* 2002;2:357–365.

112. Jimenez J, Donahay T, Schofield L, Khaw BA, Johnson LL. Smooth muscle cell proliferation index correlates with 111In-labeled antibody Z2D3 uptake in a transplant vasculopathy swine model. *J Nucl Med.* 2005;46:514–519.

24 Evaluating Vulnerable Atherosclerotic Plaque with MRI

Fabien Hyafil and Zahi A. Fayad

Despite important clinical advances in prevention and treatment of atherosclerosis during the past 20 years, coronary artery disease remains the first cause of mortality in industrialized countries.[1] Atherosclerosis affects medium- and large-diameter arteries and is characterized by a thickening of the arterial intima typically composed of a lipid core with an overlying fibrous cap. Angiography remains the gold standard for diagnosis and quantification of atherosclerotic plaques that result in flow-limiting arterial stenoses but offers only an indirect view of atherosclerosis burden.[2] Positive remodeling of the arterial wall—a process in which the vessel dilates to limit the narrowing of the lumen in presence of atherosclerotic plaques—leads to a clear underestimation of the true extension of atherosclerosis disease with angiography.[3]

High-resolution magnetic resonance imaging (MRI) has emerged as a very promising imaging technique to detect atherosclerotic plaques. Thanks to advances in both hardware and software, MRI now offers an inframillimetric resolution of the arterial wall, allowing for direct evaluation of atherosclerosis burden. Moreover, MRI does not expose patients to ionizing radiation and seems therefore well suited to monitor the extension of atherosclerotic disease and follow its evolution under antiatherosclerotic treatments.

However, symptomatic atherosclerotic plaques are mostly characterized by their specific composition rather than by their size or impact on the vessel lumen. Acute ischemic events (acute coronary syndromes, strokes) are most frequently caused by the endothelial disruption of atherosclerotic plaques (superficial intimal erosion or fibrous cap rupture), triggering the formation of an intraluminal thrombus.[4] These atherosclerotic plaques are typically described as containing a large lipid core representing more than half of the plaque volume, a thin fibrous cap ($<65\,\mu m$), and a heavy infiltrate of inflammatory cells (macrophages and lymphocytes). On the postulate that early identification of such lesions could preclude ischemic events, imaging techniques amied at the detection of vulnerable plaques, at high risk of acute thrombosis, are growing at a rapid pace. The most useful techniques will combine high spatial resolution with the detection of biological activities in atherosclerotic plaques.

In this chapter, we will describe the strategies to detect vulnerable atherosclerotic plaques with MRI. Multicontrast MRI can discriminate the components of atherosclerotic plaques with different intrinsic relaxivity properties. In addition, analysis of the accumulation intra-vascular MR contrast agents in atherosclerotic plaques allows for a better identification of the cellular composition of plaques. Finally, using an approach similar to nuclear imaging, novel specific contrast agents are developed by binding a probe targeting a molecule or biological activity characteristic of vulnerable plaques to a moiety that modifies the contrast on MRI. This latter approach opens the field of molecular imaging to MRI.

Assessment of Atherosclerosis Burden with Cardiovascular MRI

High-Resolution MRI of Atherosclerotic Plaques

The small size of the vessels requires the acquisition of high spatial and contrast resolutions for atherosclerosis imaging. Atherosclerotic plaques are detected with cardiovascular MRI (CMR) using high-resolution black-blood fast-spin echo MR sequences, obtained by nulling the signal of the flowing blood through preparatory pulses. Black-blood sequences improve the contrast between atherosclerotic plaques and the lumen and therefore offer better delineation of the contours of the plaque. New black-blood techniques[5,6] that have recently been introduced for the simultaneous acquisition of multiple slices allow for the analysis of a full-length arterial segment with a reduced total examination time. Using these techniques, clinical studies demonstrated that CMR provides excellent quantitative capabilities for the measurement of total plaque volume with an error in vessel wall area measurement as low as 2.6% for the aorta[7] and 3.5% for the carotids.[8] Similar low measurement errors in plaque area and volume (4% to 6%) were reported by others,[9,10] proving that plaque area and volume can be accurately assessed with CMR. In the future, 3.0 Tesla whole-body MR systems could further increase the spatial resolution of this technique and reduce acquisition times.

Correlation with Cardiovascular Risk Factors

The evaluation of the prevalence of atherosclerosis disease is still based on cardiovascular risk factors and probability scores measured from population studies. However, the accuracy of these probability scores could vary among different populations and even more among individuals. CMR now offers a precise imaging tool to evaluate directly the presence and extension of atherosclerosis disease in an individual. Hence, recent studies have compared, in different populations, the correlation between cardiovascular risk factors and atherosclerosis detected with CMR. For example, in asymptomatic subjects from the Framingham Heart Study (FHS), FHS coronary risk score was strongly associated with asymptomatic aortic atherosclerosis detected by CMR.[11] In this study, prevalence and extension of aortic atherosclerosis significantly increased with age and predominated in the abdominal aorta.

However, in a subset study[12] from the Multiethnic Study of Atherosclerosis (MESA), 196 participants (99 Afro-americans, 97 Caucasians; 98 men, 98 women) without symptomatic cardiovascular disease were recruited from 6 study centers in the United States. Aortic wall thickness measured with CMR increased with age but varied also by ethnic origin and sex. Men and Afro-american participants had the greatest wall thickness in this study, emphasizing the differences in the prevalence of atherosclerosis among different populations. Longitudinal sections of the aorta of a normal subject and an atherosclerotic patient are shown in Figure 24.1.

In a recent study[13] of 102 patients undergoing coronary angiography, aortic atherosclerotic plaques were detected with a higher frequency in patients with active smoking and high levels of low-density lipoprotein (LDL)-cholesterol, but the extension of atherosclerotic plaques in the aorta correlated mainly with age and high blood pressure. Only atherosclerotic plaques located in the thoracic aorta were associated with coronary artery disease.

These studies prove the strong correlation in an individual between cardiovascular risk factors and the incidence of aortic atherosclerosis detected with CMR, even if some differences can be observed among different populations. CMR demonstrated also the various effects of each cardiovascular risk factor on the location and extension of atherosclerosis in the aorta. Hence, CMR improves the direct evaluation of atherosclerosis burden in an individual and therefore may allow to monitor the effects of antiatherosclerotic treatments on aortic plaques.

Monitoring of Antiatherosclerotic Treatments

Efficacy of antiatherosclerotic treatments are currently evaluated by their beneficial effects on the lipid profile. However, CMR now provides precise measurements of total atherosclerotic plaque volume and seems therefore an interesting imaging tool to study directly the effect of lipid-lowering therapy on atherosclerotic plaques. In 51 patients with carotid and aortic atherosclerosis, CMR was performed to measure the effects of lipid-lowering therapy (statins) on plaque regression. This work[8] was the first to demonstrate that lipid-lowering therapy is associated with significant regression of established atherosclerotic lesions in humans. In an experimental rabbit study, Corti et al[14] demonstrated the beneficial effects of statins on atherosclerosis volume measured by MRI and the additional antiatherogenic benefits of combining a PPARγ agonist with simvastatin. Finally, a recent clinical study[15] using CMR has compared, the effect of 2 different dosages of the same statin on aortic plaque progression after 12 months. Treatment with the higher dosage of statin (atorvastatin, 20 mg) resulted in significant regression of atherosclerotic plaques in the thoracic aorta and slower plaque progression in the abdominal aorta. In contrast, patients treated with the lower dosage of statin (atorvastatin, 5 mg) had a significant progression of atherosclerotic plaques in both the thoracic and abdominal aorta. The plot showing the correlation between the

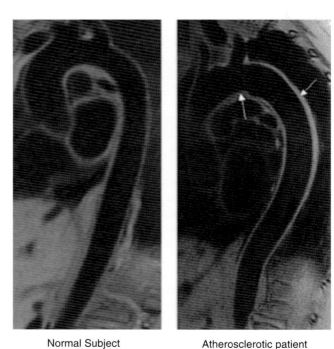

Normal Subject   Atherosclerotic patient

FIGURE 24.1. Longitudinal black-blood sections of the aorta (candy-cane view) of a normal subject (left panel) and an atherosclerotic patient (right panel). Atherosclerotic plaque can been seen in the aortic arch and thoracic aorta (arrows).

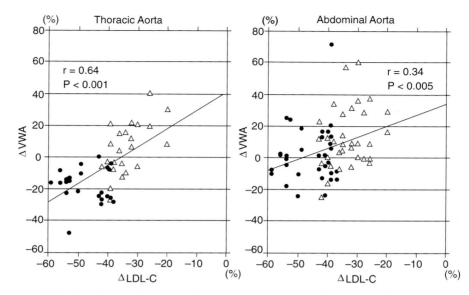

FIGURE 24.2. Correlations between the percent reduction in low-density lipoprotein-cholesterol (LDL-C) levels and the percent change in vessel wall area (VWA). The change in VWA in thoracic aortic plaques correlated well with the degree of LDL-C reduction ($r = 0.64$). A weak correlation was found in abdominal plaques ($r = 0.34$). Solid circles, 20-mg dose; open triangles, 5-mg dose. (Adapted from Yonemura A, et al. (15) with permission from The American College of Cardiology Foundation.)

reduction of LDL levels and the change in the vessel wall area in both the thoracic and abdominal aorta is presented in Figure 24.2.

These recent studies demonstrate that CMR is powerful tool to serially and noninvasively assess the regression of atherosclerotic lesion size under lipid-lowering therapies. More prospective studies are needed to determine whether there is a correlation between atherosclerotic plaque evolution measured with CMR and the occurence of acute ischemic events.

Detection of Vulnerable Atherosclerotic Plaques

Multicontrast MRI

Signal intensities detected with MRI are influenced by the relaxation times of protons (T1 and T2) and the proton density present in the different components of atherosclerotic plaques. The timing of the excitation pulses of an MR sequence will determine the weight of T1 and T2 relaxation times or proton density in the image contrast. Multicontrast MRI is based on successive T1-, T2-, and proton-density-weighted sequences. Analysis of signal intensities detected on each of these sequences allows differentiate the atherosclerotic plaque components (lipid core, fibrous tissue, hemorrhage, and calcification) by their different intrinsic relaxation properties on MRI.[16] Development of dedicated softwares, that analyze the signal intensities of multicontrast MRI on a pixel-by-pixel basis, has further improved the identification of atherosclerotic plaque components. An example of multicontrast MRI showing different plaque components and automatic segmentation of these plaques using a k-means cluster algorithm is shown in Figure 24.3.

Multicontrast MRI studies have focused mostly on carotid atherosclerotic plaques. The superficial location of carotid arteries and their relative absence of motion represent less of a technical challenge than imaging the aorta or the coronary arteries. In this location, multicontrast MRI could also be compared to corresponding

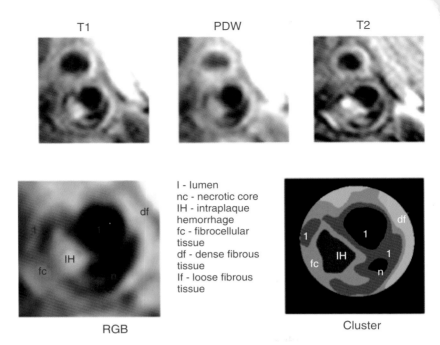

FIGURE 24.3. Multicontrast MR images of a carotid artery. Top row shows T1-weighted (T1), proton-density-weighted (PDW), and T2-weighted (T2) images of the same atherosclerotic plaque. The bottom left panel shows the RGB color composite image obtained by mapping the T1-weighted image to the red, the PD-weighted image to the green, and the T2-weighted image to the blue channel, respectively. The bottom right panel shows the plaque segmented automatically into its various components using an automated k-means cluster analysis algorithm. Intraplaque hemorrhage (IH), necrotic core (nc), loose fibers (lf), dense fibers (df), and the fibrous cap (fc) can be clearly differentiated. (l), lumen.

histology of atherosclerotic plaques from endarteriectomy specimens. For example, Yuan et al[17] demonstrated that *in vivo* multicontrast CMR of human carotid arteries had a sensitivity of 85% and specificity of 92% for the identification of a lipid core and acute intraplaque hemorrhage. Cai et al[18] confirmed the good agreement between the identification of plaque components obtained by multicontrast MRI of carotid arteries and the histologic classification of the American Heart Association (AHA) used for atherosclerotic plaques. Furthermore, in a case-controled study, Zhao et al[19] studied the effect of statins on the composition of carotid plaques and demonstrated a substantial reduction of the lipid content in plaques (with no substantial overall plaque area reduction) in patients treated for 10 years with an aggressive lipid-lowering regimen compared with untreated controls. Another recent study[20] evaluated the association between fibrous cap rupture of carotid plaques detected with multicontrast MRI and the history of recent transient ischemic attack or stroke. Ruptured caps (70%) were detected in carotid atherosclerotic plaques with a much higher frequency than plaques with a thick fibrous cap (9%) in symptomatic patients.

Recent histopathological studies[21,22] suggest that intraplaque hemorrhage may play a role in plaque rupture and also represent a potent atherogenic stimulus. Therefore, research has being directed toward the detection of intraplaque hemorrhage with multicontrast MRI. A first study[23] proved that multicontrast MRI can accuretely detect intraplaque hemorrhages in carotid atherosclerotic plaques using T2*-weighted sequences. Interestingly, a recent study[24] seems to confirm that the detection of these hemorrhages in carotid atherosclerotic plaques with MRI was associated with an accelerated increase of plaque volume in the next 18 months.

In summary, multicontrast MRI allows for the detection of the different components of atherosclerotic plaques with high accuracy and is particulary promising for the study of carotid atherosclerotic plaques. However, this technique requires a high MR signal and prolonged acquisition times, that nowadays limits its application to other arterial territories than the carotid arteries.

Contrast-Enhanced MRI

For a better identification of atherosclerotic plaque components, research is being directed toward the association of contrast agents to multicontrast MRI. Recent investigations have focused on neovessels as an important factor contributing to atherosclerotic plaque vulnerability. The extension of neovessels was associated with increased inflammatory infiltrate in atherosclerotic plaques[25] and was greater in the carotid endarterectomy specimens of symptomatic patients than in asymptomatic ones.[26] Gadolinium chelates represent the most commonly used MR contrast agents for angiographies. These paramagnetic agents, shorten the T1 relaxation time of protons, increase the luminal signal on MRI after intravenous injection and therefore could be good candidates for measuring plaque neovasculature. A recent study[27] demonstrated a correlation between the increase in signal intensity in carotid atherosclerotic plaques with gadolinium-enhanced MRI and the extent of neovessels in plaques on histology. However, gadolinium chelates have a low molecular weight and distribute rapidly into the extracellular fluid. Quantification of neovessels with gadolinum chelates will require the development of new kinetic modeling of the biodistribution of these contrast agents in atherosclerotic plaques. Alternatively, MR contrast agents that remain within the blood or diffuse more slowly in the extracellular space are currently in development.[28,29]

Novel intra-vascular MR contrast agents have also been found to accumulate in atherosclerotic plaques. For example, gadofluorine M is a lipophilic, macrocyclic, water-soluble, gadolinium chelate complex with a perfluorinated side chain. Sirol et al[30] and others[31] demonstrated that gadofluorine M enhanced only the aortic wall of Watanabe heritable hyperlipidemic rabbits but not the aorta of control rabbits. A strong correlation was found between the intensity of signal enhancement after the injection of gadofluorine with MRI in atherosclerotic plaques and the extension of lipid-rich areas on corresponding histological sections. This suggests a high affinity of gadofluorine M for lipid-rich plaques (see Figure 24.4). Since the lipid core often represents more than half the area of vulnerable atherosclerotic plaques, gadofluorine M could strongly improve the detection of these plaques with MRI.

Another class of contrast agent is represented by iron oxide nanoparticles (USPIO, SPIO), which are removed from the circulation by the reticuloendothelial system and accumulate in macrophages present in atherosclerotic plaques.[32–34] Macrophages play a pivotal role in the progression of atherosclerosis to a symptomatic disease[35] by

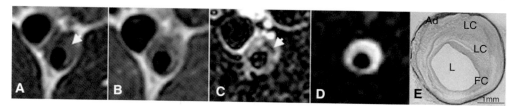

FIGURE 24.4. High-resolution in vivo MR images of a rabbit aorta. T1-weighted (A), proton-density-weighted (B), and T2-weighted (C) images were used to characterize the atherosclerotic plaque. The white arrows show the different areas of the atherosclerotic plaque (fibrous cap in T1-weighted images [A] and large lipid core in T2-weighted images [C]). Panel D displays the same atherosclerotic lesion enhanced 24 hours after gadofluorine injection via the rabbit ear vein. Gadofluorine, as previously reported by Sirol et al, improves in vivo atherosclerotic plaque detection. The corresponding histopathological section stained with combined Masson and Elastic Trichrom (CME) is shown in panel E (magnification, 4×). Ad, adventitia, FC, fibrous cap; L, lumen; LC, lipid core. (Adapted from Yonemura A, et al. (15) with permission from The American College of Cardiology Foundation.)

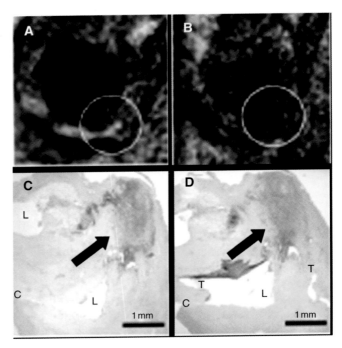

FIGURE 24.5. Corresponding in vivo MR images of the internal carotid artery with T2*-weighted gradient echo image before the administration of USPIO (A), and 24 hours later (B). A signal decrease is observed in the atherosclerotic plaque on the T2*-weighted image 24 hours after the injection of USPIO (white circle, B) compared to the pre-contrast image. On histologic sections from endarteriectomy specimens of patients imaged with USPIO-enhanced MRI, USPIO accumulated in atherosclerotic carotid plaques as shown with Perl's staining (C, blue coloring, black arrow) and colocalized with macrophages on CD 68 immunostaining (D, red coloring, black arrow). L, lumen; C, surgical cut; T, tears. (Adapted by permission from Kooi, et al. Accumulation of ultra small super paramagnetic particles of iron oxide in human atherosclerotic plaques can be detected by in vivo magnetic resonance imaging. Circulation 2003;107:2453–8.)

secreting locally abundant quantities of fibrous cap–degrading matrix metalloproteinases (MMP), proinflammatory cytokines, and tissue factor, which are involved in acute plaque destabilization and thrombus formation. Iron oxide contrast agents have superparamagnetic properties; that is, they decrease T2* relaxation time by generating heterogeneities in the local magnetic field; and can be detected on MRI as signal voids with T2*-weighted sequences. Accumulation of iron oxide nanoparticles in the macrophages present in atherosclerotic plaques can be detected as a focal decrease of the MR signal on T2*-weighted sequences. Kooi et al[33] studied 11 symptomatic patients scheduled for carotid endarterectomy with USPIO-enhanced MRI and found a 24% decrease in signal intensity on corresponding T2*-weighted sequences and uptake of USPIO on histology in 75% of ruptured or rupture-prone lesions (see Figure 24.5).

Several intra-vascular contrast agents have been found to accumulate in atherosclerotic plaques and can be detected with MRI, either by an increase (gadolinium-based contrast agents) or by a decrease (iron-oxide-based contrast agents) of the MR signal. More clinical studies are needed to confirm the potential of these contrast agents for the detection of vulnerable atherosclerotic plaques.

Molecular MRI

The ability to target molecules with specific contrast agents and MRI may greatly enhance detection and characterization of biological activities present in atherosclerotic lesions. Contrast agents linked to antibodies or peptides that target specific plaque components or molecules localized in vulnerable atherosclerotic plaque are currently in development for MR imaging.[36] For example, the scavenger receptor plays a key role in the uptake of LDL particles into macrophages. We developed a novel contrast agent formed of an antibody directed against the scavenger receptor bound to micelles containing a high payload of gadolinium molecules that allowed us to detect macrophages in atherosclerotic plaques of mice. Winter et al[37] recently demonstrated in a rabbit model of atherosclerosis that regions of neovascularization in plaques had a 47% increase in signal intensity on MRI after the injection of $\alpha_v\beta_3$-targeted nanoparticles. Many other specific MR contrast agents aimed at the detection of vulnerable plaques are currently tested targeting molecules such as oxidized low-density lipoprotein (oxLDL), endothelial integrins, matrix metalloproteinases, and extracellular matrix proteins such as tenascin-C. These targets are highlighted in a recent paper by Choudhury et al[38] and illustrated in Figure 24.6.

Intraluminal thrombosis represents the final step of the evolution of vulnerable atherosclerotic plaque and could represent another interesting target for new MR-specific contrast agents. Histologic studies have demonstrated that superficial thrombus surimposed on a ruptured atherosclerotic plaque characterizes plaques at high risk of ischemic events.[39] A recent work[40] analyzed the histology of intracoronary thrombus aspirated in 211 patients admitted for an acute myocardial infarction and

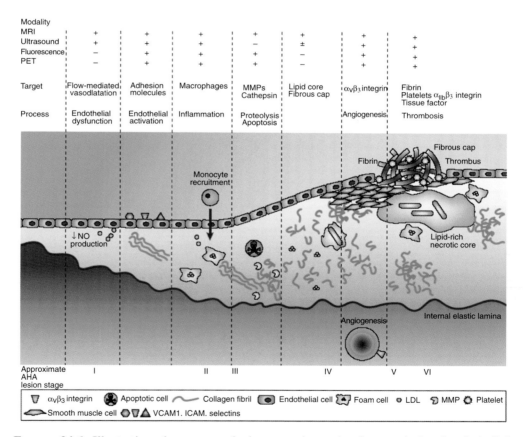

FIGURE 24.6. Illustration of processes of atherogenesis ranging from prelesional endothelial dysfunction (left) through monocyte recruitment to the development of plaques complicated by thrombosis (right). The mechanisms are grossly simplified but focus on components (e.g., cell adhesion molecules, macrophages, connective tissue elements, lipid core, fibrin), and processes (e.g., apoptosis, proteolysis, angiogenesis, thrombosis) in atherosclerotic plaques that have been imaged or that present useful potential imaging targets. Symbols indicate the feasibility (+ or −) of imaging using each of the modalities listed. (Adapted with permission from Nature Reviews Drug Discovery (reference 38) copyright 2004 Macmillan Magazines Ltd., (www.nature.com/reviews).

found that at least 50% of these thrombi were days or weeks old. Interestingly, a new fibrin-specific MR contrast agent has recently been designed. With this agent, thrombus resulting from plaque rupture has been identified using fibrin-specific MR contrast agents in a rabbit carotid crush injury model. In the 25 arterial thrombi induced by carotid crush injury, Botnar et al[41] demonstrated a sensitivity and specificity of 100% for in vivo thrombus detection using MRI. Sirol et al[42] recently used the same fibrin-specific MR contrast agent in 12 guinea pigs to demonstrate that the signal intensity of the thrombus was increased by more than 4-fold. The detection of thrombi was clearly improved from 42% identification of the thrombus before the injection of this contrast agent to 100% detection after injection. The ability to identify components of thrombus with molecular MRI may enable enhanced detection and characterization of both luminal thrombus and components of thrombus organized in an old atherothrombotic lesion (see Figure 24.7). Therefore, selection of targets pivotal in the coagulation cascade, such as fibrin, factor XIII, integrins on the surface of platelets, and tissue factor, is necessary to identify the areas of old or active thrombus formation.

Recently we developed a new class of MR contrast agent based on a recombinant high-density lipoprotein (rHDL) molecule that incorporates gadolinium-DTPA phospholipids.[43] This imaging agent has a small diameter of 7 nm to 12 nm, allowing for its diffusion in atherosclerotic plaques and, by using endogenous transport molecules, it does not trigger any immune reaction. Atherosclerotic plaques had a 35% increase of MR

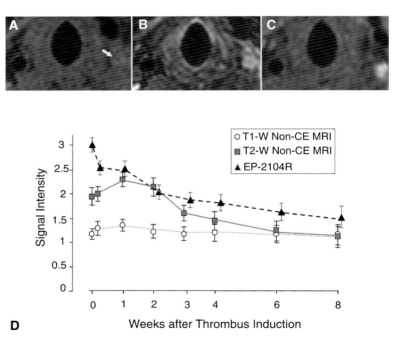

D

FIGURE 24.7. Transverse MR images of a rabbit carotid artery, 1 week after thrombus induction, using a double inversion recovery turbo-spin echo (2IR-TSE) sequence. T1-weighted (A) and T2-weighted (B) images were obtained without any injection of contrast agent. White arrow indicates location of the thrombus. (C) displays the T1-weighted images obtained 30 minutes after the injection of the fibrin-specific contrast agent (EP-2104R). (D) displays the thrombus relative signal intensity changes (mean ± SE) over time for T1-W (white circles) T2-W (gray squares) and post–EP-2104R injection (black triangles). The gadolinium-based, fibrin-targeted MR contrast agent (EP-2104R) demonstrated a significant enhancement of the thrombus compared to T1-W images ($p < 0.001$). (Adapted with permission from Sirol M et al. Chronic thrombus detection using *in vivo* magnetic resonance imaging and fibrin-targeted contrast agent. Circulation 2005;112:1594–600. Figure 2.)

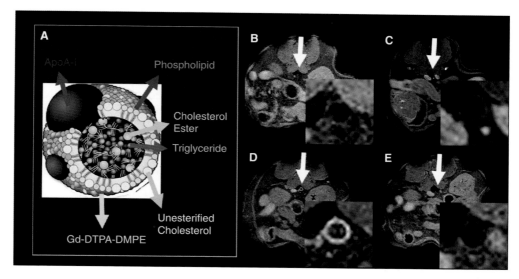

FIGURE 24.8. (A) The scheme represents the reconstituted HDL-like particle, phospholipid-based contrast agent (Gd-DTPA-DMPE) with the different components of the recombinant HDL-like MRI contrast agent. Transverse in vivo MR images of the abdominal aorta in an 8-week-old mouse at 9.4 Teslas before (B) and at 1 hour (C), 24 hours (D), and 48 hours (E) after the injection of recombinant HDL-like nanoparticles are displayed. The insets denote a magnification of the aortic region. (Adapted with permission from Frias JC et al. Recombinant HDL-like nanoparticles: a specific contract agent for MRA and atherosclerotic plaques. J Am Chem Soc. 2004;126:16316–16317. (43) Copyright 2004 American Chemical Society.)

signal intensity 24 hours after the injection of these rHDL in ApoE knockout mice. Furthermore, fluorescent rHDL colocalized with macrophages present in atherosclerotic plaques with confocal microscopy. Figure 24.8 demonstrates the enhancement of atherosclerotic plaques after the injection of rHDL.

In the future, the development of specific contrast agents for MRI will allow for in vivo imaging of biological activities present in human atherosclerotic plaques and will improve our understanding of the pathophysiology of atherosclerotic plaque rupture and subsequent intraluminal thrombosis. However, targeting very specific molecules or activities goes often along with lower concentrations of contrast agents in tissues. Therefore, novel contrast agents, highly efficient in enhancing the MR signal, will be needed in order for MRI to pursue its growth in the field of molecular imaging.

Summary Points

- Thanks to the absence of ionizing radiation, CMR could represent the imaging technology of choice for the noninvasive detection and monitoring of atherosclerosis progression.
- High image quality and sensitivity to small changes in plaque size of CMR have already permitted serial monitoring of atherosclerotic plaque progression and regression in the aorta and carotid arteries. However, reduced acquisition times and improvement in spatial resolution are needed to extend these studies to coronary arteries.
- More prospective studies would also be useful to confirm the link between the evolution of atherosclerosis plaque volume measured with CMR and the incidence of acute clinical events.
- Histologic studies have evidenced that acute ischemic events are frequently triggered by the rupture or erosion of vulnerable atherosclerotic plaques. These vulnerable plaques are characterized by their specific cellular and biological composition rather than by their volume. Therefore, imaging techniques have shifted from an anatomical to a functional evaluation of atherosclerotic plaques. Development of

contrast agents, which either accumulate or target vulnerable plaques, could allow MRI to combine precise atherosclerosis detection and identification of vulnerable plaques.

- The development of molecular imaging of atherosclerosis will improve our understanding of the key steps that lead from stable atherosclerotic plaque to an acute ischemic event and help to identify the most pertinent target for the detection of vulnerable atherosclerotic plaques.
- However, recent clinical studies[44,45] underscored the multiple locations of vulnerable and ruptured atherosclerotic plaques and the diffuse inflammation of the arterial tree in patients with acute ischemic events compared to stable patients. Therefore, the initial concept of detecting seldom high-risk atherosclerotic plaques with imaging could shift to a more global identification of vulnerable atherosclerotic patients, at high risk of acute clinical events, wherever the arterial location.[46]
- In the future, anatomical and molecular imaging of atherosclerosis should improve the individual evaluation of cardiovascular risk and help to optimize antiatherosclerotic therapies to reduce the incidence of acute thrombotic events.

Acknowledgments

This work was partially supported by the Fédération Française de Cardiologie, Paris, France (FH), and NIH/NHLBI HL071021 and HL078667 (ZAF).

References

1. Yusuf S, Reddy S, Ounpuu S, Anand S. Global burden of cardiovascular diseases: part I: general considerations, the epidemiologic transition, risk factors, and impact of urbanization. *Circulation.* 2001;104:2746–2753.
2. Topol EJ, Nissen SE. Our preoccupation with coronary luminology. The dissociation between clinical and angiographic findings in ischemic heart disease. *Circulation.* 1995;92: 2333–2342.
3. Glagov S, Weisenberg E, Zarins CK, Stankunavicius R, Kolettis GJ. Compensatory enlargement of human atherosclerotic coronary arteries. *N Engl J Med.* 1987;316:1371–1375.
4. Libby P. Current concepts of the pathogenesis of the acute coronary syndromes. *Circulation.* 2001;104:365–372.
5. Mani V, Itskovich VV, Szimtenings M, et al. Rapid extended coverage (REX) simultaneous multislice black blood vessel wall imaging. *Radiology.* 2004;232:281–288.
6. Itskovich VV, Mani V, Mizsei G, et al. Parallel and nonparallel simultaneous multislice black-blood double inversion recovery techniques for vessel wall imaging. *J Magn Reson Imaging.* 2004;19:459–467.
7. Summers RM, Andrasko-Bourgeois J, Feuerstein IM, et al. Evaluation of the aortic root by MRI: insights from patients with homozygous familial hypercholesterolemia. *Circulation.* 1998;98:509–518.
8. Corti R, Fayad ZA, Fuster V, et al. Effects of lipid-lowering by simvastatin on human atherosclerotic lesions: a longitudinal study by high-resolution, noninvasive magnetic resonance imaging. *Circulation.* 2001;104:249–252.
9. Kang X, Polissar NL, Han C, Lin E, Yuan C. Analysis of the measurement precision of arterial lumen and wall areas using high-resolution MRI. *Magn Reson Med.* 2000;44: 968–972.
10. Chan SK, Jaffer FA, Botnar RM, et al. Scan reproducibility of magnetic resonance imaging assessment of aortic atherosclerosis burden. *J Cardiovasc Magn Reson.* 2001;3:331–338.
11. Jaffer FA, O'Donnell CJ, Larson MG, et al. Age and sex distribution of subclinical aortic atherosclerosis: a magnetic resonance imaging examination of the Framingham Heart Study. *Arterioscler Thromb Vasc Biol.* 2002;22:849–854.
12. Li AE, Kamel I, Rando F, et al. Using MRI to assess aortic wall thickness in the multiethnic study of atherosclerosis: distribution by race, sex, and age. *AJR Am J Roentgenol.* 2004;182:593–597.

13. Taniguchi H, Momiyama Y, Fayad ZA, et al. In vivo magnetic resonance evaluation of associations between aortic atherosclerosis and both risk factors and coronary artery disease in patients referred for coronary angiography. *Am Heart J.* 2004;148:137–143.

14. Corti R, Osende JI, Fallon JT, et al. The selective peroxisomal proliferator-activated receptor-gamma agonist has an additive effect on plaque regression in combination with simvastatin in experimental atherosclerosis: in vivo study by high-resolution magnetic resonance imaging. *J Am Coll Cardiol.* 2004;43:464–473.

15. Yonemura A, Momiyama Y, Fayad ZA, et al. Effect of lipid-lowering therapy with atorvastatin on atherosclerotic aortic plaques detected by noninvasive magnetic resonance imaging. *J Am Coll Cardiol.* 2005;45:733–742.

16. Toussaint JF, LaMuraglia GM, Southern JF, Fuster V, Kantor HL. Magnetic resonance images lipid, fibrous, calcified, hemorrhagic, and thrombotic components of human atherosclerosis in vivo. *Circulation.* 1996;94:932–938.

17. Yuan C, Mitsumori LM, Ferguson MS, et al. In vivo accuracy of multispectral magnetic resonance imaging for identifying lipid-rich necrotic cores and intraplaque hemorrhage in advanced human carotid plaques. *Circulation.* 2001;104:2051–2056.

18. Cai JM, Hatsukami TS, Ferguson MS, Small R, Polissar NL, Yuan C. Classification of human carotid atherosclerotic lesions with in vivo multicontrast magnetic resonance imaging. *Circulation.* 2002;106:1368–1373.

19. Zhao XQ, Yuan C, Hatsukami TS, et al. Effects of prolonged intensive lipid-lowering therapy on the characteristics of carotid atherosclerotic plaques in vivo by MRI: a case-control study. *Arterioscler Thromb Vasc Biol.* 2001;21:1623–1629.

20. Yuan C, Zhang SH, Polissar NL, et al. Identification of fibrous cap rupture with magnetic resonance imaging is highly associated with recent transient ischemic attack or stroke. *Circulation.* 2002;105:181–185.

21. Kolodgie FD, Gold HK, Burke AP, et al. Intraplaque hemorrhage and progression of coronary atheroma. *N Engl J Med.* 2003;349:2316–2325.

22. Burke AP, Farb A, Malcom GT, Liang Y, Smialek JE, Virmani R. Plaque rupture and sudden death related to exertion in men with coronary artery disease. *JAMA.* 1999;281:921–926.

23. Chu B, Kampschulte A, Ferguson MS, et al. Hemorrhage in the atherosclerotic carotid plaque: a high-resolution MRI study. *Stroke.* 2004;35:1079–1084.

24. Takaya N, Yuan C, Chu B, et al. Presence of intraplaque hemorrhage stimulates progression of carotid atherosclerotic plaques: a high-resolution magnetic resonance imaging study. *Circulation.* 2005;111:2768–2775.

25. Kumamoto M, Nakashima Y, Sueishi K. Intimal neovascularization in human coronary atherosclerosis: its origin and pathophysiological significance. *Hum Pathol.* 1995;26:450–456.

26. Mofidi R, Crotty TB, McCarthy P, Sheehan SJ, Mehigan D, Keaveny TV. Association between plaque instability, angiogenesis and symptomatic carotid occlusive disease. *Br J Surg.* 2001;88:945–950.

27. Kerwin W, Hooker A, Spilker M, et al. Quantitative magnetic resonance imaging analysis of neovasculature volume in carotid atherosclerotic plaque. *Circulation.* 2003;107:851–856.

28. Lauffer RB, Parmelee DJ, Dunham SU, et al. MS-325: albumin-targeted contrast agent for MR angiography. *Radiology.* 1998;207:529–538.

29. Port M, Meyer D, Bonnemain B, et al. P760 and P775: MRI contrast agents characterized by new pharmacokinetic properties. *Magma.* 1999;8:172–176.

30. Sirol M, Itskovich VV, Mani V, et al. Lipid-rich atherosclerotic plaques detected by gadofluorine-enhanced in vivo magnetic resonance imaging. *Circulation.* 2004;109:2890–2896.

31. Barkhausen J, Ebert W, Heyer C, Debatin JF, Weinmann H-J. Detection of atherosclerotic plaque with gadofluorine-enhanced magnetic resonance imaging. *Circulation.* 2003;108:605–609.

32. Hyafil F, Laissy JP, Mazighi M, et al. Ferumoxtran-10-enhanced MRI of the hypercholesterolemic rabbit aorta: relationship between signal loss and macrophage infiltration. *Arterioscler Thromb Vasc Biol.* 2006;26:176–181.

33. Kooi ME, Cappendijk VC, Cleutjens KB, et al. Accumulation of ultrasmall superparamagnetic particles of iron oxide in human atherosclerotic plaques can be detected by in vivo magnetic resonance imaging. *Circulation.* 2003;107:2453–2458.

34. Trivedi RA, U-King-Im JM, Graves MJ, et al. In vivo detection of macrophages in human carotid atheroma: temporal dependence of ultrasmall superparamagnetic particles of iron oxide-enhanced MRI. *Stroke*. 2004;35:1631–1635.

35. Libby P, Ridker PM, Maseri A. Inflammation and atherosclerosis. *Circulation*. 2002;105: 1135–1143.

36. Lipinski MJ, Fuster V, Fisher EA, Fayad ZA. Targeting of biological molecules for evaluation of high-risk atherosclerotic plaques with magnetic resonance imaging. *Nat Clin Pract Cardiovasc Med*. 2004;1:48–55.

37. Winter PM, Morawski AM, Caruthers SD, et al. Molecular imaging of angiogenesis in early-stage atherosclerosis with alpha(v)beta3-integrin-targeted nanoparticles. *Circulation*. 2003;108:2270–2274.

38. Choudhury RP, Fuster V, Fayad ZA. Molecular, cellular and functional imaging of atherothrombosis. *Nat Rev Drug Discov*. 2004;3:913–925.

39. Virmani R, Kolodgie FD, Burke AP, Farb A, Schwartz SM. Lessons from sudden coronary death: a comprehensive morphological classification scheme for atherosclerotic lesions. *Arterioscler Thromb Vasc Biol*. 2000;20:1262–1275.

40. Rittersma SZ, van der Wal AC, Koch KT, et al. Plaque instability frequently occurs days or weeks before occlusive coronary thrombosis: a pathological thrombectomy study in primary percutaneous coronary intervention. *Circulation*. 2005;111:1160–1165.

41. Botnar RM, Perez AS, Witte S, et al. In vivo molecular imaging of acute and subacute thrombosis using a fibrin-binding magnetic resonance imaging contrast agent. *Circulation*. 2004;109:2023–2029.

42. Sirol M, Aguinaldo JGS, Graham G, et al. Fibrin-targeted contrast agent for improvement of in vivo acute thrombus detection with magnetic resonance imaging. *Atherosclerosis*. 2005;182:79–85.

43. Frias JC, Williams KJ, Fisher EA, Fayad ZA. Recombinant HDL-like nanoparticles: a specific contrast agent for MRI of atherosclerotic plaques. *J Am Chem Soc*. 2004;126: 16316–16317.

44. Rioufol G, Finet G, Ginon I, et al. Multiple atherosclerotic plaque rupture in acute coronary syndrome: a three-vessel intravascular ultrasound study. *Circulation*. 2002;106: 804–808.

45. Mauriello A, Sangiorgi G, Fratoni S, et al. Diffuse and active inflammation occurs in both vulnerable and stable plaques of the entire coronary tree: a histopathologic study of patients dying of acute myocardial infarction. *J Am Coll Cardiol*. 2005;45:1585–1593.

46. Naghavi M, Libby P, Falk E, et al. From vulnerable plaque to vulnerable patient: a call for new definitions and risk assessment strategies: part II. *Circulation*. 2003;108:1772–1778.

25 Evaluating Gene and Cell Therapy

Ahmad Y. Sheikh and Joseph C. Wu

Cardiac imaging modalities such as computed tomography (CT), magnetic resonance imaging (MRI), single photon emission computed tomography (SPECT), positron emission tomography (PET), and ultrasound have seen major advances over the past 3 decades. In the clinical setting, these modalities can provide outstanding data regarding organ structure and physiologic function. However, as molecular medicine transitions from bench to bedside in the forms of gene and cellular therapies, novel, noninvasive imaging technologies need to be developed to monitor and evaluate the efficacy of these treatments at the genetic and biochemical levels. This need has given rise to a new and rapidly evolving discipline called "molecular imaging."[1]

In its broadest sense, molecular imaging can be defined as the characterization, visual representation, and quantification of biological processes at the cellular and subcellular levels within intact living organisms.[2] The field remains in its infancy at present and to a large extent is limited to the laboratory environment. Notable exceptions are in the disciplines of oncology, neurology, and cardiology, which have started to make the transition from basic science to clinical application.

This chapter introduces the field of cardiovascular molecular imaging with specific emphasis on PET and its utility in evaluating gene and cellular therapy. The chapter is divided into the following sections: (1) background of cardiovascular molecular imaging, (2) specific imaging techniques, (3) PET reporter genes and probes, and (4) recent cardiac gene and cell therapy studies and the role of PET. Because the field may be new to many, we have simplified much of the discussion of technical details to make the context more appealing to a broad range of readers with different backgrounds.

Background of Cardiovascular Molecular Imaging

Traditionally, researchers have monitored cardiac gene transfer by using reporter constructs such as β-galactosidase (β-gal),[3] green fluorescent protein (GFP),[4] and chloramphenicol-acetyl transferase (CAT).[5] Cellular transplant therapies have employed similar techniques as well as newer approaches such as TaqMan reverse transcriptase polymerase chain reaction (RT-PCR),[6] Y-chromosome paint probes,[7] and antibodies specific to various stem cell types.[8] All these established traditional techniques, however, require invasive biopsies, postmortem tissue sampling, or both for analysis. Molecular imaging offers distinct advantages by allowing for noninvasive, quantitative, and repetitive imaging of targeted macromolecules and biological processes in living organisms.[9] Although a vast array of molecular imaging techniques is available, they all require two fundamental elements: (1) a molecular probe that can signal confirmation of gene expression by detecting messenger ribonucleic acid (mRNA) transcripts or proteins and (2) a method to monitor these probes or events. Presently, the two most widely used strategies are direct and indirect imaging.

Direct Molecular Imaging

Direct molecular imaging involves direct probe-target interaction. Targets can include receptors, enzymes, or mRNA. For *probe-receptor imaging*, radiolabeled monoclonal antibodies binding to tumor cell–specific surface antigens have been used for the past 2 decades.[10] A recent example of cardiac application involved imaging $\alpha_v\beta_3$ integrin receptor expressed during angiogenesis after myocardial infarction (MI) by using ^{111}In-RP748, a radiolabeled quinolone targeted at $\alpha_v\beta_3$.[11] For *probe-enzyme imaging*, the most well known cardiac application is 18F-fluorodeoxyglucose (^{18}F-FDG), used to assess for myocardial tissue viability. After transport across an intact cell membrane, the ^{18}F-labeled glucose analogue undergoes phosphorylation by hexokinase and is retained intracellularly in proportion to the rate of cellular glycolysis.[12] The radioactive ^{18}F undergoes positron annihilation into 2 high-energy gamma rays (511 keV), which can be detected as coincidence events by PET. For *probe-mRNA imaging*, radiolabeled antisense oligonucleotide (RASON) probes can be used.[13,14] RASON probes are typically 12 to 35 nucleotides long and are complementary to a small segment of the target mRNA. However, the RASON approach is limited at this point due to (1) a low number of target mRNA (~1000 copies) per cell compared to proteins (>10,000 copies), (2) limited tracer penetration across the cell membrane, (3) poor intracellular stability, (4) slow washout of unbound oligonucleotide probes, and (5) low target-to-background ratios.[15] Despite these limitations, antisense imaging continues to improve, as demonstrated by Hnatowich and colleagues, who have further addressed issues of delivery and targeting in both in vitro and small animal models.[16,17] On the other hand, direct imaging of DNA (2 copies) within the nuclear membrane has proved exceedingly difficult and is not yet feasible. In addition, knowing the *activity* of gene expression (as reflected in mRNA transcripts or protein levels) rather than the *number* of DNA copies is more relevant for biological research. The main disadvantage of direct imaging is that it requires synthesizing a customized probe for the product (e.g., receptor, enzyme, or mRNA) of every therapeutic gene of interest, which can be time-consuming and is not generalizable to most applications.

Indirect Molecular Imaging

Indirect molecular imaging using reporter genes has been only recently validated. The concept of imaging reporter-gene expression is illustrated in Figure 25.1. A reporter gene is first introduced into target tissues by viral or nonviral vectors. Using molecular biology techniques, the promoter or regulatory regions of genes can be cloned into different vectors to drive reporter-gene mRNA transcription. Promoter activity can be "constitutive" (always on), "inducible" (turned on or off), or "tissue specific" (expressed only in the heart, liver, or other organs).[18] Translation of mRNA leads to a reporter protein that can interact with the reporter probe. This interaction may be enzyme or receptor based (as discussed under Ideal Reporter Gene and Reporter Probe). Probe signals can then be detected by various imaging modalities such as an optical charged coupled device (CCD) camera, PET, or MRI.

Clearly, the main advantage of the reporter-gene system is its flexibility and multitasking capability. By altering various components, the reporter gene can provide information about the regulation of DNA by upstream promoters, intracellular protein trafficking, and the efficiency of vector transduction on cells. Likewise, the reporter

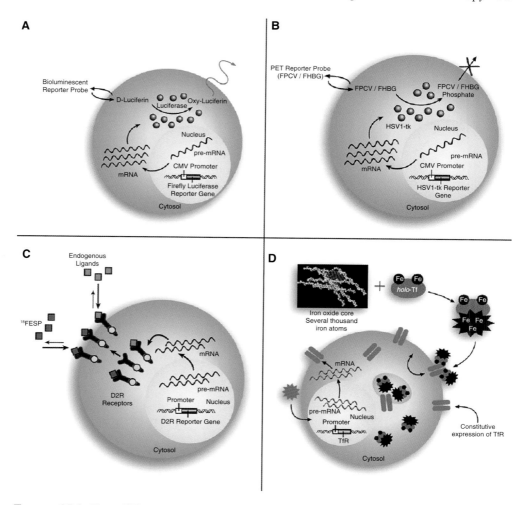

FIGURE 25.1. Four different strategies of imaging reporter gene/reporter probe. (A) Enzyme-based bioluminescence imaging. Expression of the firefly luciferase reporter gene leads to the firefly luciferase reporter enzyme, which catalyzes the reporter probe (D-Luciferin) that results in a photochemical reaction. This yields low levels of photons that can be detected, collected, and quantified by a charge-coupled device (CCD) camera. (B) Enzyme-based PET imaging. Expression of the herpes simplex virus type 1 thymidine kinase (HSV1-tk) reporter gene leads to the thymidine kinase reporter enzyme (HSV1-TK), which phosphorylates and traps the reporter probe ^{18}F-FHBG intracellularly. Radioactive decay of ^{18}F isotopes can be detected using PET. (C) Receptor-based PET imaging. The ^{18}F-FESP is a reporter probe that interacts with the dopamine 2 receptor (D2R) to result in probe trapping on or in cells expressing the D2R gene. (D) Receptor-based MRI imaging. Overexpression of engineered transferrin receptors (TfR) results in increased cell uptake of the transferrin-monocrystalline iron oxide nanoparticles (Tf-MION). These changes result in a detectable contrast change on MRI. (Reprinted from Wu JC, et al. Molecular imaging of cardiovascular gene products. J Nucl Cardiol; 11:491–505, Copyright 2004, with permission from the American Society of Nuclear Cardiology.)

probe itself does not have to be changed to study a new biological process, saving time and resources required for synthesis, testing, and validation of new reagents. However, the main disadvantage of indirect imaging is that it remains a surrogate marker for the physiologic process of interest, as opposed to a direct measure of receptor density, mRNA copies, or intracellular enzymatic activity, which might be more clinically relevant. It should be noted that, in the case of monitoring cellular survival and trafficking (e.g., cardiac cellular transplant), this is less of a concern since the focus is on detecting the presence of a population of cells.

Ideal Reporter Gene and Reporter Probe

With both the direct and indirect molecular imaging techniques, the ideal reporter gene or reporter probe should have the following characteristics: (1) The chromosomal integration or episomal expression of reporter gene should not adversely affect the cellular metabolism or physiology. (2) The reporter gene product should not elicit a host immune response. (3) The size of the promoter-enhancer elements and reporter gene should be small enough to fit into a delivery vehicle. (4) Transfection (e.g., plasmid) or transduction (e.g., lentivirus or adeno-associated virus) using the delivery vector should not be cytotoxic to the cells. (5) The reporter probe should be stable in vivo and reach the target site despite natural biological barriers (e.g., blood-vessel wall

TABLE 25.1. Summary of Common Reporter Genes and Reporter Probe for Molecular Imaging Platforms and Comparison of Imaging Modalities

Imaging Modality	Reporter Gene	Reporter Probe	Mechanisms
BLI	Firefly luciferase (Fluc)	D-luciferin	Firefly luciferase-luciferin reaction in presence of Mg^{2+} and ATP
	Renilla luciferase (hRl)	Coelenterazine	Renilla luciferase-coelenterazine reaction
FLI	Green fluorescence protein (GFP)	N/A	Excitation-emission fluorescence
	Red fluorescence protein (RFP)	N/A	Excitation-emission fluorescence
MRI	Engineered transferin receptor (TfR)	Transferrin-conjugated superparamagnetic iron oxide nanoparticles (Tf MION)	Receptor-ligand interaction
	β-galactosidase (β-Gal)	EgadMe	Hydrolysis of β-glycoside bond
	Tyrosinase	Synthetic metallomelanins ^{111}In, Fe	Metal binding to melanin
PET	Herpes simplex virus type 1 thymidine kinase (HSV1-tk)	[124]FIAU	Phosphorylation
		^{18}F-FHPG	Phosphorylation
		^{18}F-PCV	Phosphorylation
	Herpes simplex virus type 1 mutant thymidine kinase (HSV1-sr39tk)	^{18}F-FHBG	Phosphorylation
		[18]FPCV	Phosphorylation
	Dopamine 2 receptor (D2R)	^{18}F-FESP	Receptor-ligand
	Mutant dopamine 2 receptor (D2R80A)	^{18}F-FESP	Receptor-ligand
SPECT	HSV1-tk	[131]FIAU	Phosphorylation
	Human sodium iodide symporter (hNIS)	[123]Iodide or [99m]technetium	Active symport
Ultrasound	—	—	—
CT	—	—	—
BLI	3–5 mm	Seconds– minutes	1–2 cm	10^{-15}–10^{-17}	Visible light	μg–mg
FLI	2–3 mm	Seconds– minutes	<1 cm	10^{-9}–10^{-12}	Visible light or near infrared	μg–mg
MRI	25–100 μm	Minutes–hours	No limit	10^{-3}–10^{-5}	Radiowaves	μg–mg
PET	1–2 mm	Seconds– minutes	No limit	10^{-11}–10^{-12}	High-energy gamma rays	ng
SPECT	0.5–1.5 mm	Minutes	No limit	10^{-10}–10^{-11}	Lower-energy γ rays	ng
Ultrasound	50–500 μm	Seconds– minutes	mm– cm	Not known	High-frequency ultrasound	μg–mg
CT	50–200 μm	Minutes	No limit	Not known	X-rays	Not available

or blood-brain barrier). (6) The reporter probe should accumulate only within cells that express the reporter gene to yield a high signal-to-background ratio. (7) Afterward, the reporter probe should clear rapidly from the circulation to allow repetitive imaging within the same living subject. (8) The reporter probe or its metabolites should not be cytotoxic to the cells. (9) The image signals should correlate well with true levels of reporter gene mRNA and protein in vivo. (10) The reporter gene and reporter probe should be potentially applicable for human imaging in the future.[15] At present, no single reporter-gene or reporter-probe assay meets all these criteria. Thus, the optimal choice of reporter-gene and reporter-probe assay will depend on the particular application, organ system, and imaging modality available at a given institution (Table 25.1).

Imaging Techniques

Of the numerous molecular imaging modalities available for monitoring genetic and cellular activity, radionuclide-based assays (e.g., PET, SPECT, planar scintigraphy) are the most useful clinically. A number of other devices are being used to monitor biological processes in animal models of diseases. Considerable efforts have been made toward the development of miniaturized, small-animal imaging systems such as CCD cameras for bioluminescence/fluorescence, ultrasound, SPECT/PET, and MRI (Figure 25.2). Given the vast array of imaging tools available for biological research, a brief discussion highlighting the strengths and weaknesses of each modality is warranted.

Optical Imaging

Bioluminescence imaging utilizes the photogenic properties of various luciferase genes cloned from different organisms, such as firefly (*Photinus pyralis*), jellyfish (*Aequorea*), coral (*Renilla*), and dinoflagellates (*Gonyaulx*). In the case of the firefly, the firefly luciferase enzyme (FL) converts its substrate (D-luciferin) to oxyluciferin via an ATP-dependent pathway. This process emits low levels of photons (2–3 eV), which can be detected and counted by an ultrasensitive CCD camera (e.g., Xenogen IVIS system).[19] Unlike bioluminescence, fluorescence imaging does not require injection of a reporter substrate but relies on an excitation wavelength that produces an emission wavelength for measurement.[20] Recent technological advances (e.g., eXplore Optix system) have allowed the measurement, quantification, and visualization of fluorescence intensity in small living animals using the time-domain approach.[21] In general, optical-based imaging is a relatively low-cost endeavor (i.e., typically $100–200,000 versus $500,000–2 million for small animal PET and MRI systems) with the capacity for high throughput (i.e., several mice can be scanned once). However, the aforementioned techniques suffer from low spatial resolution, inability to monitor multiple physiologic processes, and photon attenuation/scatter within deep tissues.[22] Moreover, optical imaging has yet to be extrapolated into clinical usage. Novel intravascular catheter devices capable of detecting bioluminescence signals, fluorescence signals, or both from deeper tissues or organs may be possible, but the general practicality of "invasive imaging" remains to be seen.

Magnetic Resonance Imaging

Unlike optical imaging, MRI has the advantage of a very high spatial resolution (25 to 100 μm) and the ability to measure more than one physiological parameter at once by using different radiofrequency pulse sequences.[23] This makes MR a very attractive option for imaging reporter-gene expression. The imaging signal is generated as a result of spin relaxation effects, which can be altered by atoms with high magnetic moments (e.g., gadolinium and iron). One particularly useful MR imaging signal amplification system is based on the cellular internalization of superparamagnetic

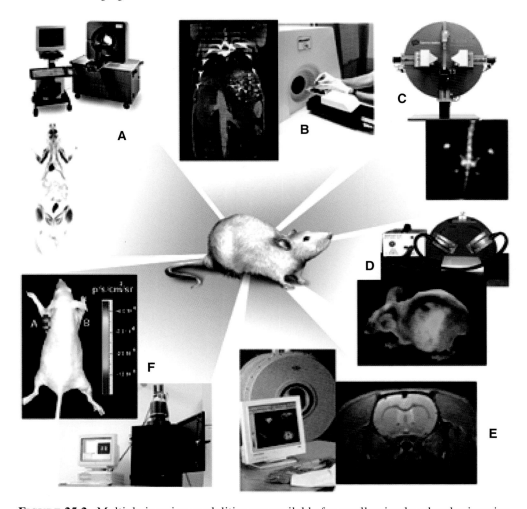

FIGURE 25.2. Multiple imaging modalities are available for small animal molecular imaging. (A) Small animal PET whole-body coronal image of a rat injected with ^{18}F-FDG, showing uptake of tracer in tissues including muscles, heart, brain, and bladder due to renal clearance. (B) Small animal CT coronal image of a mouse abdomen after injection of intravenous iodinated contrast medium. (C) Small animal SPECT coronal image of a mouse abdomen and pelvis regions after injection of ^{99m}Tc-methylene diphosphonate, showing spine, pelvis, tail, vertebrae, and femurs due to accumulation of tracer in bone. (D) Optical fluorescence image of a mouse showing GFP-expressing tumors that have spread to the liver, abdomen, spine, and brain. (E) Small animal MRI coronal T2-weighted image of a mouse brain. (F) Optical bioluminescence image of a mouse with a subcutaneous xenograft expressing renilla luciferase (Rluc) in the left shoulder region, after tail-vein injection of the reporter substrate coelentrazine. Images were obtained using a cooled CCD camera. The color image of visible light is superimposed on a photographic image of the mouse with a scale in photons per second per square centimeter per steradian (sr). (Reproduced with permission from Reference 9.)

probes such as monocrystalline iron oxide nanoparticles (MION) and cross-linked iron oxide (CLIO).[24] MIONs or CLIOs can be linked to a variety of biomolecules to produce injectable probes for targets such as hematopoietic and neural progenitor cells,[25,26] activated thrombotic factor XIII,[27] and endothelial cell surface markers such as E-selectin.[28] These studies hold promise for in vivo imaging in humans, given the widespread availability of clinical MR scanners, the nontoxic and biodegradable properties of intravenous superparamagnetic particles, and the precedent of similar preparations already in clinical use.[29] However, persisting residual signals from superparamagnetic particles may hinder the capacity for quantitative and repetitive imaging. MR is also several log of orders less sensitive (10^{-3} to 10^{-5} molar) for detection of reporter probes compared to optical bioluminescence imaging (10^{-15} to 10^{-17}) or PET (10^{-11} to 10^{-12}) imaging.[9] Therefore, further strategies for robust signal amplification will be necessary before this modality can be of practical use for imaging cardiac gene expression and detecting small numbers of transplanted cells.

Ultrasound

The scope of ultrasound for cardiac molecular imaging remains limited, largely due to the few options available for acoustically compatible molecular probes. Targeted contrast agents have been constructed by linking ligands of interest to liposomes, perfluorocarbon nanoparticles, and encapsulated microbubbles,[30] but these agents are relatively large (>250nm), precluding efficient tissue penetration. While ultrasound-based molecular imaging may play an increasing role in endothelial imaging, its utility as a molecular cardiac imaging modality to track gene or cell therapy remains to be seen.

Computed Tomography

Like ultrasound, CT is quite limited in its application as a true molecular imaging modality. Development of radiopaque probes that can accumulate in sufficient quantities for meaningful assessment of physiologic processes has proven difficult. Compared to MRI, CT-based images exhibit poor soft-tissue contrast, necessitating iodinated contrast media in addition to any probes that might be used. Presently, CT is best reserved for use as an adjunct anatomical imaging modality that can complement functional information obtained by other molecular imaging techniques, such as PET and optical imaging. In the future, improved probes may increase the applicability of CT imaging.

Radionuclide Imaging

Radionuclide probes are the first example of molecular probes used in the clinical setting; this technology represents the evolutionary roots of molecular imaging as it is known today. PET, SPECT, and planar scintigraphy have all been used to detect radionuclide-labeled probes. However, PET exhibits several advantages compared to other modalities. First, PET is more sensitive than SPECT and MRI for detection of probe activity. This may allow monitoring of gene delivery by vectors with relatively low transfection efficiencies (e.g., plasmid) or weak promoters (e.g., tissue specific), as well as detection of low numbers of cells (e.g., cardiac stem cell transplants). Second, PET imaging is more quantitative (unlike MRI) and allows for dynamic imaging with tracer kinetic modeling for analysis of rate constants underlying the biochemical processes.[31] Third, as many PET tracers have a short half-life (e.g. ~110min for ^{18}F), daily repetitive imaging of tracer retention by targeted tissues is possible. Fourth, PET imaging is tomographic (unlike two-dimensional images from optical imaging), and thus a relatively precise location of probe signal can be identified within the heart. This is especially apt in the basic research environment, as current generations of small animal PET scanners have a resolution of 1^3–2^3 mm^3 compared to ~6^3 mm^3 for clinical PET scanners.[32] Finally, studies performed in these small animal PET scanners can potentially be scaled up to patients using clinical PET scanners with relative ease.[33]

PET Reporter Genes and Probes

Of all the imaging techniques discussed, radionuclide imaging represents the most promising approach for clinical imaging of biological processes. It has several desirable characteristics, including robust detection sensitivity, quantitative capacity, tomographic resolution, and clinically available scanners. Translation into the clinical setting is well under way, with significant progress over the last few years. The first phase I/II clinical trial was published in 2001.[34] This study involved 5 patients (age range, 49 to 67 years) with recurrent glioblastomas who were infused intratumorally with liposome complex containing herpes simplex virus type 1 thymidine kinase (HSV1-tk). After vector administration, only 1 of 5 patients had specific [124]I-FIAU-associated radioactivity observed within the infused tumor. No specific FIAU-accumulation was observed in the other 4 patients, in whom tumor histology showed a significantly lower number of proliferating tumor cells. These data indicate that a certain critical number of the thymidine kinase-gene transduced tumor cells per voxel (threshold) must be present for accumulation of FIAU and detection by PET. This study was limited by pharmacokinetic issues related to the blood-brain-barrier and clearance of [124]I-FIAU radiotracer.

Recently, a more detailed clinical trial involving PET imaging of gene expression was completed in Spain.[35] In this study, 7 patients (age range, 51 to 78 years) with hepatocellular carcinomas underwent intratumoral injection of recombinant adenovirus carrying the cytomegalovirus promoter driving HSV1-tk (Ad-CMV-HSV1-tk). Successful PET imaging was achieved by using 9-(4-fluoro-3-hydroxymethylbutyl)guanine (^{18}F-FHBG) as the PET reporter probe with very good signal-to-background ratio. Anatomic and metabolic correlation was obtained by fusion PET/CT imaging (Figure 25.3). Repeated imaging was also possible in this study because of the relatively short half-life of [18]F (~110 min). The HSV1-tk, in addition to serving as a reporter gene, can be used to destroy tumor cells by exploiting its ability to convert a nontoxic prodrug such as valganciclovir into a phosphorylated, cytotoxic compound.

These two studies demonstrate the principle of using PET reporter gene to assess novel therapeutic strategies and monitor clinical responses in human subjects. The PET reporter probe ^{18}F-FHBG has been shown to have favorable characteristics such as in vivo stability, rapid blood clearance, low background signal, and acceptable radiation dosimetry in humans.[36,37] ^{18}F-FHBG has recently been approved by the FDA as an investigational new drug (IND). It is hoped that with further validation, similar studies can be performed in patients with cardiovascular diseases using a variety of PET reporter genes and PET reporter probes as discussed in the following paragraphs.

The most common enzyme-based reporter gene is the HSV1-tk.[38,39] Unlike the mammalian thymidine kinase enzyme, the viral thymidine kinase enzyme (HSV1-TK) acts on a broad range of substrates. The HSV1-TK can phosphorylate thymidine analogue probes such as FIAU and guanosine analogue probes such as FHBG. Once phosphorylated, the reporter probes are trapped intracellularly and the radioisotope ([124]I or ^{18}F) attached to the compounds can be detected as coincidence events by PET imaging. The main advantage of ^{18}F versus [124]I is its shorter half-life ($T_{1/2}$ ~110 minutes vs 4.2 days), which allows for repetitive imaging on a daily basis.

The second version of HSV1-tk is a mutant form (HSV1-sr39tk) that differs from HSV1-tk by 7 nucleotide substitutions leading to 5 different nonpolar amino acids.[40] The HSV1-sr39TK enzyme phosphorylates acycloguanosine derivatives (e.g., fluorinated ganciclovir and penciclovir as reporter probes) effectively while minimizing interaction with endogenous thymidine kinase.[41] Dynamic imaging in animal tumor models using the HSV1-sr39tk/^{18}F-FHBG combination also appears to be more sensitive compared to HSV1-tk/^{14}C-FIAU. Whereas the ^{18}F-FHBG is well retained in HSV1-sr39tk-expressing cells (C6-stb-sr39tk+) 4 hours following injection, ^{14}C-FIAU is rapidly cleared from HSV1-tk-expressing cells (MH3924A-stb-tk+).[42] A more recent study suggests that [^{3}H]2'-fluoro-2'-deoxyarabinofuranosyl-5-ethyluracil ([^{3}H]-FEAU) may exhibit the most robust affinity for either HSV1-tk or HSV1-sr39tk reporter genes, although further work is clearly warranted to assess optimal combinations of reporter genes and probes.[43]

The third version of the HSV1-tk gene is called truncated thymidine kinase (HSV1-ttk). It has a deletion of the first 135 base pairs that contain a nuclear localization

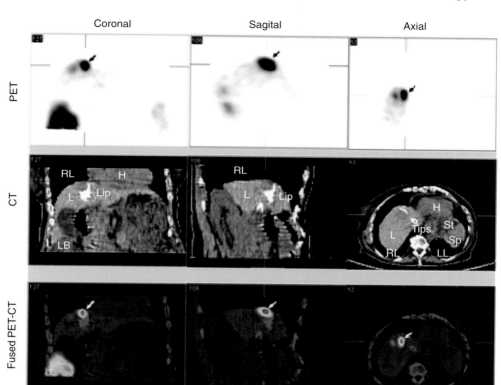

FIGURE 25.3. PET/CT imaging of HSV1-tk transgene expression in humans. Columns show the 5-mm thick coronal, sagittal, and transaxial slices, respectively, from an ^{18}F-FHBG PET/CT study in a patient. All sections are centered on the treated tumor lesion and show ^{18}F-FHBG accumulation at the tumor site (arrows). Anatomic and metabolic correlation can be obtained by fused PET/CT imaging. The white spots on the liver seen on the CT images correspond to lipiodol (arrowheads) retention after transarterial embolization of the tumor and a transjugular intrahepatic portosystemic shunt (star). Tracer signal can be seen in the treated lesion (arrows), while no specific accumulation of the tracer can be seen in necrotic, lipiodol-retaining regions around it. H, heart; L, liver; LB, large bowel; RL, right lung; Sp, spleen. (Reproduced with permission from the American Gastroenterological Association from Penvelas I, et al. (35).)

signal.[44] This deletion leads to increased cytoplasmic localization of the HSV1-tTK enzyme, resulting in better image signal activity due to higher interaction rates between HSV1-tTK and the FHBG reporter probe.[45] The 135-base-pair-deletion mutant also lacks the cryptic testis-specific transcriptional start point and thus overcomes the problem of male sterility in transgenic mice carrying the HSV1-tk gene.[46] Finally, a "humanized" version of HSV1-tk with more robust enzyme activity and attenuated immunogenicity is being evaluated for suicide- and reporter-gene purposes. In general, the main advantage of enzyme-based reporter genes is that the imaging sensitivity can be greatly enhanced by the enzymatic amplification of the reporter probe signal.

Several receptor-based PET reporter genes have also been described, two of which are discussed here. The first is the dopamine 2 receptor (D2R), a 415-amino-acid protein with a 7-transmembrane-spanning domain found in substantial levels primarily in the striatum.[47] The D2R gene has been used as a PET reporter gene, both in an adenoviral delivery vector and in stably transfected tumor cell xenografts.[48] The location, magnitude, and duration of D2R reporter-gene expression can be monitored by PET detection of D2R-dependent sequestration of injected 3-(2'-^{18}F-fluoroethyl)-spiperone (^{18}F-FESP) probe, a high-affinity D2R ligand. The second is the somatostatin type 2 receptor (SSTr2), which is expressed primarily in the pituitary gland. When it is used as a reporter gene, the location of SSTr2 expression can be monitored by systemic injection of a technetium-99m-labeled SSTr2 peptide probe (^{99m}Tc-P829) and subsequent imaging with a conventional gamma camera.[49] Another promising approach involves the human sodium/iodide symporter (hNIS) gene, which is expressed in the thyroid gland. The accumulation of radioactive iodine isotopes (^{123}I and ^{131}I) has been used in nuclear medicine for the diagnosis and targeted therapy of thyroid pathology.[50] Overall, the main advantage of receptor-based reporter genes is that they are cloned from endogenous genes: D2R from striatum, SSTr2 from pituitary, and hNIS from the thyroid gland. These endogenous genes will minimize host immune response and increase the chances of prolonged gene expression.

Recent Cardiac Gene and Cell Therapy Studies

Evaluating Gene Therapy

Gene transfer has been heralded as the most promising therapy of molecular medicine in the 21st century. It is usually defined as the transfer and expression of DNA to somatic cells of an individual with a resulting therapeutic effect.[51] In cardiovascular diseases, gene therapy offers an exciting new approach to express therapeutic factors locally in the myocardium. In general, the successful application of gene therapy requires 3 essential elements: (1) a vector for gene delivery, (2) targeted delivery of the vector to the target tissue, and (3) a therapeutic gene to be expressed in a particular patient population.

Historically, the field of cardiac angiogenesis attracted much attention from the cardiovascular community in the late 1990s, as most animal studies and phase 1 non-randomized trials uniformly showed positive results. However, recent phase 2 randomized trials such as the VIVA (Vascular Endothelial Growth Factor in Ischemia for Vascular Angiogenesis),[52] FIRST (FGF Initiating Revascularization Trial),[53] AGENT (Adenovirus Fibroblast Growth Factor Angiogenic Gene Therapy),[54] and KAT (Kuopio Angiogenesis Trial)[55] have demonstrated neither consistent nor substantial efficacy. In retrospect, several lessons can be learned from these trials. They showed that angiogenesis is a complex process regulated by the interaction of various growth factors and likely cannot be effectively induced or augmented by the transient injection of a single protein or gene.[56] Strikingly, for the aforementioned studies, there was no available method of assessing gene expression in vivo, and hence, the investigators were blinded as to whether the lack of symptomatic improvement was a result of transient gene expression, poor delivery technique, or host inflammatory response.

In the first proof-of-principle study using in vivo cardiac PET imaging, adenovirus carrying mutant thymidine kinase reporter gene (Ad-CMV-HSV1-sr39tk; 1×10^9 pfu) was injected intramyocardially.[57] The reporter probe ^{18}F-FHBG was injected intravenously before PET imaging. Cardiac reporter gene expression was robust but transient (~2 weeks total duration), presumably due to host cellular immune responses against the adenoviral vector.[58] The kinetics of cardiac transgene expression varied significantly among different animals, suggesting that the efficiency of gene transfer differed due to interindividual response. Leakage into the systemic circulation allowed the adenovirus to bind to coxsackie-adenovirus receptors (CAR) on hepatocytes, leading to expression at an unintended target site.[59] With PET imaging, the transgene expression could be localized tomographically at the anterolateral wall along the short, vertical, and horizontal axes, as shown in Figure 25.4.

In a follow-up study, Inubushi et al examined the quantitative aspects of the HSV1-sr39tk and ^{18}F-FHBG system.[60] Myocardial ^{18}F-FHBG accumulation was visualized with viral titers down to 1×10^7 particle-forming units (pfu) but not with $<1 \times 10^6$ pfu

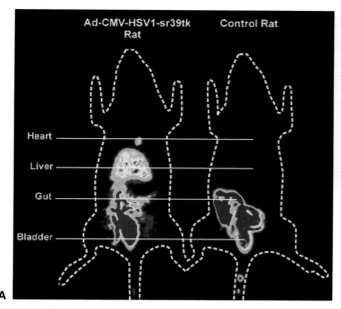
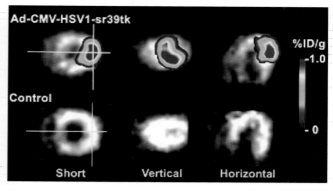

Figure 25.4. Small animal PET imaging of cardiac reporter gene expression. (A) At day 4, whole-body small animal PET image of a rat shows focal cardiac ^{18}F-FHBG activity at the site of intramyocardial Ad-CMV-HSV1-sr39tk injection. Liver ^{18}F-FHBG activity is also seen due to systemic adenoviral leakage with transduction of hepatocytes. Control rat injected with Ad-CMV-Fluc shows no ^{18}F-FHBG activity in both cardiac and hepatic regions. Significant gut and bladder activities are seen for both study and control rats due to route of ^{18}F-FHBG clearance. (B) Tomographic views of cardiac small animal PET images. The ^{13}N-NH₃ (grayscale) images of perfusion are superimposed on ^{18}F-FHBG images (color), demonstrating HSV1-sr39tk reporter-gene expression. ^{18}F-FHBG activity is seen in the anterolateral wall for the study rat compared to background signal in the control rat. Perpendicular lines represent the axis for vertical and horizontal cuts. Color scale is expressed as %ID/g. (Reproduced with permission from Reference 57.)

of HSV1-sr39tk. For comparison, most clinical trials use an adenoviral dosage of 1×10^{10} to 1×10^{12} pfu.[51] There was a good correlation between the percentage injected dose (%ID) for myocardial ^{18}F-FHBG accumulation calculated from PET images and ex vivo HSV1-sr39TK enzyme activity ($r^2 = 0.79$, $p < 0.0001$). This suggests that noninvasive imaging can be used in parallel or in lieu of traditional postmortem biochemical assays. More recently, gamma camera imaging of cardiac transgene expression using adenoviral-mediated expression of human sodium iodide symporter (Ad-CMV-hNIS) and ^{123}I or ^{99m}Tc as reporter probes was shown to be a practical and effective alternative to HSV1-tk and HSV1-sr39tk imaging.[61]

In most of the studies discussed above, however, transient cardiac gene expression and unintended target-site expression within the liver were noticed. These observations suggest that ischemic heart patients who underwent intracoronary infusion of adenovirus carrying either fibroblast growth factor (FGF)[54] or vascular endothelial growth factor (VEGF)[55] in clinical trials likely encountered these two issues.

The feasibility of transferring imaging results from a small animal PET scanner to a clinical PET scanner (ECAT EXACT scanner, Siemens/CTI) has been demonstrated in a porcine model. Bengel et al showed that myocardial tissues infected with adenovirus expressing HSV1-tk had significantly higher [124]I-FIAU retention during the first 30 minutes following injection.[62] The FIAU uptake correlated with ex vivo images, autoradiography, and immunohistochemistry for reporter gene product after euthanasia. However, the signal-to-background ratio at the site of HSV1-tk injection was only ~1.25 during the first 30 minutes following delivery. Afterward, there was significant washout at 45 to 120 minutes postinjection, and the [124]I-FIAU retention became similar to control myocardial regions. Thus, the combination of HSV1-tk/

FIAU may be less ideal than HSV1-sr39tk/FHBG for imaging cardiac transgene expression,[63] consistent with data from the oncology literature.[42]

The described cardiac studies nicely demonstrate the concepts and feasibility of utilizing reporter gene–based PET imaging. However, to effectively monitor and guide gene therapy, the PET reporter gene must be linked to a therapeutic gene of interest such as VEGF or FGF. To first demonstrate that the expression of two linked genes can have high fidelity, Chen et al constructed a bicistronic adenoviral vector whereby a CMV-driven receptor-based PET receptor gene (a mutant D2R, or D2R80a) was coupled to an enzyme-based PET reporter gene (HSV1-sr39tk) using an internal ribosomal entry site (IRES).[64] After injecting Ad-CMV-D2R80a-IRES-HSV1-sr39tk into the rat myocardium, longitudinal imaging with PET reporter probes ^{18}F-FESP and ^{18}F-FHBG, respectively, revealed a good correlation between the two linked PET reporter genes ($r^2 = 0.73; p < 0.001$). These results suggest that, if one of the PET reporter genes is replaced with a therapeutic gene, a correlated expression would likely exist and allow for indirect monitoring of the therapeutic gene. Besides the IRES system, other techniques of linking a therapeutic gene to a reporter gene also are available, including the use of two separate delivery vectors,[65] fusion of reporter genes,[45] bidirectional transcription,[66] and a dual-promoter approach, as described in the next paragraph.

The first proof-of-principle study using PET imaging to track therapeutic gene expression was conducted by Wu et al, in which adenovirus with a CMV promoter driving a VEGF$_{121}$ therapeutic gene and a second CMV promoter driving HSV1-sr39tk reporter gene was constructed.[67] The two expression cassettes are separated by poly adenine sequences (Ad-CMV-VEGF$_{121}$-polyA-CMV-HSV1-sr39tk-polyA). The adenovirus was injected into the myocardium of adult rats that had undergone left anterior descending artery ligation to create an MI model. Control animals received adenovirus without an expression cassette (Ad-null) instead. Reporter gene expression was limited to approximately 2 weeks due to the host *cellular* immune response (Figure 25.5). Repeat adenoviral injections into the same ischemic territory at 2 months did not induce any reporter-gene expression due to the host *humoral* immune response.[58] Evaluating vascular patterns at 10 weeks using immunohistochemical staining for CD31 and smooth muscle actin revealed significantly higher mean capillary (747 ± 104 vs 450 ± 101 per mm^2) and small blood vessel (8.1 ± 0.8 vs 5.1 ± 1.2 per mm^2) densities in the VEGF-treated group versus control ($p < 0.05$ for both). Functional assessment was also carried out: left ventricular ejection fraction showed mild improvement in the VEGF-treated study group (43.4 ± 8.1% at baseline to 47.3 ± 12.5% at week 10) compared with the control group (47.5 ± 9.3% to 45.2 ± 8.4%), but this did not reach statistical significance. The VEGF-treated study animals also showed an encouraging trend toward lower ^{13}N-NH$_3$ perfusion defects (15.2 ± 3.1% to 13.8 ± 2.6%) and ^{18}F-FDG metabolism deficits (12.7 ± 4.3% to 11.5 ± 4.6%), but these changes were also not statistically significant. As expected, the control group did not show any significant changes in perfusion (14.0 ± 4.0% to 15.3 ± 4.1%) or metabolism (13.4 ± 2.3% to 15.1 ± 3.0%) scores (p = NS).

Taken together, these results suggest that the microscopic level of neovasculature induced by VEGF did not translate into significant changes in clinically relevant physiological parameters such as myocardial contractility, perfusion, and metabolism under the study conditions tested. Nonetheless, important lessons can be learned from these animal studies as well as clinical trials.

For cardiac gene therapy to be successful, biological issues related to pharmacokinetics and functional and physiological effects of gene expression will need to be fully understood before expecting clinical efficacy.[68] Future effective application of gene therapy will be contingent on (1) a better understanding of the mechanics of gene delivery and incorporation of target genes into the host and (2) monitoring of therapeutic gene expression directly or via reporter-gene constructs integrated into the delivery vector. To this end, molecular imaging, and more specifically PET imaging, holds great promise as an effective clinical tool for following genetic therapy.

Cardiac Cell Therapy

In recent years, stem cell therapy has rivaled gene therapy as a promising treatment modality for ischemic heart disease. Several phase 1 clinical studies have shown that the implantation of skeletal myoblasts (SKM),[69] endothelial progenitor cells (EPC),[70] or bone marrow stem cells (BMSC)[71] into the infarcted myocardium can improve function. The mechanisms by which stem cells achieve this effect are not completely known. Possible mechanisms include stem cells secreting paracrine factors, providing a mechanical scaffold, and recruiting other peripheral and resident cardiac stem cells.[72] However, the analysis of stem cell therapy, like that of gene therapy, relies primarily on postmortem histology to identify their presence. The ability to study stem cell survival and proliferation in the context of the intact living body rather than postmortem histology would yield better insight into stem cell biology and physiology.

In the first proof-of-principle study using reporter genes to track cardiac cell survival, Wu et al transduced embryonic rat H9c2 cardiomyoblasts with adenovirus carrying either firefly luciferase or HSV1-sr39tk reporter gene before injecting into the rat myocardium (Figure 25.6).[73] Cell survival was monitored noninvasively by optical bioluminescence or small animal PET imaging. Cell signal activity was quantified in units of photons per second per square cm per steradian (photons/s/cm^2/sr) or percentage injected dose of ^{18}F-FHBG per gram tissue (%ID/g), respectively. In both cases, drastic reductions in signal activity were seen within the first 1 to 4 days due to acute donor cell death from inflammation, ischemia, and apoptosis. Interestingly, this pattern of cell death was consistent with other reports using traditional ex vivo assays such as TUNEL apoptosis,[74] classical histology,[75] and TaqMan RT-PCR.[6] All these ex vivo techniques required large numbers of animals to be sacrificed at different time points.

Given that several types of reporter genes and reporter probes are now available, it should be possible in the future to perform multimodality imaging of stem cell transplantation. For example, preliminary studies have demonstrated the feasibility of imaging murine embryonic stem cells transplanted into the rat myocardium.[76] These cells were genetically manipulated to express a triple fusion reporter that consists of red fluorescence protein for FACS analysis and single-cell fluorescence microscopy, firefly luciferase for high-throughput bioluminescence imaging, and thymidine kinase for small animal PET imaging (Figure 25.7). Similar studies are also under way evaluating BMSC implantation into the murine heart, where the implanted cells are harvested from transgenic mice that constitutively express both GFP and firefly luciferase (unpublished data). These multireporter-gene approaches allow for multimodal evaluation of stem cell survival kinetics and differentiation in the host myocardium. Finally, reporter-gene imaging may be helpful for evaluating other issues relevant to stem cell biology, such as imaging stem cell survival, proliferation, and differentiation.

The first steps toward using molecular imaging technology to track cardiac cell therapy in humans have already been taken. In a recent study by Hofmann et al, PET imaging was used to track ^{18}F-FDG-labeled autologous bone marrow used to treat acute MI in 9 patients.[36] Unselected bone marrow cells were radiolabeled with 100 MBq ^{18}F-FDG and infused into the infarct-related coronary artery (3 patients), or injected into the antecubital vein (3 patients). In an additional group of 3 patients, a CD34$^+$-enriched population of bone marrow cells was delivered by intracoronary infusion. In

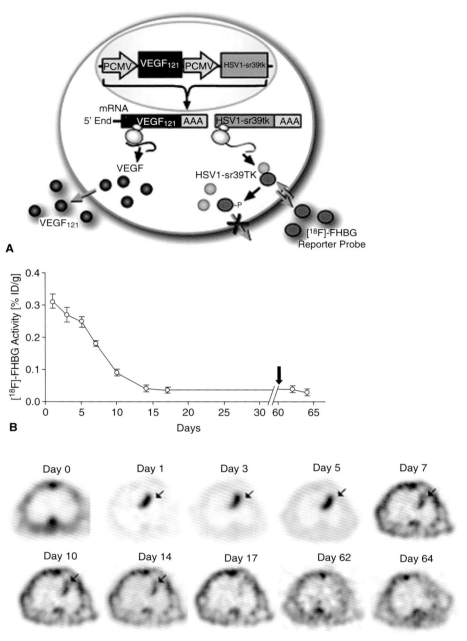

A

B

C

Day 0   Day 1   Day 3   Day 5   Day 7

Day 10   Day 14   Day 17   Day 62   Day 64

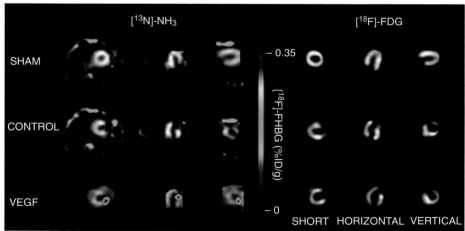

D

FIGURE 25.5. Small animal PET imaging of cardiac angiogenic gene therapy. (A) Schematic of Ad-CMV-VEGF$_{121}$-CMV-HSV1-sr39tk-mediated gene expression. Two separate gene cassettes with CMV promoters driving the expression of a VEGF$_{121}$ therapeutic gene and an HSV1-sr39tk reporter gene separated by polyA tails. The translated product of VEGF$_{121}$ is soluble and excreted extracellularly, whereas the translated product of HSV1-sr39tk (HSV1-sr39TK) traps ^{18}F-FHBG intracellularly by phosphorylation. (B) Noninvasive imaging of the kinetics of cardiac transgene expression. Gene expression peaked at day 1 and rapidly decreased thereafter. A second injection (arrow) of Ad-CMV-VEGF$_{121}$-CMV-HSV-sr39tk at day 60 yielded no detectable signal on day 62 and day 64. Error bars represent mean ± standard error of the mean. (C) A representative rat scanned longitudinally with transaxial ^{18}F-FHBG PET images shown at similar slice levels of the chest cavity. The grayscale is normalized to the individual peak activity of each image. In this rat, myocardial ^{18}F-FHBG accumulation was visualized at the anterolateral wall (arrow) from day 1 to day 14 but not day 17, 62, or 64. (D) In vivo gene, perfusion, and metabolism imaging with PET. At day 2, representative images showing normal perfusion (^{13}N-NH$_3$) and metabolism (^{18}F-FDG) in a sham rat, anterolateral infarction in a control rat (Ad-null), and anterolateral infarction in a VEGF-treated study rat (Ad-CMV-VEGF$_{121}$-CMV-HSV1-sr39tk) in short, vertical, and horizontal axis (grayscale). The color scale is expressed as % ID/g for ^{18}F-FHBG uptake. As expected, both the sham and control animals had background ^{18}F-FHBG signal only (blue) that outlined the shape of the chest cavity. In contrast, the study rat showed robust HSV1-sr39tk reporter-gene activity near the site of injection. (A–D, Reproduced with permission from Reference 67.)

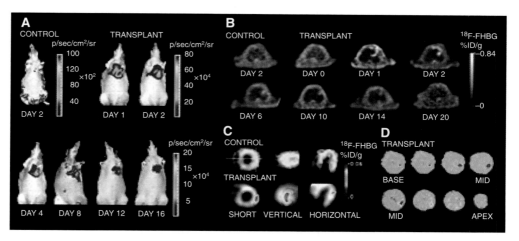

FIGURE 25.6. Optical bioluminescence and small animal PET imaging of cardiac cell transplantation in living animals. (A) Study rat transplanted with embryonic H9c2 cardiomyoblasts (3×10^6) emits significant cardiac bioluminescence activity at days 1, 2, 4, 8, 12, and 16 ($p < 0.05$ vs control). Control rat shows background signal only. (B) The location, magnitude, and duration of cell survival are determined by longitudinal imaging of ^{18}F-FHBG activity (grayscale) within the same rat. (C) Tomographic views of cardiac PET images shown in short, vertical, and horizontal axes. At day 2, study rat transplanted with embryonic cardiomyoblasts expressing HSV1-sr39tk shows significant ^{18}F-FHBG uptake (color) superimposed on ^{13}N-NH$_3$ images (grayscale). Control rat shows homogeneous ^{13}N-NH$_3$ perfusion but background ^{18}F-FHBG uptake. (D) Autoradiography of the same study rat at day 2 confirms trapping of ^{18}F by transplanted cells at the lateral wall at finer spatial resolution (~50 μm). (Reproduced with permission from Reference 73.)

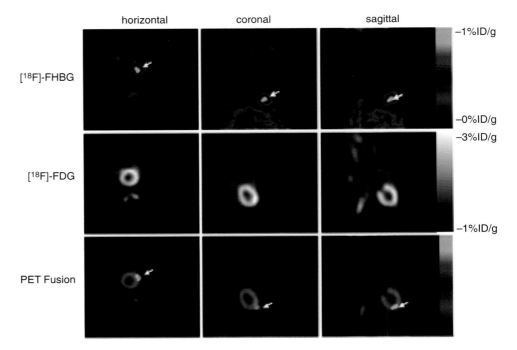

FIGURE 25.7. Preclinical validation of tracking transplanted embryonic stem (ES) cells using a small animal PET scanner. After cell transplant, animals underwent ^{18}F-FHBG reporter-probe imaging (top row) for detection of cell survival and ^{18}F-FDG imaging (middle row) for assessment of myocardial metabolic activity. Note that background bone uptake of free fluoride is seen in both images. Fusion of the two images (bottom row) shows the exact location of transplanted embryonic stem cells carrying the triple fusion reporter gene (arrow) at the anterolateral wall. The small animal PET imaging provides horizontal, coronal, and sagittal views. Similar studies should be feasible using human clinical PET scanners in the future. (Reprinted from Cao F, et al. In vivo visualization of embryonic stem cell survival, proliferation, and migration after cardiac delivery. Circulation 2006;113:1005–1014, with permission.)

all groups, cells were administered 5 to 10 days following coronary stenting, and PET imaging was carried out 50 to 75 minutes after the procedure. PET successfully detected ^{18}F signals in all groups, with higher intramyocardial signal in the intracoronary versus intravenous delivery groups. Of the two groups receiving intracoronary infusion, the CD34$^+$-enriched population had a higher myocardial signal than unselected BMSC (1.3% to 2.6% vs 14% to 39%, $p < 0.005$), suggesting enhanced homing to the injured myocardial milieu associated with CD34$^+$ stem cells (Figure 25.8).

Although conducted in a small number of patients, this study nicely demonstrates a potential means to track stem cell therapy on a short-term basis. The fact that a differing myocardial signal between groups was observed is encouraging, as it helps validate the sensitivity of clinical PET scanning for tracking cellular delivery and homing. The major limitation of this technique is its inability to track long-term survival kinetics and cellular trafficking following therapy, as the half-life of ^{18}F-FDG is only ~110 minutes. Furthermore, the PET signals do not provide information regarding cell proliferation because the radiotracers cannot be "passed" on from mother to daughter cells. It would be most useful, for example, to observe changes in myocardial stem cell populations over weeks and correlate their late-phase survival or proliferation with functional improvement. In the future, genetically engineered constructs (e.g., VEGF therapeutic gene linked to the TK reporter gene) integrated into the transplanted stem cells may allow for such measurements using a variety of the molecular imaging techniques discussed.

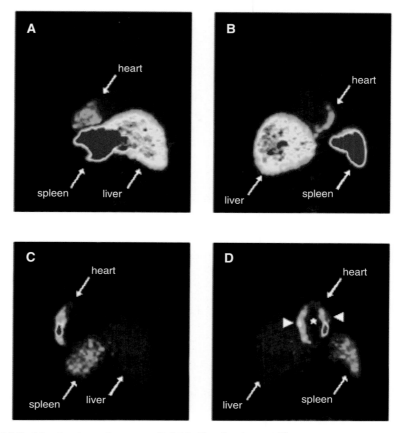

FIGURE 25.8. Monitoring of myocardial biodistribution of ^{18}F-FDG-labeled bone marrow cells in humans. Left posterior oblique (A) and left anterior oblique (B) views of the chest and upper abdomen of a patient, 65 minutes after transfer of ^{18}F-FDG-labeled, unselected bone marrow cells into the left circumflex coronary artery. Bone marrow cell homing is detectable in the lateral wall of the heart (infarct center and border zone), liver, and spleen. Left posterior oblique (C) and left anterior oblique (D) views of the chest and upper abdomen of another patient, 70 minutes after transfer of ^{18}F-FDG-labeled, CD34$^+$-enriched bone marrow cells into the left anterior descending coronary artery. Homing of CD34$^+$-enriched cells is detectable in the anteroseptal wall of the heart, liver, and spleen. CD34$^+$ cell homing is most prominent in the infarct border zone (arrowheads), but not in the infarct center (asterisk). (Reproduced with permission from Reference 36.)

Summary Points

- PET imaging has emerged as a valuable tool for monitoring gene delivery and, more recently, evaluating cellular therapy.
- Although the field is in its infancy, PET-based molecular imaging in humans is likely to grow rapidly as "molecular medicine" tailored to individual patients becomes a clinical reality in the future.
- Successful therapies will be predicated on a sound understanding of the pharmacokinetics and functional and biological aspects of gene therapy and cellular delivery.
- Cardiac molecular imaging is an important tool that can help achieve these goals.

References

1. Herschman HR. Molecular imaging: looking at problems, seeing solutions. *Science.* 2003;302:605–608.
2. Blasberg RG, Tjuvajev JG. Molecular-genetic imaging: current and future perspectives. *J Clin Invest.* 2003;111:1620–1629.
3. Schröder G, Risch K, Nizze H, et al. Immune response after adenoviral gene transfer in syngeneic heart transplants: effects of anti-CD4 monoclonal antibody therapy. *Transplantation.* 2000;70:191–198.
4. Hajjar RJ, Schmidt U, Matsui T, et al. Modulation of ventricular function through gene transfer in vivo. *Proc Natl Acad Sci U S A.* 1998;95:5251–5256.
5. Kass-Eisler A, Falck-Pedersen E, Alvira M, et al. Quantitative determination of adenovirus-mediated gene delivery to rat cardiac myocytes in vitro and in vivo. *Proc Natl Acad Sci U S A.* 1993;90:11498–11502.
6. Muller-Ehmsen J, Whittaker P, Kloner RA, et al. Survival and development of neonatal rat cardiomyocytes transplanted into adult myocardium. *J Mol Cell Cardiol.* 2002;34:107–116.
7. Herzog EL, Chai L, Krause DS. Plasticity of marrow-derived stem cells. *Blood.* 2003;102:3483–3493.
8. Shim WS, Jiang S, Wong P, et al. Ex vivo differentiation of human adult bone marrow stem cells into cardiomyocyte-like cells. *Biochem Biophys Res Commun.* 2004;324:481–488.
9. Massoud TF, Gambhir SS. Molecular imaging in living subjects: seeing fundamental biological processes in a new light. *Genes Dev.* 2003;17:545–580.
10. Verel I, Visser GW, van Dongen GA. The promise of immuno-PET in radioimmunotherapy. *J Nucl Med.* 2005;46(suppl 1):164S–171S.
11. Meoli DF, Sadeghi MM, Krassilnikova S, et al. Noninvasive imaging of myocardial angiogenesis following experimental myocardial infarction. *J Clin Invest.* 2004;113:1684–1691.
12. Schelbert HR. 18F-deoxyglucose and the assessment of myocardial viability. *Semin Nucl Med.* 2002;32:60–69.
13. Shi N, Boado RJ, Pardridge WM. Antisense imaging of gene expression in the brain in vivo. *Proc Natl Acad Sci U S A.* 2000;97:14709–14714.
14. Tavitian B, Terrazzino S, Kuhnast B, et al. In vivo imaging of oligonucleotides with positron emission tomography. *Nat Med.* 1998;4:467–471.
15. Gambhir SS, Barrio JR, Herschman HR, Phelps ME. Imaging gene expression: principles and assays. *J Nucl Cardiol.* 1999;6:219–233.
16. Nakamura K, Fan C, Liu G, et al. Evidence of antisense tumor targeting in mice. *Bioconjug Chem.* 2004;15:1475–1480.
17. Hnatowich DJ, Nakamura K. Antisense targeting in cell culture with radiolabeled DNAs—a brief review of recent progress. *Ann Nucl Med.* 2004;18:363–368.
18. Wu JC, Tseng JR, Gambhir SS. Molecular imaging of cardiovascular gene products. *J Nucl Cardiol.* 2004;11:491–505.
19. Contag PR, Olomu IN, Stevenson DK, Contag CH. Bioluminescent indicators in living mammals. *Nat Med.* 1998;4:245–247.
20. Lippincott-Schwartz J, Patterson GH. Development and use of fluorescent protein markers in living cells. *Science.* 2003;300:87–91.
21. Ramjiawan B, Ariano RE, Mantsch HH, Maiti P, Jackson M. Immunofluorescence imaging as a tool for studying the pharmacokinetics of a human monoclonal single chain fragment antibody. *IEEE Trans Med Imaging.* 2002;21:1317–1323.
22. Wu JC, Sundaresan G, Iyer M, Gambhir SS. Noninvasive optical imaging of firefly luciferase reporter gene expression in skeletal muscles of living mice. *Mol Ther.* 2001;4:297–306.
23. Bogdanov A, Weissleder R. In vivo imaging of gene delivery and expression. *Trends Biotechnol.* 2002;20:S11–S18.
24. Weissleder R, Moore A, Mahmood U, et al. In vivo magnetic resonance imaging of transgene expression. *Nat Med.* 2000;6:351–355.
25. Kircher MF, Allport JR, Graves EE, et al. In vivo high resolution three-dimensional imaging of antigen-specific cytotoxic T-lymphocyte trafficking to tumors. *Cancer Res.* 2003;63:6838–6846.
26. Lewin M, Carlesso N, Tung CH, et al. Tat peptide-derivatized magnetic nanoparticles allow in vivo tracking and recovery of progenitor cells. *Nat Biotechnol.* 2000;18:410–414.

27. Jaffer FA, Tung CH, Wykrzykowska JJ, et al. Molecular imaging of factor XIIIa activity in thrombosis using a novel, near-infrared fluorescent contrast agent that covalently links to thrombi. *Circulation.* 2004;110:170–176.

28. Kang HW, Josephson L, Petrovsky A, Weissleder R, Bogdanov A Jr. Magnetic resonance imaging of inducible E-selectin expression in human endothelial cell culture. *Bioconjug Chem.* 2002;13:122–127.

29. Bulte JW, Kraitchman DL. Iron oxide MR contrast agents for molecular and cellular imaging. *NMR Biomed.* 2004;17:484–499.

30. Dayton PA, Ferrara KW. Targeted imaging using ultrasound. *J Magn Reson Imaging.* 2002;16:362–377.

31. Schelbert HR, Inubushi M, Ross RS. PET imaging in small animals. *J Nucl Cardiol.* 2003;10:513–520.

32. Tai YC, Chatziioannou AF, Yang Y, et al. MicroPET II: design, development and initial performance of an improved microPET scanner for small-animal imaging. *Phys Med Biol.* 2003;48:1519–1537.

33. Phelps ME. Inaugural article: positron emission tomography provides molecular imaging of biological processes. *Proc Natl Acad Sci U S A.* 2000;97:9226–9233.

34. Jacobs A, Voges J, Reszka R, et al. Positron-emission tomography of vector-mediated gene expression in gene therapy for gliomas. *Lancet.* 2001;358:727–729.

35. Penuelas I, Mazzolini G, Boan JF, et al. Positron emission tomography imaging of adeno-viral-mediated transgene expression in liver cancer patients. *Gastroenterology.* 2005;128: 1787–1795.

36. Hofmann M, Wollert KC, Meyer GP, et al. Monitoring of bone marrow cell homing into the infarcted human myocardium. *Circulation.* 2005;111:2198–2202.

37. Yaghoubi S, Barrio JR, Dahlbom M, et al. Human pharmacokinetic and dosimetry studies of [(18)F]FHBG: a reporter probe for imaging herpes simplex virus type-1 thymidine kinase reporter gene expression. *J Nucl Med.* 2001;42:1225–1234.

38. Gambhir SS, Barrio JR, Wu L, et al. Imaging of adenoviral-directed herpes simplex virus type 1 thymidine kinase reporter gene expression in mice with radiolabeled ganciclovir. *J Nucl Med.* 1998;39:2003–2011.

39. Tjuvajev JG, Finn R, Watanabe K, et al. Noninvasive imaging of herpes virus thymidine kinase gene transfer and expression: a potential method for monitoring clinical gene therapy. *Cancer Res.* 1996;56:4087–4095.

40. Black ME, Newcomb TG, Wilson HM, Loeb LA. Creation of drug-specific herpes simplex virus type 1 thymidine kinase mutants for gene therapy. *Proc Natl Acad Sci U S A.* 1996;93:3525–3529.

41. Gambhir SS, Bauer E, Black ME, et al. A mutant herpes simplex virus type 1 thymidine kinase reporter gene shows improved sensitivity for imaging reporter gene expression with positron emission tomography. *Proc Natl Acad Sci U S A.* 2000;97:2785–2790.

42. Min JJ, Iyer M, Gambhir SS. Comparison of [18F]FHBG and [14C]FIAU for imaging of HSV1-tk reporter gene expression: adenoviral infection vs stable transfection. *Eur J Nucl Med Mol Imaging.* 2003;30:1547–1560.

43. Kang KW, Min JJ, Chen X, Gambhir SS. Comparison of [14C]FMAU, [3H]FEAu, [14C]FIAU, and [3H]PCV for monitoring reporter gene expression of wild type and mutant herpes simplex virus type 1 thymidine kinase in cell culture. *Mol Imag Biol.* 2005;7:296–303.

44. Degreve B, Johansson M, De Clercq E, Karlsson A, Balzarini J. Differential intracellular compartmentalization of herpetic thymidine kinases (TKs) in TK gene-transfected tumor cells: molecular characterization of the nuclear localization signal of herpes simplex virus type 1 TK. *J Virol.* 1998;72:9535–9543.

45. Ray P, De A, Min JJ, Tsien RY, Gambhir SS. Imaging tri-fusion multimodality reporter gene expression in living subjects. *Cancer Res.* 2004;64:1323–1330.

46. Cohen JL, Boyer O, Salomon B, et al. Fertile homozygous transgenic mice expressing a functional truncated herpes simplex thymidine kinase delta TK gene. *Transgenic Res.* 1998;7:321–330.

47. Missale C, Nash SR, Robinson SW, Jaber M, Caron MG. Dopamine receptors: from structure to function. *Physiol Rev.* 1998;78:189–225.

48. MacLaren DC, Gambhir SS, Satyamurthy N, et al. Repetitive, non-invasive imaging of the dopamine D2 receptor as a reporter gene in living animals. *Gene Ther.* 1999;6: 785–791.

49. Zinn KR, Buchsbaum DJ, Chaudhuri TR, Mountz JM, Grizzle WE, Rogers BE. Non-invasive monitoring of gene transfer using a reporter receptor imaged with a high-affinity peptide radiolabeled with 99mTc or 188Re. *J Nucl Med.* 2000;41:887–895.

50. Kaminsky SM, Levy O, Salvador C, Dai G, Carrasco N. The Na+/I− symporter of the thyroid gland. *Soc Gen Physiol Ser.* 1993;48:251–262.

51. Yla-Herttuala S, Alitalo K. Gene transfer as a tool to induce therapeutic vascular growth. *Nat Med.* 2003;9:694–701.

52. Henry TD, Annex BH, McKendall GR, et al. The VIVA trial: Vascular endothelial growth factor in Ischemia for Vascular Angiogenesis. *Circulation.* 2003;107:1359–1365.

53. Simons M, Annex BH, Laham RJ, et al. Pharmacological treatment of coronary artery disease with recombinant fibroblast growth factor-2: double-blind, randomized, controlled clinical trial. *Circulation.* 2002;105:788–793.

54. Grines CL, Watkins MW, Helmer G, et al. Angiogenic Gene Therapy (AGENT) trial in patients with stable angina pectoris. *Circulation.* 2002;105:1291–1297.

55. Hedman M, Hartikainen J, Syvanne M, et al. Safety and feasibility of catheter-based local intracoronary vascular endothelial growth factor gene transfer in the prevention of post-angioplasty and in-stent restenosis and in the treatment of chronic myocardial ischemia: phase II results of the Kuopio Angiogenesis Trial (KAT). *Circulation.* 2003;107:2677–2683.

56. Dor Y, Djonov V, Abramovitch R, et al. Conditional switching of VEGF provides new insights into adult neovascularization and pro-angiogenic therapy. *Embo J.* 2002;21:1939–1947.

57. Wu JC, Inubushi M, Sundaresan G, Schelbert HR, Gambhir SS. Positron emission tomography imaging of cardiac reporter gene expression in living rats. *Circulation.* 2002;106:180–183.

58. Yang Y, Li Q, Ertl HC, Wilson JM. Cellular and humoral immune responses to viral antigens create barriers to lung-directed gene therapy with recombinant adenoviruses. *J Virol.* 1995;69:2004–2015.

59. Guzman RJ, Lemarchand P, Crystal RG, Epstein SE, Finkel T. Efficient gene transfer into myocardium by direct injection of adenovirus vectors. *Circ Res.* 1993;73:1202–1207.

60. Inubushi M, Wu JC, Gambhir SS, et al. Positron-emission tomography reporter gene expression imaging in rat myocardium. *Circulation.* 2003;107:326–332.

61. Miyagawa M, Beyer M, Wagner B, et al. Cardiac reporter gene imaging using the human sodium/iodide symporter gene. *Cardiovasc Res.* 2005;65:195–202.

62. Bengel FM, Anton M, Richter T, et al. Noninvasive imaging of transgene expression by use of positron emission tomography in a pig model of myocardial gene transfer. *Circulation.* 2003;108:2127–2133.

63. Miyagawa M, Anton M, Haubner R, et al. PET of cardiac transgene expression: comparison of 2 approaches based on herpesviral thymidine kinase reporter gene. *J Nucl Med.* 2004;45:1917–1923.

64. Chen IY, Wu JC, Min JJ, et al. Micro-positron emission tomography imaging of cardiac gene expression in rats using bicistronic adenoviral vector-mediated gene delivery. *Circulation.* 2004;109:1415–1420.

65. Yaghoubi SS, Wu L, Liang Q, et al. Direct correlation between positron emission tomographic images of two reporter genes delivered by two distinct adenoviral vectors. *Gene Ther.* 2001;8:1072–1080.

66. Sun X, Annala AJ, Yaghoubi SS, et al. Quantitative imaging of gene induction in living animals. *Gene Ther.* 2001;8:1572–1579.

67. Wu JC, Chen IY, Wang Y, et al. Molecular imaging of the kinetics of vascular endothelial growth factor gene expression in ischemic myocardium. *Circulation.* 2004;110:685–691.

68. Pislaru S, Janssens SP, Gersh BJ, Simari RD. Defining gene transfer before expecting gene therapy: putting the horse before the cart. *Circulation.* 2002;106:631–636.

69. Menasche P, Hagege AA, Vilquin JT, et al. Autologous skeletal myoblast transplantation for severe postinfarction left ventricular dysfunction. *J Am Coll Cardiol.* 2003;41:1078–1083.

70. Assmus B, Schachinger V, Teupe C, et al. Transplantation of Progenitor Cells and Regeneration Enhancement in Acute Myocardial Infarction (TOPCARE-AMI). *Circulation.* 2002;106:3009–3017.

71. Wollert KC, Meyer GP, Lotz J, et al. Intracoronary autologous bone-marrow cell transfer after myocardial infarction: the BOOST randomised controlled clinical trial. *Lancet.* 2004;364:141–148.

72. Wollert KC, Drexler H. Clinical applications of stem cells for the heart. *Circ Res.* 2005;96:151–163.

73. Wu JC, Chen IY, Sundaresan G, et al. Molecular imaging of cardiac cell transplantation in living animals using optical bioluminescence and positron emission tomography. *Circulation.* 2003;108:1302–1305.

74. Zhang M, Methot D, Poppa V, Fujio Y, Walsh K, Murry CE. Cardiomyocyte grafting for cardiac repair: graft cell death and anti-death strategies. *J Mol Cell Cardiol.* 2001; 33:907–921.

75. Murry CE, Wiseman RW, Schwartz SM, Hauschka SD. Skeletal myoblast transplantation for repair of myocardial necrosis. *J Clin Invest.* 1996;98:2512–2523.

76. Cao F, Lin S, Xie X, et al. In vivo visualization of embryonic stem cell survival, proliferation, and migration after cardiac delivery. *Circulation.* 2006;113:1005–1014.

26 Imaging of Angiogenesis

Lawrence W. Dobrucki and Albert J. Sinusas

Since recognition of the key role of angiogenic factors in tumor growth more than 3 decades ago, physiological and pathological vascular development has been implicated in a number of pathological states including inflammation (e.g., coronary atherosclerotic plaque), diabetic retinopathy, peripheral vascular disease, and ischemic heart disease.[1]

Despite the recent advances in medical technology, therapy, and revascularization techniques for coronary artery disease, there is still a relatively large population of patients suffering from advanced coronary disease and myocardial ischemia that cannot be adequately managed by a combination of maximal antianginal medication, angioplasty, or coronary artery bypass surgery. Therefore, therapeutic stimulation of vascular growth in the management of myocardial ischemia seems to be a useful strategy in treating such patients. Indeed, a number of clinical trials from the past decade have examined the role of physiological regulators of blood vessel growth to promote vascular development to treat peripheral vascular disease and ischemic heart disease.[2]

The clinical studies of angiogenesis have demonstrated a mixed or inconsistent therapeutic benefit, and the assessment of therapeutic effect was focused predominantly on the physiologic consequences of the intervention. In spite of this, there is a tremendous need for development of noninvasive, targeted approaches for direct evaluation of the molecular events associated with angiogenesis. Furthermore, imaging of angiogenesis in a clinical setting allows individualized patient selection and monitoring of the therapeutic intervention.

New Vessel Formation

Vessel formation is governed by 3 distinct mechanisms. Early in development, blood vessels form from endothelial progenitor cells that differentiate and proliferate within a previously avascular tissue to build a primitive tubular network. This process, known as *vasculogenesis*, was initially described during embryonic development of the aorta and major veins as well as the capillary plexus connecting these major vessels.[3] This initial vessel network matures through both pruning and vessel enlargement; endothelial cells integrate tightly with smooth muscle cells or pericytes and extracellular matrix (ECM) in the process of *angiogenic remodeling*.[3] *Angiogenesis* or *angiogenic sprouting* is a different process, responsible for most new vessel formation in the adult, stimulated mainly by tissue hypoxia.[4] It involves the sprouting of new capillaries by cellular outgrowth from preexisting vessels into a previously avascular tissue.[5] In contrast, *arteriogenesis* is defined as the process of remodeling of newly formed or de novo growth of collateral conduits in response to local changes in shear stress.[1] Controversy remains whether arteriogenesis represents collateral development de novo (like angiogenesis) or whether it represents remodeling and enlargement of preexisting vascular channels. Studies of rodent hindlimb ischemia clearly defined arteriogenesis as remodeling of preexisting vessels.[6] It remains uncertain whether extensive preexisting collaterals are present in humans, although some functional studies in patients demonstrate the existence of collateral flow with the onset of temporary coronary occlusion.[5]

Hypoxia-induced angiogenesis is the best understood of the neovascularization processes in molecular terms. A number of ongoing clinical trials have been directed at stimulation of the angiogenic processes in conditions of ischemic heart and peripheral circulation diseases. However, the noninvasive evaluation of angiogenesis has been difficult.

Mechanism of Angiogenesis

The angiogenic process involves a cascade of events, illustrated in Figure 26.1. These include degradation of the basal membrane surrounding the parental vasculature, local proliferation and migration of vascular smooth muscle and endothelial cells, participation of blood-derived macrophages and circulating stem cells, and coalescence of endothelial cells to form tubular structures.[2,3]

An expanding number of local and circulating mediators and angiogenic factors are involved in this process, including vascular endothelial growth factor (VEGF), the most critical initiator of vascular formation by angiogenic sprouting. The angiogenic response is also modified by angiopoietin-1 (Ang-1), which is required for further remodeling and maturation of newly formed vessels, as well as by ephrin-B2, which is important in distinguishing arterial from venous vessels.[3] Moreover, the composition of ECM and intercellular adhesion molecules (e.g., integrins) also modulate angiogenesis.[7]

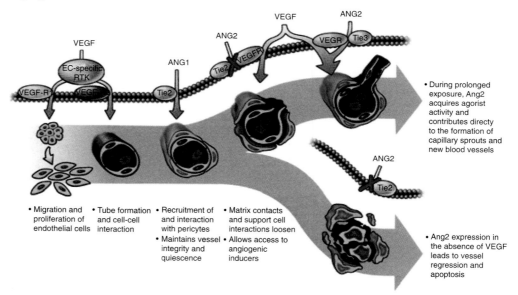

FIGURE 26.1. Regulation of angiogenesis. VEGF, vascular endothelial growth factor; VEGF-R1, VEGF receptor-1; VEGF-R2, VEGF receptor-2; EC-specific RTK, endothelial cell specific receptor tyrosine kinase; Ang-1, angiopoietin-1; Ang-2, angiopoietin-2; Tie2, angiopoietin receptor. (Reproduced from Fam NP, et al. Clinician guide to angiogenesis. Circulation. Nov 25 2003;108(21):2613–8, with permission.)

Hypoxia, defined as an imbalance between oxygen supply and demand in tissue, is one of the most potent stimulators of angiogenesis. In turn, angiogenesis provides increased perfusion and oxygenation through new vessel growth as a natural adaptation process to hypoxia. Early cellular responses to hypoxia are initiated by hypoxia-inducible factor 1α (HIF-1α).[5,8,9] HIF-1α as a transcriptional factor induces, among others, genes directly involved in angiogenesis, including the well-characterized VEGF, inducible nitric oxide synthase, lactate dehydrogenase, erythropoietin, and angiopoietins.[8]

The VEGF family consists of 5 closely related genes (VEGF-A, VEGF-B, VEGF-C, VEGF-D, and PlGF), which have overlapping abilities to interact with a set of cell-surface receptor tyrosine kinases (VEGFR-1 and VEGFR-2). VEGFR-2 seems to mediate the major growth and permeability actions of VEGF, as demonstrated in mice that lack VEGFR-2 and consequently have a complete absence of vasculature.[9,10] On the other hand, VEGFR-1 may have a negative role in suppressing signaling through VEGFR-2, as demonstrated in mice that lack VEGFR-1 and as a result have excess formation of endothelial cells that coalesce into abnormally disorganized tubules.[3]

In response to a hypoxic event, VEGF expression is induced, causing endothelial cell migration, proliferation, and development of leaky, immature, and unstable vessels (Figure 26.1). In contrast, Ang-1, which is a ligand for Tie2 receptor tyrosine kinase, stabilizes and protects the adult vasculature through recruitment of pericytes and the reestablishment of basement membrane. In transgenic animals, embryos lacking Ang-1 or Tie2 develop a normal vasculature that fails to undergo normal remodeling.[11] In mature vessels, Ang-1 inhibits endothelial cell activation, thus hindering the angiogenic response in the onset of hypoxia. Angiopoietin-2 (Ang-2) possesses a similar high affinity for Tie2 receptor, like Ang-1; however, it can either activate or antagonize Tie2.[3] Studies of transgenic mice lacking Ang-2 led to the hypothesis that Ang-2 is a key destabilizing factor involved in initiating angiogenic remodeling. Indeed, Ang-2 blocks Ang-1-Tie2 signaling, allowing endothelial cells to revert to a more plastic and destabilized state of developing vessels. These vessels then could be prone to two fates. Under certain conditions, in the absence of VEGF, Ang-2 expression may lead to vessel regression. On the other hand, destabilized vessels would be more sensitive to angiogenic changes induced by growth factors (e.g., VEGF), which would facilitate the formation of capillary sprouts.[1,3,9]

The studies presented above give a brief insight into the process of angiogenesis that involves a number of specific factors and events. More important, it is evident that a specific angiogenic program to regulate these factors both spatially and temporally is required for efficient neovascularization. Supporting the clinical potential of both VEGF and Ang-1, it is essential to know that VEGF administration can promote formation of only leaky and unstable vessels, whereas Ang-1 can protect adult vasculature from vascular leakage, thus facilitating the maturation and stabilization of newly formed vessels.[1,3]

Therapeutic Angiogenesis

Early therapeutic strategies directed toward random delivery of a single growth factor to stimulate the development of an entirely new functional network of vessels appear somewhat naive in spite of recent advances in the field.

Most clinical trials targeting angiogenesis focus on inhibiting the process (e.g., in cancer patients); however, more recently new applications have emerged in which angiogenesis is therapeutically promoted (e.g., ischemic cardiac disease). To stimulate angiogenesis in the heart, a number of angiogenic factors have been used in both animal studies and human clinical trials using different routes of administration, including direct injection of the agent or adenoviral gene transfer. In the onset of

TABLE 26.1. Summary of Selected Clinical Trials of Therapeutic Angiogenesis

Trial	N	Patients	Intervention	Follow-up	Outcome/Conclusions
FIRST (CAD)	337	Chronic angina Ineligible for revascularization	Intracoronary rFGF2	90 d to 6 m	Both exercise time and nuclear perfusion changes nonsignificant
VIVA (CAD)	178	Chronic angina Ineligible for revascularization	Intracoronary $VEGF_{165}$	60 and 90 d	Both nuclear perfusion and angiography nonsignificant Angina class improvement in high-dose VEGF group at day 120
AGENT (CAD)	79	Chronic angina Multivessel CAD	Intracoronary Ad5-FGF4	4 and 12 wk	Exercise treadmill testing results nonsignificant
REVASC (CAD)	71	Chronic angina Ineligible for revascularization	Intramuscular $Ad5-VEGF_{121}$	12 and 26 wk	Improvements in exercise treadmill time at 26 wk, exercise time to angina at 12 and 26 wk, total exercise time at 12 and 26 wk
KAT (CAD)	103	Chronic angina Suitable for revascularization	Intracoronary $VEGF_{165}$	6 m	Improved perfusion in adenovirus group
EUROINJE CT ONE (CAD)	80	Stable severe angina Ineligible for revascularization	Intramyocardial $phVEGF_{165}$	3 m	Nuclear perfusion nonsignificant Improvement in regional wall motion
TRAFFIC (PVD)	190	Chronic claudication	Intraarterial rFGF2	90 d	Improvement in exercise time at 90 d
RAVE (PVD)	105	Chronic claudication	Intramuscular $Ad5-VEGF_{121}$	12 and 26 wk	No improvement in exercise time or quality of life

peripheral vascular diseases, similar approaches have been used to stimulate angiogenic process in ischemic limbs. However, despite claims of success in early small trials, to date all double-blinded randomized clinical trials of stimulated angiogenesis have been somewhat disappointing, showing no clear benefit over placebo in patients with severe ischemic conditions.

Six large, randomized placebo-controlled clinical trials of therapeutic myocardial revascularization have been reported to date (Table 26.1). The efficacy of intracoronary administration of recombinant human $VEGF_{165}$ ($rhVEGF_{165}$) was tested in the VIVA trial (VEGF in Ischemia for Vascular Angiogenesis). Patients with severe, chronic angina pectoris unsuitable for angioplasty were randomized to receive placebo or low-dose or high-dose $rhVEGF_{165}$ by a single intracoronary infusion, followed by repeated intravenous infusions on days 3, 6, and 9. Only the high-dose treatment with $rhVEGF_{165}$ showed significant ($p < 0.05$) improvement in angina class at day 120, but it was not accompanied by improvement in myocardial perfusion.

Identical proangiogenic compound ($VEGF_{165}$) was used in two other large clinical trials for the treatment of myocardial ischemia: the Kuopio Angiogenesis Trial (KAT) and more recently the Euroinject One Trial.[12] KAT evaluated intracoronary administration of $VEGF_{165}$ after angioplasty by adenoviral gene transfer in the prevention of restenosis. Treated patients demonstrated no improvement in restenosis rate; however, myocardial perfusion improved significantly, which suggests a potential advantage of gene therapy in reaching a clear clinical benefit. In the Euroinject One Trial, patients with stable angina and no option for revascularization were injected with either plasmid gene transfer of $VEGF_{165}$ or placebo plasmid in the myocardial region that showed stress-induced myocardial perfusion defect as assessed by SPECT imaging with technetium-99 (^{99m}Tc)-labeled sestamibi or tetrofosmin. At the endpoint of this study (at 3 months), no differences among groups were found with respect to clinical and perfusion characteristics. Although myocardial perfusion did not improve, regional wall motion significantly improved after the VEGF gene transfer, suggesting an anti-ischemic effect.

Direct intramyocardial injection of replication-defective adenovirus containing the $VEGF_{121}$ gene via a minithoracotomy was used in the REVASC trial (Randomized Evaluation of VEGF for Angiogenesis in Severe Coronary disease). This study showed a sustained clinical improvement after gene therapy.

Other trials assessed the therapeutic efficacy of fibroblast growth factor-2 (FGF2). Single-bolus intracoronary injection was used in the double-blind, randomized, placebo-controlled FIRST study (FGF2 Initiating Revascularization Support Trial). This study demonstrated no significant differences between the groups assessed with nuclear perfusion and in terms of the quality of life. The approach to achieve sustained local levels of a fibroblast growth factor by the FGF4 gene transfer was used in the AGENT trial (Angiogenic GENe Therapy). Efficacy assessment suggested a tendency to have greater improvements in exercise time but with no statistical significance.

In recent years, new therapies have been introduced in patients with peripheral vascular disease (PVD) to stimulate peripheral angiogenesis, which involve administration of growth factors delivered directly or through a gene transfer. Two major randomized, double-blind, placebo-controlled trials have evaluated the use of both FGF2 and $Ad-VEGF_{121}$ in the therapy of patients with PVD. The TRAFFIC trial (Therapeutic Angiogenesis with Recombinant Fibroblast growth Factor-2 for Intermittent Claudication) demonstrated that a single infusion of FGF2 protein significantly increased walking time and improved ankle-brachial index at 90 days. The second trial, RAVE (Regional Angiogenesis with Vascular Endothelial growth factor), evaluated intramuscular delivery of adenoviral $VEGF_{121}$ but demonstrated no significant difference in standard clinical endpoints and clinical benefit.

Assuming that therapeutic angiogenesis is useful in the management of peripheral vascular disease or ischemic heart disease, then either the optimal dose and route of delivery of angiogenic growth factors have not been established or our tools to evaluate these therapies are inadequate. Current approaches use gene therapy to deliver a proangiogenic agent over a sustained period in the target tissue. In addition, because of the lack of a direct biologic marker of angiogenesis, the evaluation of therapeutic angiogenesis in clinical trials is focused on standard clinical endpoints, including the assessment of quality of life, exercise time, symptoms, and survival. Some studies have used nuclear imaging to evaluate only physiologic consequences of the therapy; therefore, there is a need to develop noninvasive imaging strategies for direct evaluation of molecular events associated with angiogenesis.

Imaging of Angiogenesis: Nontargeted Approaches

Imaging of Angiogenesis and the Assessment of Physiologic Consequences

The ability to monitor the effects of therapeutic angiogenesis has been a long-standing challenge. This can be achieved either by assessment of functional effects or by direct monitoring of blood vessel growth. The major consequence of angiogenic process is restoration of perfusion and tissue oxygenation, which in turn diminishes the effects of myocardial or peripheral ischemia. Therefore, the efficacy of therapeutic angiogenesis can be assessed by the evaluation of standard physiologic parameters such as regional myocardial perfusion, regional ventricular function, and metabolism. Alternatively, molecular imaging of angiogenesis and angiogenic markers as well as direct, angiographic visualization of new vasculature have received noticeable attention recently.[5]

Imaging of Perfusion

Effective therapeutic angiogenesis should restore myocardial perfusion (at stress and rest) as well as improve regional left ventricular function; therefore, in many clinical trials standard nuclear perfusion imaging was used. Assuming that the idea of improved perfusion due to angiogenic therapy is valid, remarkably little effect was observed with this imaging modality in treated patients despite symptomatic improvement. This raises concerns about the spatial resolution of single photon emission computed tomography (SPECT) imaging, stress protocols, choice of imaging modality, as well as perfusion tracer kinetics. Moreover, because angiogenesis may cause alterations in the microvascular structure, function, and permeability, imaging approaches that use diffusible tracers may be confounded.

Changes in perfusion are routinely assessed by either SPECT or positron emission tomography (PET) imaging. More recently, magnetic resonance imaging (MRI) has been applied as an alternative to SPECT and PET imaging. As described in Chapters 5 and 12, PET perfusion agents generally track flow better than SPECT agents do, particularly at high, stressor-induced flows. In addition, PET imaging provides better sensitivity and an established approach for attenuation correction that gives a greater potential for image quantification. However, PET imaging is an expensive technique, requiring on-site radionuclide generated by either a cyclotron or a generator, and the experience with PET in clinical coronary artery disease (CAD) trials in the United States is limited. MRI emerges as a novel technique providing great spatial resolution and high sensitivity to flow changes. Despite those advantages, validation studies are scarce, and experience with the use of MRI perfusion in large clinical trials is somewhat limited.

Imaging of Hypoxia

Hypoxia, defined as an imbalance between oxygen delivery and oxygen demand in a given tissue, is one of the most potent inducers of angiogenesis. In other words, angiogenesis per se is an adaptation to hypoxia, providing increased perfusion and oxygen through new vessel growth. Hypoxia imaging may offer a new approach for assessment of myocardial ischemia and therapeutic angiogenesis. ^{99m}Tc-labeled nitroimidazoles have been used as scintigraphic tracers for hypoxia imaging. The assessment of tissue oxygenation with nitroimidazoles may be a useful indicator of the balance of flow and oxygen consumption that would permit the evaluation of angiogenic therapies.

The proposed mechanism of hypoxic tissue retention of nitroimidazoles has been described elsewhere.[13,14] Briefly, nitroimidazoles diffuse through cell membrane and undergo reduction to form $R\text{-}NO_2^-$ radical anion. In the normooxic conditions, reduced nitroimidazole undergoes oxidation yielding superoxide and noncharged nitroimidazole, which may diffuse back into vascular space. In contrast, in the onset of hypoxia, $R\text{-}NO_2^-$ radical undergoes further reduction to nitroso-compounds that may bind to amines and remain trapped within the cell.

Several investigators have evaluated the potential of radiolabeled imidazoles for imaging of hypoxia with both SPECT and PET. Experimental studies have shown a potential of the positron-emitting ^{18}F-labeled misonidazole to detect hypoxic tissue. However, the wide use of this approach has been limited by both the availability of PET technology and the slow clearance of the radiotracer from blood and liver, which may complicate clinical imaging of the cardiovascular system. Initial studies have shown the uptake of misonidazole in hypoxic myocardium independent of a reduction in flow. Moreover, reoxygenation did not reverse this retention, suggesting irreversible binding.[15,16]

More recently, ^{99m}Tc-labeled nitroimidazoles have been introduced as an alternative approach for imaging of regional myocardial hypoxia using both in vitro and in vivo preparations.[14] Shi et al performed SPECT ^{99m}Tc-labeled nitroimidazole (BMS-181321) imaging in an open-chest canine model of partial coronary occlusion and pacing-induced demand ischemia.[17] BMS-181321 was preferentially retained in ischemic but viable myocardium; however, unfavorably high liver uptake might limit its use in clinical myocardial imaging. Other researchers also noted a significant hepatic uptake of BMS-181321.[18,19]

BMS-194796 (currently called BRU-59-21) is a more hydrophilic nitroimidazole derivative of BMS-181321 that has demonstrated superior properties for hypoxia imaging and improved heart-to-liver uptake ratios relative to BMS-181321.[18,19]

Preliminary studies with BRU-59-21 showed a twofold increase in radiotracer retention in low-flow ischemic regions after 2 minutes of total coronary occlusion in the open-chest dog. The significant liver uptake still, however, poses an important disadvantage for clinical imaging of myocardial hypoxia. Therefore, further chemical modifications of nitroimidazoles may be necessary to improve retention in hypoxic tissue and to optimize target-to-background activity ratios.

Imaging of Angiogenesis: Targeted Approaches

Molecular Targeted Imaging

The linking of noninvasive imaging of biological markers with a therapeutic intervention is attractive for approaches that rely on the selective delivery of bioactive molecules to the site of disease. The same binding molecule used for the delivery of agents can facilitate their detection using either radionuclides or fluorophores. Molecular imaging is defined as the in vivo characterization and measurement of biological processes at both the cellular and molecular levels. Targeted nuclear imaging originated from the concept of molecular imaging being defined in terms of a probe-target interaction, where the probe localization and signal magnitude are directly related to the interaction with the target epitope or peptide.

Availability of Biological Targets

Imaging cell-specific surface antigens with radiolabeled monoclonal antibodies represents some of the earliest molecular imaging applications still used in both experimental and clinical nuclear medicine research. Moreover, monoclonal antibodies are at present the only clinically proven class of high-affinity binding molecules, which can be generated against virtually any marker of disease. Slow elimination from the blood and predominant accumulation in the liver are main disadvantages of using antibodies for imaging applications, which typically prefer rapidly clearing antibody fragments. To overcome these limitations, new recombinant fragments that retain high affinity for target antigens and rapid blood clearance are being developed by genetic engineering. In the addition, the generation of monoclonal antibodies by hybridoma technology as well as identification of disease-associated antigens has stimulated preclinical and clinical studies of imaging of angiogenesis.[20]

Regulatory peptides represent another group of ligands for targeting angiogenesis. These ligands are small, readily diffusible molecules that express a broad range of receptor-mediated actions. Studies in animals with integrin-binding RGD-containing (Arg-Gly-Asp) peptides have demonstrated the feasibility of this approach to track angiogenesis.[2,21–24] However, quantitative biodistribution studies are critical in order for confirmation of these initial promising observations.

Aptamers, defined as single-stranded nucleic acids capable of adopting a complex three-dimensional structure, are an alternative class of molecules that can be generated against a variety of target antigens. This approach is based on the generation of large libraries of single-stranded nucleic acids, which can be panned for their binding to a target antigen. The potential of aptamers for tumor angiogenesis imaging has been investigated recently.[20]

Targeted imaging of biological markers is essential for understanding and tracking the temporal changes of the angiogenic process. However, it is critical to identify potential targets for imaging of angiogenesis. The recently identified targets generally fall into three principal categories: endothelial cell markers, nonendothelial cells involved in angiogenesis, and markers of the extracellular matrix. During the recent decade, most effort has been invested in the targeted imaging of endothelial cell markers of angiogenesis, which include VEGF receptors, integrins ($\alpha_v\beta_3$ and $\alpha_v\beta_5$), FGF receptors (Syndecan-4), and CD13.[2] More recently, agents (inhibitors of matrix metalloproteinases, MMPs) targeted at the process of postischemic myocardial remodeling are being developed, which have a potential to identify which patients are likely to develop heart failure as well as which are likely to respond to angiogenic therapy.[25,26]

Instrumentation

The advent of new molecular imaging strategies directed at the noninvasive evaluation of angiogenesis would be impossible without the revolution in imaging technology that has occurred during recent years. Table 26.2 illustrates the differences among the current most commonly used imaging modalities. Newer high-resolution computed tomography (CT), as well as ultrasound-based approaches, represents medical imaging techniques that provide primarily anatomical images. Due to the popularity and low cost of ultrasound instrumentation, efforts in recent years have been devoted toward development of ultrasound probes to study biochemical processes at a molecular level.[24,27–29] However, these probes are still in an early stage of development, tend to remain intravascular, and may have limited sensitivity. MRI also offers very high spatial resolution and unlimited depth penetration, which suggests that this might be a more ideal approach for molecular imaging. Unfortunately, MRI techniques suffer from a lack of widely available MRI-compatible molecular probes and relatively low sensitivity. To overcome the limited sensitivity of MRI, novel strategies have been employed. These include MRI signal amplification based on the cellular internalization of highly paramagnetic probes such as iron oxide or gadolinium nanoparticles. Indeed, there are a limited number of studies using paramagnetic nanoparticles to track biological processes, such as angiogenesis.[30,31]

Among the many imaging modalities available, nuclear imaging is particularly suited for targeted imaging because of its superior sensitivity, which requires only a trace amount of the probe (in the range of nanograms), and an overall clinical availability. Both PET and SPECT permit a relatively precise localization of radiotracer retention; however, both modalities suffer from a lack of anatomical information. Accordingly, nuclear imaging systems have been combined with a modality that provides high spatial resolution anatomic information. Indeed, the introduction of hybrid systems (PET/CT and SPECT/CT) has greatly enhanced the performance and accuracy of nuclear imaging. The CT component of these hybrid systems is used to relate tracer signal to anatomical landmarks and correct for nonuniform attenuation.

Molecular Probes and Applications

With the development of novel therapies for the treatment of ischemic heart disease directed at the stimulation of angiogenesis, noninvasive targeted imaging strategies offer far more than analysis of standard physiologic changes. The future for noninvasive imaging of angiogenesis and the remodeling process rests on the development of

TABLE 26.2. Advantages and Disadvantages of Different Imaging Modalities Used in Clinical Imaging

Modality	Spatial Resolution	Sensitivity (mol/L)	Advantages	Disadvantages
PET	1–2 mm	10^{-11}–10^{-12}	Emission directly proportional to concentration of radiolabeled probe Superior sensitivity for molecular imaging	Very short half-life tracers Limited availability Expensive instrument
SPECT	0.5–2 mm	10^{-10}–10^{-11}	Emission directly proportional to concentration of radiolabeled probe Superior sensitivity for molecular imaging	Exposure to ionizing radiation Accuracy limited by attenuation of low-energy photons
Ultrasound	0.05–0.5 mm	—	Inexpensive, widely available No ionizing radiation	Limited penetration depth Lack of molecular probes
CT	0.05–0.2 mm	—	Absorption directly proportional to concentration of contrast agent	Exposure to ionizing radiation Contrast agent toxicity
MRI	0.02–0.1 mm	10^{-3}–10^{-5}	No ionizing radiation Variety of available contrast agents Low toxicity of contrast agents	Low sensitivity Susceptible to motion Lack of molecular probes

targeted biological markers. As outlined below, the potential for targeted nuclear imaging of the VEGF receptors and $\alpha_v\beta_3$ integrin has been demonstrated in animal models of postinfarct angiogenesis (Table 26.3).

Imaging of VEGF Receptors

As described earlier, the VEGF receptor represents a specific marker of hypoxic stress within the tissue and therefore may provide a target for imaging of ischemia-mediated angiogenesis. VEGF was identified as a fundamental mediator of angiogenesis in the tumor environment; therefore, the initial efforts for targeted imaging of VEGF receptors come from cancer studies. Most of the studies used radiolabeled monoclonal antibody constructs or VEGF isoforms.

Collingridge et al developed a novel PET tracer based on human monoclonal antibody (VG76e) labeled with positron-emitting iodine-124 (^{124}I). Li et al developed a SPECT tracer constructed by labeling VEGF$_{165}$ isoform with ^{123}I. Both groups have demonstrated high specificity in binding and feasibility for in vivo imaging of angiogenesis in tumor.[32,33]

Other investigators verified the practicability of VEGF-targeted tracers for imaging ischemia-induced angiogenesis. Lu et al have demonstrated feasibility of molecular imaging of angiogenesis with indium-111 (^{111}In)-labeled VEGF$_{121}$ in a rabbit model of hindlimb ischemia.[35] The planar images showed a focal uptake in ischemic hindlimb that was confirmed by the immunohistochemistry of VEGFR-1 and VEGFR-2 receptors. Although no capillary-density measurements to confirm angiogenesis were performed, this study successfully utilized a naturally occurring ligand (VEGF isoform) as a radiolabeled probe. Advantages of this approach include specificity of $VEGF_{121}$ for hypoxia-inducible VEGF receptors and the lack of immunogenicity associated with the use of antibodies as targeting ligands. Despite favorable blood clearance, ^{111}In-$VEGF_{121}$ was strongly retained in the liver and kidneys, which limits its use in myocardial imaging. Moreover, this approach depends strongly on total $VEGF_{121}$ receptor density.

More recently, Blankenberg et al described a novel imaging construct comprised of a standard ^{99m}Tc-labeled protein noncovalently bound to a "docking tag" fused to a "targeting protein."[41] The assembly of this complex was based on interactions between "adapter protein" (human 109-amino acid, HuS), "docking tag" (15-amino-acid fragments of ribonuclease I, Hu-tag), and $VEGF_{121}$. Planar and SPECT images performed in mice implanted with mammary adenocarcinoma cells demonstrated significant uptake of ^{99m}Tc-HuS/Hu-$VEGF_{121}$ within subcutaneous tumor. This study suggested that it was possible to identify tumor neovasculature in lesions as small as several millimeters in soft tissue. Moreover, this approach can be adapted for in vivo delivery of other targeting proteins of interest without affecting their bioactivity.[41]

VEGF receptor imaging could complement routine clinical perfusion imaging by providing additional information relevant to hypoxic stress. Dual isotope imaging with ^{99m}Tc or ^{111}In-labeled VEGF-targeted probe and thallium-201 (^{201}Tl) chloride or ^{99m}Tc-sestamibi perfusion tracers could be useful for identifying sites of ongoing angiogenesis and regions at risk of ischemic injury.[2] Moreover, targeted approaches for VEGF imaging could improve the evaluation of therapeutic angiogenesis and the selection of sites for local delivery of proangiogenic agents. Despite successful applications of VEGF-targeted imaging approaches in cancer models, further studies in clinical models of myocardial ischemia will be required to validate this imaging concept in clinical practice.

TABLE 26.3. Selected Targeted Molecular Imaging Applications Using Endothelial Markers of Angiogenesis

Marker	Probe	Modality	Application	References
VEGF	^{124}I-VG76e	PET	Tumor angiogenesis	Collingridge et al[32]
$VEGF_{165}$	^{123}I-VEGF165	SPECT	Tumor angiogenesis	Li et al[33,34]
$VEGF_{121}$	^{111}In-VEGF121	SPECT	Peripheral limb angiogenesis	Lu et al[35]
$\alpha_v\beta_3$	Gd-LM609	MRI	Tumor angiogenesis	Sipkins et al[36]
$\alpha_v\beta_3$	^{111}In-RP748	SPECT	Tumor angiogenesis Myocardial angiogenesis	Harris et al[37] Meoli et al[38]
$\alpha_v\beta_3$	^{123}I-RGD	SPECT	Myocardial angiogenesis	Johnson et al[39]
$\alpha_v\beta_3$	^{125}I-c(RGD(I)yV)	SPECT	Peripheral limb angiogenesis	Lee et al[40]
$\alpha_v\beta_3$	^{99m}Tc-NC100692	SPECT	Peripheral limb angiogenesis	Hua et al[23]
$\alpha_v\beta_3$	Targeted microbubbles	ECHO	Tumor angiogenesis	Leong-Poi et al[24]

Imaging of $\alpha_v\beta_3$ Integrin

Endothelial cell adhesion and migration are two of the most important processes associated with the onset of angiogenesis. The $\alpha_v\beta_3$ integrin (vitronectin receptor) has a critical role in mediating cell-matrix adhesion and cell migration, and thus angiogenesis. This integrin mediates the adhesion of cells to a large number of ECM proteins by recognizing the conserved amino acid triplet RGD (Arg-Gly-Asp).[42] The $\alpha_v\beta_3$ integrin is minimally expressed on normal resting blood vessels and significantly upregulated in angiogenic vessels;[36] therefore, it represents a potential novel target for imaging angiogenesis, whereas RGD peptide could be considered as a molecular probe. Initial imaging studies involved monoclonal antibody against $\alpha_v\beta_3$ integrin (LM609) as a paramagnetic contrast agent in MR imaging;[3] however, these studies have been limited by slow blood clearance of the tracer.

Radiolabeled tracers based on cyclic RGD peptides with high affinity for the $\alpha_v\beta_3$ integrin have been synthesized and characterized by Haubner et al.[43] This preliminary work supported the potential for radiolabeled targeting of $\alpha_v\beta_3$ for imaging angiogenesis. Despite successful imaging of tumor angiogenesis and favorable clearance from the blood, these compounds are cleared predominantly through the hepatobiliary system, which may complicate angiogenesis imaging in the heart.

Lee et al were the first to report the potential of ^{123}I-labeled RGD peptide for targeted imaging of the peripheral angiogenesis in a murine model of hindlimb ischemia.[40] Shortly after this initial report, Hua and coworkers demonstrated the potential of a ^{99m}Tc-labeled peptide (NC100692, GE Healthcare, UK) for targeted imaging of the peripheral angiogenesis in murine model of hindlimb ischemia using high-resolution pinhole planar and microSPECT imaging.[23] The ^{99m}Tc-NC100692 was injected at multiple times after surgical right femoral artery occlusion, and both pinhole planar and microSPECT imaging were performed to evaluate temporal changes in angiogenic process within the ischemic limb. The nuclear imaging results were confirmed by both tissue gamma well counting and immunohistochemistry. There was a 2.5-fold increase in the radiotracer uptake in ischemic hindlimb compared to contralateral control leg as assessed by nuclear imaging (Figure 26.2). The dual-immunofluorescence staining of tissue samples with both endothelial cell marker (CD31) and fluorescent analog of NC100692 confirmed colocalization of radiotracer uptake within angiogenic endothelial cells. In addition, isolectin staining of tissue samples taken from control and ischemic hind limb confirmed ongoing angiogenesis by significant temporal increase in capillary density. These observed temporal changes in murine hindlimb angiogenesis were also confirmed by Leong-Poi et al by using contrast-enhanced ultrasound and microbubbles targeted at endothelial integrins.[24]

These preliminary experimental studies suggest that radiolabeled $\alpha_v\beta_3$-targeted RGD-based agents may be valuable noninvasive markers of angiogenesis after ischemic injury. Indeed, ^{99m}Tc-labeled NC100692 was used to evaluate myocardial angiogenesis in transgenic animals (with no gene for matrix metalloproteinase-9, MMP-9) subjected to surgical myocardial infarction.[44] Lindsey et al demonstrated that relative NC100692 activity in myocardial segments with diminished perfusion (0% to 40% nonischemic) was higher in MMP-9 knockout than in wild-type mice; therefore, the targeted strategies to inhibit MMP-9 early post-MI (to prevent from left ventricle remodeling) will likely not impair the angiogenic response (Figure 26.3).

To overcome limitations in the imaging of myocardial angiogenesis associated with a significant liver uptake, new tracers selective for $\alpha_v\beta_3$ integrin have been developed. Harris and coworkers recently reported the high affinity and selectivity of an ^{111}In-labeled quinolone (^{111}In-RP748, Bristol-Myers-Squibb, USA) for the $\alpha_v\beta_3$ integrin and feasibility for tumor angiogenesis imaging.[37] The same construct has been evaluated by Sadeghi et al for in vitro endothelial cell culture.[45] These investigators have demonstrated that RP748 and its homologues bind preferentially to the activated $\alpha_v\beta_3$ on endothelial cells in vitro and exhibit favorable binding characteristics for in vivo

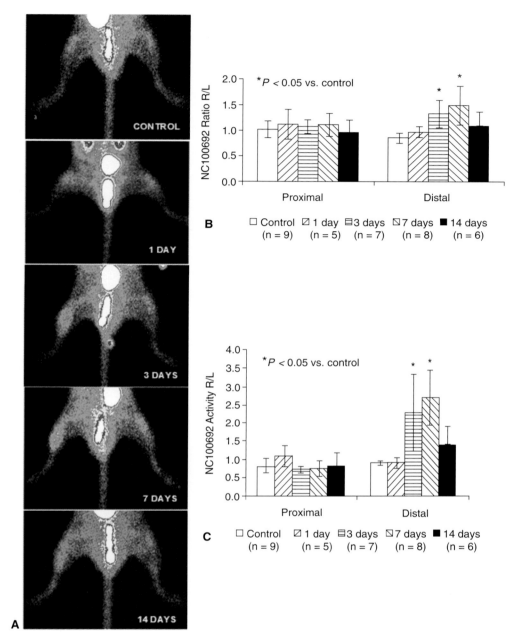

FIGURE 26.2. (A) In vivo planar pinhole images of control animals and at variable time points after femoral occlusion. Mice were injected with ^{99m}Tc-NC100692 intravenously. Hot spots were shown on days 3 and 7 and decreased on day 14. (B) Imaging analysis showed a significant ($p < 0.05$) increase in radiotracer ischemic-to-nonischemic retention ratio on days 3 and 7 versus the control group in the ischemic hind limb distal to the occlusion. This was confirmed by gamma well counting of ratio of radiotracer activity in ischemic to nonischemic contralateral hind limb (C). (Reprinted with permission from Reference 23.)

imaging. They found an approximately 15-fold increase in RP748 affinity for $\alpha_v\beta_3$ integrin on endothelial cells in the presence of Mn^{2+} activator, compared with nonactivated cells. Moreover, the same group demonstrated feasibility of RP748 imaging to track the proliferative process associated with carotid artery injury.[45] These findings may potentially lead to the development of noninvasive imaging strategies for vascular cell proliferation–associated states (i.e., postangioplasty restenosis).

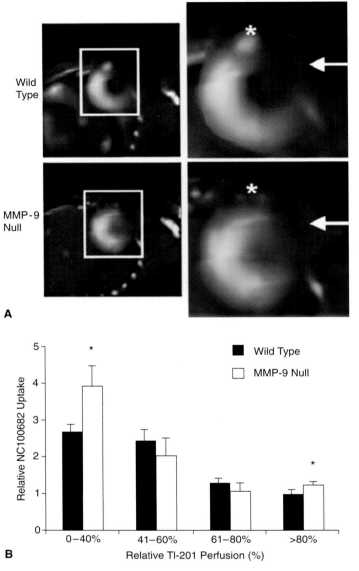

FIGURE 26.3. (A) Representative in vivo dual isotope ^{201}Tl and ^{99m}Tc-NC100692 microSPECT/ CT images are shown for wild-type and MMP-9-null mice. MicroSPECT short axis (SA) images are shown in standard format, coregistered with microCT images. The ^{99m}Tc-NC100692 microSPECT images are displayed in red color scale and fused with [201]Tl (green scale) and CT (grayscale) images to define uptake of the $\alpha_v\beta_3$ targeted radiotracer relative to the ^{201}Tl perfusion defect and anatomic structures within the chest. The areas boxed in white in the images on the left are enlarged in the images on the right. White solid arrows indicate regions of increased ^{99m}Tc-NC100692 uptake in anterior-lateral infarct territory. White asterisks indicate ^{99m}Tc-NC100692 activity associated with angiogenesis at the thoracotomy site. ^{99m}Tc-NC100692 activity is also seen in the liver. (B) By well counting, the relative uptake of the ^{99m}Tc-labeled $\alpha_v\beta_3$ peptide NC100692 was higher in MMP-9 null mice ($N = 7$), compared to wild-type mice ($N = 10$), in the infarct region (0% to 40% nonischemic region). *$p < 0.05$ for wild-type versus MMP-9 null. (Reprinted with permission from Reference 44.)

Studies by Meoli et al demonstrated the potential of ^{111}In-RP748 for in vivo SPECT imaging of myocardial angiogenesis.[38] These investigators used a canine model of myocardial infarction that is known to produce nontransmural infarction and peri-infarct ischemia. They reported favorable kinetics of ^{111}In-RP748 and observed a focal uptake of the radiotracer within the infarct region. This uptake was found to be associated with activation of the $\alpha_v\beta_3$ integrin. To interpret the ^{111}In-RP748 hot-spot SPECT images, perfusion images with ^{99m}Tc-sestamibi were acquired and coregistered. Representative in vivo and ex vivo dual-isotope SPECT images of dog hearts subjected to myocardial infarction are shown in Figure 26.4. These studies demonstrated that 3 weeks post–myocardial infarction, ^{111}In-RP748 was selectively retained in regions of injury-induced angiogenesis where ^{99m}Tc-sestamibi perfusion was reduced. To confirm that ^{111}In-RP748 tracks ischemia-induced angiogenesis, the same group performed an additional series of rat studies in which ^{111}In-RP748 uptake in the

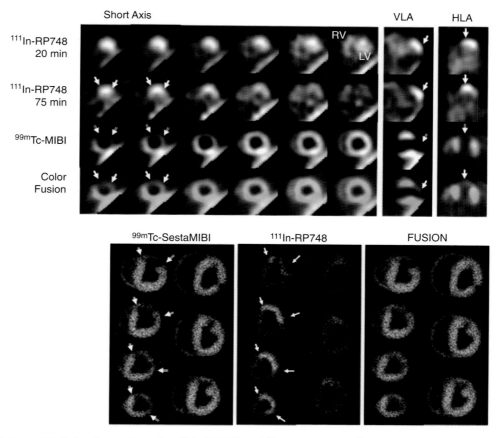

FIGURE 26.4. In vivo and ex vivo ^{111}In-RP748 and ^{99m}Tc-sestamibi (^{99m}Tc-MIBI) images from dogs with chronic infarction. (Top) Serial in vivo ^{111}In-RP748 SPECT short axis (SA), vertical long axis (VLA), and horizontal long axis (HLA) images in a dog 3 weeks after left anterior descending (LAD) artery infraction at 20 minutes and 75 minutes after injection in standard format. ^{111}In-RP748 SPECT images were registered with ^{99m}Tc-MIBI perfusion images (third row). The 75-minutes ^{111}In-RP748 SPECT images were colored red and fused with ^{99m}Tc-MIBI images (green) to better demonstrate localization of ^{111}In-RP748 activity within the heart (color fusion, bottom row). White arrows indicate region of increased ^{111}In-RP748 uptake in anterior wall. This corresponds to the anteroapical ^{99m}Tc-sestamibi perfusion defect. (Bottom) Ex vivo ^{99m}Tc-sestamibi (left) and ^{111}In-RP748 (center) images of myocardial slices from a dog 3 weeks after LAD occlusion, with color fusion image on the right. Short axis slices are in the standard orientation. Arrows indicate anterior location of nontransmural perfusion defect region and corresponding area of increased ^{111}In-RP748 uptake. (Reprinted with permission from Reference 38.)

myocardium was correlated with the uptake of a ^{99m}Tc-labeled nitroimidazole (BRU-5921) retained in hypoxic myocardium and perfusion defect assessed with ^{201}Tl chloride.[46]

The value of the $\alpha_v\beta_3$-targeted-imaging approach for assessment of myocardial angiogenesis was recently confirmed by another group of investigators, which injected a ^{123}I-labeled RGD peptide in pigs with chronic ischemia treated with direct intramyocardial injection of phVEGF$_{165}$.[39]

Other imaging modalities have been used to noninvasively assess angiogenesis. However, most of the work on imaging of myocardial angiogenesis was done using SPECT tracers. A limited number of studies utilized PET tracers or RGD-based ultrasound contrast agents; however, they have been restricted to the assessment of tumor angiogenesis. With the increasing availability of PET scanners there is also a considerable interest in developing novel positron-emitting tracers targeted at $\alpha_v\beta_3$ to noninvasively track angiogenesis in the clinical setting.[47]

Chen et al synthesized and applied a positron emitter copper-64 (^{64}Cu)-labeled PEGylated dimeric RGD peptide radiotracer for lung cancer imaging in mice.[21] The radiotracer revealed rapid blood clearance via renal system and minimum nonspecific activity accumulation in normal tissue. PEGylation improved tumor-targeting efficacy and reduced biliary excretion. Unfortunately, lower receptor binding affinity as compared to the dimeric RGD peptide, resulted in decreased tumor uptake. Although this agent is an excellent PET tracer for integrin-positive tumor imaging, biodistribution data strongly suggest that peptide ligands of this class may be promising for imaging integrin expression in the myocardium.

More recently, the general advantage of the glycosylation approach in designing peptide-based tracers with favorable imaging properties for clinical applications has been confirmed. ^{18}F-galacto-RGD, a glycosylated cyclic pentapeptide (Arg-Gly-Asp-DPhe-Val), was synthesized and characterized by Haubner et al. This tracer also showed high affinity and selectivity for the $\alpha_v\beta_3$ integrin and receptor-specific accumulation in $\alpha_v\beta_3$-positive tumors as well as rapid predominantly renal elimination.[22] The radiotracer uptake was correlated with the measurement of $\alpha_v\beta_3$ integrin expression assessed by Western blotting and immunohistochemistry of human $\alpha_v\beta_3$ (LM609) and murine β_3. In addition to the microPET imaging in mice, these investigators performed initial evaluation of tumor angiogenesis in humans. In all patients, rapid renal excretion was observed, resulting in fast tracer elimination from blood and low background activity. On average, a 9-fold higher activity accumulation was found in the tumor than in muscle.

To further improve the retention of $\alpha_v\beta_3$ radioligands, multimeric (composed of several identical subunits) RGD peptides were recently introduced. Although all work was done in tumor imaging, these multimeric RGD peptides showed increased binding affinities in vitro and improved tracer accumulation compared with the monomeric compounds, which shows promise for its use in imaging of myocardial angiogenesis.[22]

Summary Points

- Molecular imaging of angiogenesis can be used in both preclinical development and clinical applications. The validation of potential disease targets in vivo and the distribution of new tagged drugs at the desired site represent the main advantages of molecular imaging in preclinical development.
- In clinical applications, molecular imaging of angiogenesis can distinguish patient populations that would likely respond to angiogenic therapy from nonresponders. Furthermore, disease progression and response to therapy can be tracked in patients with faster feedback than currently available techniques.
- Angiogenesis manifests phenotypically in many disease pathways, which, if successfully modulated, would allow targeting of a great number of pathological processes

in patients. The modulation of angiogenesis currently attracts considerable scientific and business interest, and this trend is likely to rise. In addition, the sequencing of the human genome and the wide use of transgenic animals in basic science have resulted in the identification of many new potential therapeutic targets. Therefore, the imaging technology, which has already demonstrated promise in evaluation of angiogenesis, may prove useful for prognostication and early assessment of therapeutic efficacy.[48]

- The scientific community should be aware that too often the excitement of scientific curiosity can lead to a lack of practical focus. Developing new strategies in imaging of angiogenesis can successfully be accomplished only through close collaboration of multidisciplinary teams with a wide range of expertise. Moreover, we need to consider other alternatives, including nonimaging biomarkers, and "gene chips." These approaches belong to the new group of decision-making tools that may cost only a fraction of what imaging costs. Imaging may provide far more useful clinical data; however, awareness of competing technologies is required when developing novel imaging strategies.

- The future of noninvasive imaging of angiogenesis rests on two pathways: advancement of imaging technology and the further development of novel targeted biologic markers of angiogenesis. Indeed, the introduction of hybrid systems for imaging of small animals (microSPECT/CT and microPET/CT) greatly enhanced the performance and accuracy of nuclear imaging. CT is now available in clinical SPECT and PET scanners and can be used for anatomical localization as well as for attenuation and partial volume correction.

- Additionally, novel targets of angiogenesis continue to be identified, and new selective tracers remain under development. The interactions of integrins with the ECM are critical for vascular formation. MMPs are responsible for degradation of the myocardial ECM, and a clear cause-effect relationship between MMPs and angiogenesis has been demonstrated in experimental animal models. In light of this fact, recent effort has been placed on developing PET and SPECT tracers for MMP activity modeled after selective MMP inhibitors.[25,26]

- In our development of approaches for imaging of angiogenesis, we need to keep in mind practical and important clinical applications. Congestive heart failure (CHF) is one of these important clinical problems. Previous studies suggest that CHF may result from myocardial ischemia in the presence or absence of obstructive epicardial coronary artery disease.[10,49] Therefore, both targeted imaging of $\alpha_v\beta_3$ integrin and MMPs may be useful in the noninvasive imaging of angiogenesis and remodeling of the ECM and could be useful in the setting of CHF to track efficacy of therapeutic intervention directed at augmentation of microvascularity and restoring normal cardiac function.

- Targeted imaging of angiogenesis may become routine in clinical cardiovascular nuclear medicine laboratories in conjunction with standard imaging of physiological parameters. These hybrid imaging approaches will likely play a critical role for both diagnostic and prognostic purposes, as well as for evaluation of gene therapy strategies.

References

1. Fam NP, Verma S, Kutryk M, Stewart DJ. Clinician guide to angiogenesis. *Circulation.* 2003;108:2613–2618.
2. Sinusas AJ. Imaging of angiogenesis. *J Nucl Cardiol.* 2004;11:617–633.
3. Yancopoulos GD, Davis S, Gale NW, Rudge JS, Wiegand SJ, Holash J. Vascular-specific growth factors and blood vessel formation. *Nature.* 2000;407:242–248.
4. Ito WD, Arras M, Scholz D, Winkler B, Htun P, Schaper W. Angiogenesis but not collateral growth is associated with ischemia after femoral artery occlusion. *Am J Physiol.* 1997; 273(pt 2):H1255–H1265.

5. Simons M. Angiogenesis: where do we stand now? *Circulation*. 2005;111:1556–1566.
6. Helisch A, Schaper W. Arteriogenesis: the development and growth of collateral arteries. *Microcirculation*. 2003;10:83–97.
7. Brooks PC, Clark RA, Cheresh DA. Requirement of vascular integrin alpha v beta 3 for angiogenesis. *Science*. 1994;264:569–571.
8. Lee SH, Wolf PL, Escudero R, Deutsch R, Jamieson SW, Thistlethwaite PA. Early expression of angiogenesis factors in acute myocardial ischemia and infarction. *N Engl J Med*. 2000;342:626–633.
9. Papetti M, Herman IM. Mechanisms of normal and tumor-derived angiogenesis. *Am J Physiol Cell Physiol*. 2002;282:C947–C970.
10. Carmeliet P, Ferreira V, Breier G, et al. Abnormal blood vessel development and lethality in embryos lacking a single VEGF allele. *Nature*. 1996;380:435–439.
11. Suri C, Jones PF, Patan S, et al. Requisite role of angiopoietin-1, a ligand for the TIE2 receptor, during embryonic angiogenesis. *Cell*. 1996;87:1171–1180.
12. Kastrup J, Jorgensen E, Ruck A, et al. Direct intramyocardial plasmid vascular endothelial growth factor-A165 gene therapy in patients with stable severe angina pectoris. A randomized double-blind placebo-controlled study: the Euroinject One trial. *J Am Coll Cardiol*. 2005;45:982–988.
13. Nunn AD. The biology of technetium based hypoxic tissue localising compounds. In: Machulla H-J, ed. *Imaging of Hypoxia*. Dordrecht, The Netherlands: Kluwer Academic Publishers; 1999:19–45.
14. Sinusas A. The potential for myocardial imaging with hypoxia markers. *Semin Nucl Med*. 1999;29:330–338.
15. Martin GV, Caldwell JH, Graham MM, et al. Noninvasive detection of hypoxic myocardium using fluorine-18-fluoromisonidazole and positron emission tomography. *J Nucl Med*. 1992;33:2202–2208.
16. Shelton ME, Dence CS, Hwang DR, Welch MJ, Bergmann SR. Myocardial kinetics of fluorine-18 misonidazole: a marker of hypoxic myocardium. *J Nucl Med*. 1989;30:351–358.
17. Shi CQ, Sinusas AJ, Dione DP, et al. Technetium-99m-nitroimidazole (BMS181321): a positive imaging agent for detecting myocardial ischemia. *J Nucl Med*. 1995;36:1078–1086.
18. Rumsey W, Patel B, Kuczynski B, et al. Comparison of two novel technetium agents for imaging ischemic myocardium. *Circulation*. 1995;92(suppl I):I-181.
19. Rumsey WL, Kuczynski B, Patel B, et al. SPECT imaging of ischemic myocardium using a technetium-99m-nitroimidazole ligand. *J Nucl Med*. 1995;36:1445–1450.
20. Brack SS, Dinkelborg LM, Neri D. Molecular targeting of angiogenesis for imaging and therapy. *Eur J Nucl Med Mol Imaging*. 2004;31:1327–1341.
21. Chen X, Sievers E, Hou Y, et al. Integrin alpha v beta 3-targeted imaging of lung cancer. *Neoplasia*. 2005;7:271–279.
22. Haubner R, Weber WA, Beer AJ, et al. Noninvasive visualization of the activated alphavbeta3 integrin in cancer patients by positron emission tomography and [18F]Galacto-RGD. *PLoS Med*. 2005;2:e70.
23. Hua J, Dobrucki LW, Sadeghi MM, et al. Noninvasive imaging of angiogenesis with a 99mTc-labeled peptide targeted at alphavbeta3 integrin after murine hindlimb ischemia. *Circulation*. 2005;111:3255–3260.
24. Leong-Poi H, Christiansen J, Heppner P, et al. Assessment of endogenous and therapeutic arteriogenesis by contrast ultrasound molecular imaging of integrin expression. *Circulation*. 2005;111:3248–3254.
25. Su H, Spinale FG, Dobrucki LW, et al. Evaluation of myocardial matrix metalloproteinase (MMP) mediated post-MI remodeling with a novel radiolabeled MMP inhibitor. *J Nucl Cardiol*. 2004;11:S20.
26. Su H, Spinale F, Dobrucki L, et al. Noninvasive targeted imaging of matrix metalloproteinase activation in a murine model of postinfarction remodeling. *Circulation*. 2005;112:3157–3167.
27. Leong-Poi H, Christiansen J, Klibanov AL, Kaul S, Lindner JR. Noninvasive assessment of angiogenesis by ultrasound and microbubbles targeted to alpha(v)-integrins. *Circulation*. 2003;107:455–460.
28. Dayton PA, Pearson D, Clark J, et al. Ultrasonic analysis of peptide- and antibody-targeted microbubble contrast agents for molecular imaging of alphavbeta3-expressing cells. *Mol Imaging*. 2004;3:125–134.

29. Blankenberg FG. Molecular imaging: The latest generation of contrast agents and tissue characterization techniques. *J Cell Biochem.* 2003;90:443–453.
30. Winter PM, Morawski AM, Caruthers SD, et al. Molecular imaging of angiogenesis in early-stage atherosclerosis with alpha(v)beta3-integrin-targeted nanoparticles. *Circulation.* 2003;108:2270–2274.
31. Winter PM, Caruthers SD, Kassner A, et al. Molecular imaging of angiogenesis in nascent Vx-2 rabbit tumors using a novel alpha(nu)beta3-targeted nanoparticle and 1.5 tesla magnetic resonance imaging. *Cancer Res.* 2003;63:5838–5843.
32. Collingridge DR, Carroll VA, Glaser M, et al. The development of [(124)I]iodinated-VG76e: a novel tracer for imaging vascular endothelial growth factor in vivo using positron emission tomography. *Cancer Res.* 2002;62:5912–5919.
33. Li S, Peck-Radosavljevic M, Koller E, et al. Characterization of (123)I-vascular endothelial growth factor-binding sites expressed on human tumour cells: possible implication for tumour scintigraphy. *Int J Cancer.* 2001;91:789–796.
34. Li S, Peck-Radosavljevic M, Kienast O, et al. Iodine-123-vascular endothelial growth factor-165 (123I-VEGF165). Biodistribution, safety and radiation dosimetry in patients with pancreatic carcinoma. *Q J Nucl Med Mol Imaging.* 2004;48:198–206.
35. Lu E, Wagner WR, Schellenberger U, et al. Targeted in vivo labeling of receptors for vascular endothelial growth factor: approach to identification of ischemic tissue. *Circulation.* 2003;108:97–103.
36. Sipkins D, Cheresh D, Kazemi M, Nevin L, Bednarski M, Li K. Detection of tumor angiogenesis in vivo by alphaVbeta3-targeted magnetic resonance imaging. *Nat Med.* 1998;4:623–626.
37. Harris TD, Kalogeropoulos S, Nguyen T, et al. Design, synthesis, and evaluation of radiolabeled integrin alpha v beta 3 receptor antagonists for tumor imaging and radiotherapy. *Cancer Biother Radiopharm.* 2003;18:627–641.
38. Meoli DF, Sadeghi MM, Krassilnikova S, et al. Noninvasive imaging of myocardial angiogenesis following experimental myocardial infarction. *J Clin Invest.* 2004;113:1684–1691.
39. Johnson LL, Haubner R, Schofield L, Bouchard M, Schwaiger M. Radiolabeled RGD peptide to image angiogenesis in swine model of hibernating myocardium. *Circulation.* 2003;108(Suppl. S):405.
40. Lee KH, Jung KH, Song SH, et al. Radiolabeled RGD uptake and alphav integrin expression is enhanced in ischemic murine hindlimbs. *J Nucl Med.* 2005;46:472–478.
41. Blankenberg FG, Mandl S, Cao YA, et al. Tumor imaging using a standardized radiolabeled adapter protein docked to vascular endothelial growth factor. *J Nucl Med.* 2004;45:1373–1380.
42. Lee PC, Kibbe MR, Schuchert MJ, et al. Nitric oxide induces angiogenesis and upregulates alpha(v)beta(3) integrin expression on endothelial cells. *Microvasc Res.* 2000;60:269–280.
43. Haubner R, Wester H, Reuning U, et al. Radiolabeled alpha(v)beta3 integrin antagonists: a new class of tracers for tumor targeting. *J Nucl Med.* 1999;40:1061–1071.
44. Lindsey ML, Escobar GP, Dobrucki LW, et al. Matrix metalloproteinase-9 gene deletion facilitates angiogenesis following myocardial infarction. *Am J Physiol Heart Circ Physiol.* 2006;290:H232–H239.
45. Sadeghi MM, Krassilnikova S, Zhang J, et al. Detection of injury-induced vascular remodeling by targeting activated alphavbeta3 integrin in vivo. *Circulation.* 2004;110:84–90.
46. Meoli D, Bourke B, Hu L, Brown L, Sinusas A. Regional hypoxia correlates with radiolabeled targeted markers of myocardiol angiogenesis in ischemic rat model. *J Nucl Med.* 2002;43(Suppl. S):8P.
47. Lewis MR. Radiolabeled RGD peptides move beyond cancer: PET imaging of delayed-type hypersensitivity reaction. *J Nucl Med.* 2005;46:2–4.
48. Dzik-Jurasz A. Angiogenesis imaging in man: a personal view from the pharmaceutical industry. *Br J Radiol.* 2003;76(special number 1):S81–S82.
49. Isner JM, Losordo DW. Therapeutic angiogenesis for heart failure. *Nat Med.* 1999;5:491–492.

Part VI
Case Illustrations of Cardiac PET and Integrated PET/CT

Sharmila Dorbala, Zelmira Curillova, and Marcelo F. Di Carli

Case 1   *Normal Vasodilator Stress PET/CT Study*

Clinical History

A 52-year-old female with dyslipidemia and a family history of ischemic heart disease was referred for evaluation of nonanginal chest pain.

Electrocardiogram

The patient's resting electrocardiogram (ECG) showed sinus bradycardia.

Medications

Atorvastatin, Paroxetine, Fexonfenadine, Atenolol

Study Protocol

Myocardial perfusion PET study following the IV administration of 60 mCi of rubidium-82 (^{82}Rb) at rest and during peak dipyridamole stress, respectively. Gated myocardial perfusion PET images were obtained at rest and during peak stress.

Vasodilator stress was achieved with a standard IV infusion of dipyridamole (0.142 mg/kg/min) for 4 minutes. The heart rate increased from 47 beats per minute (bpm) at rest to a peak heart rate of 61 bpm, and the blood pressure increased from 119/43 mm Hg at rest to 131/63 mm Hg at peak hyperemia. The infusion was terminated due to the completion of the dipyridamole protocol. The clinical response to dipyridamole was nonischemic. The ECG response to dipyridamole was nonischemic. There were no arrhythmias during the dipyridamole infusion. Imaging parameters were described in Chapters 10 and 11.

Breath-hold-gated cardiac CT was performed using a 16-channel CT scanner with a 0.5-second rotation time. Quantitative coronary calcium scores were calculated according to the method described by Agatston.

Findings

  A. Image quality:
    1. Emission images: Excellent.
    2. Transmission images: Excellent.
    3. Registration of transmission and emission images: Good. Figure 1 demonstrates good registration in both the axial (A) and coronal (B) slices.
  B. Rest-stress ^{82}Rb perfusion images: The images demonstrated normal left ventricle (LV) size. They also demonstrated normal right ventricle (RV) size with normal RV tracer uptake at rest. There were no regional perfusion defects seen on the stress or rest images (Figure 2).
  C. Gated PET images: Demonstrated a rest LV ejection fraction (LVEF) of 78% and end systolic volume index (ESVI) 7 mL/m^2. The LVEF during peak stress was 83%. The LV volumes appeared normal. There were no regional wall motion abnormalities. The images demonstrated normal regional wall thickening. The RV function appeared normal.
  D. Ancillary findings: There was a small calcified pleural granuloma in the right lower lobe. There was no pleural effusion or thickening.

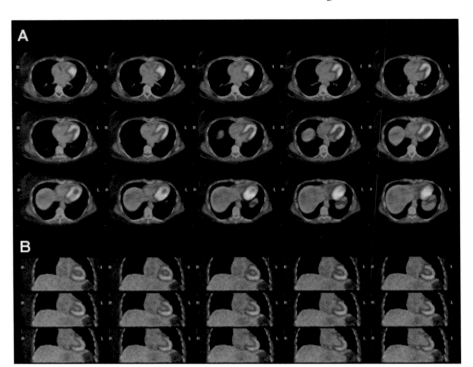

FIGURE 1. Fused emission (^{82}Rb) and CT transmission images in axial (A) and coronal (B) slices demonstrating good registration between the two data sets.

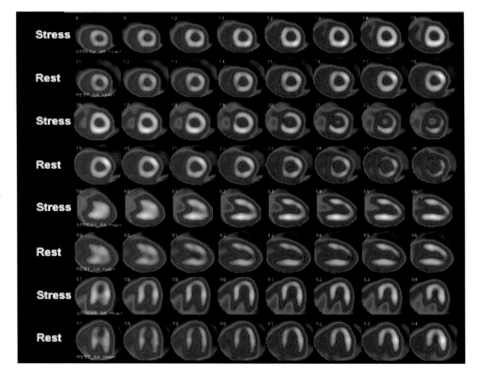

FIGURE 2. Dipyridamole stress and rest ^{82}Rb images in corresponding short axis, vertical long, and horizontal long axis slices. The short axis slices represent progression from the apical (left) to the basal (right) part of the heart and are oriented with the anterior wall on the top, the lateral wall to the right, the inferior wall at the bottom, and the interventricular septum to the left. The vertical long axis slices represent progression from the septum (left) to the lateral (right) wall and are oriented with the anterior wall on the top, the inferior wall at the bottom, and the LV apex to the right. The horizontal long axis slices represent progression from the inferior (left) to the anterior (right) wall and are oriented with the septal wall on the left, the lateral wall to the right, and the LV apex on the top. The images demonstrate normal myocardial perfusion throughout the LV.

E. Cardiac CT: The Agatston coronary calcium score was 0. This score is less than the 10th percentile rank for women age 50 to 55.

Final Impression

These combined PET/CT results are normal and suggest no evidence of calcified or hemodynamically significant coronary artery disease (CAD).

Discussion

This study demonstrates the typical features of a normal ^{82}Rb myocardial perfusion study, as described in Chapters 10 and 11. Rest and stress perfusion images demonstrate normal homogeneous radiotracer distribution. Note the lack of the usual anterior wall attenuation artifacts typically seen with single photon emission computed tomography (SPECT) imaging in women. The cavity size of the stress images is typically the same or smaller than at rest. There is an increase in ejection fraction from rest to peak stress, even with vasodilator stress.

Follow-up

Aggressive risk-factor modification for primary prevention of CAD.

Case 2   *Normal Dobutamine Stress PET/CT Study*

Clinical History

A 62-year-old female with hypertension, dyslipidemia, and a family history of ischemic heart disease was referred for evaluation of dyspnea.

Electrocardiogram

Normal sinus rhythm and nonspecific ST-T wave abnormalities.

Medications

Lisinopril, Hydrochlorothiazide, Pravachol, Asprin/dipyridamole, Nabumetone

Study Protocol

Myocardial perfusion PET study following the intravenous (IV) administration of 60mCi of ^{82}Rb at rest and during peak dobutamine stress, respectively. Gated myocardial perfusion PET images were obtained at rest and during peak stress using a prescan delay of 90 seconds.

Cardiac stress was achieved with a standard IV infusion of dobutamine (to a peak of 40 mcg/kg/min) with no additional Atropine. The heart rate increased from 85 bpm at rest to a peak heart rate of 158 bpm (100% of age-predicted heart rate [APHR]), and the blood pressure increased from 149/83 mm Hg at rest to 165/90 mm Hg at peak stress (rate-pressure product [RPP] of 26070). The infusion was terminated due to the completion of the dobutamine protocol. The clinical response to dobutamine was nonischemic. The blood pressure response was normal. The ECG response to dobutamine was nonischemic. There were no arrhythmias during the dobutamine infusion.

Coronary calcium score was assessed as defined in Case 1.

Findings

A. **Image quality:**
   1. Emission images: Excellent.
   2. Transmission images: Excellent.
   3. Registration of transmission and emission images: Good.
B. **Rest-stress ^{82}Rb perfusion images:** The images demonstrated normal LV size. They also demonstrated normal RV size with normal RV tracer uptake at rest. There were no regional perfusion defects seen on the stress or rest images (Figure 3).
C. **Gated PET images:** Demonstrated a rest LVEF of 60%. The LVEF during peak stress was 74%. The LV volumes appeared normal. There were no regional wall

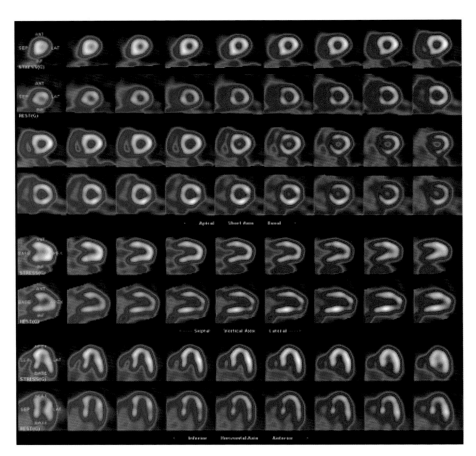

FIGURE 3. Dobutamine stress and rest ^{82}Rb images in corresponding short axis, vertical long axis, and horizontal long axis slices. The short axis slices represent progression from the apical (left) to the basal (right) part of the heart and are oriented with the anterior wall on the top, the lateral wall to the right, the inferior wall at the bottom, and the interventricular septum to the left. The vertical long axis slices represent progression from the septum (left) to the lateral (right) wall and are oriented with the anterior wall on the top, the inferior wall at the bottom, and the LV apex to the right. The horizontal long axis slices represent progression from the inferior (left) to the anterior (right) wall and are oriented with the septal wall on the left, the lateral wall to the right, and the LV apex on the top. The images demonstrate normal myocardial perfusion throughout the LV.

motion abnormalities. The patient demonstrated normal regional wall thickening. The RV function appeared normal.

D. Ancillary findings: None.

E. Gated cardiac CT: There is moderate coronary artery calcification. The Agatston coronary calcium score was 301. This score is greater than the 90th percentile rank for women aged 61 to 65 years.

Final Impression

The combined PET/CT results show moderate calcified coronary atherosclerosis without evidence of flow-limiting CAD.

Discussion

This study demonstrates the typical features of a normal rest and peak dobutamine ^{82}Rb myocardial perfusion study as described in Chapters 10 and 11. Rest and stress perfusion images demonstrate normal homogeneous radiotracer distribution. Because images are obtained during peak dobutamine infusion, the cavity size is significantly smaller on the stress compared to the rest images.

Follow-up

Aggressive risk-factor modification for secondary prevention of coronary artery disease.

Case 3   *Misregistration Artifact*

Clinical History

A 60-year-old male with hypertension was referred for evaluation of nonanginal chest pain.

Electrocardiogram

Normal.

Medications

Atenolol, Hydrochlorothiazide, Aspirin

Study Protocol

As defined in Case 1, except that a gated noncontrast CT for coronary calcium score was not obtained. The clinical and ECG responses to stress were nonischemic.

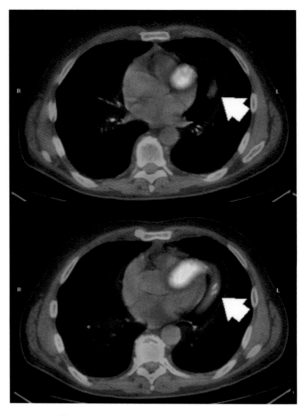

FIGURE 4. Fused emission (^{82}Rb) and CT transmission images in axial slices demonstrating severe misregistration between the two data sets, with the anterolateral wall on the ^{82}Rb images overlapping the lung field on the CT transmission images (arrows).

Findings

A. Image quality:
1. Emission images: Excellent.
2. Transmission images: Excellent.
3. Registration of transmission and emission images: Inadequate. The axial images demonstrate severe misregistration (Figure 4), with the anterolateral wall on the emission images overlapping the lung field on the CT transmission images (arrows).

B. Rest-stress ^{82}Rb perfusion images: A large perfusion defect of severe intensity in the mid- and basal anterior and anterolateral wall, showing complete reversibility (Figure 5).

C. Gated PET images: Demonstrated normal regional wall motion and wall thickening on gated rest images.

D. Ancillary findings: None.

Final Impression

Uninterpretable stress myocardial perfusion PET study.

Discussion

The reversible defect in the anterolateral wall could represent artifact from misregistration of emission and transmission images. However, true ischemia in the distribution of a diagonal coronary artery cannot be excluded. Inspection of the PET and CT transmission images demonstrates significant misregistration between the two. The pattern of misregistration, with the emission images moved cephalad in relation to transmission images (Figure 4), is usually the result of differences in breathing patterns between the short CT transmission (~10–15 seconds) and longer (~5 minutes) [82]Rb PET images. As discussed in Chapters 1, 3, and 10, this type of misregistration often results in undercorrection of PET images in regions with significant overlap with the lung, which has a very low attenuation coefficient. Quality control of the emission and transmission images is crucial for recognizing motion artifacts.

Follow-up

The stress PET study was repeated on the following day. Unlike the previous study, the new one demonstrated adequate registration of PET and CT transmission images (Figure 6), resulting in a normal myocardial perfusion stress study (Figure 7). Gated PET images revealed normal wall motion. LVEF was 60% at rest and increased to 76% during peak stress.

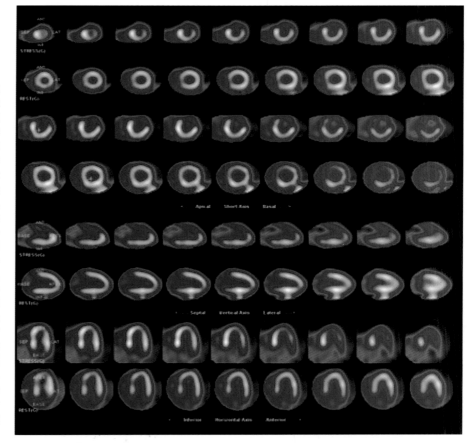

FIGURE 5. Dipyridamole stress and rest [82]Rb images in corresponding short axis, vertical long axis, and horizontal long axis slices. The short axis slices represent progression from the apical (left) to the basal (right) part of the heart and are oriented with the anterior wall on the top, the lateral wall to the right, the inferior wall at the bottom, and the interventricular septum to the left. The vertical long axis slices represent progression from the septum (left) to the lateral (right) wall and are oriented with the anterior wall on the top, the inferior wall at the bottom, and the LV apex to the right. The horizontal long axis slices represent progression from the inferior (left) to the anterior (right) wall and are oriented with the septal wall on the left, the lateral wall to the right, and the LV apex on the top. The stress images demonstrate a large and severe perfusion defect throughout the anterolateral wall, showing complete reversibility.

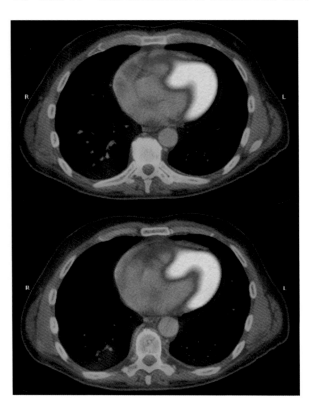

FIGURE 6. Fused emission (^{82}Rb) and CT transmission images in axial slices now demonstrate good registration between the two data sets.

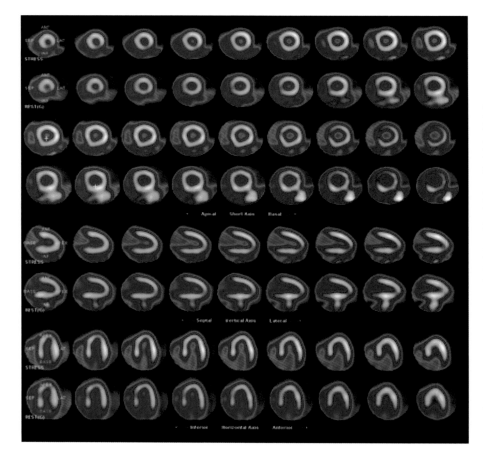

FIGURE 7. Dipyridamole stress and rest ^{82}Rb images in corresponding short axis, vertical long axis, and horizontal long axis slices. The short axis slices represent progression from the apical (left) to the basal (right) part of the heart and are oriented with the anterior wall on the top, the lateral wall to the right, the inferior wall at the bottom, and the interventricular septum to the left. The vertical long axis slices represent progression from the septum (left) to the lateral (right) wall and are oriented with the anterior wall on the top, the inferior wall at the bottom, and the LV apex to the right. The horizontal long axis slices represent progression from the inferior (left) to the anterior (right) wall and are oriented with the septal wall on the left, the lateral wall to the right, and the LV apex on the top. The images now demonstrate normal myocardial perfusion throughout the LV.

Case 4   *Attenuation Correction Artifact*

Clinical History

A 74-year-old man with diabetes, dyslipidemia, peripheral arterial disease, and known ischemic dilated cardiomyopathy was referred for preoperative evaluation prior to peripheral bypass surgery. He had a prior history of myocardial infarction with stenting of the left circumflex coronary artery and an automatic implantable cardiac defibrillator (AICD).

Electrocardiogram

Normal sinus rhythm and left bundle branch block (LBBB).

Medications

Metoprolol, Lisinopril, Furosemide, Aspirin, Insulin

Study Protocol

As defined in Case 1, except that a gated noncontrast CT for coronary calcium score was not obtained. The clinical and ECG responses to stress were nonischemic.

Findings

A. Image quality:
   1. Emission images: Excellent.
   2. Transmission images: Intense beam-hardening artifact from AICD wires in the inferoseptal region (arrow on Figure 8).
   3. Registration of transmission and emission images: Good.

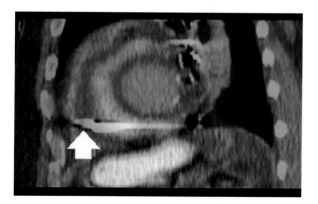

FIGURE 8. Fused emission (^{82}Rb) and CT transmission images in sagittal slices demonstrating good registration between the two data sets. The arrow points to the AICD wire, resulting in beam hardening on the CT images.

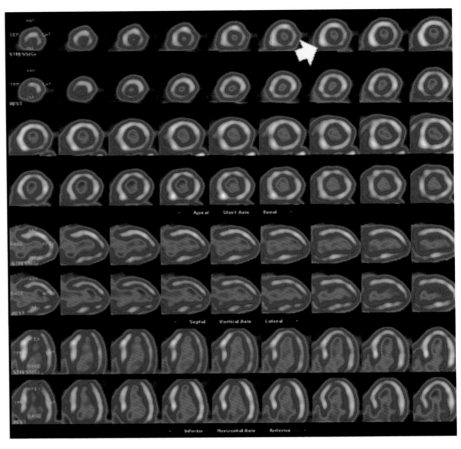

FIGURE 9. Dipyridamole stress and rest ^{82}Rb images in corresponding short axis, vertical long axis, and horizontal long axis slices. The short axis slices represent progression from the apical (left) to the basal (right) part of the heart and are oriented with the anterior wall on the top, the lateral wall to the right, the inferior wall at the bottom, and the interventricular septum to the left. The vertical long axis slices represent progression from the septum (left) to the lateral (right) wall and are oriented with the anterior wall on the top, inferior wall at the bottom, and the LV apex to the right. The horizontal long axis slices represent progression from the inferior (left) to the anterior (right) wall and are oriented with the septal wall on the left, the lateral wall to the right, and the LV apex on the top. There is a hot spot in the inferoseptal wall, more pronounced on the stress images (arrow), resulting from the overcorrection of the emission images due to metal artifact from the AICD.

B. Rest-stress ^{82}Rb perfusion images: No regional perfusion defects were seen (Figure 9). There is a hot spot in the inferoseptal wall more pronounced on the stress images (arrow).

C. Gated PET images: Demonstrated a rest LVEF fraction of 26% that remained unchanged at peak stress, 27%. The LV volumes appeared severely dilated. There were severe global wall motion abnormalities. The RV function appeared normal.

D. Ancillary findings: None.

Final Impression

The PET images demonstrate no evidence of flow-limiting CAD. However, there is evidence of severe LV systolic dysfunction.

Discussion

As discussed in Chapters 1, 3, and 10, metallic devices in the heart, usually with increased density and attenuation coefficient, result in overcorrection of the adjacent region of the emission images, frequently leading to hot spots. Although theoretically possible, in our practice we have noticed that these artifacts do not typically mask significant ischemia. Metallic valves, AICDs, and pacemaker wires are the usual culprits, with stents and CABG clips less likely to cause these artifacts. Metallic heart valves are usually too far basal to cause any impact on the images. These are cases in which a traditional gamma-ray transmission can be more helpful.

Follow-up

None.

Case 5   *High-Risk PET/CT Scan*

Clinical History

A 61-year-old woman with risk factors of hypertension, dyslipidemia, diabetes, a family history of ischemic heart disease, and obesity was referred for risk stratification after a non-ST segment elevation myocardial infarction.

Electrocardiogram

Sinus bradycardia, first-degree AV block, poor R-wave progression, and nonspecific T-wave abnormalities.

Medications

Metoprolol, Amlodipine, Captopril, Isosorbide mononitrate, Aspirin, Atorvastatin, Fenofebrate, Enoxaparin

Study Protocol

As defined in Case 1. The clinical and ECG responses to stress were nonischemic.

Findings

A. **Image quality:**
   1. Emission images: Good.
   2. Transmission images: Excellent.
   3. Registration of transmission and emission images: Excellent.
B. **Rest-stress ^{82}Rb perfusion images:** There was transient dilatation of the LV during stress. There was a large and severe perfusion defect involving the mid- and apical anterior, apical inferior, apical septal, and apical lateral walls, and the LV apex, showing near-complete reversibility. In addition, there was a medium-size and

severe perfusion defect involving the mid- and basal inferior and basal inferoseptal walls, showing complete reversibility (Figure 10).

C. Gated PET images: Demonstrated a rest LVEF of 56% that decreased during peak stress to 51%. The LV volumes appeared transiently enlarged during peak stress. There was severe hypokinesis of the mid- and apical anterior walls and the LV apex, as well as the basal inferoseptal and inferior walls, with concordant reduction in wall thickening. The RV function appeared normal.

D. Ancillary findings: None.

E. Gated cardiac CT: There was extensive coronary artery calcification. The Agatston coronary calcium score was 1367 (Figure 11). This score is greater than the 90th percentile rank for women age 61 to 65 years.

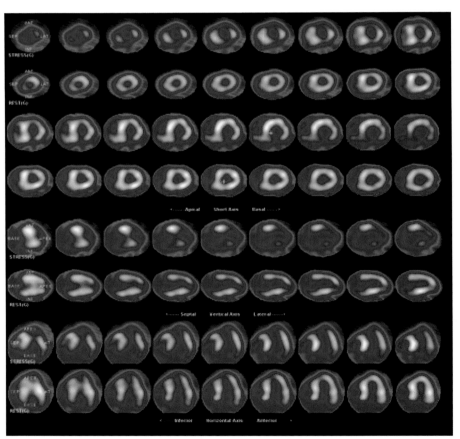

FIGURE 10. Stress and rest ^{82}Rb images in corresponding short axis, vertical long axis, and horizontal long axis slices. The short axis slices represent progression from the apical (left) to the basal (right) part of the heart and are oriented with the anterior wall on the top, the lateral wall to the right, the inferior wall at the bottom, and the interventricular septum to the left. The vertical long axis slices represent progression from the septum (left) to the lateral (right) wall and are oriented with the anterior wall on the top, the inferior wall at the bottom, and the LV apex to the right. The horizontal long axis slices represent progression from the inferior (left) to the anterior (right) wall and are oriented with the septal wall on the left, the lateral wall to the right, and the LV apex on the top. The images demonstrate transient LV dilatation and increased radiotracer uptake in the right ventricle during stress. In addition, there are large and severe perfusion defects involving the apical LV segments, the mid-anterior wall, as well as the mid- and basal inferior and basal inferoseptal walls, showing complete reversibility.

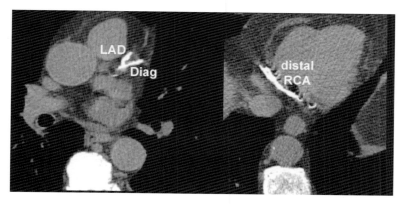

FIGURE 11. Axial CT images demonstrating extensive calcification of the distal left main, proximal left anterior descending (LAD), first diagonal branch (Diag), and distal right coronary (Distal RCA) arteries.

Final Impression

There was evidence of extensive calcified coronary plaque burden.

The PET images demonstrate extensive areas of severe stress-induced ischemia throughout the mid-left anterior descending (LAD) and posterior descending artery (PDA) territories.

Transient ischemic dilation of the left ventricle and decrease in LVEF during peak stress suggest significant ischemic burden or severe multivessel CAD or both.

Discussion

This patient has large and severe perfusion defects that are reversible and consistent with ischemia in two coronary territories. As discussed in Chapter 11, transient dilation of the left ventricle and decrease in LVEF during peak stress suggest severe multivessel CAD.

Follow-up

Coronary angiography demonstrated 3-vessel CAD with 100% stenosis of the proximal LAD, 95% ostial stenosis of a ramus branch, 45% stenosis of the proximal RCA, and 100% stenosis of the mid-RCA with a right dominant circulation. The patient underwent CABG.

Case 6   *High-Risk PET/CT Scan*

Clinical History

An 83-year-old male with hypertension and obesity was referred for a dipyridamole myocardial perfusion PET study to evaluate for nonanginal chest pain and dyspnea.

Electrocardiogram

Normal sinus rhythm, first-degree atrioventricular (AV) block, and LBBB

Medications

Acebutolol, Aspirin, Ranitidine, Epogen

Study Protocol

Imaging protocol: As defined in Case 1. The clinical and ECG responses to stress were nonischemic.

Findings

A. **Image quality:**
  1. Emission images: Excellent.
  2. Transmission images: Excellent.
  3. Registration of transmission and emission images: Good.
B. **Rest-stress ^{82}Rb perfusion images:** Transient dilatation of the LV was noted. A small defect of moderate intensity was noted in the mid- and basal inferolateral wall (arrow) that was completely reversible (Figure 12).
C. **Gated PET images:** Demonstrated a rest LVEF of 58% that declined during peak stress to 39%. The LV volumes appeared moderately dilated. There was infero-

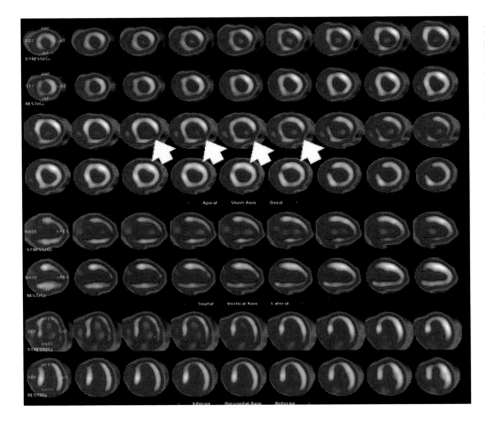

FIGURE 12. Stress and rest ^{82}Rb images in corresponding short axis, vertical long axis, and horizontal long axis slices. The short axis slices represent progression from the apical (left) to the basal (right) part of the heart and are oriented with the anterior wall on the top, the lateral wall to the right, the inferior wall at the bottom, and the interventricular septum to the left. The vertical long axis slices represent progression from the septum (left) to the lateral (right) wall and are oriented with the anterior wall on the top, the inferior wall at the bottom, and the LV apex to the right. The horizontal long axis slices represent progression from the inferior (left) to the anterior (right) wall and are oriented with the septal wall on the left, the lateral wall to the right, and the LV apex on the top. The images demonstrate transient dilatation of the LV during stress, with a small perfusion defect of moderate intensity in the mid- and basal inferolateral wall (arrow), showing complete reversibility.

lateral wall hypokinesis during peak stress, which improved at rest. The RV function appeared normal.

D. Ancillary findings: None.

E. Gated cardiac CT: There is extensive coronary artery calcification, including proximal left main coronary artery. The Agatston coronary calcium score was 2902. This score is greater than the 90th percentile rank for men older than 71 years.

Final Impression

Extensive calcified coronary plaque burden. Moderate dipyridamole-induced perfusion defect in the distribution of the left circumflex coronary artery (LCX) territory. However, a decrease in LVEF at peak stress and transient LV dilatation suggest significant multivessel CAD.

Discussion

In contrast to the previous case, this patient has a small perfusion defect with moderate ischemia in a single-vessel distribution. Although PET is a sensitive means for identification of obstructive CAD, it is somewhat limited for delineating the extent of underlying anatomic disease due to balance reduction in myocardial perfusion in the setting of multivessel CAD. High-risk scan features including transient left ventricular dilatation during peak stress and/or a decline in LVEF during peak stress are helpful to correctly identify patients with multivessel CAD.

Follow-up

Coronary angiography demonstrated 3-vessel coronary artery disease with 90% stenosis of left main coronary artery, 60% stenosis of LAD, 80% ostial stenosis of a ramus branch, and 80% stenosis of the proximal LCX artery in a left dominant circulation. Patient underwent CABG.

Case 7   *Assessing Myocardial Viability with PET/CT Study*

Clinical History

An 80-year-old female with history of diabetes, dyslipidemia, ischemic dilated cardiomyopathy, and remote anterior myocardial infarction was referred for evaluation of troponin elevation in the setting of massive gastrointestinal bleed and anemia.

Electrocardiogram

Normal sinus rhythm and intraventricular conduction delay (IVCD).

Medications

Carvedilol, Lisinopril, Furosemide, Atorvastatin, Enoxaparin, Insulin

Study Protocol

Imaging protocol: Gated rest study with 60 mCi of ^{82}Rb and a prescan delay of 120 seconds. No stress imaging was performed.

FDG study: After rest perfusion imaging, the patient received 50 gm of oral glucose followed by 20 IU of regular insulin IV to optimize myocardial glucose utilization. The patient received 12 mCi of FDG intravenously, and 60 minutes later (to allow for trapping of FDG in the myocardium) gated PET images were acquired.

Findings

A. **Image quality:**
   1. Emission images: Excellent.
   2. Transmission images: Excellent.
   3. Registration of transmission and emission images: Excellent.
B. **Rest ^{82}Rb perfusion and ^{18}FDG images:** Severe LV dilatation and radiotracer uptake in the right ventricle. A large defect of severe intensity in the mid-anterior wall, anterolateral wall, and anteroseptal wall, the entire apical portion of the ventricle and LV apex, showing a matched reduction in FDG uptake in all hypoperfused LV segments (PET match, Figure 13).
C. **Gated PET images:** Demonstrated a rest LVEF of 35%. The LV volumes appeared severely dilated. The mid-anterior wall, anterolateral wall, anteroseptal wall, and the entire apical portion of LV and LV apex were akinetic, with reduced regional wall thickening. The RV function appeared normal.
D. **Ancillary findings:** None.
E. **Gated cardiac CT:** There is extensive coronary artery calcification. The Agatston coronary calcium score was 2095. This score is greater than the 90th percentile rank for women older than 71 years.

Final Impression

A large region of myocardial scar in the LAD coronary territory. There are large areas of viable myocardium in the distribution of the left circumflex and RCA coronary territories. Severe LV systolic dysfunction.

Discussion

The various patterns of perfusion and metabolism correlations are described in Chapter 18. This case illustrates the classic "PET match pattern," reflecting myocardial scar and, consequently, a low probability for improvement in LV function if revascularization is performed.

Follow-up

Due to patient's significant medical comorbidities, large region of myocardial scar in the LAD coronary distribution, and lack of symptoms, she was managed medically without coronary angiography or revascularization.

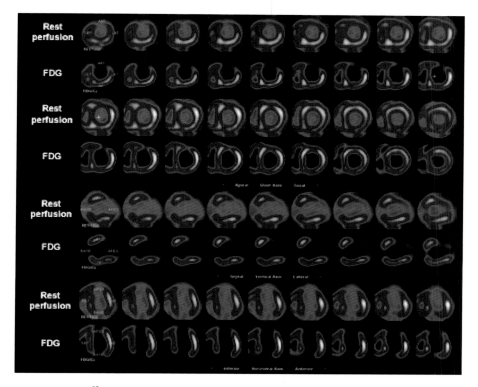

FIGURE 13. Rest ^{82}Rb and FDG images in corresponding short axis, vertical long axis, and horizontal long axis slices. The short axis slices represent progression from the apical (left) to the basal (right) part of the heart and are oriented with the anterior wall on the top, the lateral wall to the right, the inferior wall at the bottom, and the interventricular septum to the left. The vertical long axis slices represent progression from the septum (left) to the lateral (right) wall and are oriented with the anterior wall on the top, the inferior wall at the bottom, and the LV apex to the right. The horizontal long axis slices represent progression from the inferior (left) to the anterior (right) wall and are oriented with the septal wall on the left, the lateral wall to the right, and the LV apex on the top. The images demonstrate severe LV dilatation and radiotracer uptake in the right ventricle. There is a large and severe perfusion defect involving the mid-anterior, anterolateral, and anteroseptal walls, all the apical LV segments, and the LV apex, showing concordant reduction in FDG uptake (so-called PET match).

Case 8   Assessing Myocardial Viability with PET/CT Study

Clinical History

A 68-year-old female with known CAD and severe LV dysfunction was evaluated for myocardial viability for potential coronary revascularization.

Electrocardiogram

Normal sinus rhythm and IVCD.

Medications

Lopressor, Captopril, Lasix, Furosemide, Atorvastatin

Study Protocol

Imaging protocol: Gated rest study with 60 mCi of ^{82}Rb and a prescan delay of 120 seconds. No stress imaging was performed.

FDG study: After rest perfusion imaging, the patient received 25 gm of oral glucose followed by 9 units of regular insulin IV to optimize myocardial glucose utilization. The patient received 12 mCi of FDG intravenously, and 60 minutes later (to allow for trapping of FDG in the myocardium) gated PET images were acquired.

Findings

A. **Image quality:**
   1. Emission images: Excellent rubidium and FDG images.
   2. Transmission images: Excellent.
   3. Registration of transmission and emission images: Excellent.
B. **Rest ^{82}Rb perfusion and ^{18}FDG images:** The images demonstrated severe LV dilatation. They also demonstrated normal RV size with increased RV tracer uptake at rest. The rest perfusion images demonstrated a large and severe perfusion defect involving the mid- and apical anterior, anteroseptal, anterolateral, and apical inferior walls, with relatively preserved FDG uptake (PET mismatch). In addition, there was a moderate-sized and severe perfusion defect throughout the lateral wall, also showing preserved FDG uptake (PET mismatch) (Figure 14).
C. **Gated PET images:** Demonstrated a rest LVEF of 21% and ESVI 70 mL/m^2 with severely enlarged LV volumes. There was severe global LV systolic dysfunction, with akinesis of the apical LV segments and the LV apex. The RV function appeared normal.
D. **Ancillary findings:** None.

Final Impression

A large region of viable but hibernating myocardium throughout the mid-LAD and left circumflex coronary artery territories.

Discussion

Overall, the total amount of scar was calculated at ~5% of the LV mass. Severe global LV systolic dysfunction was seen with advanced remodeling. The overall likelihood of a significant improvement in LV function following revascularization is high.

Follow-up

Coronary angiogram revealed 60% left main stenosis, 95% LAD stenosis, and 100% left circumflex stenosis with severe mitral regurgitation. The patient underwent coronary artery bypass surgery with mitral annuloplasty.

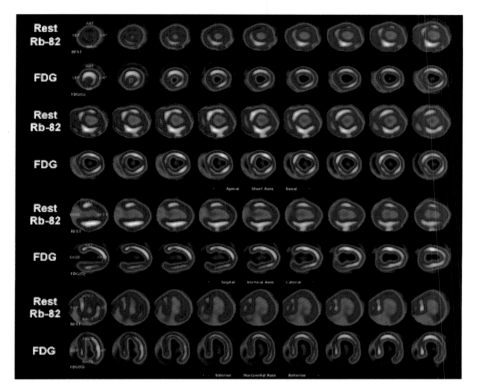

FIGURE 14. Rest ^{82}Rb and FDG images in corresponding short axis, vertical long axis, and horizontal long axis slices. The short axis slices represent progression from the apical (left) to the basal (right) part of the heart and are oriented with the anterior wall on the top, the lateral wall to the right, the inferior wall at the bottom, and the interventricular septum to the left. The vertical long axis slices represent progression from the septum (left) to the lateral (right) wall and are oriented with the anterior wall on the top, the inferior wall at the bottom, and the LV apex to the right. The horizontal long axis slices represent progression from the inferior (left) to the anterior (right) wall and are oriented with the septal wall on the left, the lateral wall to the right, and the LV apex on the top. The images demonstrate severe LV dilatation and increased radiotracer uptake in the right ventricle, reflecting increased pulmonary pressure. There is a large and severe perfusion defect involving the mid- and apical anterior, anteroseptal, anterolateral, lateral, and apical inferior walls and the LV apex, with relatively preserved FDG uptake (so-called PET mismatch).

Case 9   *Troubleshooting Myocardial Viability Assessment with PET/CT*

Clinical History

A 47-year-old male with hypertension, dyslipidemia, diabetes, a family history of ischemic heart disease, obesity, and prior CABG was referred for a PET study for evaluation of chest pain and dyspnea.

Electrocardiogram

Sinus bradycardia and nonspecific T wave abnormalities.

Medications

Metoprolol, Enalapril, Furosemide, Aspirin, Pravachol, Insulin

Study Protocol

Imaging protocol: As defined in Case 1, except that a gated noncontrast CT for coronary calcium score was not obtained. The clinical and ECG responses to stress were nonischemic.

FDG study: After perfusion imaging, the patient received 50 gm of oral glucose and 28 units of regular insulin IV to optimize myocardial glucose utilization. The patient received 12 mCi of FDG intravenously, and 60 minutes later (to allow for trapping of FDG in the myocardium) gated PET images were acquired.

Findings

A. Image quality:
   1. Emission images: Excellent rubidium images. Limited FDG images.
   2. Transmission images: Excellent.
   3. Registration of transmission and emission images: Good.

B. Rest-stress ^{82}Rb perfusion and ^{18}FDG images: There is a medium-sized defect of severe intensity throughout the lateral and inferolateral walls. Limited FDG images with patchy FDG uptake in the apical anterior wall and parts of the inferior wall (Figure 15).

C. Gated PET images: Demonstrated a rest LVEF of 30%. The LV volumes appeared moderately dilated. There was moderate global hypokinesis with akinesis of the inferolateral wall and reduced wall thickening. The RV function appeared normal.

D. Ancillary findings: None.

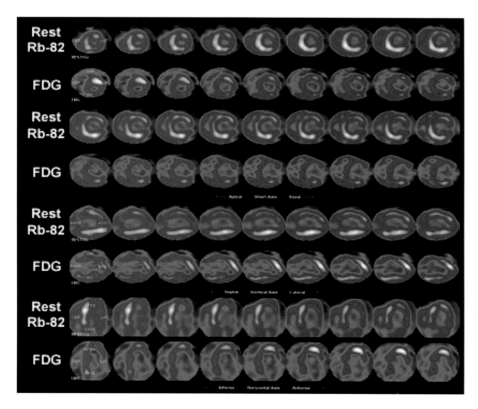

FIGURE 15. Rest ^{82}Rb and FDG images in corresponding short axis, vertical long, and horizontal long axis slices. The short axis slices represent progression from the apical (left) to the basal (right) part of the heart and are oriented with the anterior wall on the top, the lateral wall to the right, the inferior wall at the bottom, and the interventricular septum to the left. The vertical long axis slices represent progression from the septum (left) to the lateral (right) wall and are oriented with the anterior wall on the top, the inferior wall at the bottom, and the LV apex to the right. The horizontal long axis slices represent progression from the inferior (left) to the anterior (right) wall and are oriented with the septal wall on the left, the lateral wall to the right, and the LV apex on the top. There is a medium-size perfusion defect of severe intensity throughout the lateral and inferolateral walls. The FDG images are technically limited, demonstrating patchy uptake in the apical anterior wall and parts of the inferior wall.

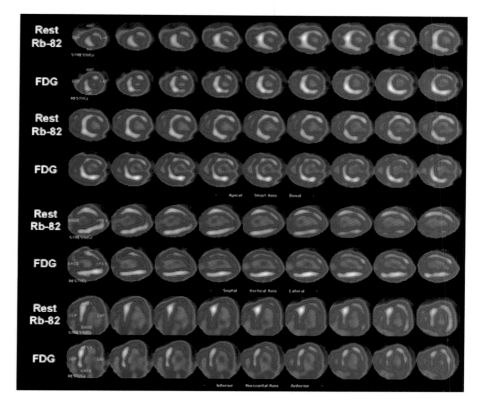

FIGURE 16. Repeat FDG images after administration of additional 4 IU of regular insulin IV, with significant improvement in myocardial uptake. These images now demonstrate a concordant reduction of both perfusion and FDG uptake throughout the inferolateral wall (so-called PET match).

Final Impression

A moderate-sized area of scar in the LCX/obtuse marginal (OM) territory. Severe LV systolic dysfunction, which appears to be disproportionate to the size of prior infarction.

Discussion

This case illustrates difficulties with FDG imaging seen in patients with insulin resistance. As described in Chapter 18, overcoming insulin resistance is critical for good-quality FDG images. Uptake of FDG in ischemic territories is independent from availability of insulin, and hence the presence of insulin resistance does usually interfere with identification of ischemic but viable myocardium. However, improper FDG uptake in normal myocardium can limit quantification of the magnitude of tissue viability.

Follow-up

FDG images were repeated after administration of an additional 4 IU of regular insulin IV, with significant improvement in myocardial uptake of FDG (Figure 16). These images demonstrate a concordant reduction of both perfusion and FDG throughout the inferolateral wall without evidence of residual viability (PET match).

Case 10 · *Integrating Calcium Scoring with Myocardial Perfusion PET*

Clinical History

A 45-year-old asymptomatic male with coronary risk factors of hyperlipidemia and family history of premature CAD (brother with myocardial infarction at age 45) was referred for evaluation of preclinical atherosclerosis. His calculated Framingham risk score suggested intermediate risk.

Electrocardiogram

Normal.

Medications

Metoprolol, Asprin, Zocor

Study Protocol

As defined in Case 1. The clinical and ECG responses to stress were nonischemic.

Findings

A. **Image quality:**
  1. Emission images: Excellent.
  2. Transmission images: Excellent.
  3. Registration of transmission and emission images: Good.
B. **Rest-stress ^{82}Rb perfusion images:** The images demonstrated normal LV size. They also demonstrated normal RV size with normal RV tracer uptake at rest. There were no regional perfusion defects seen on the stress or rest images (Figure 17).
C. **Gated PET images:** Demonstrated a rest LVEF of 64%. The LVEF during peak stress was 68%. The LV volumes appeared normal. There were no regional wall motion abnormalities. The patient demonstrated normal regional wall thickening. The RV function appeared normal.
D. **Ancillary findings:** None.
E. **Gated cardiac CT:** There is severe coronary artery calcification involving the left main (LM), LAD, and LCX coronary arteries (Figure 18). The Agatston coronary calcium score was 1140. This score is greater than the 90th percentile rank for men age 45 years.

Final Impression

Evidence of extensive calcified coronary plaque burden. However, the stress PET results suggest no flow-limiting coronary stenosis.

FIGURE 17. Dipyridamole stress and rest [82]Rb images in corresponding short axis, vertical long axis, and horizontal long axis slices. The short axis slices represent progression from the apical (left) to the basal (right) part of the heart and are oriented with the anterior wall on the top, the lateral wall to the right, the inferior wall at the bottom, and the interventricular septum to the left. The vertical long axis slices represent progression from the septum (left) to the lateral (right) wall and are oriented with the anterior wall on the top, the inferior wall at the bottom, and the LV apex to the right. The horizontal long axis slices represent progression from the inferior (left) to the anterior (right) wall and are oriented with the septal wall on the left, the lateral wall to the right, and the LV apex on the top. There is normal relative myocardial perfusion on both the rest and stress images.

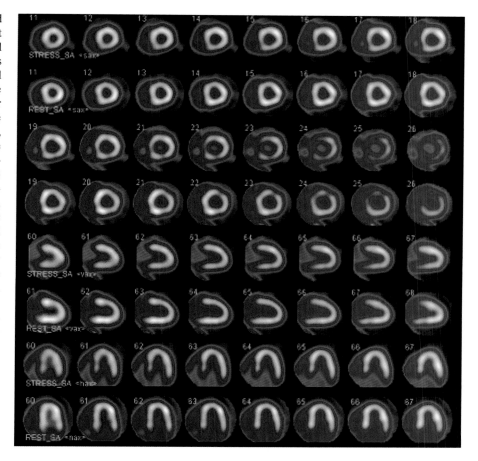

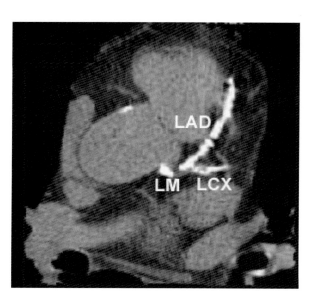

FIGURE 18. Axial CT image demonstrating extensive calcification of the distal left main (LM), left anterior descending (LAD), and proximal left circumflex (LCX) coronary arteries.

Discussion

Approximately half of asymptomatic individuals with high coronary artery calcium scores (Agatston score >400) have ischemic myocardial perfusion defects. Although extremely sensitive, however, a high coronary artery calcium score is not specific for identification of flow-limiting stenoses. A recent expert panel on appropriateness of SPECT myocardial perfusion imaging has recommended myocardial perfusion imaging as appropriate for further assessment of these patients.

Follow-up

Based on the combined results, the patient was managed medically with aggressive risk-factor modification.

Case 11   *Integrating Myocardial Perfusion and LV Function Assessments to Identify High-Risk Patients*

Clinical History

A 68-year-old male with coronary risk factors of hypertension and diabetes was evaluated for progressive anginal symptoms prior to thoracic surgery for mesothelioma.

Electrocardiogram

Normal.

Medications

Aspirin, Atorvastatin, Metformin

Study Protocol

Imaging protocol: Gated stress followed by gated rest study with two separate injections of 60 mCi of ^{82}Rb and a prescan delay of 90 seconds.
Stress protocol: Standard Adenosine (0.142 mg/kg/min) for 6 minutes without ischemic symptoms or ECG changes.
Gated cardiac CT (coronary CT angiography): A breath-hold cardiac CT study performed on a 16-slice CT scanner with a rotation time of 0.5 second using a total of 120 mL of Ultravist 370. The patient was premedicated with 10 mg of IV Lopressor prior to the study with an average heart rate of 62 bpm prior to the scan.

Findings

A. Image quality:
   1. Emission images: Excellent.
   2. Transmission images: Excellent.

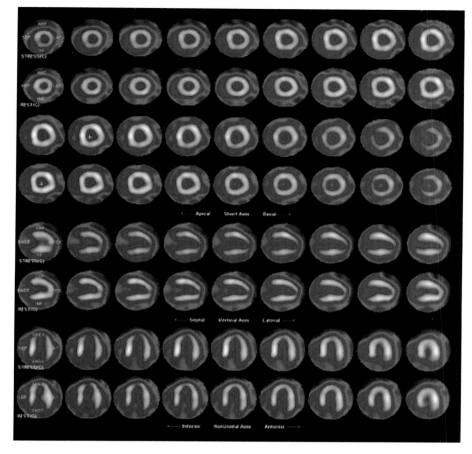

FIGURE 19. Adenosine stress and rest ⁸²Rb images in corresponding short axis, vertical long axis, and horizontal long axis slices. The short axis slices represent progression from the apical (left) to the basal (right) part of the heart and are oriented with the anterior wall on the top, the lateral wall to the right, the inferior wall at the bottom, and the interventricular septum to the left. The vertical long axis slices represent progression from the septum (left) to the lateral (right) wall and are oriented with the anterior wall on the top, the inferior wall at the bottom, and the LV apex to the right. The horizontal long axis slices represent progression from the inferior (left) to the anterior (right) wall and are oriented with the septal wall on the left, the lateral wall to the right, and the LV apex on the top. There is normal relative myocardial perfusion on both the rest and stress images.

    3. Registration of transmission and emission images: Good.

    4. CT coronary angiogram: Excellent.

B. Rest-stress ⁸²Rb perfusion images: The images demonstrated normal LV size and normal tracer uptake in the lungs. They also demonstrated normal RV size with normal RV tracer uptake at rest. There were no regional perfusion defects seen on the stress or rest images (Figure 19).

C. Gated PET images: Gated PET images revealed normal wall motion and wall thickening at rest with an LVEF of 63% that declined to 50% during peak stress with mild-moderate global hypokinesis.

D. Gated cardiac CT: Figure 20 demonstrated selected multiplane reformat cardiac CT images. Left dominant coronary anatomy with normal coronary ostial location.

    Left main coronary artery: The distal LM coronary artery demonstrates a 9.4-mm calcified plaque with severe luminal narrowing (80%) (see cross section highlighted in red square box).

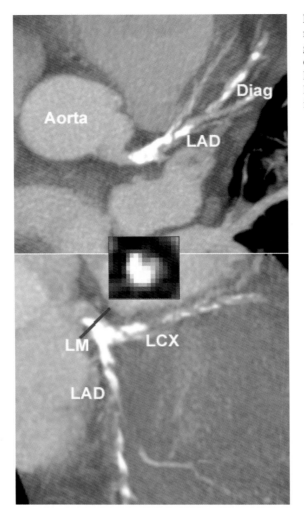

FIGURE 20. Selected multiplanar reformats of the CT coronary angiogram demonstrating extensive calcified coronary plaque in the left main (LM), left anterior descending (LAD), and left circumflex (LCX) coronary arteries. Diag, first diagonal branch.

Left anterior descending artery: The proximal and mid-LAD coronary artery is severely calcified in its proximal segment and small in caliber. One diagonal branch was seen with a 44-mm calcified plaque resulting in >75% luminal narrowing.

Left circumflex coronary artery: The proximal OM branch showed 70% stenosis.

E. Ancillary findings: Noncontrast images showed evidence of mesothelioma in the left lung.

Final Impression

Severe LM coronary artery stenosis with significant balanced ischemia.

Discussion

This is an example of a patient with no perfusion defects but a decline in LVEF during peak stress, suggesting significant left main or 3-vessel CAD. A CT coronary angiogram reveals severe calcified CAD with tight distal LM stenosis. As discussed in Chapter 14, extensive calcification can overestimate the degree of luminal narrowing due to blooming artifact on the CT images. The combined procedure helped identify significant left main stenosis noninvasively.

Follow-up

Invasive coronary angiography confirmed left dominant system with 70% distal LM, 80% ostial LAD stenosis, and 70% LCX stenosis. Patient had progressive anginal symptoms necessitating intra-aortic balloon pump in the catheterization laboratory and underwent CABG surgery.

Case 12 Integrating Myocardial Perfusion and CT Coronary Angiography to Diagnose and Manage High-Risk Patients

Clinical History

A 56-year-old male with dyslipidemia was evaluated for typical anginal symptoms.

Past Medical History

The patient underwent an exercise treadmill test in May 2005 and exercised for 11:45 minutes to a maximal heart rate of 143 bpm and a maximal blood pressure of 180 mm Hg. He experienced mild chest pain and arm tingling without ECG changes. A technetium-99m (^{99m}Tc)-sestamibi study performed at an outside hospital was reported as a fixed inferior wall defect with a diagnosis of inferior wall scar versus diaphragmatic attenuation. Despite maximal medical therapy, the patient continued to have ongoing symptoms but declined coronary angiography. Hence, he was referred for a rest-stress ^{82}Rb PET with CT coronary angiography.

Electrocardiogram

Normal.

Medications

Aspirin, Zocor, Atorvastatin

Study Protocol

Imaging protocol: Rest-gated stress study with two separate injections of 60 mCi of ^{82}Rb and a prescan delay of 120 seconds.

Stress protocol: Standard dobutamine infusion to a maximum of 40 mcg/kg/min. The maximal heart rate was 104 bpm (73% age predicted maximal heart rate) with a maximal RPP of 17745. The patient tolerated the infusion well without symptoms or ECG changes.

Gated cardiac CT (coronary CT angiography): A breath-hold cardiac CT study was performed on the 64-slice CT scanner with a rotation time of 0.33 second using a total of 85 mL of Ultravist 370. The patient was premedicated with 15 mg of IV Lopressor and 0.4 mg of SL nitroglycerin prior to the study with an average heart rate of 66 bpm prior to the scan.

Findings

A. Image quality:
   1. Emission images: Excellent.
   2. Transmission images: Excellent.
   3. Registration of transmission and emission images: Excellent.
   4. CT coronary angiogram: Excellent.
B. Rest-stress ^{82}Rb perfusion images: Normal left ventricular size. There was a small but severe perfusion defect involving the mid- and basal inferior and the basal inferoseptal walls, showing complete reversibility (Figure 21).

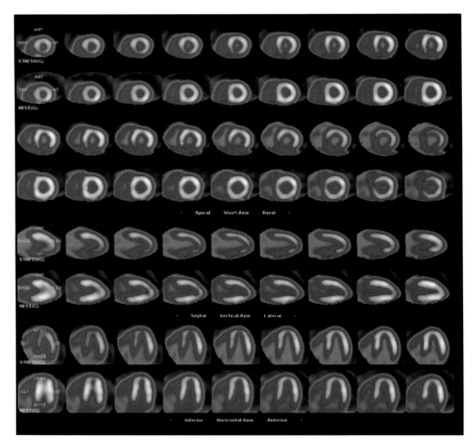

FIGURE 21. Dobutamine stress and rest ^{82}Rb images in corresponding short axis, vertical long axis, and horizontal long axis slices. The short axis slices represent progression from the apical (left) to the basal (right) part of the heart and are oriented with the anterior wall on the top, the lateral wall to the right, the inferior wall at the bottom, and the interventricular septum to the left. The vertical long axis slices represent progression from the septum (left) to the lateral (right) wall and are oriented with the anterior wall on the top, the inferior wall at the bottom, and the LV apex to the right. The horizontal long axis slices represent progression from the inferior (left) to the anterior (right) wall and are oriented with the septal wall on the left, the lateral wall to the right, and the LV apex on the top. The stress images demonstrate a medium-size and severe perfusion defect involving the mid- and basal inferior and basal inferoseptal walls, showing complete reversibility.

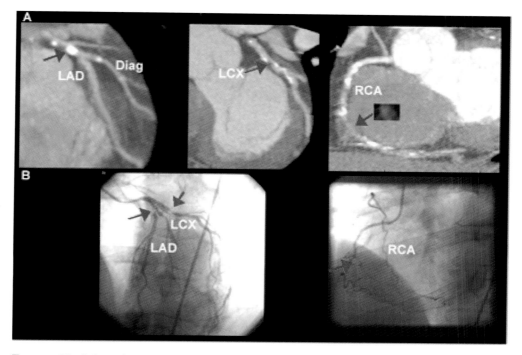

FIGURE 22. Selected curved multiplanar reformats of the CT coronary angiogram (A) and corresponding views of the catheter-based coronary angiogram (B). The CT images demonstrate a severely calcified plaque in the proximal left anterior descending (LAD; arrow in left upper panel), and severe noncalcified plaques in the proximal left circumflex (LCX; arrow in mid upper panel), and mid-right coronary artery (RCA; arrow, right upper panel), correlating with areas of significant stenoses in the conventional coronary angiogram. Diag, first diagonal branch.

C. **Gated PET images:** Gated PET images demonstrate inferior wall hypokinesis during peak stress with an EF of 61% that remained unchanged at rest.

D. **Gated Cardiac CT:** Figure 22 demonstrates selected multiplanar reformatted cardiac CT images (A) and corresponding views of catheter-based coronary angiography (B). Right dominant coronary anatomy with normal coronary ostia.

Left main coronary artery: A small calcified plaque with 20% stenosis.

Left anterior descending: The proximal LAD coronary artery shows a long complex mixed plaque with 70% stenosis. The mid-LAD distal to the takeoff of the second diagonal branch shows a small discrete calcified plaque with >70% stenosis. The distal LAD is visualized but too small in caliber to define stenosis. The first diagonal branch is small in caliber but patent. The second diagonal branch is a good-caliber vessel with a 50% stenosis.

Left circumflex coronary artery: The proximal LCX shows a 50% to 70% stenosis. The first and second OM branches are patent without stenosis.

Right coronary artery: The proximal RCA shows two sequential plaques with 50% and 70% stenosis. The mid-RCA shows a total occlusion (arrow). The distal RCA shows a long complex plaque with 90% stenosis. The acute marginal, posterior descending, and first posterolateral branches are well visualized and without angiographic stenosis.

E. **Ancillary findings:** None.

Final Impression

Severe hemodynamically significant 3-vessel CAD.

Discussion

Severe angiographic stenosis of the RCA that was flow limiting on the stress PET study. Extensive areas of calcified and noncalcified coronary atherosclerosis in the LAD and LCX coronary arteries without evidence of stress-induced perfusion abnormalities on stress PET. However, the lack of increase in LVEF during peak stress was suggestive of significant 3-vessel CAD. The integrated PET/CTA study was useful in defining the anatomic extent and physiologic significance of CAD.

Follow-up

The patient underwent CABG with left internal mammary artery (LIMA) to left anterior descending artery, a vein graft to the RCA, and another vein graft to the LCX.

Case 13 — Integrating Myocardial Perfusion and CT Coronary Angiography to Diagnose and Manage Patients with Suspected CAD

Clinical History

A 73-year-old male with dyslipidemia, family history of premature CAD, and smoking was referred for evaluation prior to esophageal surgery.

Electrocardiogram

Normal.

Medications

Atenolol, Zocor, Asprin

Study Protocol

Imaging protocol: Rest-gated stress PET study with two separate injections of 60 mCi of ^{82}Rb and a prescan delay of 120 seconds.

Stress protocol: Standard Adenosine infusion (142 mcg/kg/min). The patient tolerated the infusion well without symptoms or ECG changes.

Gated cardiac CT (coronary CT angiography): A breath-hold cardiac CT study was performed on the 64-slice CT scanner with a rotation time of 0.33 second using a total of 85 mL of Ultravist 370. The patient also received 5 mg of IV Lopressor and 0.4 mg of SL nitroglycerin prior to the study with an average heart rate of 58 bpm prior to the scan.

Findings

A. Image quality:
1. Emission images: Excellent.
2. Transmission images: Excellent.
3. Registration of transmission and emission images: Excellent.
4. CT coronary angiogram: Excellent.

B. Rest-stress ^{82}Rb perfusion images:
Normal left ventricular size. A medium-sized defect of severe intensity in the mid- and basal antero-lateral walls with significant but not complete reversibility (Figure 23).

C. Gated PET images:
Gated PET images demonstrate a rest EF of 33% with global hypokinesis of the left ventricle worse in the inferior wall.

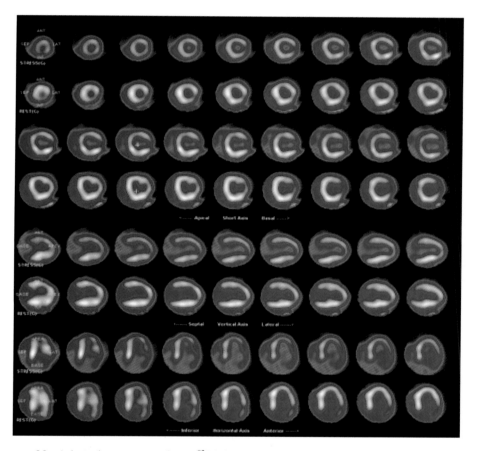

FIGURE 23. Adenosine stress and rest ^{82}Rb images in corresponding short axis, vertical long axis, and horizontal long axis slices. The short axis slices represent progression from the apical (left) to the basal (right) part of the heart and are oriented with the anterior wall on the top, the lateral wall to the right, the inferior wall at the bottom, and the interventricular septum to the left. The vertical long axis slices represent progression from the septum (left) to the lateral (right) wall and are oriented with the anterior wall on the top, the inferior wall at the bottom, and the LV apex to the right. The horizontal long axis slices represent progression from the inferior (left) to the anterior (right) wall and are oriented with the septal wall on the left, the lateral wall to the right, and the LV apex on the top. The images demonstrate a medium-size defect of severe intensity in the mid- and basal antero-lateral walls with significant but not complete reversibility.

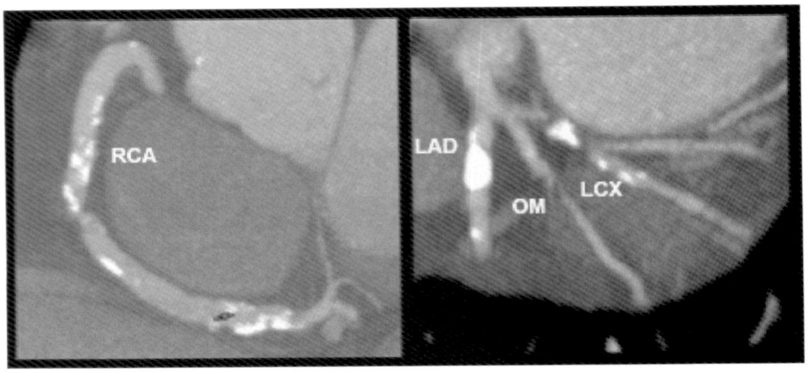

FIGURE 24. Selected curved multiplanar reformats of the CT coronary angiogram demonstrating severe calcified coronary plaque in the proximal left anterior descending (LAD) and left circumflex (LCX), and obtuse marginal (OM) coronary arteries (right panel). The right coronary artery (RCA; left panel) is ectatic with extensive calcifications and a significant stenosis in its mid-segment.

D. Gated cardiac CT: Selected curved multiplanar reformatted cardiac CT images (Figure 24). Right dominant coronary anatomy with normal coronary ostia.
Left main: No stenosis.
Left anterior descending: The proximal and mid-LAD coronary artery shows two discrete calcified plaques with 40% and 50% stenosis in cross section (not shown), respectively. The first diagonal branch shows a 30% stenosis. No other diagonal branches were seen. The distal LAD and the first septal perforator branch were well visualized and without stenosis.
Left circumflex coronary: The proximal LCX shows a calcified plaque with >90% stenosis after the takeoff of the first OM branch. The first and the second OM each have a calcified plaque with 20% and 80% stenosis, respectively. The distal LCX was too small in caliber to adequately characterize.
Right coronary: The proximal RCA was normal. The mid- and distal RCA were ectatic with diffuse disease. The PDA and one right posterolateral branch were well seen but too small to adequately characterize.
E. Ancillary findings: None.

Final Impression

Hemodynamically significant LCX CAD.

Catheter Coronary Angiogram Findings

Right dominant. No left main disease. No significant LAD disease. Proximal LCX showed a 100% lesion with left-to-left collaterals. Mid-RCA showed a discrete 70% stenosis and a 90% stenosis of the ostial PDA.

Discussion

The CTA results show severe 2-vessel angiographic coronary artery stenosis. However, the stress PET images demonstrated physiologically significant disease only in the LCX coronary artery. The presence of left-to-left collateral flow led to misinterpretation of the total occlusion of LCX on the CT images, but PET images correctly diagnosed this to be most hemodynamically significant. Thus the combined information from both studies was complementary in making a diagnosis and appropriate management decisions.

Follow-up

Percutaneous intervention of the LCX was attempted but unsuccessful. RCA was stented using a drug-eluting stent.

Case 14   *Normal PET/CT with Incidental CT Findings*

Clinical History

A 65-year-old female with hypertension, family history of premature CAD, and prior chest radiation therapy was evaluated for atypical chest pain.

Electrocardiogram

Normal.

Medications

Lopressor, Verapamil, Irbesartan, Hydrallazine

Study Protocol

Imaging protocol: Gated rest followed by gated stress study with two separate injections of 60 mCi of ^{82}Rb and a prescan delay of 120 seconds.

Stress protocol: Standard dipyridamole infusion (0.14 mg/kg/min) for 4 minutes without symptoms or ECG changes.

Findings

A. Image quality:
1. Emission images: Excellent.
2. Transmission images: Excellent.
3. Registration of transmission and emission images: Good.

B. Rest-stress ^{82}Rb perfusion images: Normal left ventricular size. There were no rest or stress myocardial perfusion defects.

C. Gated PET images: Demonstrated a rest LVEF of 70%. There were no regional wall motion abnormalities. The RV function appeared normal.

D. Ancillary findings: The CT transmission images demonstrated a focal cystic lesion in the right breast measuring $11 \times 11 \times 9$ mm (Figure 25).

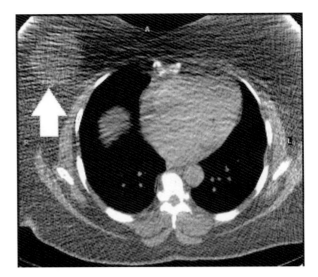

FIGURE 25. Axial CT transmission image demonstrating an incidental focal cystic lesion in the right breast measuring. $11 \times 11 \times 9$ mm.

Final Impression

The PET images demonstrate no evidence of flow-limiting CAD. However, there is evidence of a large breast cyst on the CT scan at the site of recent surgery for breast cancer and confirms findings described on a prior breast ultrasound.

Discussion

It is important to systematically review all the imaging data. In this case, the CT transmission images demonstrated clinically relevant extracardiac findings.

Follow-up

None.

Case 15   *Normal PET/CT with Incidental CT Findings*

Clinical History

A 56-year-old female with hypertension, dyslipidemia, and a family history of premature CAD was evaluated for atypical chest pain.

Electrocardiogram

Normal.

Medications

Verapamil, Irbesartan, Lopressor, Asprin

Study Protocol

Imaging protocol: Gated rest followed by gated stress study with two separate injections of 60 mCi of ^{82}Rb and a prescan delay of 120 seconds.

Stress protocol: Standard dipyridamole infusion (0.14 mg/kg/min) for 4 minutes without symptoms or ECG changes.

Findings

A. Image quality:
 1. Emission images: Excellent.
 2. Transmission images: Excellent.
 3. Registration of transmission and emission images: Good.
B. Rest-stress ^{82}Rb perfusion images: Normal left ventricular size. There was a small defect of mild intensity in the mid- and apical anterior walls with mild reversibility.
C. Gated PET images: Demonstrated a rest LVEF of 67% that was essentially unchanged at 68% during peak stress. There were no regional wall motion abnormalities. The RV function appeared normal.
D. Ancillary findings: The CT transmission images demonstrate an ill-defined, ground-glass opacity (1.2 cm) in the left upper lobe (arrow, Figure 26). Differential diagnosis includes bronchoalveolar carcinoma or inflammatory process.

Final Impression

The PET images demonstrate mild ischemia in the distribution of the mid-LAD coronary artery. In addition, the ill-defined ground-glass opacity in the left upper lobe of the lung requires further evaluation by a dedicated chest CT.

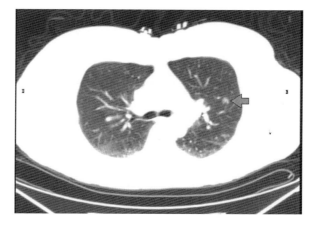

FIGURE 26. Axial CT transmission image demonstrating an ill-defined ground-glass opacity in the left upper lobe (arrow). Differential diagnosis includes bronchoalveolar carcinoma or inflammatory process.

Discussion

This case also shows relevant extracardiac findings on the CT transmission images.

Follow-up

Dedicated chest CT scan without contrast was performed. It confirmed the findings, and a 6-month follow-up study was suggested to evaluate for stability.

Case 16   *Normal PET/CT with Incidental CT Findings*

Clinical History

A 62-year-old male with hypertension was evaluated for atypical chest pain prior to consideration of renal transplantation.

Electrocardiogram

Normal.

Medications

Lopressor, Enalapril, Furosemide, Mycophenolate mofetil, Levofloxacin, Sodium polystyrene sulfonate

Study Protocol

Imaging protocol: Gated rest followed by gated stress study with two separate injections of 60 mCi of ^{82}Rb and a prescan delay of 120 seconds.
Stress protocol: Standard dipyridamole infusion (0.14 mg/kg/min) for 4 minutes without symptoms or ECG changes.

Findings

A. **Image quality:**
   1. Emission images: Excellent.
   2. Transmission images: Excellent.
   3. Registration of transmission and emission images: Good.
B. **Rest-stress ^{82}Rb perfusion images:** Normal left ventricular size. There were no rest or stress myocardial perfusion defects.
C. **Gated PET images:** Demonstrated a rest LVEF of 70%. There were no regional wall motion abnormalities. The RV function appeared normal.
D. **Ancillary findings:** The CT transmission images demonstrate innumerable hepatic cysts and ascites (Figure 27).
E. **Gated cardiac CT:** There was extensive coronary artery calcification. The Agatston coronary calcium score was 2685. This score is greater than the 90th percentile rank for men age 61 to 65 years.

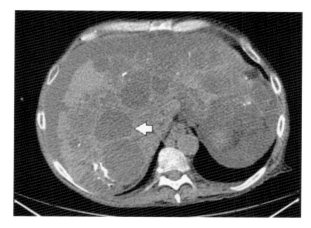

FIGURE 27. Axial CT transmission image demonstrating innumerable hepatic cysts and ascites.

Final Impression

The PET/CT images demonstrate extensive calcified coronary atherosclerosis without evidence of flow-limiting coronary stenosis. In addition, numerous hepatic cysts were seen, which is consistent with known diagnosis of polycystic disease.

Discussion

This case also shows relevant extracardiac findings on the CT transmission images.

Follow-up

None.

Case 17   *Normal PET/CT with Incidental CT Findings*

Clinical History

A 61-year-old male with diabetes was referred for a dipyridamole myocardial perfusion PET study to evaluate for dyspnea and arrhythmias.

Electrocardiogram

Normal.

Cardiac Medications

Glyburide, Enoxaparin

Study Protocol

Imaging protocol: Gated rest followed by gated stress study with two separate injections of 60 mCi of ^{82}Rb and a prescan delay of 90 seconds.

Stress protocol: Standard dipyridamole infusion (0.14 mg/kg/min) for 4 minutes without symptoms or ECG changes.

Gated cardiac CT: Quantitative coronary calcium scores were calculated according to the method described by Agatston. Breath-hold gated cardiac CT was performed using a 16-channel CT scanner with a 0.5-second rotation time.

Findings

A. Image quality:
1. Emission images: Excellent.
2. Transmission images: Excellent.
3. Registration of transmission and emission images: Good.

B. Rest-stress ^{82}Rb perfusion images: Normal left ventricular size. There no perfusion defects on the stress or rest images.

C. Gated PET images: Demonstrated a rest LVEF of 63% and ESVI 16 mL/m^2. The LVEF during peak stress was 69% with ESVI 14 mL/m^2. The LV volumes appeared normal. There were no regional wall motion abnormalities. The patient demonstrated normal regional wall thickening. The RV function appeared normal.

D. Ancillary findings: The scout and CT transmission images demonstrate a collapsed upper lobe of the right lung (Figure 28).

E. Gated cardiac CT: There is extensive coronary artery calcification. The Agatston coronary calcium score was 706. This score is between the 75th and the 90th percentile rank for men age 61 to 65 years.

Final Impression

Evidence of extensive calcified coronary plaque burden. No evidence of dipyridamole-induced perfusion abnormalities. Normal global LV systolic function. Evidence of collapsed upper lobe of the right lung.

Discussion

A dedicated chest CT scan diagnosed metastatic non–small cell lung cancer that resulted in collapse of the right upper lobe.

Follow-up

The patient underwent medical management for CAD and received chemotherapy for metastatic non–small cell lung cancer.

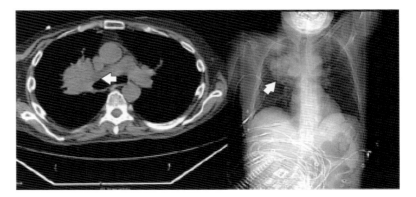

FIGURE 28. Axial CT transmission (left) and scout (right) images demonstrating a collapsed upper lobe of the right lung (arrows) corresponding to an area of known non–small cell lung cancer.

Case 18   *Normal PET/CT with Incidental CT Findings*

Clinical History

A 67-year-old female with known CAD and prior CABG was referred to us for a myocardial viability study to evaluate for recurrent chest pain. She had a history of ST elevation MI in the anterior wall (1 week prior), due to thrombotic occlusion of her saphenous vein graft (SVG) graft to LAD. A percutaneous intervention was attempted but was unsuccessful.

Electrocardiogram

Normal sinus rhythm, anterior wall MI, age indeterminate.

Cardiac Medications

Lopressor, Captopril, Aspirin, Atorvastatin

Study Protocol

Imaging protocol: Gated rest with 60 mCi of ^{82}Rb and a prescan delay of 120 seconds.
Stress protocol: Not applicable.
FDG study: The patient received 50 g of oral glucose and 20 IU of regular insulin IV to optimize myocardial glucose utilization. The patient received 11 mCi of FDG intravenously, and 60 minutes later (to allow for trapping of FDG in the myocardium) gated PET images were acquired.

Findings

- **A. Image quality:**
  1. Emission images: Excellent.
  2. Transmission images: Excellent.
  3. Registration of transmission and emission images: Good.
- **B. Rest ^{82}Rb and FDG PET images:** Normal left ventricular size. There was a large perfusion defect in the mid- to distal anterior and anteroseptal walls with a matched reduction in FDG uptake (PET match) (Figure 29). In addition, there was a small perfusion defect in the inferolateral wall with preserved FDG uptake (PET mismatch).
- **C. Gated PET images:** Demonstrated a rest LVEF of 31% with akinesis of the mid- and apical anterior and anteroseptal walls with reduced regional wall thickening.
- **D. Ancillary findings:** The CT transmission images demonstrate a focal collection in the pericardial space that is most consistent with hemopericardium (Figure 30). In addition, there is moderate bilateral pleural effusion.

Final Impression

The myocardial perfusion and FDG images demonstrate a large region of myocardial scar in the mid-LAD distribution and a small area of viable but hibernating myocardium in the left circumflex territory. There is evidence of a pericardial effusion on the CT scan, and immediate evaluation was recommended.

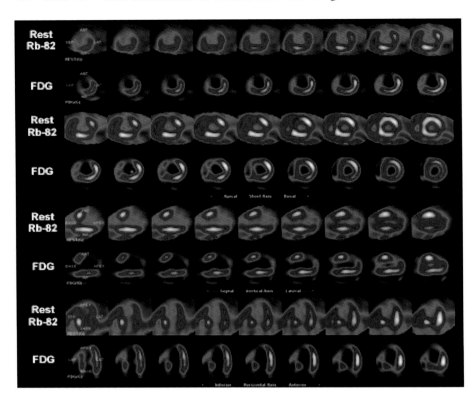

FIGURE 29. Rest ^{82}Rb and FDG images in corresponding short axis, vertical long axis, and horizontal long axis slices. The images demonstrate a large perfusion defect in the mid- to distal anterior and anteroseptal walls with a matched reduction in FDG uptake (PET match). In addition, there is a small perfusion defect in the inferolateral wall with preserved FDG uptake (PET mismatch).

Discussion

A cardiac MRI study confirmed the effusion as a hemopericardium, which was interpreted as the most likely the cause of ongoing chest pain. Localized hemopericardium was the result of a failed percutaneous intervention of the SVG to the LAD.

Follow-up

None.

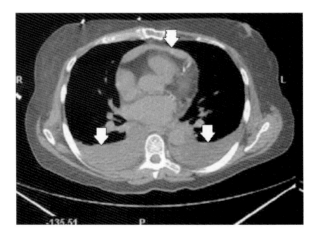

FIGURE 30. Axial CT transmission (left) and scout (right) images demonstrating a focal collection in the pericardial space that is most consistent with hemopericardium (upper arrow) and moderate bilateral pleural effusion (lower arrows).

Index

Printed in Singapore